New Insights into Musculoskeletal Disorders

New Insights into Musculoskeletal Disorders

Edited by Bran Conley

hayle
medical

New York

Hayle Medical,
750 Third Avenue, 9th Floor,
New York, NY 10017, USA

Visit us on the World Wide Web at:
www.haylemedical.com

ISBN: 978-1-63241-717-6

Trademark Notice: Registered trademark of products or corporate names are used only for explanation and identification without intent to infringe.

Cataloging-in-Publication Data

New insights into musculoskeletal disorders / edited by Bran Conley.
    p. cm.
Includes bibliographical references and index.
ISBN 978-1-63241-717-6
1. Musculoskeletal system--Diseases. 2. Musculoskeletal system--Abnormalities.
3. Musculoskeletal system--Wounds and injuries. I. Conley, Bran.
RC925 .N49 2019
616.7--dc23

Table of Contents

Preface

The pain and injuries of the human musculoskeletal system are categorized as musculoskeletal disorders. Sudden exertion from lifting something heavy, strain from awkward positions and making strenuous repetitive motions can cause such disorders. They can affect several parts of the body, including the hands, feet, neck, arms, legs, shoulders and lower back. Assessment of the patient's medical history, physical examination, lab tests, x-rays and Nordic Questionnaire are usually used by the doctors to diagnose musculoskeletal disorders. Weight loss and frequent weight lifting are quite useful in preventing musculoskeletal disorders related to the lower back and spine. The topics included in this book on musculoskeletal disorders are of utmost significance and bound to provide incredible insights to readers. It aims to shed light on some of the unexplored aspects of musculoskeletal disorders and the recent researches related to it. This book is appropriate for students seeking detailed information in this area as well as for doctors and experts.

All of the data presented henceforth, was collaborated in the wake of recent advancements in the field. The aim of this book is to present the diversified developments from across the globe in a comprehensible manner. The opinions expressed in each chapter belong solely to the contributing authors. Their interpretations of the topics are the integral part of this book, which I have carefully compiled for a better understanding of the readers.

At the end, I would like to thank all those who dedicated their time and efforts for the successful completion of this book. I also wish to convey my gratitude towards my friends and family who supported me at every step.

Editor

The efficacy and safety of combined administration of intravenous and topical tranexamic acid in primary total knee arthroplasty

Huazhang Xiong[1,2], Yi Liu[2], Yi Zeng[1], Yuangang Wu[1] and Bin Shen[1*]

Abstract

Background: The combined administration of intravenous (IV) and topical tranexamic acid (TXA) in primary total knee (TKA) knee remains controversial. The purpose of this meta-analysis was to assess the efficacy and safety of combined administration of IV and topical TXA in primary TKA.

Methods: PubMed, EMBASE, Cochrane Central Register of Controlled Trials, Web of Science, Google Search Engine and China National Knowledge Infrastructure databases were searched for randomized controlled trials (RCTs) were comparing the combined administration of IV and topical TXA following primary TKA. The primary outcomes were total blood loss, maximum hemoglobin drop, and deep venous thrombosis (DVT) and/or pulmonary embolism (PE). The second outcomes were drainage volume and transfusion requirements. Data were analyzed using RevMan 5.3.

Results: A total of 6 RCTs involving 701 patients were included in the meta-analysis. The combined group provided lower total blood loss (MD − 156.34 mL, 95% CI, − 241.51 to − 71.18; $P = 0.0003$), drainage volume (MD − 43.54 mL, 95% CI, − 67.59 to − 19.48; $P = 0.0004$), maximum hemoglobin drop (MD − 0.56 g/dl, 95% CI, − 0.93 to − 0.19; $P = 0.003$) than IV TXA alone. No significant difference were found in terms of transfusion requirements (RR 0.48, 95% CI, 0.16 to 1.44; $P = 0.19$), DVT (RR 1.01, 95% CI, 0.14 to 7.12; $P = 0.99$) and PE (RR 0.33, 95% CI, 0.01 to 7.91; $P = 0.49$) between the two group. Subgroup analyses shows that the combined group was less total blood loss in non-tourniquet ($P = 0.0008$), topical TXA dose > 1.5 g ($P < 0.00001$) and number of IV TXA ≥ 2 doses ($P = 0.005$) of TXA compared with the IV group alone.

Conclusions: The available evidence indicates combined group were associated with lower total blood loss, drainage volume, and maximum hemoglobin drop. A similar transfusion requirement was found in both groups. Subgroup analyses demonstrates that total blood loss was less in patients with non-tourniquet, topical TXA dose > 1.5 g and number of IV TXA ≥ 2 doses of TXA. There was no increase the rates of DVT and PE.

Keywords: Total knee arthroplasty, Tranexamic acid, Intravenous, Topical, Blood loss

* Correspondence: shenbin71@hotmail.com
[1]Department of Orthopaedic Surgery, West China Hospital, West China Medical School, Sichuan University, Chengdu, Sichuan Province 610041, People's Republic of China
Full list of author information is available at the end of the article

Background

Total knee arthroplasty (TKA) and total hip arthroplasty (THA) is an effective orthopedic procedure for patients with severe knee and hip diseases [1–4]. However, significant blood loss may occur due to hyper-fibrinolysis induced by surgical trauma or tourniquet. Thus, it often leads to significant postoperative anemia and transfusion requirements [5, 6]. Postoperative anemia may be an important issue associated with adverse events, including increased mortality and morbidity and prolonged hospitalization due to transfusion-related needs.

Tranexamic acid (TXA) is a synthetic lysine analog, it can competitively inhibit the activation of plasminogen and plasmin binding protein [7, 8]. Several randomized controlled trials (RCTs) [9, 10] and meta-analysis studies [11, 12] have shown that intravenous (IV) [13, 14], topical (TA) [8] or oral [15] application of TXA can successfully reduce blood loss and transfusions in primary TKA without increasing the risk of thrombosis. Recently, an increasing number of studies have focused on the issue that when compared with only IV or TA TXA, whether combination application of IV and topical TXA has additional benefits in primary TKA [16, 17]. Compared with IV TXA, TA application has the advantage of being easy to administer, it leads to 70% lower systemic absorption and thus may be a safer alternative to giving it systemically. Additionally, topical application of TXA has the advantage of inducing partial microvascular hemostasis by stopping fibrin clot dissolution in the affected area [4, 8, 11, 18]. Once topically applied, TXA is rapidly absorbed and achieves the effect of hemostasis.

Several meta-analyses [19–21] were performed to evaluate the combination of IV and topical TXA in primary TKA. However, it may have some limitations and the conclusion might have the bias: First, as they included both TKA and THA in the analysis [19, 20], they did not account for the difference in the type of surgery. It cannot draw meaningful conclusions, and we believed that stricter criteria need to be applied to determine the benefits of combining TXA in a meta-analysis. Second, these studies were also affected by many other confounding factors [19–21], such as the application of tourniquet or non-tourniquet, and different topical TXA dose or the number of IV TXA. Thus, subgroup analysis based on the application of tourniquet or non-tourniquet, and topical TXA dose (≤1.5 g or > 1.5 g) or the number of IV TXA (single or ≥ 2 doses) were conducted, resulting in more accurate conclusions. Therefore, because of this bias factor, the efficacy of the combined IV and topical TXA in primary TKA has not been clearly concluded. Currently, there have been some well-designed studies [21–24] comparing the efficacy of combined administration of IV and topical TXA versus IV-TXA alone during TKA. Thus, the authors performed a meta-analysis to assess the highest evidence-based (level I) studies in order to investigate the effectiveness and safety of combined IV and TA application of TXA versus single IV TXA after primary TKA in regarding with (1) blood loss, including total blood loss and drainage volume; (2) transfusion requirements and maximum hemoglobin drop; and (3) thromboembolic complications, including deep venous thrombosis (DVT) and/or pulmonary embolism (PE). Additionally, subgroup analyses were also conducted to evaluate the benefits of the application of tourniquet or non-tourniquet, different topical (≤1.5 g or > 1.5 g) or the number of IV TXA (single or ≥ 2 doses) for total blood loss, maximum hemoglobin drop and transfusion requirements.

Methods

The method used for this meta-analysis is based on the recommended PRISMA checklist guidelines [25]. The study was registered in the Research Registration Unique Identifying Number (review registry 249; http://www.researchregistry.com).

Search strategy

We searched the following electronic databases: PubMed (1966 to December 2017), Embase (1974 to December 2017), Cochrane Central Register of Controlled Trials (December 2017) and Web of Science (1990 to December 2017). To identify additional potential studies, we also used the Google Search Engine (December 2017) and China National Knowledge Infrastructure (December 2017). We used the following keywords to search the database above: (total knee arthroplasty OR total knee replacement OR TKA OR TKR) AND (Tranexamic acid OR TXA OR TA). A search strategy with "PubMed" as an example in a manuscript: #1 Total Knee Arthroplasty; #2 Total Knee Replacement; #3 TKA; #4 TKR; #5 #1 OR #2 OR #3 OR #4; #6 Tranexamic Acid; #7 TXA; #8 TA; #9 #6 OR #7 OR #8; #10 #5 AND #9. There is no restriction on language and region.

Inclusion criteria

The inclusion criteria for these studies were performed as follows: (1) studies were RCTs that included combined IV and topical application of TXA, and IV application of TXA; **(2) patients were performed primary unilateral TKA; and (3)** The outcomes of each RCTs included at least one of the following: blood loss, drainage volume, transfusion requirements, maximum hemoglobin drop, DVT, and PE. The studies were excluded if: (1) there were no sufficient outcomes; (2) revision **or simultaneous bilateral total knee arthroplasty. All titles and abstracts were** independently reviewed by two reviewers (XXX, XXX) to identify potential studies. These eligible studies were then obtained for inclusion based on the review of the full text. The differences were resolved by consensus after discussion, or a third reviewer was consulted if necessary.

Assessment of methodological quality

Two reviewers (XXX, XXX) assessed independently the methodological quality as described by the Cochrane Collaboration for Systematic Reviews [26]. The six items included random sequence generation, allocation sequence concealment, blinding, incomplete outcome data, selective outcome reporting, and other risks. The overall methodological quality of each included study was characterized as low (low risk of bias), high (high risk of bias), and unclear (unclear risk of bias). Additionally, the two reviewers (XXX, XXX) used the modified Jadad scale to assess the risk of bias of the included studies [27]. Studies obtaining 4 or more points (up to 8 points) is considered to be of high quality, and the differences will be resolved by consensus after discussion, and if necessary, the third reviewer was consulted (XXX).

Outcome measures

The effectiveness and safety of combined IV and TA application of TXA versus single IV TXA after primary TKA in this meta-analysis were compared. The primary outcomes were total blood loss, maximum hemoglobin drop, and deep venous thrombosis (DVT) and/or pulmonary embolism (PE). The second outcomes were drainage volume and transfusion requirements. Furthermore, Subgroup analysis was also performed based on whether the use of tourniquet and drainage tube to compare the additional benefits for blood loss.

Data extraction

Two reviewers (XXX, XXX) independently extracted outcomes from the included studies. Their data includes authors, publication year, patients, age, and the intervention method of TXA, the method of DVT prophylaxis and screening, blood transfusion criterion. **If the study reported the same patient during the different follow-up period, we chose a longer follow-up time to avoid duplication of data.**

Data synthesis

Statistical analyses of the meta-analysis were performed using RevMan 5 software (Version 5.3, the Cochrane Collaboration, UK). For continuous data, the mean differences (MD) and 95% confidence interval (CI) were calculated, such as total blood loss, drainage volume, and maximum hemoglobin drop. For dichotomous data, the risk ratio (RR) and 95% confidence interval (CI) were calculated, such as transfusion requirements, DVT or PE. The chi-squared test and I2 statistic were used to assess statistical heterogeneity. If the chi-squared test > 0.1 or the $I^2 < 50\%$, the fixed-effects model was chosen. Otherwise, a random-effects model was chosen. Publication bias was tested independently using funnel plots of total blood loss, drainage volume, maximum hemoglobin drop, transfusion requirements and DVT. If the funnel plot was symmetric, then there was a low potential for publication bias, or vice-versa.

Results

Search results

The flow chart in Fig. 1 shows the process by screening the potential studies. A total of 1689 studies were screened through the initial search, 1410 were excluded on the basis of their titles and abstracts, and then leaving 279 were read for full-text. After scanning full-text, 273 were also excluded since it did not meet inclusion criteria. Thus, 6 RCTs had been published between 2014 and 2017 used in the meta-analysis [16, 17, 22–24, 28]. These studies included 351 patients in combined administration of IV and topical TXA group (combined group) and 350patients in IV TXA group (IV TXA group). Sample size in included trials ranged from 25 to 95. Of all 6 studies, 5 studies were published in the English language [16, 17, 22–24], 1 study was published in the Chinese language [28]. Randomization was conducted in all 6 studies [16, 17, 22–24, 28]. All but 1 study [28] reported randomization method, of which 4 studies [17, 22–24] were reported using a computer-generated randomization, and in 1 [16] study reported the use of sealed envelope technique. There were 4 studies [16, 17, 22, 24] performed a clear blinding. All but two studies [17, 22] performed drainage, and the tourniquet was applied in four studies [16, 17, 23, 24]. All patients in the included studies received DVT prophylaxis of physical and chemical methods, including intermittent pneumatic compression, low-molecular-weight heparin, aspirin or rivaroxaban. Table 1 summarizes the baseline characteristics of included studies.

Table 2 summarizes the methodological quality and the risk of bias of the included studies. All 6 trials were relatively well designed, and the modified Jadad scores showed that the quality of the 6 trials was high, of which there were 2 at least 4 points, there were 3 up to 7 points. The meta-analysis used independently funnel plots of total blood loss, drainage volume, maximum hemoglobin drop, transfusion requirements and DVT to assess publication bias; the plots were generally symmetrical and shown a lower publication bias (Fig. 2 A, B, C, D, E).

Meta-analysis of blood loss

A total of five studies [16, 17, 22–24] report relevant data regarding total blood loss (326 and 325 patients in the combined group and IV group, respectively). The outcome of meta-analysis indicates that total blood loss

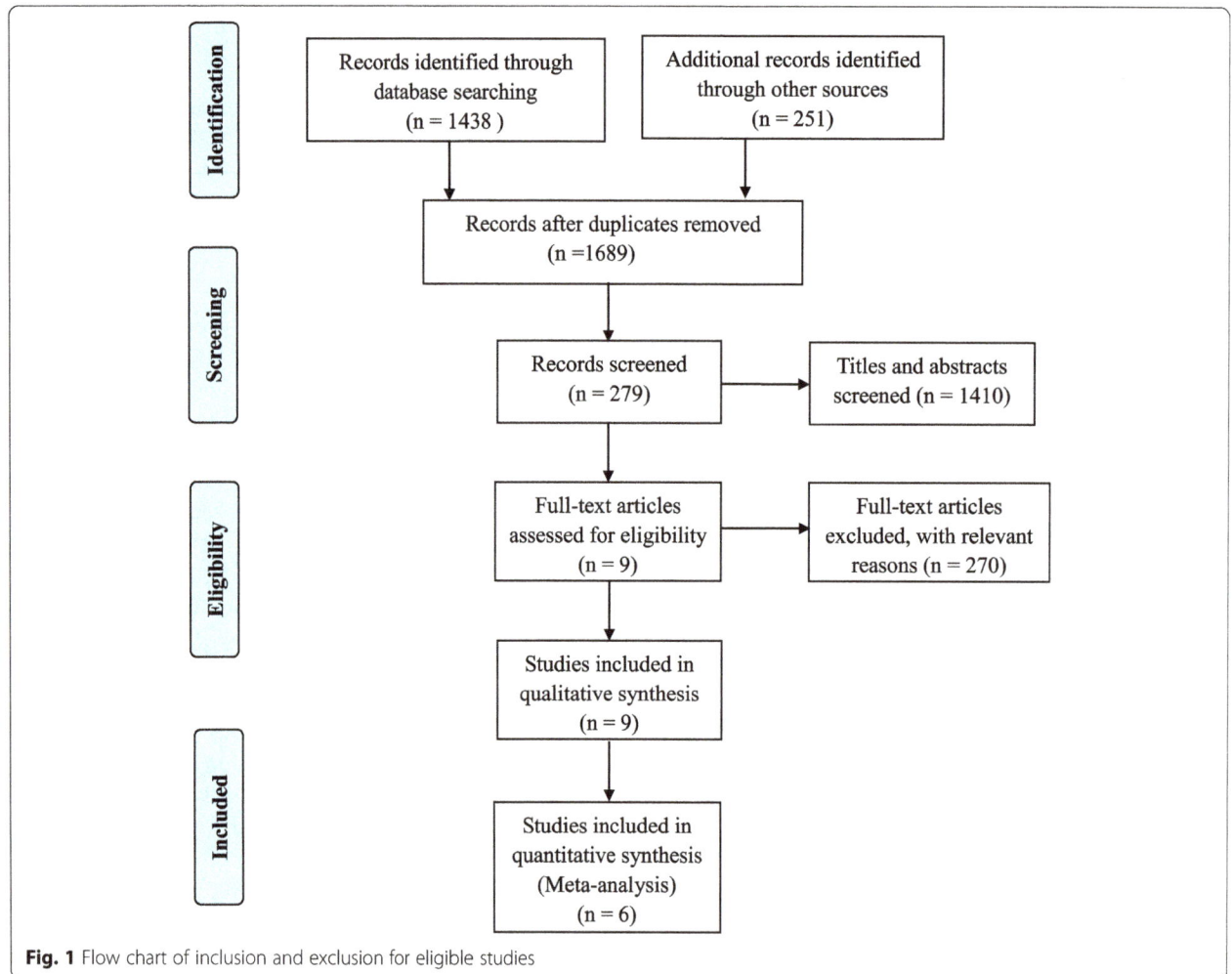

Fig. 1 Flow chart of inclusion and exclusion for eligible studies

found in the combined group significantly reduced blood loss by a mean of 156.34 mL compared with the IV group (95% CI, − 241.51 to − 71.18; $P = 0.0003$) (Fig. 3). A random-effects model was used since there was significant heterogeneity among the studies ($P = 0.002$, $I^2 = 77\%$).

Subgroup analysis was performed base on the use of tourniquet or non-tourniquet, different topical (≤1.5 g or > 1.5 g) or number of IV TXA (single or ≥ 2 doses) of TXA. The outcome revealed that there was the significant difference between the two groups in terms of tourniquet or non-tourniquet, topical TXA dose or the number of IV TXA (Table 3).

3.3 Meta-analysis of drainage volume
A total of three studies [16, 24, 28] reported relevant data regarding drainage volume (167 and 167 patients in the combined group and IV group, respectively). The outcome of meta-analysis indicates that drainage volume found in the combined group significantly reduced drainage volume by a mean of 43.54 mL

compared with the IV group (95% CI, − 67.59 to − 19.48; $P = 0.0004$) (Fig. 4). A fixed model was used since there was no significant heterogeneity among the studies ($P = 0.34$, $I^2 = 7\%$).

Meta-analysis of maximum hemoglobin drop
A total of four studies [16, 17, 23, 24] reported relevant data regarding maximum hemoglobin drop (296 and 295 patients in the combined group and IV group, respectively). The outcome of meta-analysis indicates that maximum hemoglobin drop found in the combined group significantly reduced maximum hemoglobin drop by a mean of 0.56 g/dl compared with the IV group (95% CI, − 0.93 to − 0.19; $P = 0.003$) (Fig. 5). A random-effects model was used since there was significant heterogeneity among the studies ($P < 0.00001$, $I^2 = 90\%$). Similar results were received in subgroup analysis based on the application of tourniquet or non-tourniquet, topical TXA dose or the number of IV TXA (Table 4).

Table 1 Characteristics of included studies

Author	Diagnose	No. Of patients	Age (years)	Interventions	Drainage	Tourniquet	Transfusion criteria	DVT prophylaxis	DVT screen
Huang [16]	OA	VI: 92	VI: 64.7	VI: 3 g used before inflation	Yes	Yes	70 g/L ≤ Hb ≤ 90 g/L with anemia, Hb ≤70 g/L	LMWH Rivaroxaban	Ultrasound
		Combined: 92	Combined: 65.4	Combined:1.5 g used intravenously before inflation + 1.5 g used topically					
Jain [17]	OA	VI:60	VI: 70.0	VI: 15 mg/kg 30 min before skin incision, 10 mg/kg was repeated 3 and 6 h later.	No	No	7.0 g/d L ≤ Hb ≤ 8.0 g/dL with symptomatic anemia or Hb ≤7.0 g/dL	Aspirin	Clinical+ ultrasound
		Combined:59	Combined: 68.27	Combined: Same IV dose + 2 g used before closure of arthrotomy					
Nielsen[22]	NS	VI:30	VI: 63.2	VI: 1 g used + 100 mL of saline used after closure of the capsule	No	No	Hb < 7.5 g/dL or < 10 g/dL with heart disease or Hb reduced > 25%	Rivaroxaban	Clinical
		Combined:30	Combined: 65.5	Combined: same IV dose+ 3 g used after closure of the capsule					
Lee [23]	OA	VI:93	VI: 73.4	VI: 10 mg/kg 30 min before deflation, same dose repeated 3 h later	Yes	Yes	7.0 g/dL ≤ Hb ≤ 8.0 g/dL with symptomatic anemia or Hb ≤7.0 g/dL	Rivaroxaban, Aspirin	Clinical +CT
		Combined:95	Combined: 72.1	Combined: 10 mg/kg 30 min before deflation, same dose repeated 3 h later + 2 g injected.					
Song [24]	OA	VI:50	VI: 69.2	VI: 10 mg/kg 20 min before inflation,10 mg/kg 15 min before deflation, and 10 mg/kg 3 h later.	Yes	Yes	Hb < 8 g/%	LMWH	Ultrasound + CT
		Combined:50	Combined: 70.8	Combined: Same IV dose + 1.5 g used topically after wound closure					
Liu [19]	OA	VI:25	VI: NS	VI: 1 g 10 min before inflation	Yes	Yes	Hb ≤8 g/dL	Rivaroxaban	Ultrasound
		Combined:25	Combined: NS	Combined: same VI dose + ˙ g 10 min before inflation					

Abbreviation: *OA* osteoarthritis, *VI* intravenous, **NS not stated**, *DVT* deep venous thrombosis, *Hb* hemoglobin, *LMWH* low-molecular weight heparin, *CT* computed tomographic

Table 2 Quality assessment and modified Jadad score of included 6 randomized controlled trials

Studies (years)	Random sequence generation	Allocation concealment	Blinding	Incomplete outcome data	Selective reporting	Other bias	Modified Jadad score
Huang (2014) [16]	Low	Low	Low	Low	Low	Low	8
Liu (2015) [19]	Unclear	Unclear	Unclear	Low	Low	Low	4
Jain (2016) [17]	Low	Low	Low	Low	Low	Low	7
Nielsen (2016) [22]	Low	Low	Low	Low	Low	Low	8
Lee (2017) [23]	Low	Low	Unclear	Low	Low	Low	6
Song (2017) [24]	Low	Low	Low	Low	Low	Low	7

Abbreviation: Low:low risk of bias; Unclear: unclear risk of bias; High: high risk of bias

Meta-analysis of transfusion requirements

A total of five studies [16, 17, 22–24] reported relevant data regarding transfusion requirements (326 and 325 patients in the combined group and IV group, respectively). The outcome of meta-analysis indicates that transfusion requirements found 4 of 326 patients in the combined group, compared to 9 of 325 patients in the IV group. The risk ratio (RR) shown there was no significant difference between the two group in the incidence of transfusion requirement (RR = 0.48, 95% CI, 0.16 to 1.44;$P = 0.19$) (Fig. 6). A Fixed-effects model was used since there was no significant heterogeneity among the studies ($P = 0.69$, $I^2 = 0\%$). Similar results were received from subgroup analysis based on the application of the tourniquet or non-tourniquet, topical dose and number of IV TXA (Table 4).

Meta-analysis of DVT and PE

A total of six studies [16, 17, 22–24, 28] reported relevant data regarding DVT (351 and 350 patients in the

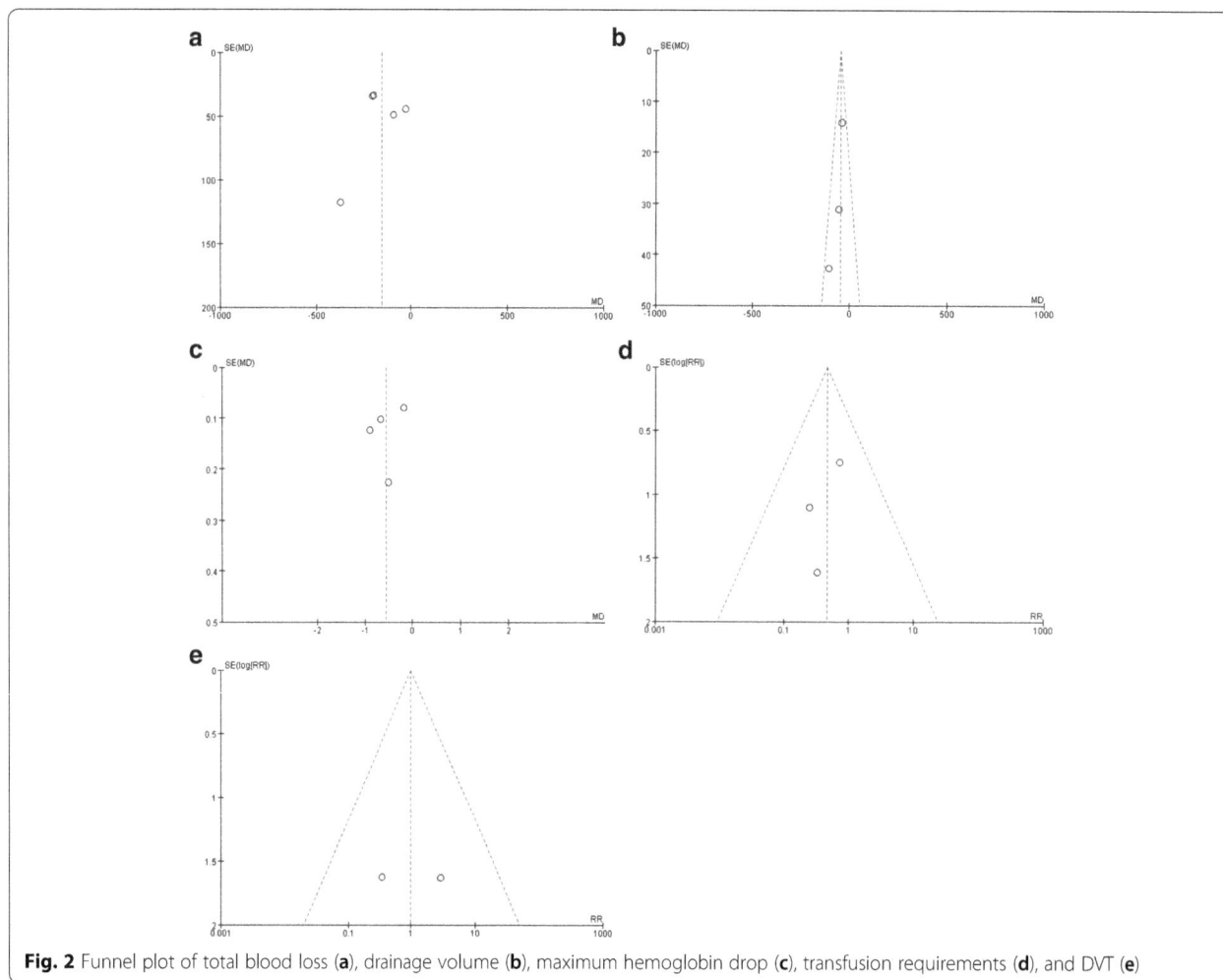

Fig. 2 Funnel plot of total blood loss (**a**), drainage volume (**b**), maximum hemoglobin drop (**c**), transfusion requirements (**d**), and DVT (**e**)

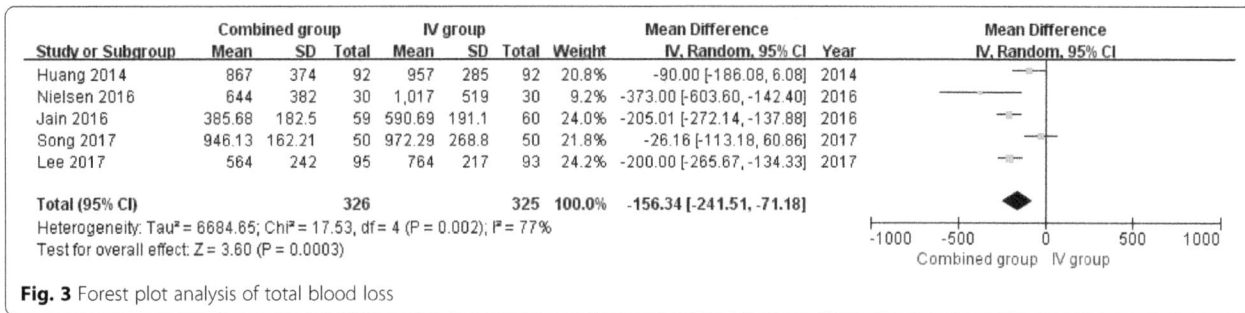

Study or Subgroup	Combined group Mean	SD	Total	IV group Mean	SD	Total	Weight	Mean Difference IV, Random, 95% CI	Year	Mean Difference IV, Random, 95% CI
Huang 2014	867	374	92	957	285	92	20.8%	-90.00 [-186.08, 6.08]	2014	
Nielsen 2016	644	382	30	1,017	519	30	9.2%	-373.00 [-603.60, -142.40]	2016	
Jain 2016	385.68	182.5	59	590.69	191.1	60	24.0%	-205.01 [-272.14, -137.88]	2016	
Song 2017	946.13	162.21	50	972.29	268.8	50	21.8%	-26.16 [-113.18, 60.86]	2017	
Lee 2017	564	242	95	764	217	93	24.2%	-200.00 [-265.67, -134.33]	2017	
Total (95% CI)			326			325	100.0%	-156.34 [-241.51, -71.18]		

Heterogeneity: Tau² = 6684.65; Chi² = 17.53, df = 4 (P = 0.002); I² = 77%
Test for overall effect: Z = 3.60 (P = 0.0003)

Fig. 3 Forest plot analysis of total blood loss

combined group and IV group, respectively). There was 1 in each of the two groups. Of which, 1 of 92 patients [16] who received combination intravenous and topical TXA developed DVT, and 1 of 60 patients [17] who received only intravenous TXA developed DVT (RR 1.01, 95% CI, 0.14 to 7.12; $P = 0.99$) (Fig. 7). All but 1 study [23] reported 1 PE found in the IVTXA (RR 0.33, 95% CI, 0.01 to 7.91; $P = 0.49$). Thus, no significant differences were found in the two groups in terms of the incidence of DVT and PE. A fixed-effects model was used, since there was no significant heterogeneity among the studies ($P = 0.34$, $I^2 = 0\%$).

Discussion

Tranexamic acid, an analog of the amino acid lysine, successfully reduces perioperative blood loss and transfusion requirements in primary TKA [5, 6, 29, 30]. TXA can be applied during the perioperative period either intravenously [13, 31], topically [8, 32], and orally [15, 33]. Recently, an increasing number of studies have focused on the issue that when compared with only intravenous or topical TXA, whether combination application of IV and topical TXA has additional benefits in primary TKA [16, 17, 22]. Thus, we performed the meta-analysis to assess the efficacy and safety of combined application versus intravenous application of TXA in TKA.

The main finding of this meta-analysis is that the combined application intravenous and topical of TXA can significantly reduce postoperative total blood loss, drainage volume, maximum hemoglobin drop compared to the application of intravenous TXA alone. Subgroup analyses showed that total blood loss was less in patients with non-tourniquet, topical TXA dose > 1.5 g and IV TXA ≥ 2 doses. No significant differences were found in the incidence of DVT and PE between the two groups.

The administration of IV TXA in TKA has been well established in a lot of literature. Akgül et al. [34] reported 20 mg/kg IV-TXA given before the skin incision in the primary TKA could decrease the total blood loss from 1166.42 mL to 634.03 mL and reduce

the drainage volume from 640.74 mL to 311.11 mL. Pitta et al. [35] performed another retrospective study involving 610 patients during 4 years, they reported the administered IV of TXA resulted in a significant decrease by 9.4% in blood loss compared to the control group in TKA, and no significantly different was found in the incidence of DVT. Compared with the safety concerns with intravenous administration, topical TXA has been a growing interest to prevent bleeding. As previously reported, it was considered to less of 70% systemic absorption and thus may be a systemic alternative. Ishida et al. [36] conducted a randomized controlled trial that injected 2000 mg/20 mL topical TXA compared with a placebo group in TKA, the results revealed that postoperative decreasing in Hb level and knee joint swelling was significantly reduced in the TXA group compared to the control group. Recently, a new strategy of combined administration of TXA was explored considering the advantages of both methods. A randomized, double-blind, placebo-controlled trial [22] of 60 patients comparing patients who received combined IV and topical TXA or IV TXA in primary TKA found that combined administration results in significantly lower total blood loss and postoperative Hb level, while the incidence of DVT was similar between the two groups. Lee et al. [23] have also found the similar results that while there were no patients in any study group received an allogeneic transfusion, the combined group had lower total blood loss than the IV-only group.

The current meta-analysis shows that combined group could effectively reduce postoperative total blood loss by about 156.34 mL compared with IV TXA alone. Similarly, subgroup analysis suggested that there is also the significant difference between the two group in terms of the use of tourniquet or non-tourniquet, topical (≤1.5 g or > 1.5 g) and the number of IV TXA (single or ≥ 2 doses). Furthermore, the meta-analysis indicates that drainage volume found in the combined group significantly reduced drainage volume by a mean of 43.54 mL compared with the IV group. Thus, the combined

Table 3 Results of meta-analysis and subgroup analyses of the included studies

Results (Combined vs. IV groups)	No.of studies / knee	P	Effect Size			Model
			MD/RR	95% CI	Heterogeneity p (I^2)	
1. Total blood loss						
All studies	5/651	0.0003	−156.34	241.51 to −71.18	0.002 (77%)	Random
Tourniquet or Non-tourniquet						
Tourniquet	3/471	0.05	− 108.68	− 217.44 to 0.08	0.005 (81%)	Random
Non-tourniquet	2/179	0.0008	− 251.30	−398.40 to − 104.19	0.17 (47%)	Fixed
Topical TXA dose						
≤ 1.5 g	2/284	0.10	−54.93	−119.43 to 9.57	0.33 (0%)	Fixed
>1.5 g	3/367	< 0.00001	− 209.39	− 255.95 to − 162.83	0.36 (1%)	Fixed
Number of IV TXA						
Single dose	2/244	0.13	−210.91	− 485.30 to 63.47	0.03 (80%)	Random
≥ 2 doses	3/407	0.005	− 147.43	−251.16 to −43.69	0.002 (84%)	Random
2. Maximum hemoglobin drop						
All studies	4/591	0.003	−0.56	−0.93 to −0.19	< 0.00001 (90%)	Random
Tourniquet or Non-tourniquet						
Tourniquet	3/472	0.05	−0.52	−1.04 to 0.00	< 0.00001 (92%)	Random
Non-tourniquet	1/119	< 0.00001	−0.68	− 0.88 to − 0.48	–	–
Topical TXA dose						
≤ 1.5 g	2/284	0.006	−0.21	−0.35 to − 0.06	0.17 (47%)	Fixed
>1.5 g	2/307	< 0.00001	−0.78	−0.99 to − 0.56	0.17 (47%)	Fixed
Number of IV TXA						
Single dose	1/184	0.03	−0.17	−0.33 to − 0.01	–	–
≥ 2 doses	3/407	< 0.00001	−0.73	−0.93 to − 0.54	0.21 (36%)	Fixed
3. Transfusion requirements						
All studies	5/651	0.19	0.48	0.16 to 1.44	0.69 (0%)	Fixed
Tourniquet or Non-tourniquet						
Tourniquet	3/472	0.70	0.75	0.17 to 3.26	–	–
Non-tourniquet	2/179	0.16	0.28	0.05 to 1.64	0.89 (0%)	Fixed
Topical TXA dose						
≤ 1.5 g	3/344	0.50	0.64	0.17 to 2.37	0.65 (0%)	Fixed
>1.5 g	2/307	0.21	0.25	0.03 to 2.21	–	–
Number of IV TXA						
Single dose	2/244	0.50	0.64	0.17 to 2.37	0.65 (0%)	
≥ 2 doses	3/407	0.21	0.25	0.03 to 2.21	–	–
4. Drainage volume	3/334	0.0004	−43.54	−67.59 to −19.48	0.34 (7%)	Fixed
5. DVT	6/701	0.99	1.01	0.14 to 7.12	0.34 (0%)	Fixed

Abbreviation: RR, risk ratio; MDs, mean differences; IV, Intravenous; DVT, deep venous thrombosis

administration of TXA could be a reasonable alternative to IV TXA alone for decreasing blood loss and drainage volume in primary TKA.

In our meta-analysis, the rate of transfusion requirements was slightly less for the combined group (1.2%) than for the IV TXA group (2.8%), but the difference was not statistically significant (RR 0.48, $P =$ 0.19). Subgroup analyses showed similar results for the tourniquet or non-tourniquet and different topical or the number of IV TXA. Huang et al. [16] performed one RCT, 1.5 g topical TXA administered combined with 1.5 g IV-TXA, and there was no statistically significant difference regarding transfusion requirements between the two groups. Another RCT

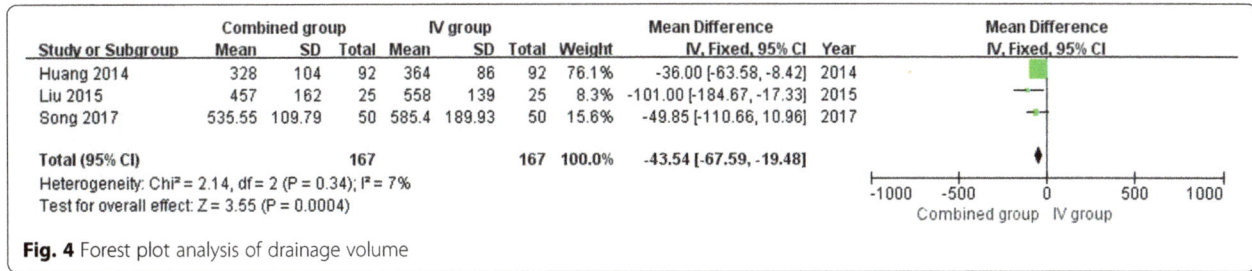

Fig. 4 Forest plot analysis of drainage volume

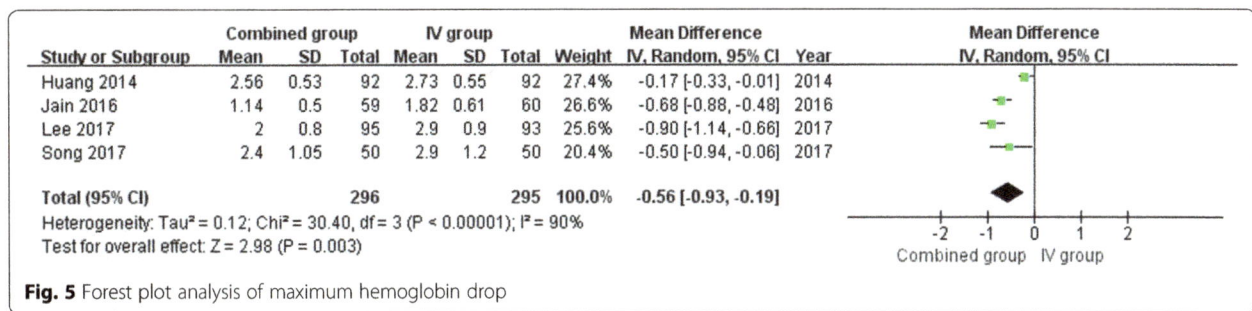

Fig. 5 Forest plot analysis of maximum hemoglobin drop

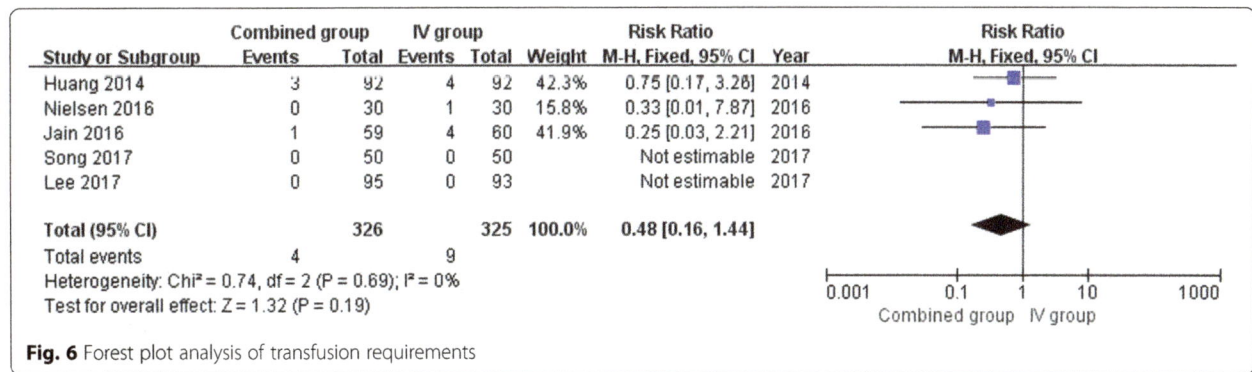

Fig. 6 Forest plot analysis of transfusion requirements

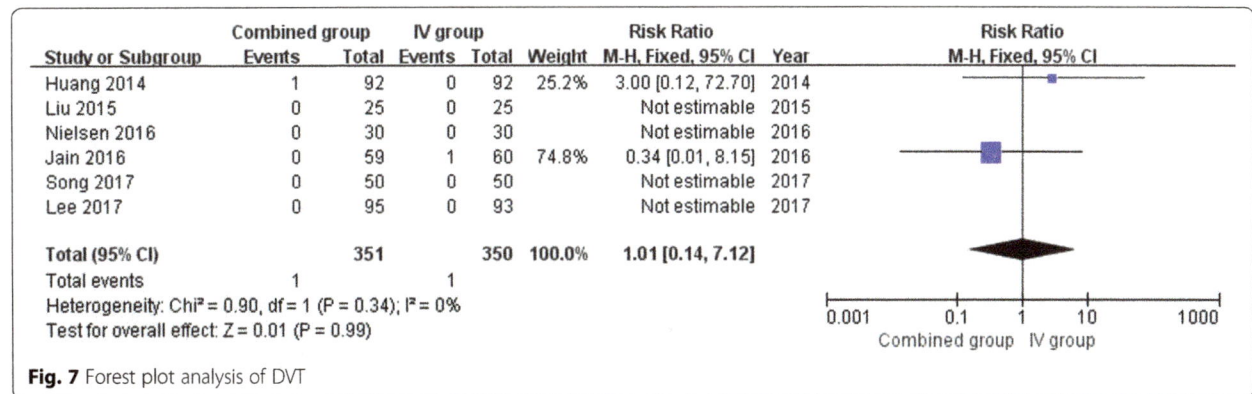

Fig. 7 Forest plot analysis of DVT

[23], 119 patients were randomized into combined group and IV group alone, the combined group provided better results than IV alone in total blood loss (590.69 ± 191.1mLvs. 385.68 ± 182.5 mL, $P <$ 0.001), but no difference in blood transfusion rate (6.6% vs. 1.6%, $P = 0.364$). The result of our meta-analysis evaluating transfusion rates was consistent with these studies.

Thromboembolic prophylaxis methods were performed in all of the studies and as follow: low-molecular-weight heparin, aspirin, and enoxaparin. As Anderson et al. [37] reported in "N Engl J Med", they found that among patients who received 5 days of rivaroxaban prophylaxis following TKA/THA, extended prophylaxis with aspirin was not significantly different from rivaroxaban in the prevention of DVT. Additionally, all thromboembolic events were detected by clinical symptomatic, routine Doppler ultrasound, or CT angiography. Finally, there was 1 in each of the two groups. The total rate of DVT was 0.03%. There was no difference in both two group ($P = 0.99$). 1 PE was found in the IV TXA group. Our findings are consistent with those of RCT [17, 23] or meta-analysis [38, 39] which found that no previous studies have reported increased rates of symptomatic DVT or PE with the combined administration of TXA in TKA.

The current study had the following strengths. First, all of the included studies have been well-designed and satisfied the defined eligibility criteria comparing the efficacy of combined TXA versus intravenous administration of TXA during TKA. Second, subgroup analysis was performed based on the use of the tourniquet or non-tourniquet and different topical or the number of IV TXA. The results showed that combined administration of TXA in TKA can effectively reduce total blood loss and maximum hemoglobin drop compared with IV TXA alone. Third, this study independently used funnel plots to assess publication bias, the plots were generally symmetrical and shown a lower publication bias. However, the meta-analysis also has limitations. First, the reported blood loss methods are not consistent, which may lead to deviations in the clinical outcome of blood loss. In addition, the method for estimating displacement is not detailed, so it cannot exclude the result deviation caused by human factors measurement. Second, the number of RCTs included was limited. Thus, more carefully and scientifically designed RCTs are needed in the future to further confirm and compare the different results. Third, due to the limited sample size of the study, our meta-analysis failed to extract adequate data pertaining to some items from these studies, such as function outcomes, patient satisfaction, and other complications, etc. Last, there was substantial heterogeneity in the meta-analysis of several outcomes, including total blood loss and drainage volume. However, taking into account the effects of the tourniquet and different topical TXA dose (≤1.5 g or > 1.5 g) or

number of IV TXA (single or ≥ 2 doses), thus subgroup analysis was performed to decrease heterogeneity.

Conclusions

This meta-analysis of currently available evidence indicates that combined administration of intravenous and topical TXA in primary TKA can significantly reduce total blood loss, drainage volume and maximum hemoglobin drop compared with IV TXA alone. The main finding, however, is that there is no significant difference in transfusion rates because this is the most clinically relevant point in this **meta-analysis.**

Abbreviations
CI: Confidence interval; DVT: DVT; IV: Intravenous; MD: Mean differences; PE: Pulmonary embolism; RCT: Randomized controlled trials; RR: Risk ratio; SD: Standard deviation;; TA: Tranexamic acid; TKA: Total knee arthroplasty; TKR: Total knee replacement; TXA: Tranexamic acid

Authors' contributions
Bin Shen conceived, designed and coordinated the experiments and drafted the manuscript. Huazhang Xiong and Yi Zeng contributed to data acquisition. Yi Zeng and Yuangang Wu analysed and interpreted the data. Huazhang Xiong and Bin Shen revised the manuscript. All authors read and approved the final manuscript.

Competing interests
The authors declare that they have no competing interests.

Author details
 Department of Orthopaedic Surgery, West China Hospital, West China Medical School, Sichuan University, Chengdu, Sichuan Province 610041, People's Republic of China. [2]Department of Orthopedic Surgery, The First Affiliated Hospital of Zunyi Medical College, Zunyi 563003, Guizhou Province, China.

References
1. Zeni JA Jr, Axe MJ, Snyder-Mackler L. Clinical predictors of elective total joint replacement in persons with end-stage knee osteoarthritis. BMC Musculoskelet Disord. 2010;11:86.
2. Levine BR, Haughom B, Strong B, Hellman M, Frank RM. Blood management strategies for total knee arthroplasty. J Am Acad Orthop Surg. 2014;22:361–71.
3. Edelstein AI, Kwasny MJ, Suleiman LI, Khakhkhar RH, Moore MA, Beal MD, et al. Can the American College of Surgeons risk calculator predict 30-day complications after knee and hip arthroplasty? J Arthroplast 2015;30:5–10.
4. Wong J, Abrishami A, El Beheiry H, Mahomed NN, Roderick Davey J, Gandhi R, et al. Topical application of tranexamic acid reduces postoperative blood loss in total knee arthroplasty: a randomized, controlled trial.J Bone Joint Surg Am 2010 ;92:2503–2513.
5. Chen JY, Chin PL, Moo IH, Pang HN, Tay DK, Chia SL, et al. Intravenous versus intra-articular tranexamic acid in total knee arthroplasty: a double-blinded randomised controlled noninferiority trial. Knee. 2016;23:152–6.
6. Wu Y, Yang T, Zeng Y, Li C, Shen B, Pei F. Clamping drainage is unnecessary after minimally invasive total knee arthroplasty in patients with tranexamic acid: a randomized, controlled trial. Medicine. 2017;96:e5804.
7. Xie J, Ma J, Kang P, Zhou Z, Shen B, Yang J, et al. Does tranexamic acid alter the risk of thromboembolism following primary total knee arthroplasty with sequential earlier anticoagulation? A large, single center, prospective cohort study of consecutive cases. Thromb Res. 2015;136:234–8.
8. May JH, Rieser GR, Williams CG, Markert RJ, Bauman RD, Lawless MW. The assessment of blood loss during Total knee arthroplasty when comparing intravenous vs Intracapsular Administration of Tranexamic Acid. J Arthroplast. 2016;31:2452–7.

9. Georgiadis AG, Muh SJ, Silverton CD, Weir RM, Laker MW. A prospective double-blind placebo controlled trial of topical tranexamic acid in total knee arthroplasty. J Arthroplast. 2013;28:78–82.

10. MacGillivray RG, Tarabichi SB, Hawari MF, Raoof NT. Tranexamic acid to reduce blood loss after bilateral total knee arthroplasty: a prospective, randomized double blind study. J. Arthroplasty. 2011;26:24–8.

11. Wang H, Shen B, Zeng Y. Comparison of topical versus intravenous tranexamic acid in primary total knee arthroplasty: a meta-analysis of randomized controlled and prospective cohort trials. Knee. 2014;21:987–93.

12. Wei Z, Liu M. The effectiveness and safety of tranexamic acid in total hip or knee arthroplasty: a meta-analysis of 2720 cases. Transfusion medicine (Oxford, England). 2015;25:151–62.

13. Charoencholvanich K, Siriwattanasakul P. Tranexamic acid reduces blood loss and blood transfusion after TKA: a prospective randomized controlled trial. Clin Orthop Relat Res. 2011;469:2874–80.

14. Tzatzairis TK, Drosos GI, Kotsios SE, Ververidis AN, Vogiatzaki TD, Kazakos KI. Intravenous vs topical tranexamic acid in Total knee arthroplasty without tourniquet application: a randomized controlled study. J Arthroplast. 2016; 31:2465–70.

15. Lee QJ, Ching WY, Wong YC. Blood sparing efficacy of oral tranexamic acid in primary Total knee arthroplasty: a randomized controlled trial. Knee surgery & related research. 2017;29:57–62.

16. Huang Z, Ma J, Shen B, Pei F. Combination of intravenous and topical application of tranexamic acid in primary total knee arthroplasty: a prospective randomized controlled trial. J Arthroplast. 2014;29:2342–6.

17. Jain NP, Nisthane PP, Shah NA. Combined Administration of Systemic and Topical Tranexamic Acid for Total knee arthroplasty: can it be a better regimen and yet safe? A randomized controlled trial. J Arthroplast. 2016;31:542–7.

18. Seo JG, Moon YW, Park SH, Kim SM, Ko KR. The comparative efficacies of intra-articular and IV tranexamic acid for reducing blood loss during total knee arthroplasty. Knee Surg Sports Traumatol Arthrosc. 2013;21(8):1869–74.

19. Shang J, Wang H, Zheng B, Rui M, Wang Y. Combined intravenous and topical tranexamic acid versus intravenous use alone in primary total knee and hip arthroplasty: a meta-analysis of randomized controlled trials. Int J Surg. 2016;36:324–9.

20. Li JF, Li H, Zhao H, Wang J, Liu S, Song Y, Wu HF. Combined use of intravenous and topical versus intravenous tranexamic acid in primary total knee and hip arthroplasty: a meta-analysis of randomised controlled trials. J Orthop Surg Res. 2017;12(1):22.

21. Wang Z, Shen X. The efficacy of combined intra-articular and intravenous tranexamic acid for blood loss in primary total knee arthroplasty: a meta-analysis. Medicine. 2017;96(42)

22. Nielsen CS, Jans O, Orsnes T, Foss NB, Troelsen A, Husted H. Combined intra-articular and intravenous tranexamic acid reduces blood loss in Total knee arthroplasty: a randomized, double-blind, placebo-controlled trial. J Bone Joint Surg Am. 2016;98:835–41.

23. Lee SY, Chong S, Balasubramanian D, Na YG, Kim TK. What is the Ideal Route of Administration of Tranexamic Acid in TKA? A Randomized Controlled Trial. Clin Orthop Relat Res. 2017;475:1987–96.

24. Song EK, Seon JK, Prakash J, Seol YJ, Park YJ, Jin C. Combined administration of IV and topical tranexamic acid is not superior to either individually in primary navigated TKA. J Arthroplast. 2017;32:37–42.

25. Moher D, Liberati A, Tetzlaff J, Altman DG. Preferred reporting items for systematic reviews and meta-analyses: the PRISMA statement. Open medicine : a peer-reviewed, independent, open-access journal. 2009;3:e123–30.

26. Higgins JP, Altman DG, Gotzsche PC, Juni P, Moher D, Oxman AD, et al. The Cochrane Collaboration's tool for assessing risk of bias in randomised trials. BMJ (Clinical research ed). 2011;343:d5928.

27. Huang Z, Ma J, Pei F, Yang J, Zhou Z, Kang P, et al. Meta-analysis of temporary versus no clamping in TKA. Orthopedics. 2013;36:543–50.

28. Liu L, Yang Z, Yao J, Xu P. Effect of local injection combined intravenous drip tranexamic acid on blood loss in total knee arthroplasty. J N Sichuan Med Coll. 2015;30:611–4.

29. Gomez-Barrena E, Ortega-Andreu M, Padilla-Eguiluz NG, Perez-Chrzanowska H, Figueredo-Zalve R. Topical intra-articular compared with intravenous tranexamic acid to reduce blood loss in primary total knee replacement: a double-blind, randomized, controlled, noninferiority clinical trial. J Bone Joint Surg Am. 2014;96:1937–44.

30. Patel JN, Spanyer JM, Smith LS, Huang J, Yakkanti MR, Malkani AL. Comparison of intravenous versus topical tranexamic acid in total knee arthroplasty: a prospective randomized study. J Arthroplast. 2014;29:1528–31.

31. Alshryda S, Sarda P, Sukeik M, Nargol A, Blenkinsopp J, Mason JM. Tranexamic acid in total knee replacement: a systematic review and meta-analysis. J Bone Joint Surg. 2011;93:1577–85.

32. Alshryda S, Sukeik M, Sarda P, Blenkinsopp J, Haddad FS, Mason JM. A systematic review and meta-analysis of the topical administration of tranexamic acid in total hip and knee replacement. The bone & joint journal. 2014;96-B:1005–15.

33. Fillingham YA, Kayupov E, Plummer DR, Moric M, Gerlinger TL, Della Valle CJ. The James a. Rand young Investigator's award: a randomized controlled trial of oral and intravenous tranexamic acid in Total knee arthroplasty: the same efficacy at lower cost? J Arthroplast. 2016;31:26–30.

34. Akgul T, Buget M, Salduz A, Edipoglu IS, Ekinci M, Kucukay S, et al. Efficacy of preoperative administration of single high dose intravenous tranexamic acid in reducing blood loss in total knee arthroplasty: a prospective clinical study. Acta Orthop Traumatol Turc 2016;50:429–431.

35. Pitta M, Zawadsky M, Verstraete R, Rubinstein A. Intravenous administration of tranexamic acid effectively reduces blood loss in primary total knee arthroplasty in a 610-patient consecutive case series. Transfusion. 2016;56: 466–71.

36. Ishida K, Tsumura N, Kitagawa A, Hamamura S, Fukuda K, Dogaki Y, et al. Intra-articular injection of tranexamic acid reduces not only blood loss but also knee joint swelling after total knee arthroplasty. Int Orthop. 2011;35: 1639–45.

37. Anderson DR, Dunbar M, Murnaghan J, Kahn SR, Gross P, Forsythe M. Aspirin or rivaroxaban for VTE prophylaxis after hip or knee arthroplasty. N Engl J Med. 2018;378(8):699–707.

38. Zhang XQ, Ni J, Ge WH. Combined use of intravenous and topical versus intravenous tranexamic acid in primary total joint arthroplasty: a meta-analysis of randomized controlled trials. International journal of surgery (London, England). 2017;38:15–20.

39. Zhao-Yu C, Yan G, Wei C, Yuejv L, Ying-Ze Z. Reduced blood loss after intra-articular tranexamic acid injection during total knee arthroplasty: a meta-analysis of the literature. Knee surgery, sports traumatology, arthroscopy : official journal of the ESSKA. 2014;22:3181–90.

2

Predicting the outcome of conservative treatment with physiotherapy in adults with shoulder pain associated with partial-thickness rotator cuff tears – a prognostic model development study

Cordula Braun[1,2,4*], Nigel C. Hanchard[1], Helen H. Handoll[1] and Andreas Betthäuser[3]

Abstract

Background: Rotator cuff disorders represent the commonest type of painful shoulder complaints in clinical practice. Although conservative treatment including physiotherapy is generally recommended as first-line treatment, little is known about the precise treatment indications for subgroups of rotator cuff disorders, particularly people with shoulder pain associated with partial-thickness tears of the rotator cuff, PTTs: "symptomatic PPTs". The aim of this study was to develop a prognostic model for predicting the outcome of a phase of conservative treatment primarily with physiotherapy in adults with symptomatic PTTs.

Methods: A prospective observational cohort study was conducted in an outpatient setting in Germany. Ten baseline factors were selected to evaluate nine pre-defined multivariable candidate prognostic models (each including between two and nine factors) in a cohort of adults with symptomatic atraumatic PTTs undergoing a three-month phase of conservative treatment primarily with physiotherapy. The primary outcome was change in the Western Ontario Rotator Cuff Index. The models were developed using linear regression and an information-theoretic analysis approach: Akaike's Information Criterion (AIC_C).

Results: Eight candidate models were analyzed using data from 61 participants. Two "best models" were identified: smoking & pain catastrophizing and disability & pain catastrophizing. However, none of the models had a satisfactory performance or precision.

Conclusions: We could not determine a prognostic model with satisfactory performance and precision. Further high-quality prognostic model studies with larger samples are needed, but should be underpinned, and thus preceded, by robust research that enhances knowledge of relevant prognostic factors.

Study registration: DRKS00004462. Registered 08 April 2014; retrospectively registered (prior to the analysis).

Keywords: Shoulder pain, Rotator cuff, Conservative treatment, Physical therapy, Prognosis, Prognostic model development

* Correspondence: braun@hs21.de
[1]School of Health and Social Care, Teesside University, Middlesbrough, UK
[2]Present address: Faculty of Health and Physiotherapy, Buxtehude, Germany
Full list of author information is available at the end of the article

Background

Painful shoulder complaints are common musculoskeletal disorders in clinical practice [1], most being attributed to rotator cuff pathology [2, 3]. Rotator cuff pathology encompasses a range of pathologies from tendinopathy to tears, which may be partial- or full-thickness [4]. Reported rates of symptomatic partial-thickness tears (PTTs), the condition of interest in this study, vary between 7% [5] and 24% [6] in shoulder pain populations. Of the four rotator cuff tendons (supraspinatus, infraspinatus, teres minor, subscapularis), the supraspinatus is by far the most often affected [7], and also usually the first to tear [8, 9]. In order to concisely label the population of interest, we use the term "symptomatic PTT" to describe people with shoulder pain in the presence of a PTT of the rotator cuff.

The clinical presentation of symptomatic PTTs is essentially that of "shoulder impingement" [7, 9, 10]. Verification of a PTT requires diagnostic imaging, commonly ultrasonography (US) or magnetic resonance imaging (MRI) [11].

Current guidelines for rotator cuff disorders [12, 13] recommend conservative treatment with medical care and physiotherapy as the first-line treatment; surgical intervention being mainly reserved for non-responders. Head-to-head comparisons of conservative and surgical interventions [14] have overall shown no clinically relevant differences. However, utilisation of surgery for rotator cuff disorders has significantly increased in many countries [15–17], with physiotherapy bypassed in some cases [18]. Both unnecessary surgery and ineffective conservative treatment are undesirable. Knowledge about a patient's likely response to conservative treatment at the point of diagnosis would save time, effort and suffering, limit exposure to the risks of surgery, and inform distribution of resources. "Understanding which patients [with rotator cuff tears] do best with non-operative treatment" has been rated a top "priority scientific research issue" ([19], p. 10).

The importance of predicting individuals' responses to particular interventions is increasingly recognized [20], with a corresponding development in prognosis research methodology [21, 22]. One aspect of prognosis research involves the identification of single, independent factors [23]. However, these are unlikely to predict outcomes satisfactorily. Multivariable prognostic models are better placed as they account for real-life clinical complexities [24, 25]. Estimates of prognosis are highly context-dependent, with relevant contextual factors being existing diagnostic and treatment practices, time and place.

Prognostic model research encompasses three key phases: development including internal validation; external validation; and evaluation of clinical impact [25]. External validation is essential before a model may be usable in practice [25]. While prospective cohort studies are generally considered the preferable design for the initial development of a prognostic model [25–27], evaluations of the clinical impact of a prognostic model ultimately require comparative studies.

Our systematic review of the evidence on prognostic models for predicting outcomes in adults undergoing physiotherapy for rotator cuff disorders showed a lack of clinically usable prognostic models and, crucially, of prognostic model research on PTTs [28]. The study's primary aim was to develop a multivariable prognostic model for the outcome of a phase of conservative treatment with physiotherapy in adults with symptomatic atraumatic PTTs. Secondary aims were to determine the incidence of tear progression and to establish participants' perceived change of their shoulder complaints over time.

Methods

The study was based on an a priori protocol and was approved by the Teesside University School of Health and Social Care Research Governance & Ethics Committee and the Ethics Commission of the Hamburg Medical Council (Germany). It was registered in the German Clinical Trials Register (reg.no DRKS00004462). The study design was informed by the most current methodological guidance available at the time of planning [21, 22]. All deviations from protocol were discussed and recorded prior to implementation [29]; the only two relevant deviations are flagged up in this section. This report complies with the items required by the TRIPOD (Transparent Reporting of a multivariable prediction model for Individual Prognosis Or Diagnosis) prediction model development checklist [30].

Study design, setting and key dates

We conducted a prospective observational single-group cohort study set in Hamburg, Germany. All recruitment and assessments took place in a single-handed medical specialist practice led by one of the authors, AB, an orthopaedic shoulder specialist and DEGUM (German Society for Ultrasonography in Medicine) certified instructor in ultrasonographic shoulder diagnosis. The physiotherapy treatment took place in 24 collaborating physical therapy practices in the broader area of Hamburg. (In our protocol, we initially considered seven collaborating practices, but expanded their number eventually to 24 to improve recruitment). Recruitment took place between December 2012 to September 2014. Follow-up ended in January 2015.

Participants

Eligible patients were adults (≥ 18 years) presenting with shoulder pain unrelated to a traumatic event (e.g. an accident) and an ultrasonographically determined PTT who had accepted advice to undergo conservative treatment with physiotherapy (see Table 1 for the full eligibility criteria). These patients typically present with clinical signs of "shoulder impingement", such as a painful arc or positive "impingement signs" [7, 9, 10]. We additionally determined the presence of a PTT by diagnostic ultrasonography, which is highly specific for detecting PTTs [31]. Our intention was to recruit patients whose shoulder pain could reasonably be linked to the presence of a PTT; however, we acknowledge that the precise link between shoulder pain and the presence of a PTT (similar to other shoulder structures) is unclear [32]. Following standard practice, the assessment involved a structured patient history, physical and ultrasonographic evaluation. The physical evaluation was based on DVSE (German Society for Shoulder and Elbow Surgery) recommendations [33]. The ultrasonographic evaluation followed DEGUM and DGOU (German Society for Orthopaedics and Trauma) standards [34]. An ultrasound unit within the highest DEGUM appliance class was used together with a linear transducer with a resolution of ≥ 10 MHZ and width of ≥ 40 mm. Diagnosis of a rotator cuff defect was based on alterations of structure and form, following the criteria of Hedtmann & Fett [35, 36]. In distinction to a PTT, a full-thickness

tear (FTT) was marked by the absence of a depiction of the rotator cuff (discontinuity of the cuff).

Treatment

Participants were followed over three months of standard conservative care with physiotherapy in one of the collaborating practices. Adjunctive medical treatment (e.g. local steroid injections), was delivered by AB where considered appropriate. The physiotherapy treatment followed a broad best-evidence protocol based on two systematic reviews [37, 38]. These reviews provided evidence supporting exercises with or without manual therapy as the first-line approach for treating patients with rotator cuff related shoulder pain including PTTs, but could not provide conclusive guidance on the optimal type or dose of treatment. Since there was no justification for restricting treatment to any specific exercises or manual techniques, the protocol was based on the broad principles that a) exercises, preferably combined with manual techniques (soft tissue and/or joint mobilisation), would be the key treatment components, and b) flexibility of the interventions and in the provision of adjunctive modalities would be allowed. In keeping with the ethos of an observational study, the specific content and amount of treatment were unregulated, i.e. individually advised. Treatment, which included the clinical follow-up appointment at three months to assess progress and need for further treatment, was delivered in compliance with German healthcare regulations and AB's standard practice. Acceptability of the physiotherapy protocol was confirmed by all collaborating physiotherapy practices. Treatment details were documented in a purpose-designed, piloted report form.

Outcomes

The primary outcome, the outcome to be predicted, was the change in 'disability' (disability and health-related quality of life) from baseline to follow-up, measured by a validated German version of the Western Ontario Rotator Cuff Index (WORC) [39, 40]: $WORC_{CHANGE}$. The WORC has been shown to be a valid, reliable and responsive patient-reported outcome measure (PROM) for use in people with rotator cuff disorders [41, 42]. It comprises 21 questions. Responses are made by putting a mark on a 100 mm visual analogue scale (VAS), with lower scores indicating less disability. Scores range from 0 to 2100 [39]. We adjusted all $WORC_{CHANGE}$ values for Regression to the Mean (RTM) using methods outlined by Linden [43]. Participants completed questionnaires at baseline and at 3 to 4 months, the study endpoint, either at AB's clinic or at home.

As both the WORC and all prognostic factors were patient-assessed, there was no blinding of participants.

Table 1 Eligibility criteria

Inclusion:
- Patients with (local) shoulder pain in the presence of an atraumatic (ultrasonographically detected) partial thickness tear
- Clinical signs of 'shoulder impingement' (e.g. painful arc, positive impingement tests)
- Adults (≥ 18 years)
- No restrictions on sex
- Agreement on conservative treatment
- Ability to speak and comprehend the German language
- Agreement to participate (signed informed consent)
- Anticipated availability for follow-up (living in area of Hamburg)
- Agreement to physiotherapy in a collaborating practice

Exclusion:
- Presence of a full thickness tear at the affected shoulder
- Previous substantial shoulder trauma (e.g. shoulder dislocation, fractures)
- Previous surgery for the affected shoulder
- Previous surgery in the shoulder area that may be causal of or contributory to the current problem (e.g. surgery for breast cancer)
- Clinically relevant glenohumeral degeneration or disease (e.g. frozen shoulder)
- Current glenohumeral septic arthritis
- Clinically relevant acromioclavicular arthritis (e.g. local tenderness, positive provocation tests)
- Clinically relevant calcific tendinitis
- Ultrasonographic evidence of long head of biceps (LHB) tendon subluxation/ dislocation
- Referred pain from the cervical spine region
- Multisite musculoskeletal pain
- Systemic disorders, diseases or comorbidities as potential sources of (the current) shoulder pain (e.g. breast cancer, rheumatoid disease, inherited disorders (e.g. Marfan syndrome, Ehlers-Danlos syndrome)), or as impairing treatment (e.g. cancer, cardiac insufficiencies)
- Neurological disorders or deficits as potential sources of (the current) shoulder pain or impairing assessment and treatment (e.g. hemiplegic shoulder)
- Worker's compensation claims
- Unwillingness or inability to give informed consent (e.g. cognitive or intellectual impairments)

Nonetheless, the WORC was completed independently and in the absence of AB and study investigators.

Secondary outcomes were tear progression, defined as the presence (yes or no) of an FTT at follow-up, and participants' perceived overall change of their shoulder problem, measured by a 7-point Global Perceived Change (GPC) scale (from -3 = "worse as ever" to $+3$ = "completely recovered"). Lastly, physical therapy-related adverse events were monitored.

Prognostic factors

Inclusion of candidate factors was restricted to factors from the baseline assessment, regardless of their type (e.g. demographic, physical). Selection was done through a systematic, three-stage approach comprising identification of factors, critical assessment of these, and a consensus phase that aimed to select a maximum of 10 factors (see Fig. 1 for an outline of the process; a full account is available in Braun 2016 ([29, Chapter 5]). The process was informed by comprehensive literature searches of several electronic databases, including Medline, Embase and Cinahl, for primary prognostic studies, prognostic systematic reviews and expert consensus studies. We screened overall around 3900 records and identified 23 primary study reports (relating to 22 studies), one systematic review and one expert consensus study as relevant sources for informing the selection of factors for our study (a list of these articles is provided in Additional file 1). We extracted and considered 36 factors altogether (these are listed in Additional file 2, which also shows for each factor whether it was included or excluded and the reasons for exclusion). We assessed the relevance of all factors to the study population and setting, their measurement properties, practicality of use, and their applicability, and excluded those that were either not relevant to the study population and setting, not sufficiently valid and reliable, or not applicable in most clinical settings. We grouped the remaining factors according to the availability of clinical evidence and expert consensus supporting their prognostic relevance; we gave preference to the selection of those factors for which there was reasonably consistent support for their prognostic relevance, either through clinical evidence from several studies, or from both clinical evidence and expert consensus. Notably, there was reasonably consistent evidence of prognostic value from several studies pertaining to clinical outcomes of conservative treatment in adults with rotator cuff disorders for only three factors: age, disability and symptom duration. We finally agreed on 10 factors: age, sex, physical demands, disability, pain, history of shoulder pain, symptom duration, diabetes, smoking and pain catastrophizing. We gave thorough attention to factor definitions and measurements (Table 2). All factors were assessed during the patients' baseline appointment with AB. Since the study was prospective, the assessment of prognostic factor information was inherently blinded to knowledge about the outcome.

Sample size

The multivariable nature of prognostic model studies makes it difficult to estimate the required sample size [26]. Indeed, no formal methods (based on either power calculations or adequate precision of estimation of effects) are available to determine the effective sample size, and recommendations for the sample size vary across the literature. Following work by Vittinghoff & McCulloch [44], we based the minimum sample size of our study on a requirement of 5 to 9 outcome events (events equate to individuals for continuous outcomes) per candidate prognostic factor in relation to the full model (i.e. the model including all 10 factors). As per our protocol, we initially planned to analyze the WORC as a binary outcome variable, but subsequently (and prior to the analysis) decided to analyze it as a continuous variable to avoid the unnecessary loss of information that would have resulted from dichotomization [45, 46]. By analyzing the WORC on a continuous scale, and setting out to study overall 10 factors, which we considered feasible, we aimed to include (5 to 9)*10 = 50 to 90 participants. Increased by 20% to allow for losses to follow-up, the recruitment target was 60 to 108 patients.

Missing data

Any missing prognostic factor and outcome data were documented. The decision about the method for dealing with missing data, including whether or not to impute

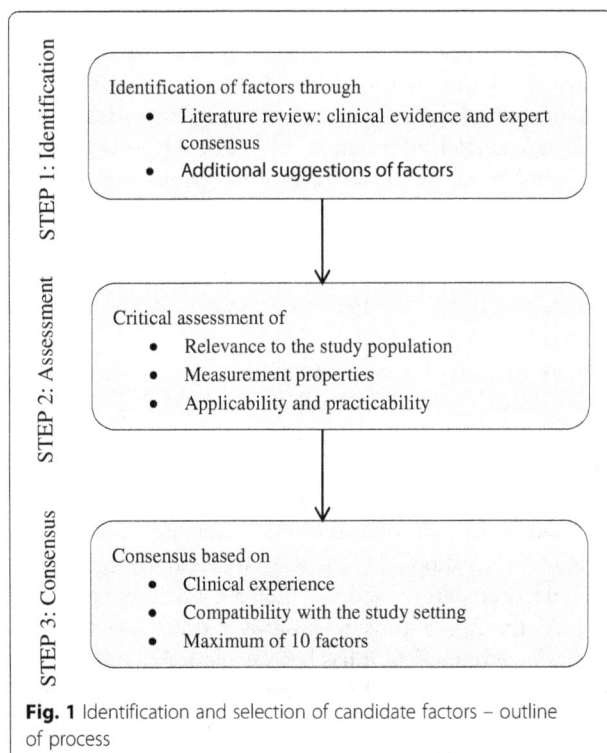

Fig. 1 Identification and selection of candidate factors – outline of process

Table 2 Candidate factors – definition and measurement

No	Predictor variable	Measure / measurement system
1	Age	Age at initial presentation (years)
2	Sex	Sex (female, male)
3	Physical demands	"Before you had your current shoulder problem, did a typical week include one or more of the following activities (yes, no): • Repetitive or prolonged use of the affected arm for strength effort (e.g. lifting, carrying or moving heavy loads, athletic sports, strength-demanding skilled manual work) • Repetitive or prolonged use of the arm above shoulder height (e.g. overhead work, overhead sports, throwing sports, work as a hairdresser)?"
4	Disability	Western Ontario Rotator Cuff Index (WORC) [39]; validated German version [40] (score)
5	Pain	"What is the worst amount of pain that you have experienced within the past week?" (100 mm visual analogue scale VAS)
6	History of shoulder pain (incl. Previous treatment)	"Prior to the current episode, have you ever seen a medical doctor or therapist for pain in this shoulder?" (yes, no)
7	Symptom duration	"For how long have you been having your current shoulder complaints?" (weeks)
8	Diabetes	"Do you have diabetes?" (yes, no)
9	Smoking	"Are you a smoker? Please tick "yes" if you regularly smoke at least once a week any amount of tobacco" (yes, no)
10	Pain catastrophizing	Pain Catastrophizing Scale (PCS) [56]; validated German version [57] (score)

any missing data, was made prior to the analysis. We considered the amount and also the potential reasons for missing values, i.e. whether the reasons for missingness appeared systematic or random. We decided to limit the replacement of missing values to those missing for the two multi-item measures, the WORC (baseline and follow-up) and the Pain Catastrophizing Scale (PCS). No standard missing rule was available for the WORC in the literature; therefore, we replaced missing WORC values by the mean of the respective domain. We replaced missing PCS values by the mean of the items that were completed, as suggested by the primary originator of the scale, Prof Michael Sullivan (personal communication 02/06/2014). We did not replace any missing values where the PCS was completely missing. As the information-theoretic analysis approach we used required identical datasets, the data were analyzed on a complete-case basis. We would have considered formal testing of the effects of missing data should the amount have been bigger and should the reasons for missingness have been of concern.

Statistical analysis methods

We intended to include all 10 candidate factors in the prognostic modelling analysis. All continuous factors, WORC and PCS scores, were analyzed as continuous measurements. All non-continuous factors were binary.

We based our analysis on an information-theoretic approach, namely on a small-sample variant of Akaike's Information Criterion (AIC) approach, AIC_C [47]. Information-theoretic approaches to model selection differ from other approaches, particularly from the widely used stepwise regression approaches, in several ways. Under the AIC approach, selection is based on the comparison of multiple candidate models, which are pre-specified based on "theory", rather than on a single global set of factors [48]. Selection is further based on an information-theoretic criterion (e.g. AIC), which provides "numerical values that represent the scientific evidence" for a model, but no "test statistics" such as p values, thus avoiding the application of arbitrary cut-offs of "statistical significance" ([47] p. 64). Reflecting the perspective that models never reflect "full reality", i.e. that they are approximations ([47], p. 27), the AIC value represents an estimator of the information that is inherently lost when a model is used to approximate full reality (Kullback-Leibler information) [48]. The AIC accounts for the number of candidate factors by 'penalizing' models with larger numbers of factors, thereby favouring parsimony ([47], p. 60–1). The model with the lowest AIC value (AIC_{MIN}) represents the closest approximation and is accordingly termed the "best model" within a set of models [47]. AIC differences ($\Delta AIC = AIC - AIC_{MIN}$) can then be calculated to rank the models by their distance to the best model [47, 48]. Burnham et al. ([48], p. 25) have proposed considering models with ΔAIC values < 4 to 7 as "plausible" alternatives to the best model, whereas models with higher ΔAIC values (> 9) have little to no support. AIC values are relative rather than absolute, and "on the scale of information" ([47], p. 84). Accordingly, their use is limited to comparing models within a defined set of models [49]. As the AIC approach will always select a best model among a set of models, it has been suggested that the worth of the best or the global (full) model be assessed, e.g. by a goodness-of-fit test, analysis of residuals or the adjusted R^2 (the percentage of variance explained) [47].

Following recommendations from the literature that the number of candidate models should usually be limited to a few [47], we decided to analyze a selection of nine candidate models. The selection of models was based on clinical and theoretical considerations, with the first model (number 1 in Table 3) including all 10 candidate prognostic factors (thus representing the "full model"). The composition of the other eight models, which included between two to eight of these factors, was based on various characteristics, as shown in Table 3. Examples of characteristics were the potential for modification (model 2) or the effort required for the assessment of prognostic factors (models 5 and 7, inclusion or exclusion of questionnaires), which would be highly relevant to clinical practitioners. The primary analysis approach was a linear regression analysis [26, 49] which we conducted in IBM SPSS Statistics 22. All continuous factors were modelled as linear. Satisfaction of the assumptions of linear regression was assessed visually for each model based on the residual plot (scatterplot of standardized residuals against standardized predicted values) [50].

We extracted the following statistics: the AIC_C value; the standard error of the estimate (SEE), as the primary measure of model precision; the adjusted coefficient of (multiple) determination (R^2_{ADJ}), as a complementary measure of model performance; the regression constant (Constant); and the unstandardized regression coefficients (B) of all factors with their 95% confidence intervals (CIs). For comparison of the different models, we extracted AIC_C, ΔAIC and SEE values.

Model validation and further analyses

We intended to compare the SEE of the best model with the estimate of the Minimal Important Difference (MID) of the WORC, which we intended to derive from the sample data, and to internally validate any model with an SEE substantially lower than the MID. We intended to conduct the following exploratory subgroup analyses: amount of physiotherapy (number of sessions); medical treatment (specifically provision of injections); and length of follow-up.

Results
Participants
Figure 2 illustrates the flow of participants. Of 82 eligible participants, 70 were included, of whom 65 (representing 65 shoulders) completed the study. The baseline characteristics and prognostic factor information of these 65 participants are presented in Table 4.

The amount of missing data was small: six values (0.4% of all values) were missing for the baseline WORC; 11 (1%) for the follow-up WORC; and six (1%) for the single-item prognostic factors. The PCS was missing completely for three participants; beyond this, only one PCS value (0.1%) was missing. The distribution appeared random, thus non-systematic. Four participants had missing prognostic factor data after replacement of missing WORC and PCS values, and were consequently, in keeping with the need for identical datasets for the AIC approach [47], excluded from the modelling. The data of 61 participants were analyzed. The

Table 3 Candidate prognostic models and key model statistics

No	Candidate model	N^* factors	Main characteristic	AIC_C	$\Delta AIC_C^\dagger$	SEE	$R^2_{ADJ}{}^\S$
1	Age + sex + physical demands + disability (WORC) + pain + history of shoulder pain + symptom duration + smoking + pain catastrophizing (PCS) (+ diabetes removed[‡])	9	Full model (all factors)	891	11	313	0.12
2	Smoking + pain catastrophizing (PCS) (+ diabetes removed[‡])	2	Potential for modification (could be modified (addressed) by some action (e.g. treatment)	880	0	314	0.11
3	Age + sex	2	Factors that cannot be modified	889	9	336	−0.02
4	Age + sex + physical demands + pain + history of shoulder pain + symptom duration + smoking (+ diabetes removed[‡])	7	Type of assessment: "no questionnaires"	899	19	344	−0.06
5	Disability (WORC) + pain catastrophizing (PCS)	2	Type of assessment: "questionnaires"	880	0	314	0.11
6	Smoking (+ diabetes removed[‡])	(1)	Type of factor: "bio(logical) factors"	Excluded from analysis due to removal of diabetes			
7	History of shoulder pain + symptom duration	2	Background (patient history)	889	9	336	−0.02
8	Pain + history of shoulder pain + symptom duration	3	Further models: pain-related factors (excluding pain catastrophizing)	889	9	335	−0.01
9	Pain + pain catastrophizing (PCS)	2	Further models: pain and attitude towards pain	882	2	318	0.09

[*]Denotes the number of factors in each model as analyzed (i.e. after removal of diabetes). [†]An ΔAIC_C value of 0 denotes the model(s) with the lowest AIC_C value(s), representing the "best" model(s) within the set of candidate models; [‡]Model initially included diabetes, which was excluded from the analyses due to its low prevalence in the sample; [§]Negative R^2 values are generally interpreted as "0"

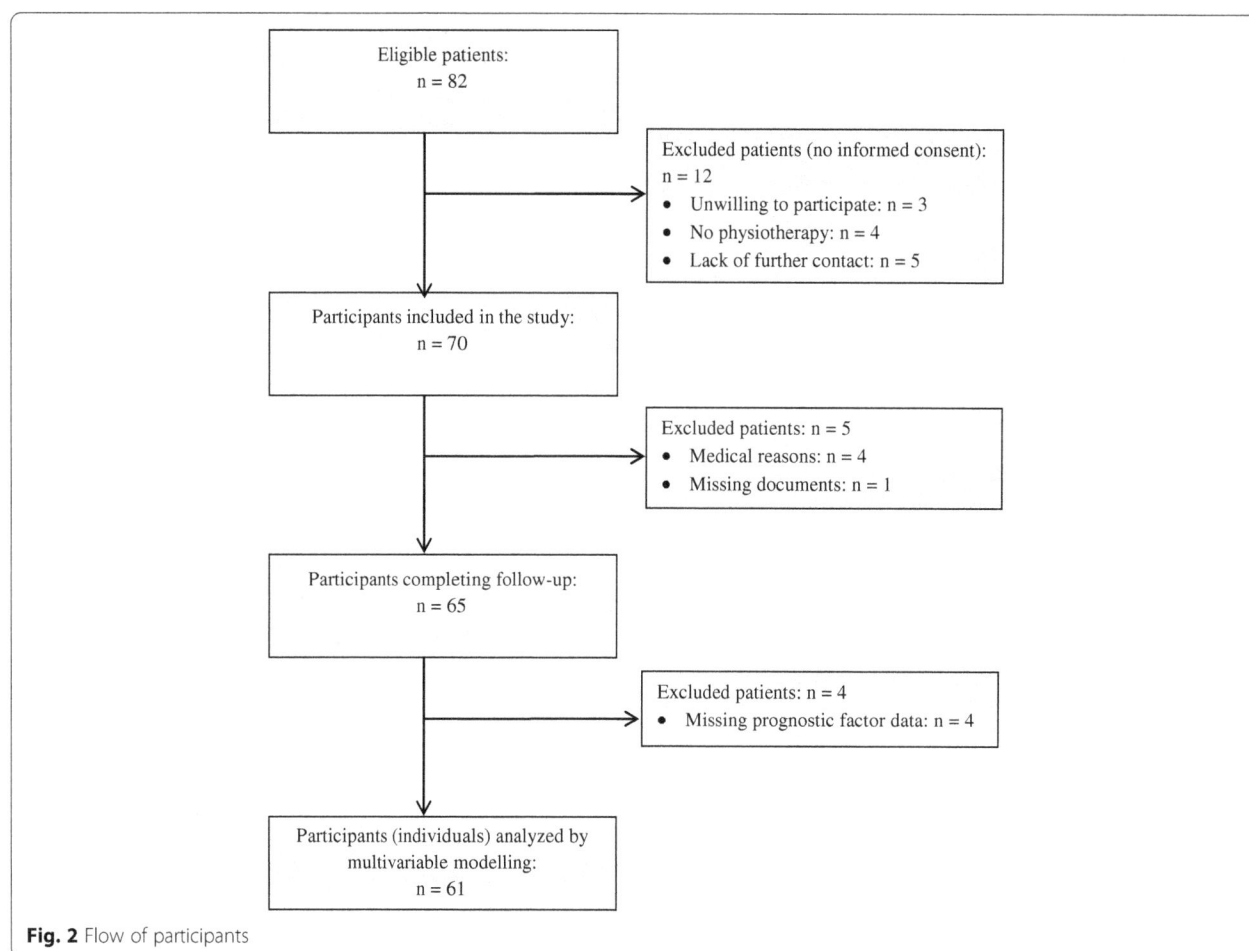

Fig. 2 Flow of participants

mean (SD) interval between completion of the base-line and follow-up WORC (and GPC) was 97 (17) days (n = 65 for WORC, 64 for GPC). The mean (SD) interval between the baseline and follow-up US assessment was 100 (13) days (n = 52).

Treatment

All participants received conservative treatment with physiotherapy. The mean (SD) number of physiotherapy sessions was 12 (6); and the mean (SD) duration of single sessions was 28 (13) minutes. A breakdown of the physiotherapy treatment content, documented by the physiotherapists, is provided in Table 5. Treatment usually included a combination of exercises and manual techniques. Consistent with physiotherapy practice in Germany, where this study took place, all physiotherapists routinely provided advice and patient education.

Thirty-seven participants (57% of 65) received some supplementary medical treatment: i.e. subacromial steroid injection (27; of these, 24 received one injection and three received two injections), elastic tape (12) or prescription of oral medication (Metamizole, 1). No participant was put on sick leave.

Outcomes

The mean (SD) unadjusted WORC$_{CHANGE}$ score (n = 65) was − 363 (361); the range was − 1248 to 372. The mean (SD) RTM-adjusted WORC$_{CHANGE}$ score was − 363 (341); the range was − 1102 to 387. Tear progression to an FTT occurred in two participants (4%, n = 52). Adverse events were reported for six participants (9%, n = 65), and related exclusively to temporary exacerbations of the shoulder symptoms. Fifty-five participants (86%, n = 64) rated their shoulder problem as improved (positive GPC ratings), five (8%) as unchanged (GPC = 0), and four (6%) as deteriorated (negative GPC ratings). The MID estimate for the WORC, which we derived from the sample data using an anchor-based approach (n = 64), was − 300 (this analysis is reported in a separate article [51]).

Prognostic modelling

There were no complexities (e.g. unit of analysis issues) in the data. We excluded diabetes from the analysis because of its very low prevalence in the sample (Table 4), and consequently excluded one two-factor model, 'diabetes & smoking' (Table 3). The ratio of the number of outcome events (individuals with data available for

Table 4 Baseline characteristics and prognostic factor data

Characteristic (n)	Measurement	Values		
Continuous prognostic factors			SD	Range
Age (65)	year	50	12	24–76
Disability (65)*	WORC_1 score	897	380	130–1660
Pain (64)	mm VAS	63	26	7–100
Symptom duration (63)	week	36	49	1–250
Pain catastrophizing (62)*†	PCS score	15	9	1–37
Categorical prognostic factors		N	%	
Sex (65)	female	25	38	
	male	40	62	
Physical demands (64)	yes	41	64	
	no	23	36	
History of shoulder pain (64)	yes	35	55	
	no	29	45	
Diabetes (65)	yes	4	6	
	no	61	94	
Smoking (64)	yes	10	16	
	no	54	84	
Additional characteristics		N	%	
Affected tendon (65)	1. supraspinatus	63	97	
	2. infraspinatus	1	2	
	3. supraspinatus + infraspinatus	1	2	
	4. any other	0	0	
Dominant arm affected (65)	yes	46	71	
	no	19	29	
Work status (64)	5. full-time	41	64	
	6. part-time	11	17	
	7. sick leave	0	0	
	8. retired	10	16	
	9. not working (other reason)	2	3	

*Includes replaced values for missing data (see section 6.6.15); †PCS data were completely missing for three cases

analysis) to the overall number of analyzed candidate factors approximated to 7 (61/9); the range across all models was, depending on the number of factors included in each model, approximately 7 to 31. The residual plots showed no strong evidence of a violation of the assumptions for linear regression for any of the models.

The key model statistics are shown in Table 2. The coefficient statistics for each model and each prognostic factor are provided with the supplementary materials (Additional file 3). Two models with the same AIC_C value (models 2 and 5) were identified as the best models. The model with the third-highest AIC_C value (model 9) had an ΔAIC_C within the range of plausible alternatives (ΔAIC_C < 7) to the best models [48]. The remaining models had ΔAIC_C values outside this range. The SEE ranged from 313 to 344, and was, for all models, higher than the

estimated MID of the WORC (300). The full model (model 1) had the highest R^2_{ADJ} (the range of all models was from − 0.06 to 0.12).

Model validation and further analyses
The performance and precision of the analyzed models did not justify internal validation; nor the planned subgroup analyses.

Discussion
Principal findings
Despite our rigorous approach and meeting our minimum sample size (relating to the full model), we did not achieve our primary aim of developing a prognostic model for the outcome of a phase of conservative treatment with physiotherapy in adults with symptomatic

Table 5 Breakdown of physiotherapy treatment

Category	Domain (n = 65)	N	%
Types of exercises	Strengthening exercises focused at rotator cuff muscles	52	80
	Scapula positioning exercises	47	72
	Stabilisation exercises	41	63
	Stretching techniques or exercises (shoulder/shoulder girdle)	36	55
	Strengthening exercises focused at shoulder girdle muscles	34	52
	Humeral head 'positioning' exercises	33	51
	Coordination exercises	25	38
	Inclusion of high load exercises (> 80% RPM[†])	5	8
	Correction of thoracic spine posture[*]	2	3
	Proprioceptive Neuromuscular Facilitation (PNF)[*]	1	2
Types of exercise equipment	Use of small equipment (e.g. elastic bands)	45	69
	Use of training machines (e.g. pulley, pull-down)	27	42
Setting of exercise treatment	Provision and supervision of supplementary home exercises	42	65
Types of manual techniques	Soft tissue techniques (shoulder or shoulder girdle)	56	86
	Manual mobilisation techniques (shoulder)	51	78
	Manual mobilisation of thoracic spine[*]	9	14
	Manual mobilisation of ribs[*]	2	3
	Manual mobilisation of cervical spine[*]	2	3
Supplementary modalities	Heat or cold applications	14	22
	Therapeutic ultrasound[*]	1	2

Interventions are listed by general category and specific domain; domains are in descending order of use; [*]recorded in "anything else?" category (physiotherapy report form); [†]RPM = one-repetition maximum

atraumatic rotator cuff PTTs. Of the eight models for which testing was appropriate, none had a satisfactory performance (R^2_{ADJ}) or precision (SEE).

Strengths and weaknesses of the study

The rigorous methodological design of our study helped to avoid various potential sources of bias. This included avoidance of statistical univariable selection techniques, which have been linked to biased predictions [52], and the analysis of continuous measurements on their continuous scale, hereby avoiding the various problems associated with the categorization of continuous measurements [45, 46]. The latter reflected our post-protocol decision to analyze the WORC on a continuous scale, instead of analyzing it as a binary outcome. By using an information-theoretic analysis approach, we purposely avoided the selection of factors within the multivariable analysis based on arbitrary cut-offs of "statistical significance", as these, in particular stepwise regression techniques, have been linked to biased predictions [52–54]. Although the outcome assessment could not be blinded to the prognostic factor information, any influence of participants' knowledge about prognostic factor information on the outcome is unlikely because the participants did not know which of the multiple baseline variables were modelled.

The ratio of outcome events to candidate factors was within the pre-specified range of 5 to 9 for the full model (and considerably higher, i.e. > 20, for some of the other models), and losses to follow-up and missing data were few. Additionally, as the reasons for missingness appeared non-systematic, we considered the data from the complete cases as representative of the whole sample. However, despite our meeting our sample size estimate, sample size is a key limitation of our study as indicated by the low precision and also by the rejection of the 'diabetes & smoking' model due to the low numbers of diabetic patients recruited. In the absence of any formal methods to determine the effective sample size, and without prior knowledge of the relationship between the candidate prognostic factors, it was difficult to estimate the sample size for our study (please see reviewer feedback on this aspect in Open Peer Review Reports). Considering the low precision of the analyzed models in our study, we conclude that a much larger sample size would have been needed to increase the chances of achieving satisfactory precision of the analyzed models.

Rigour was applied to the consideration of the clinical relevance, practicality of measurement and applicability of the study findings. All PTTs were diagnosed by US, which is highly specific (94%), but less sensitive (68%) for detecting PTTs [31]. This means that, while some

PTTs might have been missed, those identified were almost certainly true positives; hence, the study population was homogeneous in this respect. We aimed to enroll patients at a fairly similar state of health. Similarity of several baseline characteristics such as pain intensity, symptom duration and disability could not be guaranteed, as their restriction would have threatened recruitment, but was accounted for by candidate prognostic factors.

The physiotherapy protocol accommodated clinical autonomy within an evidence-based framework. Some of the study participants received adjunctive medical treatment, such as a local steroid injection. Arguably, the different treatments may have had an impact on the overall improvement of the participants during the three-month treatment period and also on the predictive performance of the analyzed models. We are confident, though, that this was not a relevant issue in our study. Consistent with our study question, we selected prognostic factors that were present at baseline before starting conservative treatment. The primary treatment was exercise-based physiotherapy within an evidence-based framework. The adjunctive treatments, which were provided to a minority of participants, included subacromial corticosteroid injections, elastic tapes and oral pain medication. The evidence on the effectiveness of these treatments for rotator cuff related shoulder pain is limited. Notably, for corticosteroid injection, which was the most often delivered adjunctive treatment, there is evidence of no relevant difference compared with physiotherapy [55]. Considering this and that the majority of the participants in our study who received injections received only one injection, we consider the likely impact of corticosteroid injections was minimal. Similar considerations apply to the other adjunctive treatments, which were received by smaller numbers of participants. In this context, we consider our decision not to perform the planned exploratory subgroup analyses, which included "medical treatment (specifically provision of injections)", was appropriate.

Although set within one country, Germany, with clinical care under one orthopaedic specialist, the study findings are broadly applicable to adults with symptomatic PTTs undergoing a three-month period of conservative treatment with exercise-based physiotherapy.

The eight analyzed models could explain only a very limited amount (up to 12%, see R^2_{ADJ} values), of the variability of the outcome, which means that most of the variability remains unexplained. This finding could be partly due to the fact that the evidence base for most of the factors identified was generally very limited. Although we cannot say what other factors may have contributed to this unexplained variability, we suggest these may be among the 36 factors listed in the supplementary table. As evidenced by their low precision (SEE), the predictions are affected by considerable uncertainty; they consequently do not provide reliable estimates of population parameters. The "natural" temptation to select out more "promising" factors, such as pain catastrophizing, which featured in the three best models, should be countered by the realization that our study was explicitly designed to explore multivariable models rather than individual factors. Thus, the presented coefficient statistics do not represent the factors' independent contributions to the predictions.

Lastly, it should be kept in mind that generally, any prognostic model that has been developed in a single population should only be considered clinically usable after it has been externally validated and, ideally, also evaluated for clinical impact [25].

Comparison with other studies

As already established, this is the first study aimed at predicting the outcome of conservative treatment with physical therapy in adults with symptomatic PTTs. Comparison with studies of adults undergoing conservative treatment with physiotherapy for rotator cuff disorders, in general, would be uninformative because of heterogeneity, not least in methodological terms [28].

Conclusions

We could not determine a prognostic model with satisfactory performance and precision. Thus, the challenge remains to develop a prognostic model with a satisfactory performance and precision for predicting the outcome of a phase of conservative treatment with physiotherapy in adults with symptomatic PTTs. Further high-quality prognostic studies are needed but should be underpinned, and thus preceded, by robust research aimed at improving knowledge of relevant factors. Consensus approaches (e.g. Delphi studies) may provide guidance about which factors to prioritize for future studies. Collaborative data collection and data sharing initiatives could enhance the realization of larger studies and applicability. Further methodological research is also needed to determine the optimal methods for developing prognostic models. Investigators of future prognostic model development studies should attend to the importance of the internal and external validation of any models with a promising performance.

Abbreviations
ΔAIC_C: AIC_C difference; ADJ, _ADJ_: Adjusted (in the context of this study: for regression to the mean, RTM); AIC: Akaike's Information Criterion;
AIC_C: Akaike's Information Criterion, small sample variant; AIC_MIN: Smallest AIC

(AIC$_c$) value; CI: Confidence interval; DEGUM: Deutsche Gesellschaft für Ultraschall in der Medizin [German Society for Ultrasound in Medicine]; DVSE: Deutsche Vereinigung für Schulter- und Ellenbogenchirurgie [German Society of Shoulder and Elbow Surgery]; FTT: Full-thickness tear (rotator cuff); GPC: Global Perceived Change; LHB: Long head of biceps; MID: Minimal Important Difference; MRI: Magnetic resonance imaging; PCS: Pain Catastrophizing Scale; PROM: Patient-reported outcome measure; PTT: Partial-thickness tear (rotator cuff); R^2: Coefficient of (multiple) determination; RTM: Regression to the mean; SD: Standard deviation; SEE: Standard error of the estimate; TRIPOD: Transparent Reporting of a Multivariable Prediction Model for Individual Prognosis or Diagnosis (checklist); US: Ultrasonography; VAS: Visual analogue scale; WORC: Western Ontario Rotator Cuff index; WORC_1: Baseline WORC; WORC_2: Follow-up WORC; WORC_change: Change of WORC score from baseline to follow-up

Acknowledgements
This study formed part of the work included in the PhD thesis (conferred December 2016) of CB at Teesside University, Middlesbrough, UK. We are grateful to all patients who participated in the study, and to all collaborating physiotherapists.

Funding
This research did not receive any grant from funding agencies in the public, commercial or not-for-profit sectors.

Authors' contributions
CB designed the study, managed the acquisition of data, analyzed and interpreted the data (with support from a statistician, who had access to the full dataset) and drafted and edited the manuscript. NCH and HHH made substantial contributions to the design of the study, the analysis and interpretation of the data, revised the manuscript for important intellectual content, and contributed to writing and editing. AB made substantial contributions to the design of the study and to the acquisition of data, contributed to the interpretation of the data, and revised the manuscript for important intellectual content. All authors read and approved the final manuscript.

Competing interests
The authors declare that they have no competing interests.

Author details
[1]School of Health and Social Care, Teesside University, Middlesbrough, UK. [2]Present address: Faculty of Health and Physiotherapy, Buxtehude, Germany. [3]schulter-zentrum.com, Hamburg, Germany. [4]Faculty of Health, Harburger Str. 6, 21614 Buxtehude, Germany.

References
1. Kooijman M, Swinkels I, van Dijk C, de Bakker D, Veenhof C. Patients with shoulder syndromes in general and physiotherapy practice: an observational study. BMC Musculoskelet Disord. 2013;14:128.
2. Östör AJK, Richards CA, Prevost AT, Speed CA, Hazleman BL. Diagnosis and relation to general health of shoulder disorders presenting to primary care. Rheumatology. 2005;44:800–5.
3. van der Windt DA, Koes BW, de Jong BA, Bouter LM. Shoulder disorders in general practice: incidence, patient characteristics, and management. Ann Rheum Dis. 1995;54:959–64.
4. Cook JL, Purdam CR. Is tendon pathology a continuum? A pathology model to explain the clinical presentation of load-induced tendinopathy. Br J Sports Med. 2009;43:409–16.
5. Reilly P, Macleod I, Macfarlane R, Windley J, Emery RJH. Dead men and radiologists don't lie: a review of cadaveric and radiological studies of rotator cuff tear prevalence. Ann R Coll Surg Engl. 2006;88:116–21.
6. Yamaguchi K, Ditsios K, Middleton WD, Hildebolt CF, Galatz LM. The demographic and morphological features of rotator cuff disease: a comparison of asymptomatic and symptomatic shoulders. J Bone Jt Surgery, Am Vol. 2006;88A:1699–704.
7. Matava MJ, Purcell DB, Rudzki JR. Partial-thickness rotator cuff tears. Am J Sports Med. 2005;33:1405–17.
8. Beaudreuil J, Bardin T, Orcel P, Goutallier D. Natural history or outcome with conservative treatment of degenerative rotator cuff tears. Joint Bone Spine. 2007;74:527–9.
9. Hedtmann A. Weichteilerkrankungen der Schulter – Subakromialsyndrome. Orthopädie und Unfallchirurgie up2date. 2009;4:85–106.
10. Finnan RP, L a C. Partial-thickness rotator cuff tears. J Shoulder Elb Surg. 2010;19:609–16.
11. Lenza M, Buchbinder R, Takwoingi Y, Johnston RV, Hanchard NC, Faloppa F. Magnetic resonance imaging, magnetic resonance arthrography and ultrasonography for assessing rotator cuff tears in people with shoulder pain for whom surgery is being considered. Cochrane Database Syst Rev. 2013;9:CD009020.
12. Tashjian RZ. AAOS clinical practice guideline: optimizing the management of rotator cuff problems. J Am Acad Orthop Surg. 2011;19:380–3.
13. Beaudreuil J, Dhénain M, Coudane H, Mlika-Cabanne N. Clinical practice guidelines for the surgical management of rotator cuff tears in adults. Orthop Traumatol Surg Res. 2010;96:175–9.
14. Ryösä A, Laimi K, Äärimaa V, Lehtimäki K, Kukkonen J, Saltychev M. Surgery or conservative treatment for rotator cuff tear: a meta-analysis. Disabil Rehabil. 2017;39(14):1357-63.
15. Colvin AC, Egorova N, Harrison AK, Moskowitz A, Flatow EL. National trends in rotator cuff repair. J Bone Joint Surg Am. 2012;94:227–33.
16. Paloneva J, Lepola V, Äärimaa V, Joukainen A, Ylinen J, Mattila VM. Increasing incidence of rotator cuff repairs--a nationwide registry study in Finland. BMC Musculoskelet Disord. 2015;16:189.
17. Svendsen SW, Frost P, Jensen LD. Time trends in surgery for non-traumatic shoulder disorders and postoperative risk of permanent work disability: a nationwide cohort study. Scand J Rheumatol. 2012;41:59–65.
18. Ylinen J, Vuorenmaa M, Paloneva J, Kiviranta I, Kautiainen H, Oikari M, et al. Exercise therapy is evidence-based treatment of shoulder impingement syndrome. Current practice or recommendation only. Eur J Phys Rehabil Med. 2013;49:499–505.
19. Butler M, Forte M, Braman J, Swiontkowski M, Kane RL. Nonoperative and Operative treatments for rotator cuff tears: future research needs: identification of future research needs from comparative effectiveness review no. 22. Rockville: Agency for Healthcare Research and Quality (US). Report No.: 13-EHC050-EF. AHRQ Future Research Needs Papers. 2013. https://www.ncbi.nlm.nih.gov/pubmed/23905196.
20. Croft P, Altman DG, Deeks JJ, Dunn KM, Hay AD, Hemingway H, et al. The science of clinical practice: disease diagnosis or patient prognosis? Evidence about "what is likely to happen" should shape clinical practice. BMC Med. 2015;13:20.
21. Cochrane Prognosis Methods Group. 2018.http://prognosismethods.cochrane.org/. Accessed 21 Apr 2018.
22. Progress. mrc prognosis research strategy partnership. 2018.http://progress-partnership.org/. Accessed 21 Apr 2018.
23. Riley RD, Hayden JA, Steyerberg EW, Moons KGM, Abrams K, Kyzas PA, et al. Prognosis research strategy (PROGRESS) 2: prognostic factor research. PLoS Med. 2013;10:e1001380.
24. Hemingway H, Croft P, Perel P, Hayden JA, Abrams K, Timmis A, et al. Prognosis research strategy (PROGRESS) 1: a framework for researching clinical outcomes. BMJ. 2013;346:e5595.
25. Steyerberg EW, Moons KGM, van der Windt DA, Hayden JA, Perel P, Schroter S, et al. Prognosis research strategy (PROGRESS) 3: prognostic model research. PLoS Med. 2013;10:e1001381.
26. Moons KGM, Royston P, Vergouwe Y, Grobbee DE, Altman DG. Prognosis and prognostic research: what, why, and how? BMJ. 2009; 338:b375.
27. Royston P, Moons KGM, Altman DG, Vergouwe Y. Prognosis and prognostic research: developing a prognostic model. BMJ. 2009;338:b604.
28. Braun C, Hanchard NC, Batterham AM, Handoll HH, Betthäuser A. Prognostic models in adults undergoing physical therapy for rotator cuff disorders: systematic review. Phys Ther. 2016;96:961–71.
29. Braun C. Predicting the outcome of physiotherapy in poeple with painful partial-thickness rotator cuff tears. A thesis submitted in partial fulfillment of the requirements of Teesside University for the award of the degree of Doctor of Philosophy (PhD) http://tees.openrepository.com/tees/handle/10149/621790 (2016). Accessed 21 Apr 2018.
30. Collins GS, Reitsma JB, Altman DG, Moons KGM. Transparent reporting of a multivariable prediction model for individual prognosis or diagnosis (TRIPOD): the TRIPOD statement. BMJ. 2015;350:g7594.
31. Roy J-S, Braën C, Leblond J, Desmeules F, Dionne CE, MacDermid JC, et al. Diagnostic accuracy of ultrasonography, MRI and MR arthrography in the characterisation of rotator cuff disorders: a systematic review and meta-analysis. Br J Sports Med. 2015;49:1316–28.

32. Khan KM, Cook JL, Maffulli N, Kannus P. Where is the pain coming from in tendinopathy? It may be biochemical, not only structural, in origin. Br J Sports Med. 2000;34:81–3.

33. DVSE. Untersuchungstechniken des Schultergelenks. Expertenevaluation auf der Basis einer Literaturanalyse. Obere Extermität. 2012;7(Suppl 1):3–68.

34. Konermann W, Gruber G. Ultraschalldiagnostik Der Bewegungsorgane. In: Kursbuch nach den Richtlinien der DEGUM und der DGOU. 2nd ed. Stuttgart: Thieme; 2007.

35. Hedtmann A, Fett H. Schultersonographie bei Subakromialsyndromen mit Erkrankungen und Verletzungen der Rotatorenmanschette (Sonography of the shoulder in subacromial syndromes with diseases and injuries of the rotator cuff). Orthopade. 1995;24:498–508.

36. Hedtmann A, Fett A. Sonographie der Rotatorenmanschette (Ultrasonographic diagnosis of the rotator cuff). Orthopade. 2002;31:236–46.

37. Braun C, Hanchard NCA. Manual therapy and exercise for impingementrelated shoulder pain. Phys Ther Rev. 2010;15:62–83.

38. Braun C, Bularczyk M, Heintsch J, Hanchard NCA. Manual therapy and exercises for shoulder impingement revisited. Phys Ther Rev. 2013;18:263–84.

39. Kirkley A, Alvarez C, Griffin S. The development and evaluation of a disease-specific quality-of-life questionnaire for disorders of the rotator cuff: the western Ontario rotator cuff index. Clin J Sport Med. 2003;13:84–92.

40. Huber W, Hofstaetter JG, Hanslik-Schnabel B, Posch M, Wurnig C. Translation and psychometric testing of the western Ontario rotator cuff index (WORC) for use in Germany. Z Orthop Ihre Grenzgeb. 2005;143:453–60.

41. Huang H, Grant JA, Miller BS, Mirza FM, Gagnier JJ. A systematic review of the psychometric properties of patient-reported outcome instruments for use in patients with rotator cuff disease. Am J Sports Med. 2015;43:2572–82.

42. St-Pierre C, Desmeules F, Dionne CE, Frémont P, MacDermid JC, Roy J-S. Psychometric properties of self-reported questionnaires for the evaluation of symptoms and functional limitations in individuals with rotator cuff disorders: a systematic review. Disabil Rehabil. 2016;38:103–22.

43. Linden A. Assessing regression to the mean effects in health care initiatives. BMC Med Res Methodol. 2013;13:119.

44. Vittinghoff E, McCulloch CE. Relaxing the rule of ten events per variable in logistic and cox regression. Am J Epidemiol. 2007;165:710–8.

45. Altman DG, Royston P. The cost of dichotomising continuous variables. BMJ. 2006;332(7549):1080.

46. Royston P, Altman DG, Sauerbrei W. Dichotomizing continuous predictors in multiple regression: a bad idea. Stat Med. 2006;25:127–41.

47. Anderson DA. Model based inference in the life sciences. In: A primer on evidence. New York: Springer science + business Media; 2008.

48. Burnham KP, Anderson DR, Huyvaert KP. AIC model selection and multimodel inference in behavioral ecology: some background, observations, and comparisons. Behav Ecol Sociobiol. 2011;65:23–35.

49. Burnham KP, Anderson DR. Model selection and multimodel inference. A practical information-theoretic approach. 2nd ed. New York: Springer; 2002.

50. Miles J, Shevlin M. Applying regression & correlation. London: Sage Publications; 2001.

51. Braun C, Handoll HH. Estimating the minimal important difference for the western Ontario rotator cuff index (WORC) in adults with shoulder pain associated with partial-thickness rotator cuff tears. Musculoskelet Sci Pract. 2018;35:30–3.

52. Harrell FE, Lee KL, Mark DB. Multivariable prognostic models: issues in developing models, evaluating assumptions and adequacy, and measuring and reducing errors. Stat Med. 1996;15:361–87.

53. Flom PL, Cassell DL. Statistics and Data Analysis: Why stepwise and similar selection methods are bad , and what you should use (statistics and data analysis): North East SAS Users Group (NESUG) Annual Conference 2007. 2007.http://www.lexjansen.com/pnwsug/2008/DavidCassell-StoppingStepwise.pdf, https://www.lexjansen.com/nesug/. Accessed 21 Apr 2018.

54. Harrell FE. Regression modeling strategies. 1st ed. New York: Springer; 2001.

55. Mohamadi A, Chan JJ, Claessen FMAP, Ring D, Chen NC. Corticosteroid injections give small and transient pain relief in rotator cuff Tendinosis: a meta-analysis. Clin Orthop Relat Res. 2017;475:232–43.

56. Sullivan MJL, Bishop SR, Pivik J. The pain Catastrophizing scale: development and validation. Psychol Assess. 1995;7:524–32.

57. Meyer K, Sprott H, Mannion AF. Cross-cultural adaptation, reliability, and validity of the German version of the pain Catastrophizing scale. J Psychosom Res. 2008;64:469–78.

3

Construction of an adherence rating scale for exercise therapy for patients with knee osteoarthritis

Jianji Wang[1,2,3], Long Yang[1,2,3], Qingjun Li[1,2,3], Zhanyu Wu[1,2,3], Yu Sun[1,2,3], Qiang Zou[1,2,3], Xuanze Li[1,2,3], Zhe Xu[1,2,3] and Chuan Ye[1,2,3,4*]

Abstract

Background: Knee osteoarthritis (KOA) is one of the most common chronic diseases in the elderly and is the primary cause of the loss of motor function and disability in this population. Exercise therapy is a core, basic and matureand treatment method of treating patients with KOA. Exercise therapy is "strongly recommended" or "recommended" in the diagnosis and treatment guidelines of osteoarthritis in many countries, and most scholars advocate exercise therapy as the preferred rehabilitation method for KOA patients. However, poor long-term adherence is a serious problem affecting the therapeutic effect of this mature treatment. The objective of this study was to construct a concise and practical adherence rating scale (ARS) based on the exercise therapy adherence prediction model in patients with knee osteoarthritis.

Methods: A binary logistic regression model was established, with the adherence of 218 cases of KOA patients as the dependent variable. The patients' general information, exercise habits, knowledge, attitude, and exercise therapy were independent variables. The regression coefficients were assigned to various variables in the model, and the ARS was constructed accordingly. Receiver operating characteristic curves and curve fitting were used to analyse the effect of the ARS in predicting the adherence and to determine the goodness of fit for the adherence. The external validity of the ARS was examined in a randomized controlled trial.

Results: The construction of the adherence model and the ARS included the following variables: age (1 point), education level (1 point), degree of social support (2 points), exercise habits (3 points), knowledge of KOA prevention and treatment (2 points), degree of care needed to treat the disease (1 point), familiarity with exercise therapy (4 points) and treatment confidence (3 points). The critical value of the total score of the ARS was 6.50, with a sensitivity of 87.20% and a specificity of 76.34%.

Conclusions: A KOA exercise therapy adherence model and a simple and practical ARS were constructed. The ARS has good internal validity and external validity and can be used to evaluate the adherence to exercise therapy in patients with KOA.

Keywords: KOA, Exercise therapy, Adherence, Randomized controlled trial, Logistic regression analysis

* Correspondence: yechuanchina@hotmail.com
[1]Department of Orthopedic Surgery, Affiliated Hospital of Guizhou Medical University, Guiyang, China
[2]Center for Bioprinting and Biomanufacturing, Guizhou Medical University, Guiyang, China
Full list of author information is available at the end of the article

Background

In disease prevention or treatment, the World Health Organization (WHO) has defined adherence as the degrees of consistency of the behaviours of the patient concerning the diet, lifestyle and medication with the health care programme developed by the medical practitioner [1–3]. Meanwhile, the WHO has indicated that, compared with the development of a new treatment, the improvement in the patient's adherence to the current mature treatment will result in greater health benefits [1]. Knee osteoarthritis (KOA) is one of the most common chronic diseases in the elderly and is the primary cause of the loss of motor function and disability in this population [4–6]. Exercise therapy is not only a mature [7] but also a core, basic and front-line treatment method of treating KOA [8–12]. Exercise therapy is "strongly recommended" [8] or "recommended" [9–12] in the diagnosis and treatment guidelines of osteoarthritis in many countries, and most scholars advocate exercise therapy as the preferred rehabilitation method for KOA patients [13, 14]. In recent years, large numbers of empirical studies have also provided evidence that exercise therapy can effectively relieve knee pain, reduce the rate of disability, improve knee function and improve the patient's quality of life [15–18]. Therefore, improving adherence to this mature exercise therapy will enable KOA patients to reap more health benefits.

Poor long-term adherence is not only a serious problem affecting the health and quality of life of the population but also increases the economic burden of chronic diseases around the world [19, 20]. In practice, exercise therapy, similar to other chronic diseases, also has a serious poor adherence problem [21–24], which directly influences the therapeutic effect of this mature treatment. Therefore, an analysis of the risk factors of patient adherence and the interventions for these risk factors and for the improvement of adherence are important measures for ensuring the efficacy of this mature treatment.

In this study, considering the current poor patient adherence and low participation rate, an adherence prediction model was established with the adherence of the KOA patients as the dependent variable and the personal information, medical history and knowledge of KOA prevention and treatment as the independent variables. The values of the variables in the model were assigned based on regression coefficients to construct the adherence rating scale (ARS). This scale is expected to be able to provide early predictions of patient adherence and its risk factors, provide the basis for the development of personalized interventions and, ultimately, enable patients to achieve the greatest health benefits from exercise therapy.

Methods

In this study, an ARS for exercise therapy for KOA patients was constructed, and the internal validity and the external validity of this ARS were detected. The design flow is shown in Fig. 1.

Construction of the ARS

Methods: The current status survey and multivariate logistic stepwise regression analysis were applied. Patients clinically diagnosed with KOA in the outpatient department of the affiliated hospital from October 2015 to July 2016 were collected as the study subjects. The sampling method was systematic random sampling, resulting in a total of 704 cases. Exercise therapy was not prescribed for 486 cases of the KOA patients and was prescribed for 218 patients. Among the 218 eligible KOA patients, there were 53 males and 165 females, with ages ranging from 38 to 80 years old. The current statuses of the 218 included patients were investigated and patients were classified into good adherence group and bad adherence group using Morisky scale to develop the adherence prediction model and the ARS.

The inclusion criteria for patients were as follows: (1) the patient diagnosis was in line with the Chinese Orthopedic Association (COA) osteoarthritis diagnosis and treatment guidelines (2007 edition) [11]; (2) the patient had performed or was performing exercises; (3) the patient provided informed consent; and (4) the patient showed clear consciousness, could correctly answer the questions and was willing to cooperate.

The exclusion criteria for patients were as follows: (1) the patient's diagnosis was associated with severe medical diseases, such as severe heart, lung and brain diseases; (2) the patient had been diagnosed with any of the following mental disorders: cerebellar lesions, mental retardation, mental illness and cognitive disorders; (3) the patient experienced any of the following peripheral neuromuscular symptoms: limb muscle weakness, poor mobility or inability to perform autonomous activities; (4) the patient had showed no treatment history of exercise therapy (exercise was not recommended by the physician); or (5) the patient was unwilling to participate in the study.

In the development of the adherence prediction model, a survey with face-to-face interviews was conducted by 12 investigators using a structured questionnaire for the study subjects. The contents of the questionnaire included (1) personal information, such as age, gender, educational level and occupation; (2) daily exercise habits, such as whether the subject played sports and the daily exercise intensity; (3) the history of KOA and its treatment; (4) the knowledge of KOA prevention and treatment and the attitude and practices associated with the disease, that is KAP; (5) family, social factors, such as family members, and social support; and (6) exercise therapy factors, such as the complexity of the exercise therapy prescription and the familiarity of

Flow chart of the technical procedures

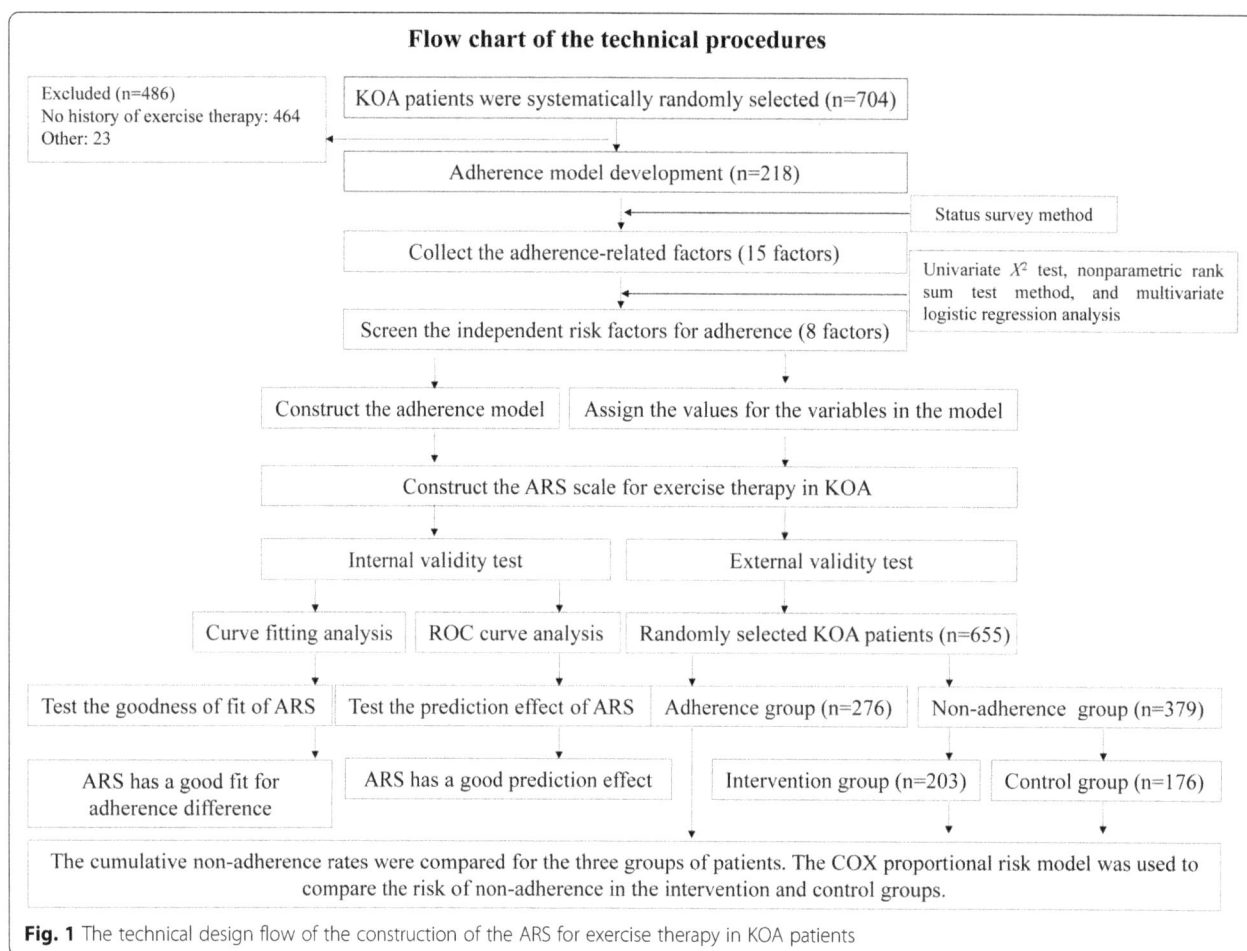

Fig. 1 The technical design flow of the construction of the ARS for exercise therapy in KOA patients

the exercise therapy. The questionnaire covered six areas and included more than 70 questions.

A binary logistic regression model was established with adherence as the dependent variable and personal information, exercise habits, exercise therapy familiarity, history of KOA and treatment history as the independent variables. While controlling some main influencing factors, the confounding factors were excluded. Other potential influencing factors were screened using univariate analysis. Factors showing $P < 0.05$ in univariate analysis and those with professional significance were included in the multivariate binary logistic regression analysis to finally determine independent influencing factors. The adherence prediction model was finally constructed.

To facilitate clinical application, this study assigned an appropriate value to each predictor based on its weight (which was calculated as the rounded number of the ratio of the regression coefficient of each factor and the minimum regression coefficient in the model) as the indicator to evaluate the adherence, thus constructing the ARS.

Testing the internal validity of the ARS
The receiver operating characteristic (ROC) curve was used to analyse the total score of the patients' adherence to exercise therapy, and the area under the curve (AUC) was calculated to evaluate the goodness of fit of the ARS, thereby determining the predictive effect of the total score on the adherence. Curve fitting was used to analyse the adherence score and the predicted possibility of the non-adherence rate correlation to assess the correlation and fitness of the ARS in distinguishing the adherence of exercise therapy.

Testing the external validity of the ARS
For the method, a randomized controlled trial (RCT) was used. Patients who were newly diagnosed with KOA in the outpatient department from August 2016 to October 2017 were randomly selected, resulting in a total of 655 cases, including 156 males and 499 females. The inclusion and exclusion criteria were the same as those described above.

First, the ARS scores were obtained for all KOA patients (grouped by the pre-determined threshold), and the patients were divided into adherence and non-adherence groups based on their scores. Second, the cases in the non-adherence group were randomly divided into intervention and control subgroups by a random number table. The cases in the adherence, control and intervention groups were followed up for nine months to observe the changes in the non-adherence and the cumulative non-adherence of each group in each month. The interventions were given to the intervention group at the beginning of the third month of the treatment. The intervention measures included the knowledge of KOA exercise therapy developed based on a measurement domain in the ARS, the specific exercise measures and psychological counselling. Regular propaganda and education were provided for the control group. Propaganda and education measures included a complete exercise prescription, verbally informing patients that KOA needs exercise therapy and adhering to exercise therapy can alleviate their disease as well as improve their quality of life.

Contents and methods of the exercise therapy

The contents of the exercise therapy and the methods of exercise used the guidelines of KOA treatment in China and other countries as references [12], which included lower limb muscle training, knee activity training and aerobic exercise. For the method used, according to the patient's physical condition and the specific circumstances, each patient was given a corresponding exercise prescription. The goodness of adherence in this study was related to the patient's individual exercise prescription.

Exercise therapy and the adherence evaluation criteria

The method of adherence evaluation employed in this study was the Morisky scale [25]. Based on the Morisky scale, an adherence scale for KOA exercise therapy was developed, including four questions: (1) Have you ever forgotten to exercise once or more during exercise therapy? (2) Do you often not take exercise seriously? (3) If the joint pain and swelling symptoms are improved, do you stop exercising or reduce the number of exercises? (4) If you feel physically uncomfortable after exercise, do you stop exercising or reduce the number of exercises? For each question, the answer of "yes" was recorded as 1 point, and the answer of "no" was recorded as 0 points. The total score of the scale was 0–4 points. A total score of 0 points indicated that the adherence was good, and a total score greater than or equal to 1 point indicated that the adherence was poor. A higher score indicated worse adherence.

Statistical methods

SPSS 19.0 statistical software was used for the data processing. The measurement data are presented as the means ± standard deviations, while the counting data are presented as frequencies. Dichotomous counting data such as gender, nature of occupation and exercise

habit were tested using χ^2 test; single-group ordered hierarchy data such as age and education level were tested using the nonparametric rank-sum test. Logistic stepwise regression analysis was used to analyse the factors influencing adherence. Differences with $P < 0.05$ were considered statistically significant.

Results
Construction of the ARS

In total, 704 cases of KOA patients were randomly selected, among which 486 cases (69.3%) were not recommended by the physician to perform exercise or did not meet the inclusion criteria, while 218 patients (30.7%) met the inclusion criteria. These 218 patients included 165 females (75.69%) and 53 males (24.31%), with an average age of 65.52 ± 15.14 years old. The shortest and longest courses of treatment for the patients were 14 and 229 days, respectively, with an average of 131.4 days.

For the univariate x^2 analysis of adherence, the x^2 test or the nonparametric rank-sum test was used to investigate the factors influencing adherence. Age, educational level, nature of the patient's occupation, social support, lifestyle, exercise habits, the knowledge of KOA prevention and treatment, the degree of care needed to treat the disease, the familiarity of the exercise therapy and the complexity of the treatment regimen may have statistically significant impacts on the adherence ($P < 0.05$). The impacts of other factors on the adherence, such as gender, the length of disease history and the number of joints, were not statistically significant, as shown in Table 1.

For the multivariate logistic regression analysis of adherence, using the factors showing P < 0.05 in the univariate analysis including age, education level, nature of occupation, social support, lifestyle, exercise habit, knowledge of KOA prevention and treatment, degree of care needed to treat the disease, familiarity of the exercise therapy and complexity of the treatment regimen, as well as medical staff-patient relationship and treatment confidence with professional significance as independent variables, and the adherence as the dependent variable, multivariate logistic regression analysis was performed. The method of gradual entering was used, with entry and exclusion criteria of 0.05 and 0.10, respectively. The results were as follows. (1) The assigned values of the multivariate regression variables and the assigned weight are shown in Tables 2 and 3, respectively. (2) Age, educational level, social support, exercise habits, the knowledge of KOA prevention and treatment, the degree of care needed to treat the disease, the familiarity of the exercise therapy and the complexity of the treatment regimen were the independent influencing factors of adherence to KOA exercise therapy, while the nature of the KOA patient's occupation could not be considered

Table 1 Univariate analysis of the influencing factors of adherence to KOA exercise therapy

Factor	Adherence		x^2/Z	P
	Good	Bad		
Gender				
Male	22	31	0.038	0.846
Female	71	94		
Age #				
< 60	60	41	−4.979	< 0.001
60–75	24	44		
> 75	9	40		
Medical history #				
< 6	29	37	−0.332	0.740
6–12	31	41		
> 12	33	47		
Number of joints #				
Unilateral	29	30	−1.263	0.207
Bilateral	31	42		
Knee + other	33	53		
Education level #				
College and above	60	25	−6.734	< 0.001
High school	19	38		
Elementary school	14	62		
Nature of occupation				
Mainly mental work	69	72	6.427	0.011
Mainly physical work	24	53		
Social support				
Good	85	77	24.804	< 0.001
Fair	8	48		
Lifestyle				
Regular	79	57	35.181	< 0.001
Irregular	14	68		
Exercise habit				
Yes	60	47	15.459	< 0.001
No	33	78		
Knowledge of KOA prevention and treatment #				
Good	57	41	−4.830	< 0.001
Fair	29	45		
Poor	7	39		
Degree of care needed to treat the disease #				
Good	54	22	−7.492	< 0.001
Fair	33	41		
Poor	6	62		
Familiarity of the exercise therapy				
Familiar	88	82	26.162	< 0.001
Not familiar	5	43		

Table 1 Univariate analysis of the influencing factors of adherence to KOA exercise therapy *(Continued)*

Factor	Adherence		x^2/Z	P
	Good	Bad		
Treatment regimen				
Simple	74	70	13.212	< 0.001
Complex	19	55		
Medical staff-patient relationship				
Good	79	100	0.888	0.346
Fair	14	25		
Treatment confidence				
Good	80	100	1.343	0.246
Poor	13	25		

Note: # analysed using the nonparametric rank-sum test

to have an independent impact on the adherence, as shown in Table 3.

Test of the internal validity of the ARS
An receiver operating characteristic (ROC) curve was used to analyse the predictive effect of the total score of the ARS on adherence. The AUC of the total adherence score was 0.903 (0.864–0.942), which was statistically significant, suggesting that the total score of the scale had a certain predictive effect on adherence. The critical value of the total score was 6.50, with a sensitivity of 87.20% and a specificity of 76.34%. The score of the adherence group was 4.43 ± 2.74, and the score of the non-adherence group was 10.91 ± 4.25, with a statistically significant difference ($t = 12.854$, $P < 0.001$) (Fig. 2).

The Morisky scale (=0 for adherence; ≥1 for non-adherence) and the ARS (< 6.5 for adherence; ≥6.5 for non-adherence) ($x^2 = 89.786$, $df = 1$, $P < 0.001$) were used to divide the study subjects into adherence and non-adherence groups. The differences between these two groups were compared, and the grouping results of the two methods were highly correlated ($x^2 = 89.786$, $df = 1$, $P < 0.001$), suggesting that the ARS had a goodness of fit for the difference of exercise therapy adherence (Fig. 3).

Test of the external validity of the ARS
There were a total of 655 KOA patients, including 156 males (23.82%) and 499 females (76.18%), with an average age of 64.28 ± 14.43 years. The subjects were divided into adherence (276 cases) and non-adherence (379 cases) groups according to their ARS scores (with a threshold of 6.5). Furthermore, the cases in the non-adherence group were randomly divided into intervention (203 cases) and control (176 cases) groups. There were no significant differences in the baselines for gender, mean age, mean follow-up time or treatment regimen among the three groups ($P > 0.05$).

Table 2 Assigned values of the multivariate regression variables for adherence to KOA exercise therapy

Variable	Assigned value
Adherence	Good = 0, poor = 1
Age	< 60 = 0, 60–75 = 1. > 75 = 2
Education level	College or above = 0, high school = 1, elementary school = 2
Nature of occupation	Mainly mental work = 0, Mainly physical work = 1
Social support	Good = 0, fair = 1
Lifestyle	Regular = 0, irregular = 1
Exercise habits	Yes = 0, no = 1
Knowledge of KOA prevention and treatment	Good = 0, fair = 1, poor = 2
Degree of care needed to treat the disease	Good = 0, fair = 1, poor = 2
Familiarity of the exercise therapy	Familiar = 0, not familiar = 1
Treatment regimen	Simple = 0, complex = 1
Medical staff-patient relationship	Good = 0, fair = 1, poor = 2
Treatment confidence	Good = 0, fair = 1, poor = 2

The relationships of the cumulative non-adherence rates at different stages of the entire treatment course among the different groups are outlined in Fig. 4. There was no significant difference between the intervention and control groups in the first and second months of the treatment ($P > 0.05$), while in the third to ninth months of the treatment, the cumulative non-adherence rates of the intervention group were significantly lower than those of the control group ($P < 0.05$). This difference is because the individualized interventions for the intervention group were provided at the beginning of the third month of the treatment, indicating that the individualized interventions were effective and could significantly improve the treatment adherence of the KOA patients. The cumulative non-adherence rates of the control group at different stages of the entire treatment course were significantly higher than those of the adherence group ($P < 0.05$), indicating that the ARS had a good distinguishing effect on the actual adherence of the KOA patients; furthermore, the validity of the ARS was demonstrated. In addition, the cumulative non-adherence

rates of the intervention group in the first two months of the treatment were higher than those of the adherence group, but the cumulative non-adherence rates in the last seven months of the treatment gradually approached those of the adherence group, though the differences were still statistically significant ($P < 0.05$), indicating that the intervention was effective, as shown in Table 4.

The COX proportional hazards model was used to compare the onset risk of non-adherence for the intervention and control groups. The hazard ratio (HR) was 0.476 (95% confidence interval (CI): 0.373–0.607), and the difference of the intervention was statistically significant ($P < 0.05$), suggesting that the intervention was effective.

Discussion

It is important to construct an ARS for KOA exercise therapy. Although the WHO has provided a theoretical framework for the influencing factors for adherence to chronic disease treatment, on the one hand, as time passes and with in-depth studies of chronic disease treatment models, the theory of adherence is also

Table 3 Coefficients of the multivariate logistic regression for adherence to KOA exercise therapy

Variable/Factor	B	SE	Wald	P	OR	95%CI	Assigned value
Age	0.563	0.285	3.905	0.048	1.757	1.005–3.072	1
Education level	0.693	0.320	4.700	0.030	2.000	1.069–3.744	1
Social support	1.036	0.509	4.146	0.042	2.819	1.040–7.643	1
Exercise habit	1.740	0.426	16.713	0.000	5.698	2.474–13.123	3
Knowledge of KOA prevention and treatment	0.906	0.281	10.384	0.001	2.473	1.426–4.290	2
Degree of care needed to treat the disease	0.714	0.348	4.205	0.040	2.043	1.032–4.042	2
Familiarity of the exercise therapy	1.978	0.635	9.716	0.002	7.229	2.084–25.077	4
Treatment regimen	1.430	0.461	9.605	0.002	4.179	1.692–10.325	3
Constant	−3.745	0.564	44.095	0.000	0.024		

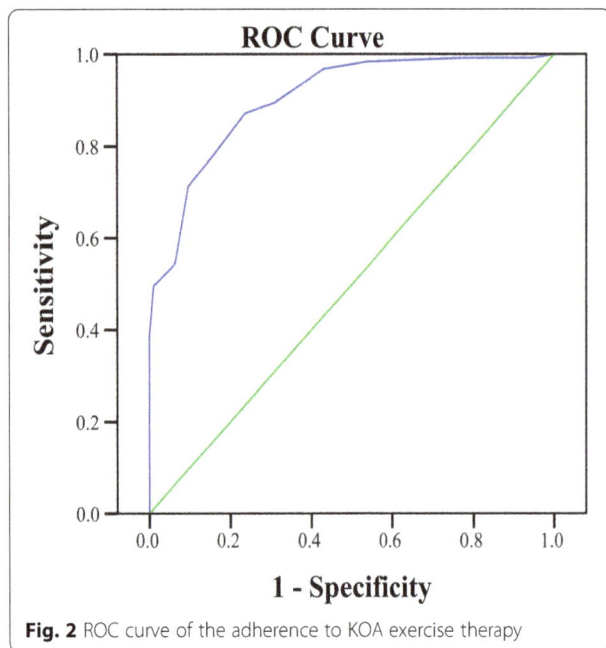

Fig. 2 ROC curve of the adherence to KOA exercise therapy

continuously developing and updating; on the other hand, the WHO adherence theory framework is constructed using generalized and universal influencing factors of chronic diseases, while specific descriptions for specific chronic diseases such as KOA exercise therapy are lacking. Therefore, this study constructed a special ARS for KOA as a specific disease.

In our study, the Morisky scale used for ARS construction was reliable in distinguishing good or bad adherence

of KOA patients. Morisky adherence scale was first proposed by Morisky et al. in 1986 [26]. It is a universal measurement scale for medication adherence, and its items have little relevance with specific diseases or drugs. The report of WHO in 2003 mentioned this scale when discussing the measurement methods of adherence. In 2008, Morisky et al. added unintentional non-adherence (e.g. forgetting) and intentional non-adherence (e.g. deterioration of disease, worrying about drug adverse reactions) items on the basis of original scale, which increased the Cronbach's α of scale to 0.83 [25]. Currently, according to disease characteristics of different specialties, researchers in different fields have constructed various adherence rating scales for the treatment of specific chronic diseases, such as scales for hypertension, pulmonary tuberculosis, acupuncture and moxibustion, and acquired immune deficiency syndrome (AIDS). Exercise therapy of KOA has general characteristics of chronic disease treatment. Therefore, we constructed the ARS for KOA exercise therapy on the basis of Morisky scale, and used this ARS to distinguish good or bad adherence of patients.

The ARS was constructed according to classical regression analysis, with good internal validity and coherence. Existing studies had mostly explored or elucidated the influencing factors for the adherence to exercise therapy. Few studies on the predictive model of risk factors for the adherence to exercise therapy and the research or application of quantitative evaluations of the variables have been reported. The eight independent variables in the adherence prediction model established in this study were obtained by screening more than 70

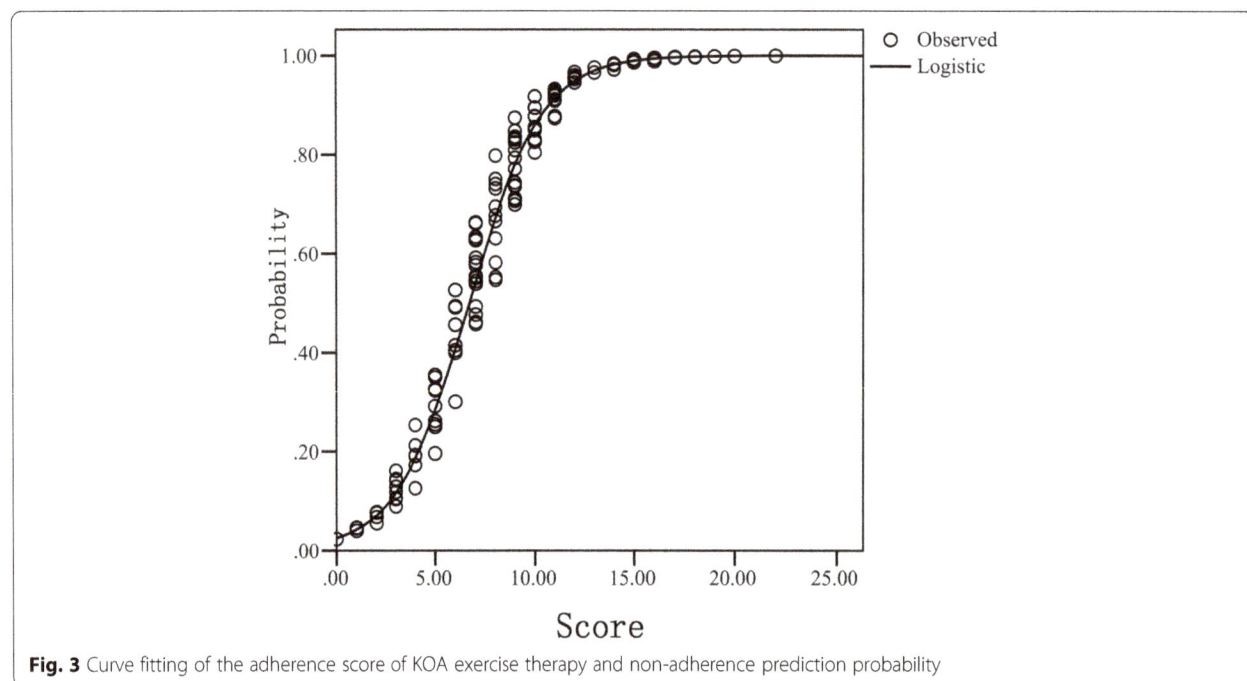

Fig. 3 Curve fitting of the adherence score of KOA exercise therapy and non-adherence prediction probability

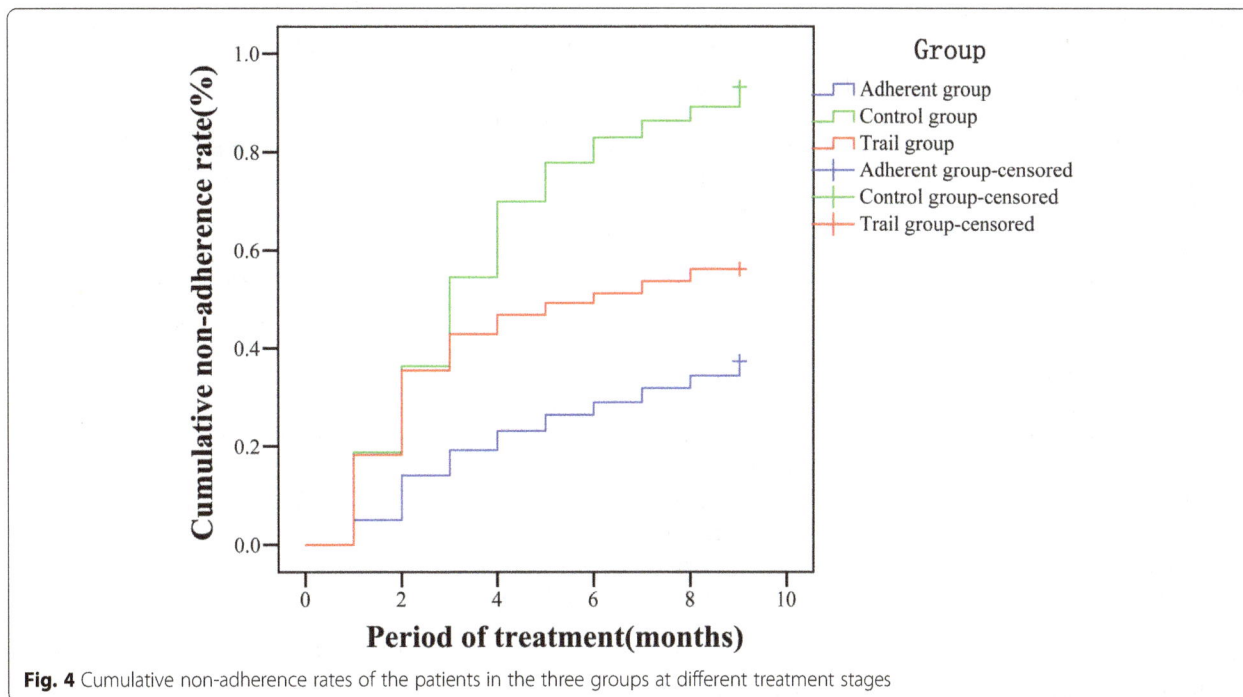

Fig. 4 Cumulative non-adherence rates of the patients in the three groups at different treatment stages

related factors; these variables covered several major measurement areas that affected adherence in the literature. Based on the adherence prediction model, the ARS was derived, and the ROC curve and curve fitting analyses were conducted for this scale. The scale had a good predictive effect and goodness of fit for the adherence. Therefore, the scale had good content validity, structural validity and distinguishing validity.

The ARS had good external validity and responsiveness. In general, an evaluation tool can be generalized and universal only after the evaluation of its external validity. To promote the ARS, this study investigated its external validity and responsiveness. In the test of external validity, interventions were given to the intervention group at the beginning of the third month to evaluate the effectiveness of intervention measures. Result showed that the cumulative non-adherence rates of intervention group after intervention were significantly lower than those of control group, indicating that the individualized interventions were effective and could

significantly improve the treatment adherence of the KOA patients. Moreover, this also indicated that the ARS had good effect in judging the non-adherence risk factors of KOA patients, because the individualized intervention measures were developed based on the non-adherence risk factors of each patient evaluated by the ARS. In conclusion, the ARS is effective in distinguishing the actual adherence of KOA patients and identifying non-adherence risk factors.

This simple ARS is more suited to clinical practice. In analyses with univariate x^2 testing and multivariate stepwise logistic regression, the adherence prediction model was ultimately determined. In general, the model can be directly used to predict the risk factors of patient adherence and to determine a given patient's adherence, but to facilitate its use in clinical practice, this study simplified the model, that is, the ARS was constructed. The advantages of the ARS are as follows: (1) it provides direct and comprehensive quantifications of the risk factors of adherence to judge the patient's adherence

Table 4 Comparison of the non-adherence rates at different time points in each group

Group	1	2	3	4	5	6	7	8	9
Adherence group ($n = 276$)	14	35	44	52	59	67	74	79	82
Control group ($n = 176$)	33*	64*	94*	119*	133*	143*	149*	155*	159*
Intervention group ($n = 203$)	37*	72*	81*Δ	88*Δ	94*Δ	99*Δ	102*Δ	105*Δ	108*Δ
x^2	25.662	38.637	64.190	97.270	114.301	125.300	128.161	130.837	138.317
P	< 0.001	< 0.001	< 0.001	< 0.001	< 0.001	< 0.001	< 0.001	< 0.001	< 0.001

Note: * Compared with the adherence group, $P < 0.05$; Δ compared with the control group, $P < 0.05$

based on the total score; and (2) it allows for the quantification of each risk factor in the model to provide the basis for the development of personalized and targeted interventions.

The core of the intervention treatment is the intervention measures. Personalized and precise interventions can effectively reduce the rate of non-adherence. The eight items in the ARS can be broadly categorized into two classes: Class 1 includes short-term intervention items, such as the degree of care needed to treat the disease, the knowledge of KOA prevention and treatment, the familiarity of the exercise therapy and the confidence of the treatment; these items can be improved through appropriate interventions in a shorter term. Class 2 includes the non-short-term intervention items, such as the education level, social support and the habits of exercise; these items cannot be improved within a short time. Therefore, two principles are recommended in the use of this scale. First, key and non-key intervention principles: the intervention should be mainly conducted for items that can be intervened. Second, the principle of individuality: the specific risk factors and the number of items for each patient are different; therefore, the development of the intervention measures should follow the principle of individuality to achieve the medical precision goals.

This study has some limitations. No multi-centre research was performed. Second, the KOA cases were from China, and the education and medical knowledge levels of some cases were associated with local economic and education levels. Therefore, the development of ARS in other countries should be cautious when promoting.

Conclusions

A KOA exercise therapy adherence model and an ARS were constructed by analyses of univariate factor x^2 testing and a multivariate logistic stepwise regression. The ARS has good internal and external validity and can be used to evaluate the adherence to exercise therapy in patients with KOA.

Abbreviations
ARS: Adherence rating scale; AUC: Area under the curve; CI: Confidence interval; HR: Hazard ratio; KOA: Knee osteoarthritis; RCT: Randomized controlled trial; ROC: Receiver operating characteristic; WHO: World Health Organization

Funding
This study was funded by the Health and Family Planning Commission of Guizhou province (gzwjkj2017-1-30), the Education Department of Guizhou Province (2017161), Science and Technology Bureau of Guiyang (20175-17) and National Natural Science Foundation (81360232), China.

Authors' contributions
WJJ are responsible for the study design. YC and WJJ gathered and reviewed the literature and data and drafted the initial manuscript. SY, ZQ and LXZ assisted with the literature search. LQJ, WZY and XZ participated in the interpretation of data and preparation of the final manuscript. All authors read and approved the final manuscript.

Competing interests
All named authors declare that they have no competing interest with respect to the research, authorship, and/or publication of this article.

Author details
[1]Department of Orthopedic Surgery, Affiliated Hospital of Guizhou Medical University, Guiyang, China. [2]Center for Bioprinting and Biomanufacturing, Guizhou Medical University, Guiyang, China. [3]Center for Tissue Engineering and Stem Cells, Guizhou Medical University, Guiyang, China. [4]China Orthopedic Regenerative Medicine Group (CORMed), Guiyang, China.

References
1. World Health Organization. Innovative care for chronic conditions. Building blocks for action: global report. Geneva: WHO; 2002.
2. Bosworth HB, Granger BB, Mendys P, et al. Medication adherence: a call for action. Am Heart J. 2011;162(3):412–24. https://doi.org/10.1016/j.ahj.2011.06.007.
3. Blackwell B. Compliance. Psychother Psychosom. 1992;58(3–4):161–9.
4. Tang X, Wang S, Zhan S, et al. The prevalence of symptomatic knee osteoarthritis in China results from the China heath and retirement longitudinal study. Arhritis Rheumatol. 2016;68(3):648–53.
5. Gabriel SE, Michaud K. Epidemiological studies in incidence, prevalence, mortality, and comorbidity of the rheumatic diseases. Arthritis Res Ther. 2009;11(3):1–16.
6. Cauley JA. Osteoporosis: fracture epidemiology update 2016. Curr Opin Rheumatol. 2017;29(2):150.
7. Smidt N, De vet HC, Bouter LM, et al. Effectiveness of exercise therapy: a best-evidence summary of systematic reviews. Aust J Physiother. 2005;51(2): 71–85.
8. Mc H, Altman RD, April KT, et al. American College of Rheumatology 2012 recommendations for the use of nonpharmacologic and pharmacologic therapies in osteoarthritis of the hand, hip, and knee. Arthritis Care Res. 2012;64(4):465–74.
9. Nelson AE, Allen KD, Golightly YM, et al. A systematic review of recommendations and guidelines for the management of osteoarthritis: the chronic osteoarthritis management initiative of the U.S. bone and joint initiative. Semin Arthritis Rheu. 2014;43(6):701–12.
10. Zhang W, Moskowitz RW, Nuki G, et al. OARSI recommendations for the management of hip and knee osteoarthritis, part II: OARSI evidence-based, expert consensus guidelines. Osteoarthr Cartilage. 2008;16(2):137–62.
11. Cutolo M, Berenbaum F, Hochberg M, et al. Commentary on recent therapeutic guidelines for osteoarthritis. Semin Arthritis Rheu. 2015;44(6):611–7.
12. Mcalindon TE, Bannuru RR, Sullivan MC, et al. OARSI guidelines for the non-surgical management of knee osteoarthritis. Osteoarthr Cartil. 2014;22(3): 363–8.
13. Roddy E, Zhang W, Doherty M, et al. Evidence-based recommendations for the role of exercise in the management of osteoarthritis of the hip or knee-the MOVE consensus. Rheumatol. 2005;44(1):67.
14. Torstensen TA, Grooten WJA, Østerås H, et al. How does exercise dose affect patients with long-term osteoarthritis of the knee? A study protocol of a randomised controlled trial in Sweden and Norway: the SWENOR study. BMJ Open. 2018;8(5):e018471. https://doi.org/10.1136/bmjopen-2017-018471.
15. Brosseau L, Taki J, Desjardins B, et al. The Ottawa panel clinical practice guidelines for the management of knee osteoarthritis. Part two: strengthening exercise programs. Clin Rehabil. 2017;31(5):596–611.
16. Hinman R. Manual physiotherapy or exercise leads to sustained reductions in pain and physical disability in people with hip and knee osteoarthritis. J Physiother. 2014;60(1):56.
17. Li Y, Su Y, Chen S, et al. The effects of resistance exercise in patients with knee osteoarthritis: a systematic review and meta-analysis. Clin Rehabil. 2016;30(10):947–59.
18. Skou ST, Roos EM. Good Life with Osteoarthritis in Denmark (GLA:D™): evidence-based education and supervised neuromuscular exercise delivered by certified physiotherapists nationwide. BMC Musculoskel Dis. 2017;18(1):72.
19. Hovstadius B, Petersson G. Non-adherence to drug therapy and drug acquisition costs in a national population - a patient-based register study. BMC Health Serv Res. 2011;11:326. https://doi.org/10.1186/1472-6963-11-326.

20. Kaona FA, Tuba M, Siziya S, et al. An assessment of factors contributing to treatment adherence and knowledge of TB transmission among patients on TB treatment. BMC Public Health. 2004;29(4):68.

21. Nour K, Laforest S, Gnuvin L, et al. Behavior change following a serf-management intervention for housebound older adults with arthritis: an experimental study. Int J Behav Nutr Phys Act. 2006;3(1):1–13.

22. Focht BC, Ganvin L, Rejeski WJ. The contribution of daily experiences and acute exercise to fluctuations in daily feeling states among older, obese adults with knee osteoarthritis. J Behav Med. 2004;27:101–21.

23. Damush TM, Perkins SM, Mikesky AE, et al. Motivational factors influencing older adults diagnosed with knee osteoarthritis to join and maintain an exercise program. J Aging Phys Act. 2005;13:45–60.

24. Thorstensson CA, Boos EM, Petersson IF, et al. How do middle-aged patients conceive exercise as a form of treatment for knee osteoarthritis? Disabil Rehabil. 2006;28:51–9.

25. Morisky DE, Ang A, Kousel-Wood M, et al. Predictive validity of a medication adherence measure in an outpatient setting. J Clin Hypertens (Greenwich). 2008;10(5):348–54.

26. Morisky DE, Green LW, Levine DM, et al. Concurrent and predictive validity of a self-reported measure of medication adherence. Med Care. 1986;24(1):67–74.

4

Subgroups of lumbo-pelvic flexion kinematics are present in people with and without persistent low back pain

Robert A. Laird[1,4*] ⓘ, Jennifer L. Keating[1] and Peter Kent[2,3]

Abstract

Background: Movement dysfunctions have been associated with persistent low back pain (LBP) but optimal treatment remains unclear. One possibility is that subgroups of persistent LBP patients have differing movement characteristics and therefore different responses to interventions. This study examined if there were patterns of flexion-related lumbo-pelvic kinematic and EMG parameters that might define subgroups of movement.

Methods: This was a cross-sectional, observational study of 126 people without any history of significant LBP and 140 people with persistent LBP ($n = 266$). Wireless motion and surface EMG sensors collected lumbo-pelvic data on flexion parameters (range of motion (ROM) of trunk, lumbar, and pelvis), speed, sequence coordination and timing, and EMG extensor muscle activity in forward bending (flexion relaxation)), and sitting parameters (relative position, pelvic tilt range and tilt ratio). Latent class analysis was used to identify patterns in these parameters.

Results: Four subgroups with high probabilities of membership were found (mean 94.9%, SD10.1%). Subgroup 1 ($n = 133$ people, 26% LBP) had the greatest range of trunk flexion, fastest movement, full flexion relaxation, and synchronous lumbar versus pelvic movement. Subgroup 2 ($n = 73$, 71% LBP) had the greatest lumbar ROM, less flexion relaxation, and a 0.9 s lag of pelvic movement. Subgroup 3 ($n = 41$, 83% LBP) had the smallest lumbar ROM, a 0.6 s delay of lumbar movement (compared to pelvic movement), and less flexion relaxation than subgroup 2. Subgroup 4 ($n = 19$ people, 100% LBP) had the least flexion relaxation, slowest movement, greatest delay of pelvic movement and the smallest pelvic ROM. These patterns could be described as standard (subgroup 1), lumbar dominant (subgroup 2), pelvic dominant (subgroup 3) and guarded (subgroup 4). Significant post-hoc differences were seen between subgroups for most lumbo-pelvic kinematic and EMG parameters. There was greater direction-specific pain and activity limitation scores for subgroup 4 compared to other groups, and a greater percentage of people with leg pain in subgroups 2 and 4.

Conclusion: Four subgroups of lumbo-pelvic flexion kinematics were revealed with an unequal distribution among people with and without a history of persistent LBP. Such subgroups may have implications for which patients are likely to respond to movement-based interventions.

Keywords: Low back pain, Subgroups, Patterns, Movement disorders, Range of movement (ROM), Flexion relaxation, Lumbo-pelvic rhythm, Velocity

* Correspondence: robert.laird@monash.edu
[1]Department of Physiotherapy, Monash University, PO Box 527, Frankston, Victoria 3199, Australia
[4]Superspine, Forest Hills, Melbourne, Australia
Full list of author information is available at the end of the article

Background

Persistent low back pain (LBP) is often described as a multidimensional problem, within a bio-psycho-social context [1, 2]. Dimensions that are thought to influence pain and function include patho-anatomic changes, cognitions and emotions, lifestyle, societal circumstances, and movement/posture [3–9]. People with LBP are quite heterogeneous within these dimensions. Identifying clinically important subgroups that are relatively homogenous within these dimensions has been a research priority [10, 11], based on a prevailing belief that better outcomes are likely when treatment is matched with subgroup-specific features.

A number of movement-based classification systems have been developed, underpinned by observations of relationships between movement and LBP, with the intention of providing subgroup-specific, targeted treatment [8, 12–15]. Different classification systems use different, albeit overlapping, combinations of examination findings to define subgroups, [16]. Examination findings include subjective reports, visual observation and pain responses to movement, but rarely include measurement of lumbo-pelvic kinematic parameters.

There is evidence that flexion-related activities are particularly important in LBP. For example, in a study on people with subacute LBP by Pengel et al. [17], the three most frequently nominated pain-related activities were sitting, bending and lifting, which all involve elements of flexion. As a consequence, there are potentially important clinical questions to be investigated in empirical measurements of flexion-related lumbo-pelvic kinematics: (i) are there different patterns in the way people perform flexion, and (ii) are any patterns more common in people with persistent LBP than in people who have never had LBP?

Studies of lumbo-pelvic kinematic parameters have identified differences in range of motion (ROM) in people with and without LBP, using between-group mean differences and their standard deviations (SD), but have generally not described subgroups based on lumbo-pelvic kinematics [18, 19]. Identifying that lumbar ROM is, on average, reduced in people with LBP [18] would suggest that improving ROM might be a treatment target. However, if some people with LBP do not have reduced lumbar ROM, a treatment strategy aimed at increasing lumbar ROM may be unhelpful. Lumbo-pelvic kinematics include a range of parameters such as trunk, lumbar and pelvic ROM, timing of regional movement, muscle activation, movement duration, movement coordination, and postural position. Using multivariable clusters of these kinematic parameters may identify different patterns of flexion that might assist in matching targeted interventions to specific lumbo-pelvic kinematic goals.

Previous work by Marras et al. [20], Dankaerts et al. [21] and Mayer et al. [22] all used kinematic analysis to validate pre-defined subgroups of people with persistent LBP but did not use kinematic data a priori to define subgroups. Marras et al. [20] quantified and matched angular data, velocity and acceleration kinematic parameters to modified Quebec classification subgroups. Dankaerts et al. [21] measured ROM and EMG parameters in two subgroups of people classified with an O'Sullivan classification system [14] and Mayer et al. [22] pre-classified people with persistent LBP into four groups based on 'normal' versus 'abnormal' lumbo-pelvic ROM and EMG of lumbar extensors during flexion.

The availability of wireless inertial and EMG sensors for use in clinical environments now enables detailed and accurate measurement of lumbo-pelvic movement. A recent study (Laird et al., 2018, unpublished) on lumbo-pelvic kinematics using data from this type of device found that, compared to people without LBP, people with persistent LBP showed a higher prevalence of smaller trunk, lumbar and pelvic ROM, slower movement, delayed pelvic versus lumbar movement and greater lumbar extensor muscle activation in the fully flexed position. That study also identified a wide range of variance for most parameters. It did not, however, investigate whether subgroups of movement patterns were evident in the data.

The current study aimed to explore (i) if patterns (subgroups) of flexion-related lumbo-pelvic kinematics could be identified in a suitably large sample of people, (ii) if patterns were present, whether they occurred with different frequency in people with and without persistent LBP, and (iii) to investigate clinical and demographic characteristics that are associated with any patterns.

Method

This cross-sectional, observational study used latent class analysis to identify subgroups in the movement patterns of flexion-related lumbo-pelvic kinematics using a previously reported dataset (Laird et al. 2018).

Study sample

Inclusion and exclusion criteria have been previously reported in detail [23]. In summary, 140 adults (18–65 years old) with persistent LBP were recruited from primary and secondary care (physiotherapy clinics and outpatient departments). Inclusion criteria were LBP > 3 months' duration, pain scores of 3 or higher (on a 0–10 point numerical rating scale), with current back +/– leg pain. Exclusion criteria were previous lumbar surgery; any invasive spinal procedures for LBP, including therapeutic injections, within the last 12 months; any serious medical or musculoskeletal issues that had the potential to affect the lumbo-pelvic region; an implanted electrical medical device; a BMI > 30 (where it becomes difficult to palpate bony landmarks); or pregnancy. Adults ($n = 126$) who had never had LBP (NoLBP group) were recruited from universities, workplaces and community groups by poster and word of mouth advertising and were eligible for inclusion if they had no significant health issues that would affect movement, and no history of any LBP episode that required visiting a health professional or taking time off either work or usual sport. All participants were screened for inclusion and exclusion initially by administrative staff and then re-checked by the assessing clinician. In addition, people in the NoLBP group were asked if they had any current LBP and excluded if they did. Demographic data can be seen in Table 1. There was a significant difference in age between the groups, as people with in the LBP group were, on average, 7 years older than those in the NoLBP group.

Data collection

Data were collected on age, sex, BMI, and for people with persistent LBP only, pain intensity (numerical rating scale 0–10 using the average of current, usual, and worst pain scores) [24], activity limitation (Roland Morris Disability Questionnaire) [25] and a study-specific, non-validated 'does flexion aggravate and extension ease' (FLAG) pain questionnaire. The FLAG is scored from 0 to 48 where higher scores indicate a greater pattern of flexion-aggravating and extension-easing pain behaviour (see Appendix). The FLAG has four questions, two that ask about flexion-aggravating activities and two that ask about extension-easing activities. Each question has two parts: the first part asks about frequency and is scored (a) never =0, rarely =1 sometimes =2, often =3, always =4; and the second part asks about intensity and is scored none =0, low =1, medium =2, and high =3. For each of the four questions, a score is calculated by multiplying frequency (0–4) by intensity responses (0–3) with possible scores of 0–12. Scores for the four questions were then summed to give an indication of the extent to which flexion aggravated and extension eased pain (maximum score = 48).

Movement data were collected using wireless inertial motion and electromyographic (EMG) sensors (ViMove hardware and software, DorsaVi, Melbourne, Australia). Participants were partially undressed, without shoes and stood in a relaxed upright position. Motion sensors were placed over T12 and S2, and EMG sensors applied 1.5 cm

Table 1 Between-group comparisons for demographic and kinematic data

Demographics	Details	NoLBP ($n = 124$)	LBP ($n = 140$)	p-value
Age (years)		34.4 ± 13.5^a	41.4 ± 12.6	$p = .0001^b$
BMI		23.6 ± 3.5	25.6 ± 4.9	$p = .0001^b$
Sex - % female		59%	57%	$p = .8250$
Pain intensity (0–10)			5.3 ± 1.5	not applicable
Activity limitation (0–100)			39 ± 21	not applicable
Kinematic parameters		No LBP ($n = 124$)	LBP ($n = 140$)	p-value
Flexion: Peak trunk flexion	Trunk flexion angular inclination (T12)	$111° \pm 16°$	$93° \pm 16°$	$p < .0000^b$
Flexion: Peak lumbar flexion	Lumbar ROM	$52° \pm 11°$	$46° \pm 12°$	$p < .0000^b$
Flexion: Peak pelvic flexion	Pelvic flexion angular inclination (S2)	$59° \pm 15°$	$48° \pm 15°$	$p < .0000^b$
Flexion: Lumbo-pelvic co-ordination	Mean Lumbar % contribution	$48 \pm 11\%$	$49 \pm 11\%$	$p = .217$
Flexion: Flexion Relaxation Response	A ratio formed by units of surface EMG activity	0.012 ± 0.32	0.25 ± 0.32	$p < .0000^b$
Sitting: Mean pelvic tilt range	Range from full anterior tilt to full posterior tilt	$29° \pm 13°$	$29° \pm 13°$	$p = .883$
Sitting: Mean pelvic tilt ratio	A ratio of pelvic tilt range/range of trunk ROM change	2.1 ± 1.3	2.4 ± 1.4	$p = .064$
Sitting: Mean relative sitting position	Max slump sit = 100%, maximum upright sit = 0%	$48 \pm 35\%$	$50 \pm 35\%$	$p = .619$
		No LBP ($n = 100$)	LBP ($n = 105$)	
Flexion: Delay at 0°	Mean delay (negative numbers indicate pelvic delay)	-0.21 ± 0.46 s	-0.36 ± 0.46 s	$p = .023^b$
Flexion: Delay at 20°	Mean delay (negative numbers indicate pelvic delay)	-0.30 ± 0.88 s	$-0.51 \pm 0.90s$	$p = .105$
Flexion: Mean movement duration	Time from start of flexion to full flexion	2.28 ± 0.94 s	3.18 ± 0.94 s	$p < .0000^b$

[a]All data represented as mean and standard deviation [b]significant p values italicised

either side of L3, using a standardized procedure. Motion sensors were calibrated to zero in the relaxed standing position.

Movements analysed

Movement and positional data were recorded for standing, flexion and sitting. People were asked to stand in their normal standing pose. They were then asked to bend (flex) towards the ground as far they could. A single practice repetition was performed. Three repetitions of flexion with a time count of 3 s in the fully flexed position were then performed, using standardized instructions from trained testers and were automatically captured by a computerized process. Patients were then instructed to sit in their usual, full slumped and full upright sitting positions with angular inclination data averaged over 5 s for each position once the position was stable. Figure 1 demonstrates the sensor placement.

Lumbo-pelvic kinematic parameter definitions

Eight flexion lumbo-pelvic kinematic parameters were assessed during a standing flexion movement including (i) trunk ROM (angular inclination of the trunk at T12), (ii) pelvic ROM (angular inclination of the pelvis at S2), each measured as maximum angular displacement, (iii) lumbar ROM measured as the difference between trunk angular displacement at T12

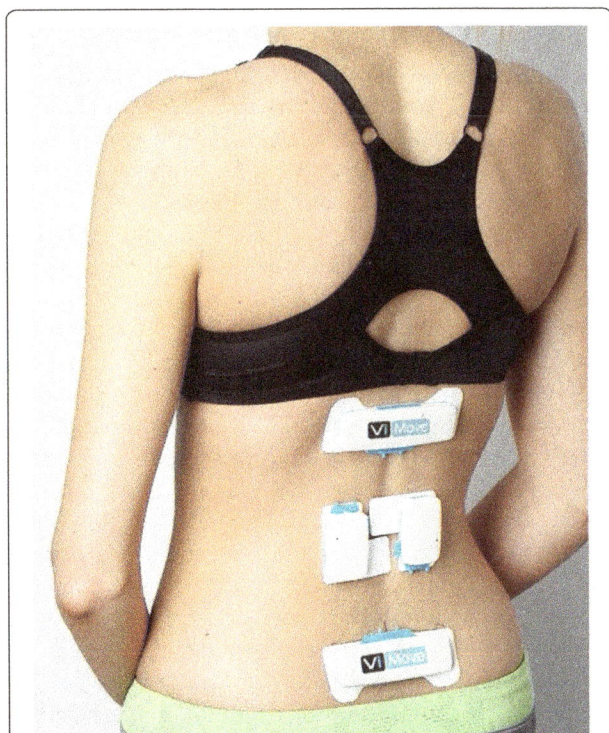

Fig. 1 Sensor placement

and pelvic angular displacement at S2, (iv) lumbo-pelvic coordination (also known as lumbo-pelvic rhythm) measured as the percentage of lumbar contribution to trunk movement, using two methods; area under the curve and peak angular displacement, (v) the flexion relaxation response (a response where lumbar extensors muscles show full relaxation in the fully flexed position in healthy individuals [26]) measured as summed EMG activity of extensor muscle activity during the fully flexed position divided by the sum of EMG activity during eccentric (standing to full flexion) and concentric (return from full flexion) phases (vi) the duration/time of eccentric flexion from the start of movement to full flexion where the beginning and end of the movement was determined by a velocity of $> 7°/sec$ then $< 7°/sec$ respectively, (vii and viii) relative timing of lumbar versus pelvic movement at the beginning of the movement and at 20° (i.e did both lumbar and pelvic regions move synchronously or was there a time-related delay in the movement of lumbar or pelvic regions at the onset of movement, or in the time it took for each region to achieve 20° of flexion).

The three sitting kinematic parameters included (i) pelvic tilt range, the difference between full posterior and full anterior pelvic tilt as measured by angular inclination at S2, (ii) a 'pelvic tilt ratio' which compared the amount of angular pelvic tilt movement to angular tilting at T12, where numbers > 1 indicate more pelvic than trunk movement and numbers < 1 indicate more trunk than pelvic movement and (iii) the 'usual' sitting position, a relative sitting position, calculated as a percentage where the slumped sitting angle (full posterior pelvic tilt) was 100% and the angle of upright sitting (full anterior tilt) was 0%. These parameters are described in detail in Additional file 1.

A summary of results for flexion and sitting can be seen in Table 1 at a group level. Due to a software version evolution between 2011 and 2014, the time related and sitting variables were only available for people measured after 2014 (LBP group = 105 and NoLBP = 100), whereas the range of movement and EMG-related data, were available for all participants.

Statistical analyses

Latent Class Analysis, a probabilistic form of unsupervised (data-driven) analysis, was used to identify potential subgroup models. Latent Class models were estimated for up to 10 subgroups, using 500 random seed points to reduce the possibility of local solutions. A co-variate consisting of the LBP/NoLBP status of each participant was included in each model to assist in post-hoc analysis but did not contribute to the subgroup modelling. The resultant models were ex-amined for the degree of contributions of each kine-matic variable and residual correlations within classes. Model fit was assessed using the Bayesian Information Criterion and informed by posterior probability diag-nostics (average posterior probability for each sub-group, classification error and odds of correct classification). We planned to choose the model with the lowest Bayesian Information Criterion score, pro-vided it reduced the criterion score by 1% or more when adding a subgroup [7]. Indicator variables that were not contributing to the discrimination of sub-groups ($r^2 < 10\%$) were removed to create more parsi-monious models that estimated fewer parameters and had more power. After the final model was chosen, participants were assigned to subgroups based on their individual posterior probability.

A post-hoc analysis of between-subgroup differences was performed, to assist in profiling and subgroup de-scription. For variables that were normally distributed, a one-way analysis of variance was used with post-hoc (unadjusted alpha level $p = .05$, Bonferroni adjusted alpha level $p = 0.0083$) t-test pairwise com-parisons. For variables that were not normally distrib-uted, a Kruskal–Wallis Test was used followed by Dunn's test for pair-wise (Bonferroni adjusted alpha level $p = .0083$) comparisons. Latent Class Analysis was undertaken using Latent GOLD 4.5 (Statistical Innovations Inc., Belmont, CA, USA) and all other statistical procedures used Stata/IC version 15 (Stata-Corp, College Station, TX, USA).

Ethics

Ethics approval was obtained from the Monash Uni-versity Human Research Ethics Committee (approval number 2016–1100) and from the Regional Commit-tees on Health Research Ethics for Southern Denmark (approval number S-20110071). All participants were given information about the study and they provided written informed consent.

Results

Selection of subgroups

Initially, latent class models included all 11 kine-matic variables but, as the sitting-related variables all contributed little to the subgroup models (all with an $r^2 < 4\%$ for each variable), we subsequently removed mean pelvic tilt range, pelvic tilt ratio and usual sitting position from further model building. The model with the lowest eligible Bayesian Infor-mation Criterion score, was the four-subgroup model. The mean (SD) probability of membership for subgroups 1 to 4 was 95.1% (10.0%), 91.2%

(13.4%), 96.7% (7.7%) and 96.6% (11.1%) respectively, which were considerably above the recommended minimum for model adequacy of 70% [27]. Collect-ively, 92.6% of participants had a posterior probabil-ity of > 80.0% of belonging to the subgroup into which they were classified and 84.0% of participants had a greater than 90.0% probability. The overall classification error of the four-subgroup model was acceptable at 5.6%.

The odds of correct classification for subgroups 1 to 4 were 19.2, 10.4, 29.4 and 28.2 respectively, well above the minimum value of 5 that is sug-gested to represent high assignment accuracy [27]. Figure 2 uses lumbo-pelvic kinematic parameters, normalised to a 0 to 1 scale, to illustrate differ-ences between subgroups. Figure 3 provides a clin-ical interpretation of the four subgroups.

Movement characteristics of the subgroups

Subgroup 1 was the largest group with 50% of the total cohort (133/266 people) and represented 78% (98/126) of the NoLBP and 25% (35/140) of the LBP groups. This cluster was characterized by the largest trunk ROM with lumbar and pelvic ROM contribut-ing in almost equal parts to trunk flexion, complete relaxation of extensor muscles in full flexion, quicker movement speed and with relatively synchronous movement of pelvic and lumbar spine at the start and also at 20° of movement.

Subgroup 2 represented 17% and 37% of the NoLBP and LBP groups respectively. Compared to subgroup 1, subgroup 2 had less trunk ROM, higher lumbar and lower pelvic angular inclination with greater acti-vation of lumbar extensor muscles, slower movement and a greater delay of pelvic motion at the start and at 20° of movement, i.e. angular inclination occurred through the lumbar spine first, followed by pelvic movement.

Subgroup 3 represented 6% and 24% of the NoLBP and LBP groups respectively. Compared to Subgroup 1, Subgroup 3 had markedly less lumbar movement but similar pelvic angular inclination and was differ-ent from Subgroup 2 with a reversed pattern of less lumbar and greater pelvic ROM and with greater lumbar extensor activity at the end of flexion than Subgroups 1 or 2. Subgroup 3 was the only group to have delayed lumbar rather than pelvic motion, i.e. angular inclination occurred at the pelvis first, followed then by movement of the lumbar spine.

Subgroup 4 contained only people with LBP (14% of the total LBP group) and also displayed the smallest trunk and pelvic angular inclination of all subgroups, but with comparable lumbar flexion ROM. Subgroup 4

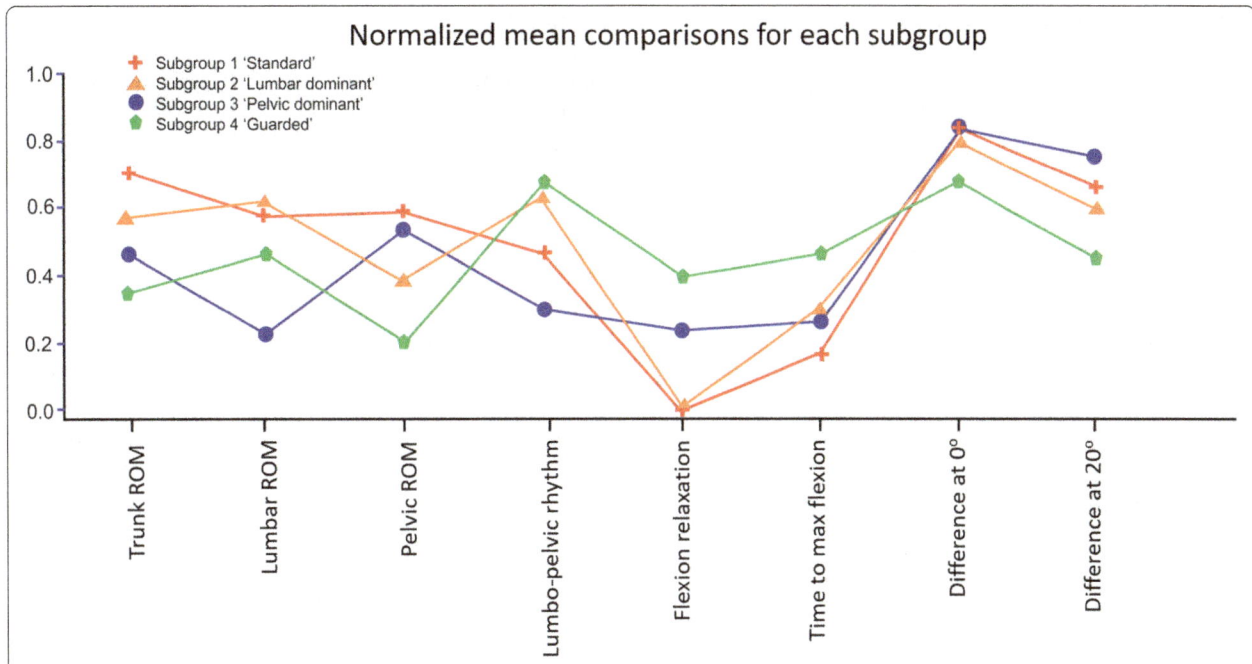

Fig. 2 Comparisons of the means for each subgroup on each kinematic parameter (scale normalised to 0–1). Figure 2 illustrates a clinical visualization for each subgroup, with angular inclination for trunk (at T12), pelvis angular inclination (at S2), lumbar movement range and lumbar extension muscle activity (with movement duration and pelvic or lumbar delay at 20° added as text below each subgroup). On the normalised scale of 0–1, 0 is the lowest score observed and 1 is the highest score

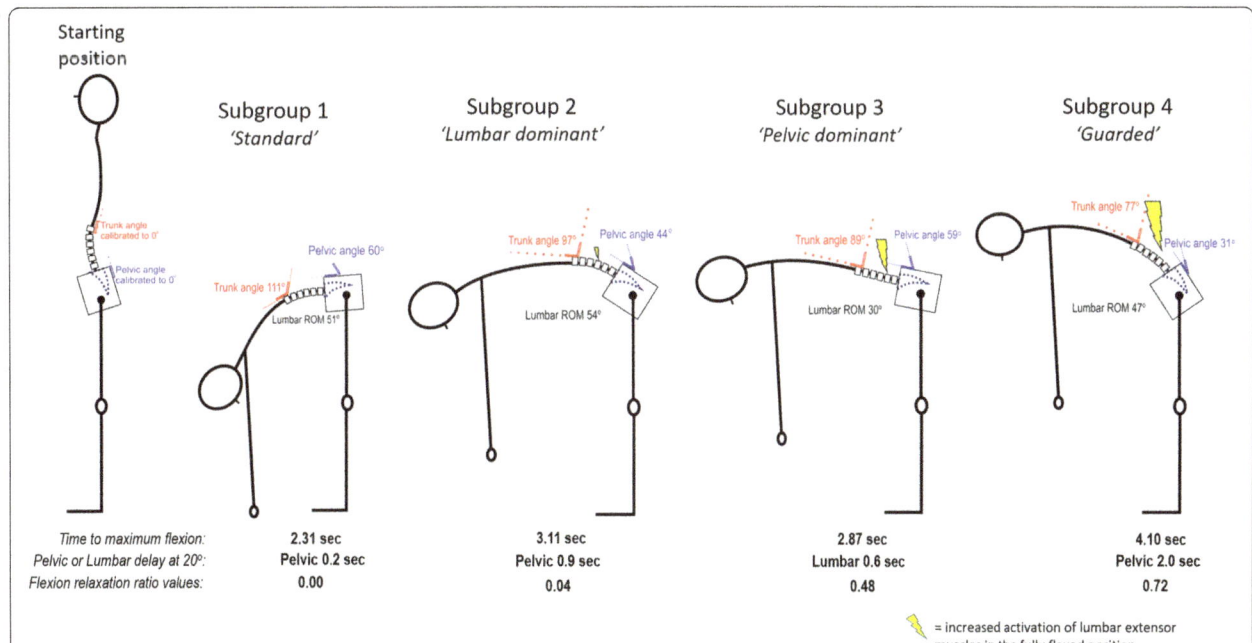

Fig. 3 Clinical visualization of mean peak kinematic parameters, temporal and muscle relaxation parameters for each subgroup. This figure illustrates the four-subgroup solution with the image describing each parameter using *normalized* means where 1 = the maximum value and 0 = 0. For ROM, higher values indicate larger ROM, for lumbo-pelvic rhythm (lumbo-pelvic coordination) higher scores indicate a larger percentage of lumbar contribution, for 'time to max flexion' larger scores indicate slower movement, for 'difference at 0° and 20°' lesser scores indicate a lag of pelvic (versus lumbar) movement with the greatest score indicating a lag of lumbar movement

had the poorest flexion relaxation response (highest amount of lumbar extensor activity in the fully flexed position), slowest movement speed and greatest pelvic delay at 20° of movement (see Fig. 3).

Between-subgroup differences

Table 2 displays post hoc analysis of between-subgroup differences. Significant differences were seen for age (Subgroup 1 versus Subgroup 3 only, $p = 0.0049$), direction-specific (flexion aggravates, extension eases) pain intensity, activity limitation, percentage of people with leg pain, and for all kinematic parameters, with most p values < 0.001.

Discussion

This study used data from a previous observational cohort study to examine whether patterns of movement could be seen in multivariable flexion-related lumbo-pelvic kinematics (eight standing flexion parameters and three sitting parameters) and if these patterns occurred equally in people with and without persistent LBP. Latent Class Analysis identified four relatively well-defined subgroups with three of the subgroups containing both NoLBP and LBP participants, and one subgroup consisting of LBP participants only. These results support the concept that people demonstrate heterogenous movement characteristics, and some of those patterns are

Table 2 Subgroup descriptions and post hoc analysis

	SubGroup 1	SubGroup 2	SubGroup 3	SubGroup 4	Difference between subgroups
Percentage of total cohort (n = 266)	50% (n = 133)	27.4% (n = 73)	15.4% (n = 41)	7.1% (n = 19)	
Percentage (and number) of people with LBP in each sub group cluster	26.3% (35)	71.2% (52)	82.9% (34)	100.0% (19)	
Posterior probability of belonging to each cluster	0.95 ± 0.10	0.91 ± 0.13	0.97 ± 0.08	0.97 ± 0.11	
Post hoc analysis – demographics					
Age	36.5 ± 13.6 [3]	37.5 ± 13.7	42.1 ± 14.8	38.1 ± 13.5	Yes
Sex (female)	60.9%	57.5%	56.1%	47.3%	No
Pain behaviour (for LBP people only)					
Pain intensity using numerical rating scale (0–10 scale)	5.2 ± 1.4	5.1 ± 1.3	5.6 ± 1.8	5.3 ± 1.5	No
'Flexion aggravates, Extension eases' pain score (0–48 scale) [a]	12.8 ± 7.3 [4]	14.5 ± 8.0 [4]	16.4 ± 8.8 [4]	22.7 ± 8.4 [1,2,3]	Yes
Activity limitation (0–100 scale)	31 ± 17 [4]	38 ± 20	42 ± 22	48 ± 26 [1]	Yes
Percentage of LBP people with leg pain [b]	36.3% [2,4]	52.0% [1,4]	21.8% [4]	76.5% [1,2,3]	Yes
Lumbo-pelvic flexion kinematic parameters					
Trunk Peak ROM (°)	111 ± 12 [2,3,4]	97 ± 17 [1,3,4]	89 ± 16 [1,2,4]	77 ± 20 [1,2,3]	Yes
Lumbar Peak ROM (°)	51 ± 9 [3]	54 ± 10 [3,4]	30 ± 8.5 [1,2,4]	47 ± 14 [2,3]	Yes
Pelvic ROM (°)	60 ± 11 [2,4]	44 ± 5 [1,4]	59 ± 15 [2,4]	31 ± 11 [1,2,3]	Yes
Percentage of lumbar contribution to trunk flexion (%)	47 ± 7 [2,3,4]	57 ± 10 [1,3]	35 ± 9 [1,2,4]	60 ± 9 [1,3]	Yes
Flexion relaxation response	0.00 ± 0.00 [2,3,4]	0.04 ± 0.05 [3,4]	0.48 ± 0.50 [1,2]	0.72 ± 0.55 [1,2]	Yes
Duration of trunk flexion (sec)	2.31 ± 0.63 [2,3,4]	3.11 ± 1.11 [1]	2.87 ± 0.70 [1]	4.10 ± 1.83 [1]	Yes
Pelvic time-lag at start of movement (sec) [c]	+ 0.17 ± 0.14 [2,4]	+ 0.42 ± 0.31 [1,3]	+ 0.13 ± 0.24 [2,4]	+ 1.10 ± 1.34 [1,3]	Yes
Pelvic time-lag at 20° of movement (sec) [c]	+ 0.22 ± 0.30 [2,4]	+ 0.86 ± 0.53 [1,4]	- 0.55 ± 0.8 [4]	+ 2.04 ± 1.74 [1,2,3]	Yes

Superscript numbers represent subgroups i.e. [3] = Subgroup3 and indicate a significant difference between the column named subgroup and the superscripted subgroup
[a] A study-specific, non-validated questionnaire based on directional pain responses where flexion aggravates and extension eases (see Appendix)
[b] Percentage calculated by number of people with leg pain in each subgroup over number of people with LBP in each subgroup
[c] positive numbers indicate a time-lag (delay) of pelvic movement, i.e. the lumbar spine moves first then the pelvis begins to move, lagging behind lumbar movement (at start and at 20° of lumbar and pelvic flexion). Negative numbers indicate a time-lag for the lumbar spine, i.e. the pelvis moves or achieves 20° of flexion earlier than the lumbar spine achieving 20°

associated with persistent LBP. These findings align with the heterogeneity reported in and across other health data such as cognitions, pain behaviour, and improvement trajectories.

The concept of movement-related subgroups is not new. Two of the movement patterns identified in this sample are similar to patterns described in other classification systems such as the flexion and 'active-extension' motor control impairment described by O'Sullivan [14, 21] with Subgroup 2 and Subgroup 3 respectively matching these descriptive groups. Several studies using pre-classified groups have identified kinematic differences between flexion and 'active extension' subgroups, and between people with LBP and healthy controls [21, 28–30]. However, in all of these studies, subgroups were pre-defined based on observation and history, without objective measurement of lumbo-pelvic kinematics, and analysed smaller samples. Where studies subsequently contrasted those subgroups using laboratory-based measurement tools, these contrasts were usually only univariate comparisons. This study differs by using multivariable clusters of lumbo-pelvic kinematic parameters to describe patterns that are seen in both NoLBP and LBP populations, in a large sample using wireless motion and surface EMG sensors that are readily available for clinical settings.

The relationship between movement and pain
Subgroups 1, 2, and 3 all included people who reported never having had LBP that warranted seeing a clinician or taking time off work or sport. The presence of people with no history of LBP in these subgroups, particularly Subgroups 2 and 3, suggest that these movement patterns can pre-exist injury or a chronic pain experience. The decreasing percentage of people with no LBP history within Subgroups 2–4 suggests that pain and movement are associated, and that identifying cause and/or consequence relationships between pain and movement is likely to be important. Subgroup 4 included only people from the LBP group. The observed reduced movement range and increased muscle activation may be protective of, or a reactive response to, pain. However, we do not know if pre-existing movement patterns, such as those seen in Subgroups 2 and 3, increase the risk of developing LBP. Further research is required to see if the presence of a particular movement pattern or specific lumbo-pelvic kinematic parameter increases the risk of LBP occurrence, delays recovery or is associated with differing trajectories of recovery.

The mean pain score did not differentiate between subgroups, a finding previously seen in other subgrouping studies [29]. However, direction-specific pain questions (does flexion aggravate and extension ease pain?) showed increasing pain scores with correspondingly reduced ROM from Subgroups 1 to 4 and increasingly reduced flexion relaxation. Clinicians often observe a pain response matched to directionally specific movement ([13, 31, 32], so this relationship between flexion aggravation pain scores and flexion kinematics is not surprising. A similar pattern of progressively increased activity limitation from Subgroups 1 to 4 was seen and is consistent with the direction-specific pain score that quantified flexion-related pain activities. Leg pain and pelvic ROM also showed the interesting and clinical plausible finding where the two subgroups that had the lowest pelvic ROM also had the largest percentage of people with a leg pain component associated with their LBP (52% and 76% for Subgroups 2 and 4 compared to 36% and 22% for Subgroups 1 and 3).

Implications for research and clinical management
The presence of relatively distinct and different patterns lends support to the concept that treatments are likely to be more effective if the treatment matches the identified deficit. For example, improving the flexion relaxation response is recommended for people with persistent LBP and may be helpful for people in Subgroups 3 and 4 but is unlikely to assist when people with persistent LBP have the flexion movement pattern seen in Subgroups 1 and 2. Similarly, improving lumbar ROM may be helpful for people in Subgroup 3, where lumbar flexion has the greatest reduction, but is less likely to be useful for people in Subgroup 4 where lumbar flexion is only slightly less than almost 80% of the NoLBP group. While there is limited evidence that individualized treatment approaches have favourable outcomes [31, 33–35], it is unknown if treatments aimed at specific kinematic subgroups have better outcomes. If these subgroups continue to be seen in other samples, matching specific treatments to subgroups based on lumbo-pelvic kinematics could be a focus for further research.

While pain and activity limitation are seen to some extent in all people with persistent LBP, this is not necessarily true for the presence of some lumbo-pelvic kinematic features. In this sample, 25% of people with persistent LBP had a 'standard' pattern of movement that was found in almost 80% of the NoLBP group, suggesting that people in this subgroup have flexion kinematics that are not obviously affected by pain and are the same as people without LBP. It is possible that other unmeasured parameters (e.g. ROM in other directions, different muscle activation patterns or strength factors) might have been problematic or it may be that movement factors are not relevant for some people with persistent LBP. This has implications for research and measuring change in movement as an outcome measure. Measuring changes to pain and activity limitation are relevant to most LBP patients but measuring change to movement may be less relevant for some people.

Strengths

Classification accuracy was high which provides greater confidence in observing subgroup patterns. The sample size was sufficiently large to observe non-predetermined patterns. An additional benefit was the inclusion of 126 people with no history of significant back pain which allowed insight into whether movement patterns could pre-exist the onset of pain.

There are clinically relevant strengths of this study. The use of single, univariable comparisons has frequently been used to contrast NoLBP and LBP groups, with varying results [18]. A strength of using multivariable lumbo-kinematic parameter analysis that uses clusters of parameters to define patterns (subgroups) of patients is that it reflects real-world clinical practice which incorporates many sources of information in decision-making. For example, including pelvic ROM as one of the flexion-related lumbo-pelvic parameters combined with the flexion relaxation response helped differentiate between Subgroups 2 and 4. Conversely, if lumbar ROM were the main measure of physical assessment without reference to other measures, the distinction between those subgroups would not be possible. Another clinically relevant strength is that the lumbo-pelvic kinematic parameters used in this study can all be measured in a typical clinical setting.

Limitations

Flexion was chosen as the focus of kinematic assessment because flexion-related activities have been previously identified as the most common pain-related activities in people with LBP [17]. Additionally, previous work has shown that flexion has greater measurement reliability and consistency compared to other directions, most likely due to the larger relative ROM, limited effect of attenuation of range on correlational indices, and lower susceptibility to skin movement artefacts [23]. However, other movement directions and parameters (i.e strength, proprioception) may also inform clinical decision-making. The inclusion of other movement-related parameters are likely to add to, and change, overall subgroup profiles. It is also possible that while flexion was not problematic for

some of the people with persistent LBP in this sample, other movement directions, e.g. extension, could have been painful for them. Also, functional tasks are often three dimensional, whereas this sample of people were tested using sagittal plane motion only. However, Marras et al. [36] and Gombatto [28] both assessed para-sagittal and three-dimensional movement, with both studies demonstrating that the sagittal plane was the movement plane where movement effects were most visible. It would both be very difficult to assemble a sample of people who had never experienced any LBP at any time point, and the results from such a group would not be broadly applicable to the general population. In addition, age can affect ROM and there was a significant difference in age only between Subgroups 1 and 3 of approximately 6 years. In our view, that difference is unlikely to account for the 21° difference of lumbar ROM seen between those subgroups. Another limitation of the study was that other pain-related parameters such as duration of pain and frequency of recurrence may have provided additional information about subgroup characteristics. Lastly, these results have not been verified in an independent sample and, until such time, the possibility that observed clusters are sample specific, must be considered.

Conclusion

Movement was studied in 140 people with and 126 people without persistent LBP, with four movement-pattern subgroups seen in flexion related lumbo-pelvic kinematics. Subgroup 1, the 'standard' group was the largest, accounting for almost 80% of NoLBP and 25% of people with LBP and 50% of the total group. Subgroup 1 ('standard' subgroup) had the greatest trunk ROM, full flexion relaxation at end range flexion, and relatively synchronous pelvic and lumbar movement. Subgroups 2 ('lumbar-dominant') and 3 ('pelvic-dominant') showed progressive loss of flexion relaxation and opposite lumbo-pelvic rhythm patterns. Subgroup 4 ('guarded' movement) had the lowest trunk and pelvic ROM, but similar lumbar ROM to the standard subgroup, had the highest extensor muscle activation in full flexion, the slowest movement, and the greatest pelvic delay. In addition, leg pain occurred more frequently in the two subgroups that had the lowest range of pelvic movement. Although mean pain intensity scores were similar across subgroups, activity limitation and the 'flexion aggravates/extension eases' pain scores progressively increased, reaching significance for the comparison between Subgroup 1 (standard) and Subgroup 4 (guarded). These results indicate that different patterns of flexion are present in people with and without persistent LBP and this has implications for both further research and treatment.

Appendix
Study specific LBP questionnaire on flexion aggravates, extension eases (FLAG questionnaire)

Low Back Pain - Aggravating activities and classifier

Pt Name:_____

* Please read each question (1-12) and place a cross in the box for the response which best describes your lower back pain. There should be a cross in section A and a cross in section B for each question (for Q 1-8).

Date:_____

	Section A						Section B				TOTAL
	0	1	2	3	4		0	1	2	3	
(*Please answer all questions)	(tick one box only in Section A)						(tick one box only in Section B)				(A X B)
	Never	Rarely	Sometimes	Often	Always		None	Low	Medium	High	
1. Is your pain aggravated by bending forward activities?	☐	☐	☐	☐	☐	If so, is the level of increase:	☐	☐	☐	☐	___
2. Is your pain aggravated by putting socks & shoes on?	☐	☐	☐	☐	☐	If so, is the level of increase:	☐	☐	☐	☐	___
3. Is your pain eased by sitting upright or sitting with back support?	☐	☐	☐	☐	☐	If so, is the level of reduction of pain:	☐	☐	☐	☐	___
4. Is your pain eased by arching backward?	☐	☐	☐	☐	☐	If so, is the level of reduction of pain:	☐	☐	☐	☐	___

Sub Total Flexion ☐

Fig. 4 The study-specific, non-validated 'does flexion aggravate and extension ease' (FLAG) pain questionnaire

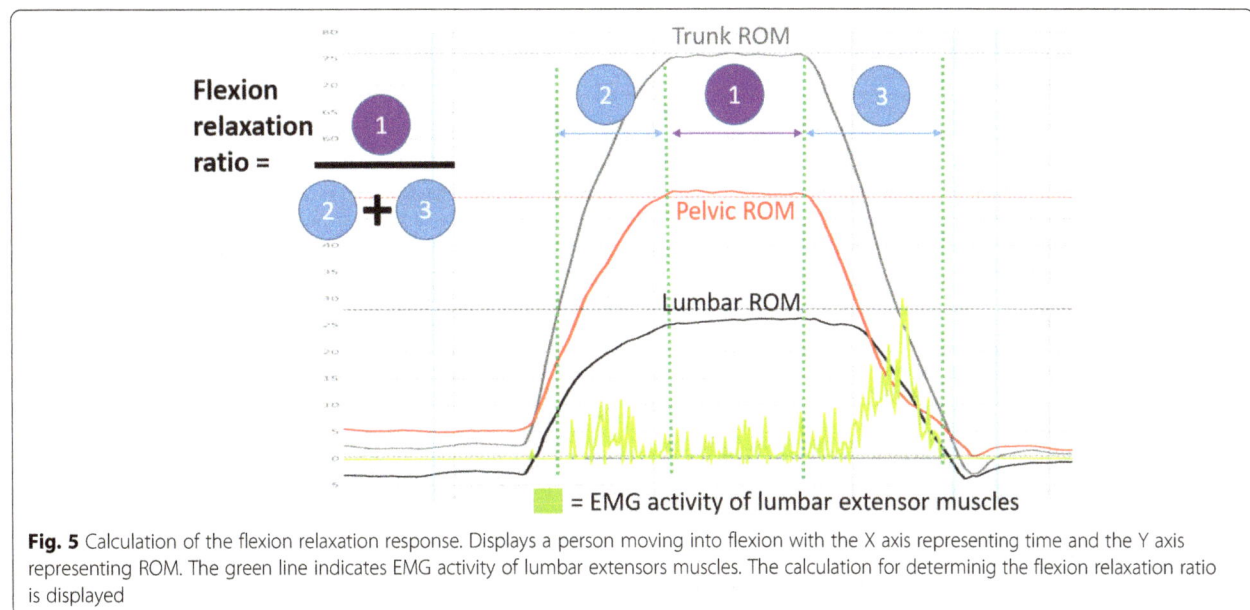

Fig. 5 Calculation of the flexion relaxation response. Displays a person moving into flexion with the X axis representing time and the Y axis representing ROM. The green line indicates EMG activity of lumbar extensors muscles. The calculation for determinig the flexion relaxation ratio is displayed

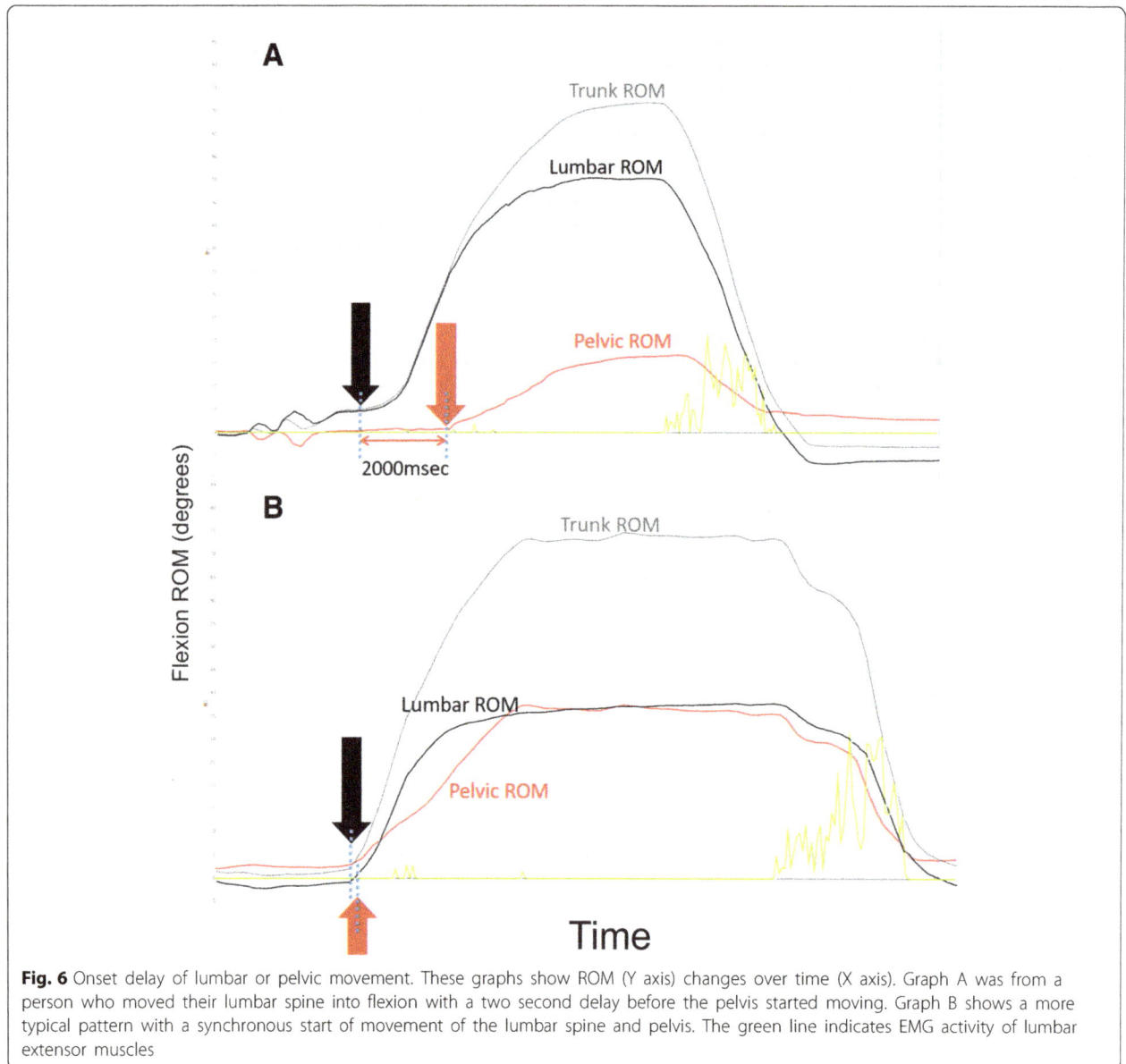

Fig. 6 Onset delay of lumbar or pelvic movement. These graphs show ROM (Y axis) changes over time (X axis). Graph A was from a person who moved their lumbar spine into flexion with a two second delay before the pelvis started moving. Graph B shows a more typical pattern with a synchronous start of movement of the lumbar spine and pelvis. The green line indicates EMG activity of lumbar extensor muscles

Abbreviations
FRR: Flexion relaxation response; LBP: Low back pain; NoLBP: Participants without low back pain; RMDQ: Roland Morris disability questionnaire; ROM: Range of motion

Funding
No funding was received for this study.
The lead author (RL) has been engaged as a consultant by DorsaVi for training clinicians in how to use the ViMove device, but otherwise has no financial interest in the company, DorsaVi, nor has received any funding for this study. DorsaVi had a 25% ownership in a private physiotherapy clinic that RL is a director. In 2012, PK received a market-rate consulting fee from DorsaVi for clinical trial design advice unrelated to the current study, but otherwise has no financial interest in the company, DorsaVi.

Authors' contributions
RL contributed to data collection. RL was the main author of this paper, leading the concept, writing, data analysis, interpretation, draft revision and gave approval of the final manuscript. JK and PK both provided concept guidance, statistical direction, analysis, draft revision and gave approval of the final manuscript. RL, JK and PK agree to be accountable for all aspects of the work in ensuring that questions related to the accuracy or integrity of any part of the work are appropriately investigated and resolved. All authors read and approved the final manuscript.

Competing interests
No benefits in any form have been, or will be, received for this study from a commercial party related directly or indirectly to the subject of this paper. This paper does not contain information about drugs. The authors do not hold stocks or shares in any company that might be directly or indirectly affected by this study. No patents have been applied for or received due to the content of this paper and there are no non-financial competing interests associated with this paper.

Author details
[1]Department of Physiotherapy, Monash University, PO Box 527, Frankston, Victoria 3199, Australia. [2]School of Physiotherapy and Exercise Science, Curtin

University, Perth, Australia. [3]Department of Sports Science and Clinical Biomechanics, University of Southern Denmark, Odense, Denmark. [4]Superspine, Forest Hills, Melbourne, Australia.

References

1. Waddell G. A new clinical model for the treatment of low-back pain. Spine. 1987;12(7):632–44.
2. Marin TJ, Van Eerd D, Irvin E, Couban R, Koes BW, Malmivaara A, Van Tulder MW, Kamper SJ. Multidisciplinary biopsychosocial rehabilitation for subacute low back pain. Cochrane Database Syst Rev. 2017;6:CD002193.
3. O'Sullivan P, Smith A, Beales D, Straker L. Understanding adolescent low back pain from a multidimensional perspective: implications for management. J Orthop Sports Phys Ther. 2017;47(10):741–51.
4. Deyo R, Bryan M, Comstock B, Turner J, Heagerty P, Friedly J, Avins A, Nedeljkovic S, Nerenz D, Jarvik J. Trajectories of symptoms and function in older adults with low back disorders. Spine. 2015;40(17):1352–62.
5. O'Sullivan PB. Diagnosis and classification of chronic low backpain disorders: maladaptive movement and motor control impairments as underlying mechanism. Manual Ther. 2005;10:242–55.
6. Sahrmann S. Movement impairment syndromes of the lumbar spine. In: Diagnosis and treatment of movement impairment syndromes. 1st ed. St. Loius: Mosby Inc; 2002. p. 5–118.
7. Kongsted A, Kent P, Hestbaek L, Vach W. Patients with low back pain had distinct clinical course patterns that were typically neither complete recovery nor constant pain. A latent class analysis of longitudinal data. Spine J. 2015;15:885–94.
8. Delitto A, Erhard RE, Bowling RW. A treatment-based classification approach to low back syndrome: identifying and staging patterns for conservative treatment including commentary by DeRosa CP and Greathouse DG with author response. Phys Ther. 1995;75(6):470–89.
9. Kongsted A, Kent P, Albert h JT, Manniche C. Patients with low back pain differ from those who also have leg pain or signs of nerve root involvement – a cross-sectional study. BMC Musculoskelet Disord. 2012;12: 236–45.
10. Borkan JMMDP, Koes BP, Reis SMD, Cherkin DCP. A report from the second international forum for primary care research on low back pain: reexamining priorities. Spine. 1998;23(18):1992–6.
11. Costa LCMP, Koes BWMDP, Pransky GMDMOH, Borkan JMDP, Maher CGMDP, Smeets RJEMMDP. Primary care research priorities in low back pain: an update. Spine. 2013;38(2):148–56.
12. McKenzie R, May S. Lumbar Spine, Mechanical Diagnosis and Therapy. 2nd ed. Waikanae: Spinal Publications Ltd; 2003.
13. Sahrmann S. Diagnosis and treatment of movement impairment syndromes. St. Louis: Mosby; 2002.
14. O'Sullivan P. Diagnosis and classification of chronic low back pain disorders: maladaptive movement and motor control impairments as underlying mechanism. Manual Ther. 2005;10(4):242–55.
15. Hodges P, Cholewicki J, Van Dieen J. Spinal control: the rehabilitation of back pain. Edinburgh: Elsevier; 2013.
16. Karayannis N, Jull G, Hodges P. Physiotherapy movement based classification approaches to low back pain: comparison of subgroups through review and developer/expert survey. BMC Musculoskelet Disord. 2012;13:24.
17. Pengel LH, Refshauge KM, Maher CG. Responsiveness of pain, disability, and physical impairment outcomes in patients with low back pain. Spine. 2004; 29(8):879–83.
18. Laird R, Gilbert J, Kent P, Keating J. Comparing lumbo-pelvic kinematics in people with and without back pain: a systematic review and meta-analysis. BMC Musculoskelet Disord. 2014;15(1):229.
19. Marras WS, Ferguson SA, Gupta P, Bose S, Parnianpour M, Kim JY, Crowell RR. The quantifications of low back disorder using motion measures: methodology and validation. Spine. 1999;24(20):2091–100.
20. Marras WS, Parnianpour M, Ferguson SA, Kim JY, Crowell RR, Bose S, Simon SR. The classification of anatomic- and symptom-based low back disorders using motion measure models. Spine. 1995;20(23):2531–46.
21. Dankaerts W, O'Sullivan P, Burnett A, Straker L, Davey P, Gupta R. Discriminating healthy controls and two clinical subgroups of nonspecific chronic low back pain patients using trunk muscle activation and lumbosacral kinematics of postures and movements: a statistical classification model. Spine. 2009;34(15):1610–8.
22. Mayer TG, Neblett R, Brede E, Gatchel RJ. The quantified lumbar flexion-relaxation phenomenon is a useful measurement of improvement in a functional restoration program. Spine. 2009;34(22):2458–65.
23. Laird R, Kent P, Keating J. How consistent are lordosis, range of movement and lumbo-pelvic rhythm in people with and without back pain? BMC Musculoskelet Disord. 2016;17:403–17.
24. Ross R, LaStayo P. Clinical assessment of pain. In: van Deusen J, Brunt D, editors. Assessment in Occupational Therapy and Physical Therapy. Philadelphia: WB Saunders Co; 1997.
25. Roland M, Fairbank J. The Roland-Morris disability questionnaire and the Oswestry disability questionnaire. Spine. 2000;25(24):3115–24.
26. McGorry RW, Lin J-H. Flexion relaxation and its relation to pain and function over the duration of a back pain episode. PLoS ONE. 2012;7(6):e39207.
27. Nagin D. Group-based modeling development. Cambridge: Harvard University Press; 2005.
28. Gombatto S, D'Arpa N, Landerholm S, Mateo C, O'Connor R, Tokunaga J, Tuttle L. Differnece in kinematics of the lumbar spine and lower extremities between poeple with and wihtout low back pain during the down phase of a pick up task, an observational study. Musculoskelet Sci Pract. 2017;28:25–31.
29. Hemming R, Sheeran L, van Deursen R, Sparkes V. Non-specific chronic low back pain: differences in spinal kinematics in subgroups during functional tasks. Eur Spine J. 2017;27(1):163–70.
30. Dankaerts W, O'Sullivan P, Burnett A, Straker L. Altered patterns of superficial trunk muscle activation during sitting in nonspecific chronic low back pain patients: importance of subclassification. Spine. 2006;31(17):2017–23.
31. Long A, Donelson R, Fung T. Does it matter which exercise? A randomized control trial of exercise for low back pain. Spine. 2004;29(23):2593–602.
32. Maitland G. Peripheral manipulation. 3rd ed. London: Butterworth-Heinemann; 1991.
33. Fersum KV, O'Sullivan P, Skouen JS, Smith A, Kvale A. Efficacy of classification-based cognitive functional therapy in patients with non-specific chronic low back pain: a randomized controlled trial. Eur J Pain. 2012;17(6):916–28.
34. Ford JJ, Hahne AJ, Surkitt LD, Chan AY, Richards MC, Slater SL, Hinman RS, Pizzari T, Davidson M, Taylor NF. Individualised physiotherapy as an adjunct to guideline-based advice for low back disorders in primary care: a randomised controlled trial. BJSM online. 2016;50(4):237–45.
35. Kent P, Laird R, Haines T. The effect of changing movement and posture using motion-sensor biofeedback, versus guidelines-based care, on the clinical outcomes of people with sub-acute or chronic low back pain-a multicentre, cluster-randomised, placebo-controlled, pilot trial. BMC Musculoskelet Disord. 2015;16:131–50.
36. Marras WS, Ferguson SA, Gupta P, Bose S, Parnianpour M, Kim JY, Crowell RR. The quantification of low back disorder using motion measures: methodology and validation. Spine. 1999;24(20):2091–100.

5

Intervertebral disc degeneration induced by long-segment in-situ immobilization: a macro, micro, and nanoscale analysis

Yan-Jun Che[1,2], Hai-Tao Li[1], Ting Liang[1], Xi Chen[1], Jiang-Bo Guo[1], Hua-Ye Jiang[1], Zong-Ping Luo[1]* and Hui-Lin Yang[1]

Abstract

Background: Cervical spine fixation or immobilization has become a routine treatment for spinal fracture, dislocation, subluxation injuries, or spondylosis. The effects of immobilization of intervertebral discs of the cervical spine is unclear. The goal of this study was to evaluate the effects of long-segment in-situ immobilization of intervertebral discs of the caudal vertebra, thereby simulating human cervical spine immobilization.

Methods: Thirty-five fully grown, male Sprague-Dawley rats were used. Rats were randomly assigned to one of five groups: Group A, which served as controls, and Groups B, C, D, and E, in which the caudal vertebrae were in-situ immobilized using a custom-made external device that fixed four caudal vertebrae (Co7-Co10). After 2 weeks, 4 weeks, 6 weeks, and 8 weeks of in-situ immobilization, the caudal vertebrae were harvested, and the disc height, the T2 signal intensity of the discs, disc morphology, the gene expression of discs, and the structure and the elastic modulus of discs was measured.

Results: The intervertebral disc height progressively decreased, starting at the 6th week. At week 6 and week 8, disc degeneration was classified as grade III, according to the modified Pfirrmann grading system criteria. Long-segment immobilization altered the gene expression of discs. The nucleus pulposus showed a typical cell cluster phenomenon over time. The annulus fibrosus inner layer began to appear disordered with fissure formation. The elastic modulus of collagen fibrils within the nucleus pulposus was significantly decreased in rats in group E compared to rats in group A ($p < 0.05$). On the contrary, the elastic modulus within the annulus was significantly increased in rats in group E compared to rats in group A ($p < 0.05$).

Conclusion: Long-segment in-situ immobilization caused target disc degeneration, and positively correlated with fixation time. The degeneration was not only associated with changes at the macroscale and microscale, but also indicated changes in collagen fibrils at the nanoscale. Long-segment immobilization of the spine (cervical spine) does not seem to be an innocuous strategy for the treatment of spine-related diseases and may be a predisposing factor in the development of the symptomatic spine.

Keywords: Intervertebral disc degeneration, Immobilization, Cervical spine, Fixation, Biomechanics, Rat model

* Correspondence: zongping_luo@yahoo.com
[1]Orthopaedic Institute, Department of Orthopaedics, The First Affiliated
Hospital of SooChow University, 708 Renmin Rd, Suzhou, Jiangsu 215006,
People's Republic of China
Full list of author information is available at the end of the article

Background

Previous studies have shown that disc degeneration is closely associated with low back pain (LBP) [1, 2]. The mechanical environment of the intervertebral disc (IVD) at least in part determines the rate of disc degeneration. However, in terms of overload and "wear and tear" theory, the mechanical environment around the nucleus pulposus (NP) and annulus fibrosus (AF) is more harsher, so that damage to the disc cannot be completely recovered [3]. In previous studies, the degeneration model of articular cartilage induced by immobilization has been clearly demonstrated [4–9], however, the IVD degeneration induced by immobilization in human spine is still controversial. Due to fractures of the cervical spine, dislocations and cervical spondylosis, in order to restore the stability of the spine (cervical spine), a cervical extension collar, brace, or Halo-vest immobilization may be required. However, after release of immobilization, complications may remain, including stiffness of the neck and restricted movement [10, 11]. It cannot be ruled out that the immobilization apparatus was a causal factor to the complications, and the underlying mechanism that is a factor in these complications has yet to be identified. In this study, three caudal vertebrae (including two discs) were fixed, this method manufactured reconstitution alterations that were similar to those found using static compression, but with less changes in configuration and synthesis [12]. Immobilization using fixation of two caudal vertebrae, including one disc, downregulated the expression of anabolic genes [13]. The hypothesis that movement increases the conveyance of nutrients and metabolites in the disc was recently investigated, and it was found that essential nutrients are transported through diffusion and convection [14]. Moreover, it was suggested that a "pumping" effect would accelerate the conveyance of molecules larger than that of sulfate ions. Several studies have shown the effect induced by short-segment immobilization (usually fixation is less than/or equal to three caudal vertebrae, including two discs). Because of the anatomical features of the cervical vertebrae (C4–7 intervertebral discs is an easier segment to degenerate or protrude), cervical spine immobilization or fixation (a brace or Halo-Vest fixator) is more inclined to overall fixation (similar to long tube fixation). However, the effect of long-segment in-situ immobilization and the underlying mechanism involved in the onset of complications remains unknown.

The purpose of this study is to identify the effect of long-segment in-situ immobilization (fixation of four caudal vertebrae, including three discs) caused by biochemical composition, gene expression, matrix reconstruction, and cellular responses, and to assess the effects of long-segment in-situ immobilization on intervertebral discs of the caudal vertebra, thereby simulating human

cervical spine immobilization. Therefore, we hypothesize: 1) intervertebral disc degeneration is induced by long-segment in-situ immobilization; 2) intervertebral disc degeneration positively correlates with immobilization time; 3) the mechanism involved in complications of cervical spine long-segment in-situ immobilization can be explained at least in part by intervertebral disc degeneration.

Methods

In this study, thirty-five fully grown, 3-month-old male Sprague-Dawley rats were used [15]. Animals were randomly assigned to one of five groups (Table 1). Group A ($n = 7$ rats, the caudal vertebrae were instrumented with K-wires only, Fig. 1a) which served as controls. In the other four groups, vertebrae were immobilized using a custom-made external device to fix four caudal vertebrae (Co7-Co10). After 2 weeks ($n = 7$ rats, Group B), 4 weeks ($n = 7$ rats, Group C), 6 weeks ($n = 7$ rats, Group D), and 8 weeks ($n = 7$ rats, Group E) of immobilization, animals were euthanized and the caudal vertebrae were harvested for further analysis. The disc space was measured using radiography [16], and MRI qualitative analysis according to the modified Pffirmann scale [17]. Next, an experienced radiologist and a senior director experienced in spines analyzed the MRI-derived data (Table 2). Histological evaluation was based on the grading system developed by Han et al. [18]. Disc anabolic (collagen I, collagen II, aggrecan) and expression of catabolic genes (MMP3, MMP13, ADAMTs-4) were measured, respectively. Four K-wires were fixed in parallel using two aluminum alloy cuboids, which do not compress or stretch the experimental disc (Fig. 1b).

Histological analysis

After immobilization for 2, 4, 6, and 8 weeks, respectively, the rats were examined by X-ray and MRI analysis. Then, the animals were euthanized by an excess of isoflurane (isoflurane, RWD Life science co. Shenzhen, China). The target discs Co7-Co8, Co8-Co9, Co9-Co10 were harvested, fixed in 10% buffered formalin solution (Shanghai Yuanye Bio-Technology Co. Ltd., Shanghai, China) for 24 h, and decalcified in 10% ethylenediaminetetraacetic acid (EDTA) (Biosharp, Hefei, China) for 30 days. The discs were then paraffin-embedded (Leica,

Table 1 Summary of study design

Group	Instrumented level (Co7-Co10)	No. of Animals
A (Control)	Instrumented with K-wires only	7
B	Imm-2 week	7
C	Imm-4 week	7
D	Imm-6 week	7
E	Imm-8 week	7

Imm indicates immobilization, *Co* indicates Coccygeal spine

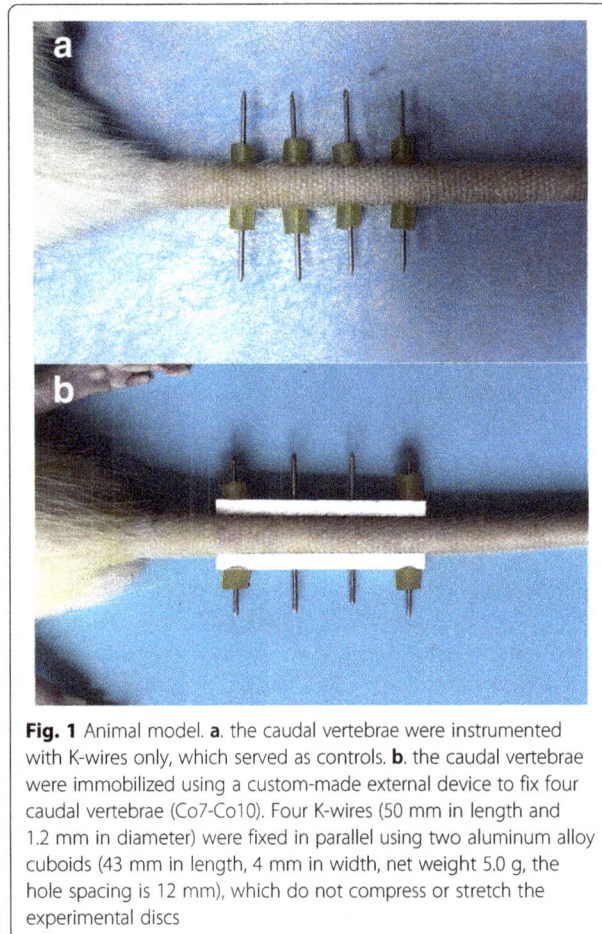

Fig. 1 Animal model. **a**. the caudal vertebrae were instrumented with K-wires only, which served as controls. **b**. the caudal vertebrae were immobilized using a custom-made external device to fix four caudal vertebrae (Co7-Co10). Four K-wires (50 mm in length and 1.2 mm in diameter) were fixed in parallel using two aluminum alloy cuboids (43 mm in length, 4 mm in width, net weight 5.0 g, the hole spacing is 12 mm), which do not compress or stretch the experimental discs

Richmond, USA), and sectioned using a histotome (Leica, Heidelberger, Germany). For histological analysis, sections (5 µm) were stained with hematoxylin/eosin (Beijing BiotoppedScience & Technology Co. Ltd., Beijing, China), whereas for AFM scanning, 10-20 µm sections were used. Histological images were visualized using a binocular microscope (XSP-2CA, Shanghai, China), and changes in the AF were assessed using a grading scale of the stained images at a magnification of 200× as described by Masuda et al. [16]. The number of cells in the NP was scored by counting from the hematoxylin/eosin stained images at a magnification of 400 ×.

Table 2 Modified Magnetic Resonance Imaging Pfirrmann Grading

Grade	Structural Changes Within NP	Signal Intensity	IVDH
I	Homogenous and bright	Hyperintense	Normal
II	Heterogeneous	Intermediate	Normal
III	Heterogeneous and gray	Intermediate	Decreased
IV	Heterogeneous and black	Hypointense	Decreased or collapsed

NP indicates nucleus pulposus, *IVDH* indicates Intervertebral Disc Height

Gene expression analysis by RT-PCR

For each specimen, (35 rats, 1 disc levels, AF and NP; $n = 70$), total RNA was extracted using TRIzol® reagent and a total of 1 µg of total RNA was reverse-transcribed using the Revert Aid First Strand cDNA Synthesis Kit (Thermo Fisher Scientific; Waltham, MA, USA). To quantify mRNA expression, an amount of cDNA that was equivalent to 50 ng of total RNA was amplified by real-time PCR using the iTaqTM Universal SYBR® Green Supermix kit (Bio-Rad, Hercules, CA, USA) [19]. Transcript levels of anabolic genes (collagen I, collagen II, aggrecan) and catabolic genes (MMP3, MMP13, ADAMTs-4) were evaluated. GAPDH served as an internal standard. Primer sequences are presented in Table 3. Rt-PCR was performed on a CFX96TM rt-PCR System (Bio-Rad, Hercules, CA, USA) following the manufacturer's guidelines. Relative transcript levels were calculated as $\chi = 2\text{-}\Delta\Delta Ct$, in which $\Delta\Delta Ct = \Delta E - \Delta C$, $\Delta E = Ctexp - CtGAPDH$, and $\Delta C = Ctct1 - CtGAPDH$ [19].

AFM imaging and nano-mechanical testing

AFM scanner (Dimension ICON, Bruker, USA) was used at atmospheric pressure [20]. The structure and the elastic modulus of individual collagen fibrils within intervertebral discs Co9-Co10 were tested at the nanoscale using AFM in week 2, 4, 6, and 8, respectively. A total of

Table 3 Primers and Probes for Real-Time RT-PCR

Target Gene	Sequence (5'→3')
GAPDH	
Forward:	AGA CAG CCG CAT CTT CTT GT
Reverse:	TAC TCA GCA CCA GCA TCA CC
Collagen I	
Forward:	ATG TTC AGC TTT GTG GAC
Reverse:	GGA TGC CAT CTT GTC CAG
Collagen II	
Forward:	CCT GGA CCC CGT GGC AGA GA
Reverse:	CAG CCA TCT GGG CTG CAA AG
Aggrecan	
Forward:	AGG ATG GCT TCC ACC AGT GC
Reverse:	TGC GTA AAA GAC CTC ACC CTC C
MMP-3	
Forward:	TCT TCC TCT GAA ACT TGG CG
Reverse:	AGT GCT TCT GAA TGT CCT TCG
MMP-13	
Forward:	GCA GCT CCA AAG GCT ACA A
Reverse:	CAT CAT CTG GGA GCA TGA AA
ADAMTS-4	
Forward:	CTT CGC TGA GTA GAT TCG TGG
Reverse:	AGT TGA CAG GGT TTC GGA TG

thirty-five collagen fibrils from each rat were tested. Both AFM imaging and nano-mechanical testing were conducted at a scanning rate of 1 Hz using a Scan Asyst-Air probe, a curvature radius of 5 nm, and a force constant of 0.4 N/m.

Statistical analysis
Experimental data are presented as the mean ± standard deviation (SD). Significant differences between study groups were obtained by using a one-way analysis of variance (ANOVA) with Fisher's Partial Least-Squares Difference (PLSD) to analyze the influence of immobilization loading and time. Statistical significance was set at $p \leq 0.05$.

Results
All 35 rats successful completed the 8 week study. At the beginning of the study, the average body weight was 400 g. Body weight increased to 405 g after 28 days, and was 411 g at the end of the study. This indicated that rats gained weight over time and that the surgery did not affect normal growth and development. The device that was used for immobilization weighted roughly 5.0 g and was well tolerated by the rats, as evidenced by their ability to lift and easily move their tails with the devices attached. Although the segments within the apparatus were largely immobilized, rats were able to move and control their tails both proximal and distal to the devices.

Histology and morphology
The intervertebral disc height progressively decreased with time. A significant decrease was observed in rats in group D and group E with time as shown in Fig. 2A. The percentage of intervertebral disc space height in groups A was significantly higher compared to that in group D and E (Fig. 2B) ($p < 0.05$). The disc thickness was significantly different between rats in group A compared to rats in group D ($p = 0.021$), group A vs group E ($p < 0.0001$), and group B vs group E ($p = 0.028$). At 8 weeks after spine immobilization, modified Pfirrmann grades of I, II, III, and IV were found in 12, 9, 14, and 0 rats, respectively. At week 6 and 8, the intervertebral disc degeneration was classified as grade III, based on the modified Pfirrmann grading system criteria. A total of 14 out of 35 discs had deteriorated between day 0 and 8 weeks after immobilization. A modified Pfirrmann grade of IV was not found in any of the animals examined.

Histological assessments were performed based on the grading system [18]. Previous studies have shown degeneration changes in immobilization IVD [12, 13, 21]. The histological changes found in this study were in line with the changes described by other groups [13, 21]. However, no significant decrease was found in the number of cells in the nucleus pulposus among rats in group A, B,

C, D, and E ($p = 0.370$). In contrast, the number of cells in the nucleus pulposus was slightly increased over time in rats in group D and E ($p > 0.05$). Moreover, the cluster formation of the nucleus pulposus cells became obvious. Cells within these clusters maintained their typical morphology with a polymorphonuclear shape, intracellular vacuoles, and stellar nuclei. Moreover, the Extracellular Matrix (ECM) progressively increased and the granules were shriveled. The inner layer of AF appear to be progressive disorders and hyperplasia (Fig. 3f-j). Round or ovoid-shaped chondrocytes infiltrated the AF, leading to the formation of cartilage-resembling tissue bordering the NP. This cartilage-resembling tissue could clearly be distinguished from the NP, displaying a different cell morphology and a matrix that was more intensely stained by hematoxylin/eosin (Fig. 3a-j). Characteristic AFM images of collagen fibrils from IVD of NP and AF for every group are presented in Fig. 4A. Within the NP, the elastic modulus of collagen fibrils progressively decreased (Fig. 4Ba), and was significantly different in rats in group A compared to rats in group E ($p < 0.001$), group A vs group D ($p < 0.05$), group B vs group E ($p < 0.05$), and group C vs group E ($p < 0.05$). Moreover, a gradual increase was found within the AF (Fig. 4Bb), and was significantly different between the elastic modulus of collagen fibrils of rats in group A compared to rats in group E ($p < 0.001$), group B vs group E ($p < 0.001$), and group C vs group E ($p < 0.05$).

Gene expression
In-situ immobilization affected the anabolic and catabolic gene expression of discs. The disc gene expression of Group A was consistent with those of the internal control discs. The trend of gene expression including downregulation of collagen II and aggrecan ($p < 0.05$ for both), upregulation of collagen I, MMP3, MMP13, ADAMTs-4 of nucleus pulposus in Group B, C, D, and E, with the exception of group A ($p < 0.05$ all) (Fig. 5A(A-F)). Moreover, downregulation of collagen I ($p < 0.05$), upregulation of collagen II of AF in Group B, C, D, and E, and with the exception of group A(all $p < 0.05$), but did not show a significant effect on gene expression levels of aggrecan, MMP3, MMP13, and ADAMTs-4 of AF in Group A, B, C, D, and E ($p > 0.05$) (Fig. 5B(A-F)).

Discussion
Abnormal mechanically conditions are crucial contributing factors in IVD degeneration, however genetic factors may also play a significant role [22, 23]. This study is the first to describe the changes in intervertebral discs in different periods of time during in-situ immobilization of caudal vertebrae in rats, based on a macro, micro, and nanoscale change analysis.

The complications of spine immobilization that are associated with halo-vest or a brace treatment have been

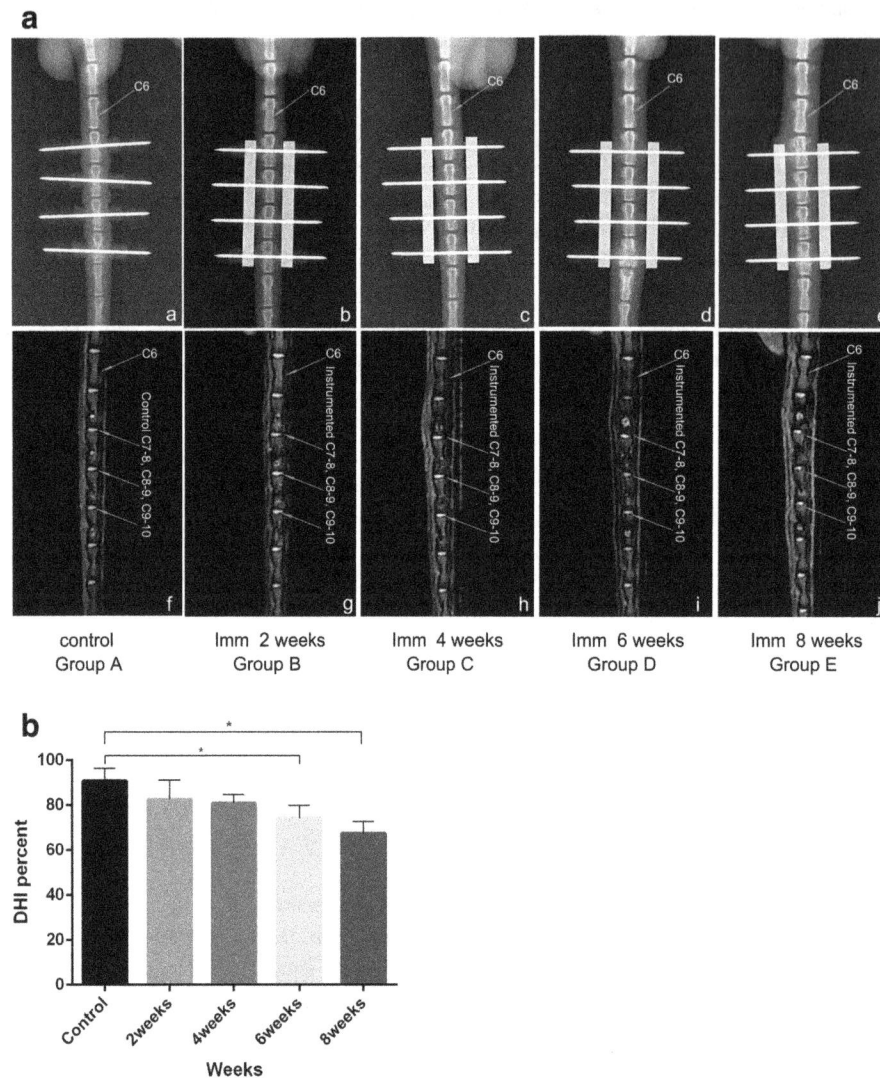

Fig. 2 A. The disc space and T2 signal intensity were measured using radiography and MRI Scans. Radiographs: (a~e) were obtained under anesthesia using a digital, self-contained cabinet x-ray machine (exposure time: 10 s, 26 kV). a (Group A) which served as controls, b~e (Group B~E) as shown in the figure, over time, progressive loss of disc height, d and e more obvious. MRI Scans: (f~j) (Scanning Sequence: FRFSE-XL, Slice thickness:1.4 mm, Interlayer Spacing: 5 mm) uses magnetic waves to create pictures to determine nucleus pulposus size and hydration status according to T2 signal intensity. Over time, the T2 signal intensity progressive decrease, as described above, i and j more serious. The IVD degeneration was classified as grade III. Imm indicates immobilization. B. The intervertebral disc height assessment based on radiographs. In control group (group A), imm-2 weeks (group B), and imm-4 weeks (group C), the intervertebral disc space height was slightly decreased, postoperatively, and this reduction was significant starting at the 6th week (group D). (*) indicates significant difference from other groups discs (*p* < 0.05)

intensively investigated [24–27]. These studies showed that complications included osteomyelitis and heterotopic ossification etc. It has not yet been analyzed how halo immobilization leads to the complications associated with intervertebral disc degeneration. In our study, we have assessed the effects of long-segment in-situ immobilization on the intervertebral disc of the caudal vertebra, thereby simulating human cervical spine immobilization. Elliott et al. [28] demonstrated a link between intervertebral discs and body weight that was similar in rats and humans. The rat-tail model was

chosen as a model [12, 29–31], in our study, the mechanical environment of the IVD that allows for precise control. Thereby we can rule out the effect of mechanical manipulation from other contributing factors.

A retrospective study in which the stress and activity of IVD degeneration was evaluated, demonstrated that mechanical intervention not only plays a role in changing the pressure or activity, however the application device also reduced the activity of the disc, which can result in IVD degeneration [21]. Our study showed that the the disc height and the MRI T2 signal strength of

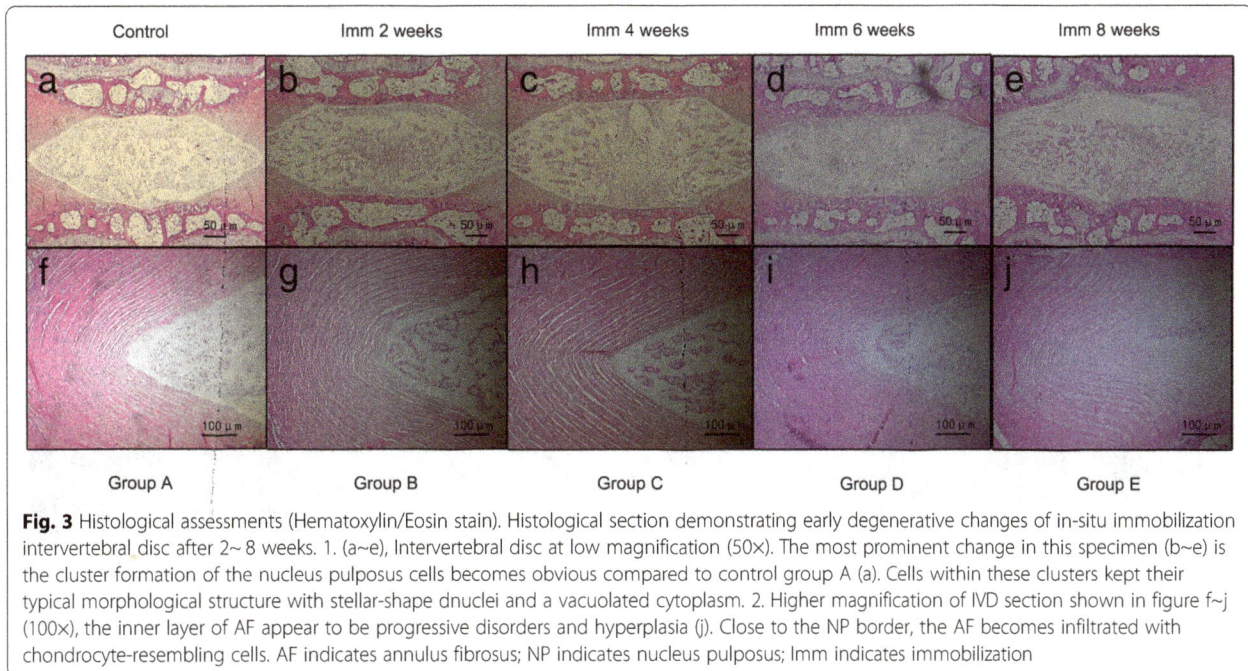

Fig. 3 Histological assessments (Hematoxylin/Eosin stain). Histological section demonstrating early degenerative changes of in-situ immobilization intervertebral disc after 2~8 weeks. 1. (a~e), Intervertebral disc at low magnification (50×). The most prominent change in this specimen (b~e) is the cluster formation of the nucleus pulposus cells becomes obvious compared to control group A (a). Cells within these clusters kept their typical morphological structure with stellar-shape dnuclei and a vacuolated cytoplasm. 2. Higher magnification of IVD section shown in figure f~j (100×), the inner layer of AF appear to be progressive disorders and hyperplasia (j). Close to the NP border, the AF becomes infiltrated with chondrocyte-resembling cells. AF indicates annulus fibrosus; NP indicates nucleus pulposus; Imm indicates immobilization

the experimental disc gradually decreased with fixation time.

Previous studies have shown that fixation triggered a degradation pattern in the IVD, such as downregulation of anabolic gene expression [13], and a decrease in glycosaminoglycan content [32]. Our findings further indicated that the effects of immobilization were more significant in the NP compared to the AF. The greatest effect was observed in group E, and combined with the loss of disc height, MRI T2 signal attenuation and IVD elastic modulus gradual decline over time, and confirmed that degeneration of IVD was not only present at the macroscale and microscale, but also at the nanoscale. These data suggested that immobilization can cause early stage degeneration of the IVD that progressed in severity over time. The long-term nature of this study that hypomobility has an effect on gene expression of the NP was more prominent compared to changes found in the AF. This discrepancy may be due to the different periods of immobilization time and abnormal mechanical conditions. In our study, we were the first to show direct evidence of metabolic response in the IVD in vivo associated with long-segment in-situ immobilization.

The AF with a highly organized structure, runs at angles of approximately 60° to the spinal column [33]. Therefore, elastic fibers perform a very crucial role in the total mechanical properties of the AF [34]. In our previous study, we demonstrated the structure and biomechanics at the nanoscale level from different regions of the AF in loaded IVD [20]. This study revealed that the elastic modulus of nucleus pulposus collagen fibrils

in group E was markedly decreased compared to group A (control group). Moreover, the elastic modulus was remarkably increased within the AF, and a significant difference was found in the elastic modulus of collagen fibrils over time. The results are consistent with the morphologic changes of NP and AF at the microscale as indicated by hematoxylin/eosin staining. Moreover, the tendency of gene expression of NP and AF were consistent with the former. Therefore, the results indicate that degradation was not only associated with the disorganization at the microscale, but also suggested modification of collagen fibrils at the nanoscale, which would directly change the mechanical environment around the cells of the AF and NP.

From what has been discussed above, in-situ immobilization creates a unique mechanical state that can cause disc degeneration. Previous studies have confirmed that too much or too little pressure/stretch contributes to a catabolism effect on intervertebral discs, in which hypomobility or excessive activities will increase the damage rate, leading to intervertebral disc on the load response of a U-shaped distribution [35]. It is generally accepted that immobilization osteoporosis (IOP) caused by partial fixation after fractures of the lower limb is a common complication in clinical therapeutics. Bed rest and immobilization time are independent predictors of low bone density in the hip [36]. According to Wolff's law, disuse osteoporosis is thought to be associated with a lack of mechanical forces [37, 38]. We believe that hypomobility or immobilization caused degeneration of muscular ligaments and facet joints in surrounding spine tissue. However, we cannot exclude

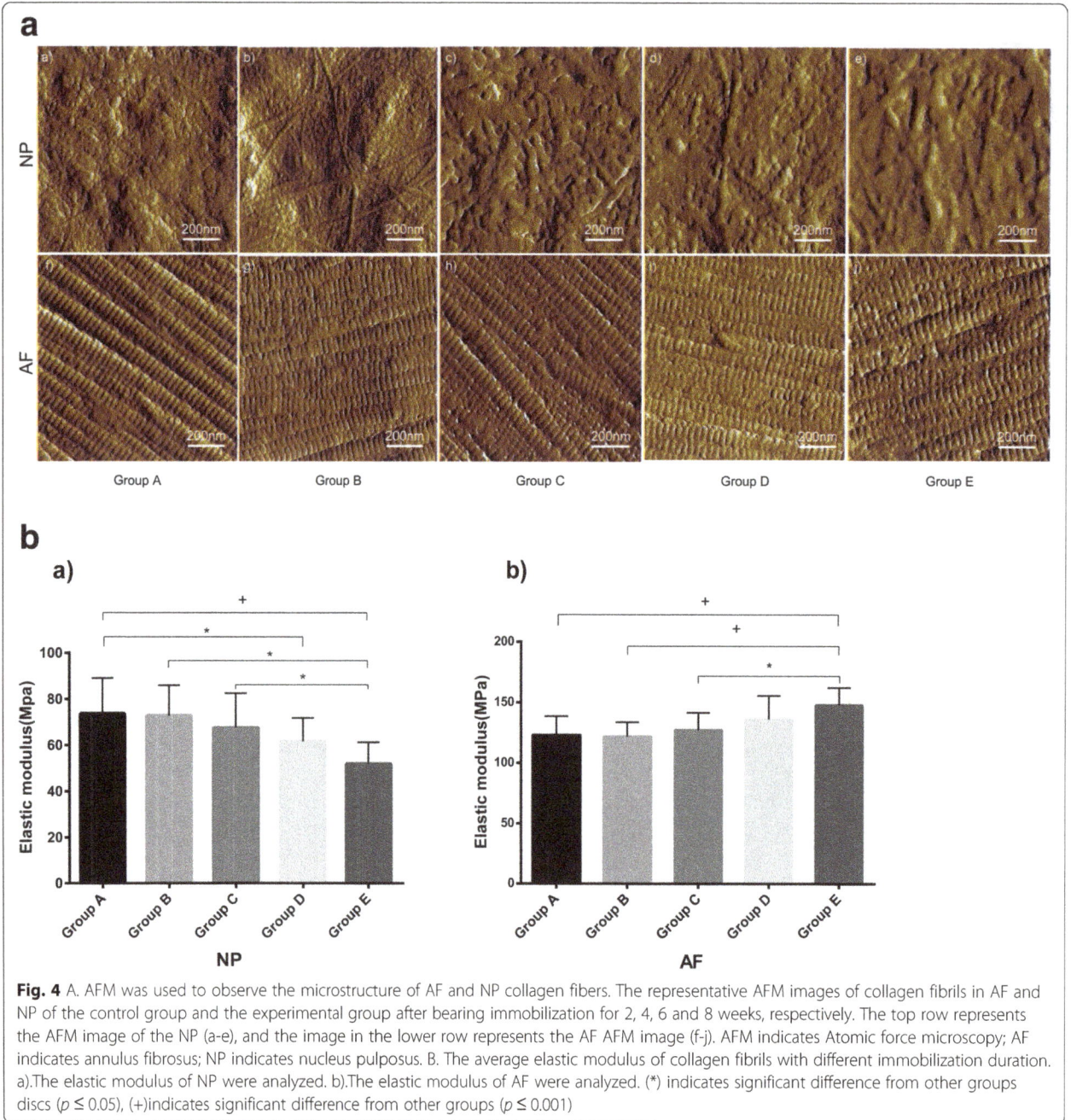

Fig. 4 A. AFM was used to observe the microstructure of AF and NP collagen fibers. The representative AFM images of collagen fibrils in AF and NP of the control group and the experimental group after bearing immobilization for 2, 4, 6 and 8 weeks, respectively. The top row represents the AFM image of the NP (a-e), and the image in the lower row represents the AF AFM image (f-j). AFM indicates Atomic force microscopy; AF indicates annulus fibrosus; NP indicates nucleus pulposus. B. The average elastic modulus of collagen fibrils with different immobilization duration. a).The elastic modulus of NP were analyzed. b).The elastic modulus of AF were analyzed. (*) indicates significant difference from other groups discs ($p \leq 0.05$), (+)indicates significant difference from other groups ($p \leq 0.001$)

the possibility that the immobilization apparatus was a factor in the degeneration. Setton et al. showed that hypomobility produced a reduced stimulus to the metabolic activity of disc cells [39]. In an unloaded condition, the IVD swells and starts to lose proteoglycans [40]. Dynamic loading of a certain magnitude, frequency, and duration has been shown to maintain the ECM balance within the disc [41–44]. Static loading induces cell death and causes disc degradation [21, 45–47]. Choi et al. [48] insisted that spine fixation and endplate injury or fracture by internal transpedicular fixation without fusion plays a crucial role

in IVD degradation. These studies suggested that hypomobility or immobilization and static loads are both not an innocuous mechanical environment to IVD, in contrast, an adverse effect was found. Ragab et al. [49] showed that cervical fusion resulted in increased strains at adjacent levels. However, long-segment cervical fusions (2 and 3-level fusions) compared to short-segment fusions (1-level fusions), increased the strain approximately 2- to 3-fold compared to the standard. These findings suggested that long-segment fusions or immobilization result in increased side effects compared to short-segment fusions or

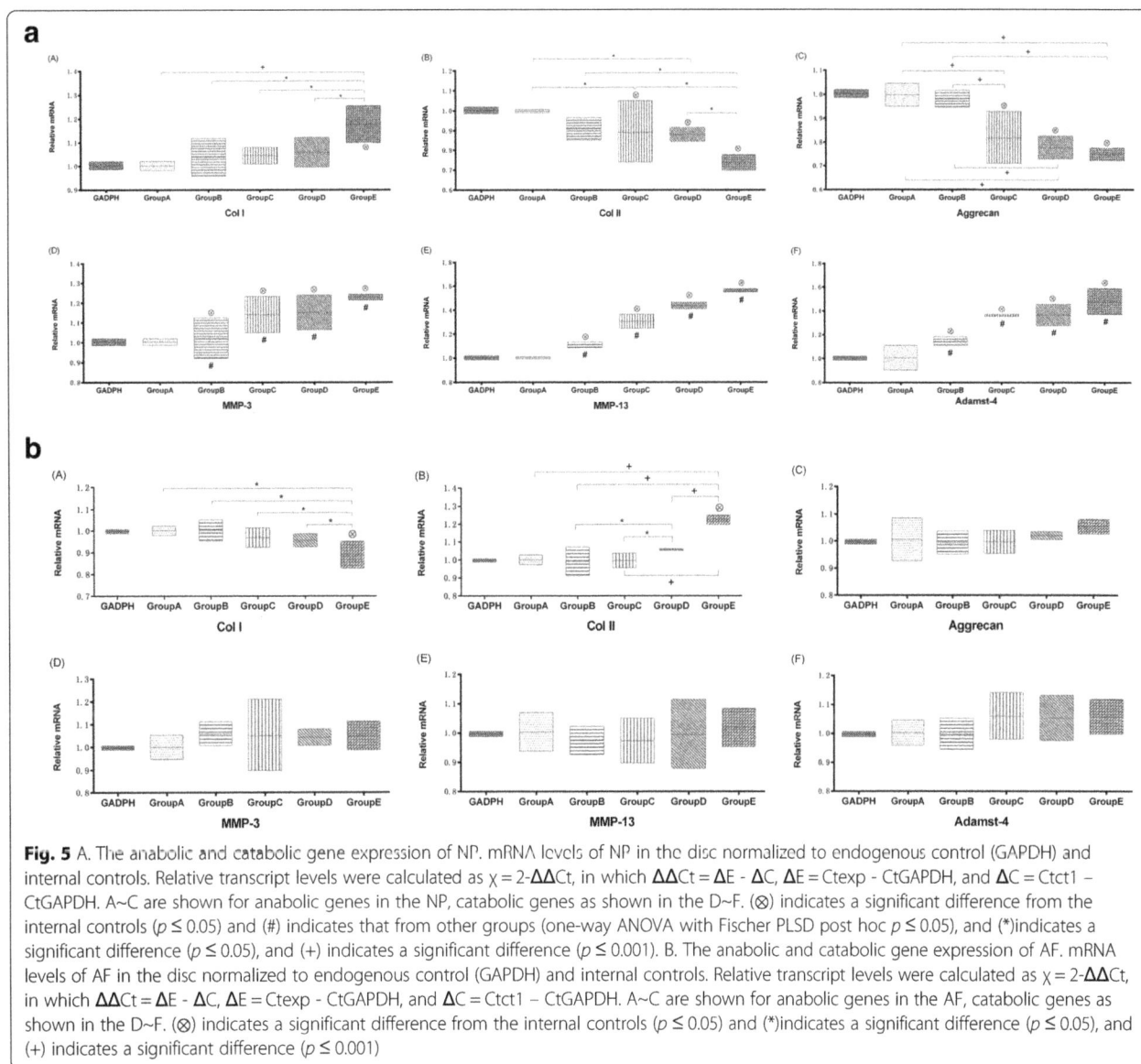

Fig. 5 A. The anabolic and catabolic gene expression of NP. mRNA levels of NP in the disc normalized to endogenous control (GAPDH) and internal controls. Relative transcript levels were calculated as $\chi = 2\text{-}\Delta\Delta Ct$, in which $\Delta\Delta Ct = \Delta E - \Delta C$, $\Delta E = Ctexp - CtGAPDH$, and $\Delta C = Ctct1 - CtGAPDH$. A~C are shown for anabolic genes in the NP, catabolic genes as shown in the D~F. ($\otimes$) indicates a significant difference from the internal controls ($p \leq 0.05$) and (#) indicates that from other groups (one-way ANOVA with Fischer PLSD post hoc $p \leq 0.05$), and (*)indicates a significant difference ($p \leq 0.05$), and (+) indicates a significant difference ($p \leq 0.001$). B. The anabolic and catabolic gene expression of AF. mRNA levels of AF in the disc normalized to endogenous control (GAPDH) and internal controls. Relative transcript levels were calculated as $\chi = 2\text{-}\Delta\Delta Ct$, in which $\Delta\Delta Ct = \Delta E - \Delta C$, $\Delta E = Ctexp - CtGAPDH$, and $\Delta C = Ctct1 - CtGAPDH$. A~C are shown for anabolic genes in the AF, catabolic genes as shown in the D~F. ($\otimes$) indicates a significant difference from the internal controls ($p \leq 0.05$) and (*)indicates a significant difference ($p \leq 0.05$), and (+) indicates a significant difference ($p \leq 0.001$)

fixation. This indicates that the long-segment in-situ immobilization triggered a degradation pattern in the IVD. Therefore, in the clinic, it should be possible to reduce spine (cervical spine) long segmental immobilization, and spine (cervical spine) immobilization time (≤6 weeks).

However, a limitation of this study was the difference between a rat tail disc and a human cervical disc in terms of biochemical composition, molecular composition, and biomechanical capabilities. We used the rat caudal vertebral model to simulate human cervical spine IVD changes. While not completely equal to human intervertebral disc changes, the rat model is the currently accepted model and was easier to build and replicate than alternatives. More importantly, it provided relevant experimental specimens and related parameters of IVD that human cervical spine cannot provide. It also provides us with detailed

experimental data and theoretical basis for further elaborating the effect of immobilisation on intervertebral disc.

Conclusions

In this study, long-segment in-situ immobilization caused target disc degeneration, and positively correlated with fixation time. These findings showed that, over time, in-situ immobilization induced a progressive decrease in the intervertebral disc space height and T2 signal intensity of IVD. In addition, downregulation of collagen II, and upregulation of collagen I, aggrecanase, collagenase, stromelysin of NP, and downregulation of collagen I, and upregulation of collagen II of AF were found. However, the effects on aggrecanase, collagenase, stromelysin of AF were not significant. These changes suggested that immobilization loading initiated a degenerative cascade, although this trend was significantly observed in the NP compared to AF. These results as well as the variation tendency of the elastic modulus of collagen fibrils within the NP and AF were confirmed. The discrepancy found with other studies, may be due to the different periods of immobilization and loading conditions. Histological analysis, including hematoxylin/eosin staining indicated that the NP and AF showed a progressive degeneration by in-situ immobilization. However, the comparison with overload conditions was moderate. This study evaluated how hypomobility of the spine may result in IVD degradation and spine lesions. The loading parameters chosen for our study were intended to imitate cervical spine long-segment in-situ immobilization in humans. The results indicated that the degeneration was not only associated with changes at the macroscale, microscale, but also indicated changes in collagen fibrils at the nanoscale, which would directly change the mechanical environment around the cells of the NP and AF. In conclusion, increasing our understanding of the pathogenesis and complications found after long-segment immobilization of the cervical spine, and how to optimize the use of external fixator devices are clearly warranted.

Abbreviations

AF: Annulus fibrosus; AFM: Atomic Force Microscope; Co: Coccygeal spine; ECM: Extracellular Matrix; EDTA: Ethylenediaminetetraacetic acid; IVD: Intervertebral disc; LBP: Low back pain; NP: Nucleus pulposus; PCR: Polymerase chain reaction

Acknowledgements

We thank Zong-Da Jin PhD, (Department of Public Health, ZheJiang medical College), and Yue Zhang PhD, (Department of Epidemiology, School of Public Health, Fudan University) for their help with the statistical analysis.

Funding

Funding for the study was provided by the National Natural Science Foundation of China (81320108018, 31570943, 31270995 and 81702146), Innovation and Entrepreneurship Program of Jiangsu Province, and the Priority Academic Program Development of Jiangsu Higher Education Institutions. The funding body did not influence the design of the study, the collection, analysis, or interpretation of the data, or the writing of the manuscript.

Authors' contributions

YJC and ZPL initiated the study design. HTL, TL, XC, JBG and HYJ participated in the data collection and data analysis. YJC and ZPL participated in the data analysis and the preparation of the manuscript. HLY was an advisor. All authors have read and approved the final manuscript.

Competing interests

The authors declare that they have no competing interests.

Author details

[1]Orthopaedic Institute, Department of Orthopaedics, The First Affiliated Hospital of SooChow University, 708 Renmin Rd, Suzhou, Jiangsu 215006, People's Republic of China. [2]Department of Orthopedics, Peace Hospital Affiliated to Changzhi Medical College, Changzhi, Shanxi, People's Republic of China.

References

1. Schwarzer AC, Aprill CN, Derby R, Fortin J, Kine G, Bogduk N. The relative contributions of the disc and zygapophyseal joint in chronic low back pain. Spine (Phila Pa 1976). 1994;19(7):801–6.
2. Buckwalter JA. Aging and degeneration of the human intervertebral disc. Spine (Phila Pa 1976). 1995;20(11):1307–14.
3. Urban JP, Roberts S. Development and degeneration of the intervertebral discs. Mol Med Today. 1995;1(7):329–35.
4. Hong SP, Henderson CN. Articular cartilage surface changes following immobilization of the rat knee joint. A semiquantitative scanning electron-microscopic study. Acta Anat (Basel). 1996;157(1):27–40.
5. Leroux MA, Cheung HS, Bau JL, Wang JY, Howell DS, Setton LA. Altered mechanics and histomorphometry of canine tibial cartilage following joint immobilization. Osteoarthr Cartil. 2001;9(7):633–40.
6. Muller FJ, Setton LA, Manicourt DH, Mow VC, Howell DS, Pita JC. Centrifugal and biochemical comparison of proteoglycan aggregates from articular cartilage in experimental joint disuse and joint instability. J Orthop Res. 1994;12(4):498–508.
7. Narmoneva DA, Cheung HS, Wang JY, Howell DS, Setton LA. Altered swelling behavior of femoral cartilage following joint immobilization in a canine model. J Orthop Res. 2002;20(1):83–91.
8. Saamanen AM, Tammi M, Jurvelin J, Kiviranta I, Helminen HJ. Proteoglycan alterations following immobilization and remobilization in the articular cartilage of young canine knee (stifle) joint. J Orthop Res. 1990;8(6):863–73.
9. Setton LA, Mow VC, Muller FJ, Pita JC, Howell DS. Mechanical behavior and biochemical composition of canine knee cartilage following periods of joint disuse and disuse with remobilization. Osteoarthr Cartil. 1997;5(1):1–16.
10. Askins V, Eismont FJ. Efficacy of five cervical orthoses in restricting cervical motion. A comparison study. Spine (Phila Pa 1976). 1997;22(11):1193–8.
11. Clancy MJ. Clearing the cervical spine of adult victims of trauma. J Accid Emerg Med. 1999;16(3):208–14.
12. Iatridis JC, Mente PL, Stokes IA, Aronsson DD, Alini M. Compression-induced changes in intervertebral disc properties in a rat tail model. Spine (Phila Pa 1976). 1999;24(10):996–1002.
13. MacLean JJ, Lee CR, Grad S, Ito K, Alini M, Iatridis JC. Effects of immobilization and dynamic compression on intervertebral disc cell gene expression in vivo. Spine (Phila Pa 1976). 2003;28(10):973–81.
14. Urban JP, Holm S, Maroudas A, Nachemson A. Nutrition of the intervertebral disc: effect of fluid flow on solute transport. Clin Orthop Relat Res. 1982; (170):296–302. PMID: 7127960.
15. Hughes PC, Tanner JM. The assessment of skeletal maturity in the growing rat. J Anat. 1970;106(Pt 2):371–402.
16. Masuda K, Aota Y, Muehleman C, Imai Y, Okuma M, Thonar EJ, Andersson GB, An HS. A novel rabbit model of mild, reproducible disc degeneration by an anulus needle puncture: correlation between the degree of disc injury and radiological and histological appearances of disc degeneration. Spine. 2005;30(1):5–14.
17. Pfirrmann CW, Metzdorf A, Zanetti M, Hodler J, Boos N. Magnetic resonance classification of lumbar intervertebral disc degeneration. Spine (Phila Pa 1976). 2001;26(17):1873–8.
18. Han B, Zhu K, Li FC, Xiao YX, Feng J, Shi ZL, Lin M, Wang J, Chen QX. A simple disc degeneration model induced by percutaneous needle puncture in the rat tail. Spine. 2008;33(18):1925–34.
19. Liu X, Zhou L, Chen X, Liu T, Pan G, Cui W, Li M, Luo ZP, Pei M, Yang H, et al. Culturing on decellularized extracellular matrix enhances antioxidant properties of human umbilical cord-derived mesenchymal stem cells. Mater Sci Eng C Mater Biol Appl. 2016;61:437–48.
20. Liang T, Zhang LL, Xia W, Yang HL, Luo ZP. Individual collagen fibril thickening and stiffening of annulus Fibrosus in degenerative intervertebral disc. Spine (Phila Pa 1976). 2017;42(19):E1104–E1111. PMID: 28146016. https://doi.org/10.1097/BRS.0000000000002085.
21. Stokes IAF, Iatridis JC. Mechanical conditions that accelerate intervertebral disc degeneration: overload versus immobilization. Spine. 2004;29(23):2724–32.
22. Walter BA, Korecki CL, Purmessur D, Roughley PJ, Michalek AJ, Iatridis JC. Complex loading affects intervertebral disc mechanics and biology. Osteoarthr Cartil. 2011;19(8):1011–8.
23. Kroeber MW, Unglaub F, Wang H, Schmid C, Thomsen M, Nerlich A, Richter W. New in vivo animal model to create intervertebral disc degeneration and to investigate the effects of therapeutic strategies to stimulate disc regeneration. Spine (Phila Pa 1976). 2002;27(23):2684–90.

24. Baum JA, Hanley EN Jr, Pullekines J. Comparison of halo complications in adults and children. Spine (Phila Pa 1976). 1989;14(3):251–2.

25. Kang M, Vives MJ, Vaccaro AR. The halo vest: principles of application and management of complications. J Spinal Cord Med. 2003;26(3):186–92.

26. Hossain M, McLean AN, Fraser MH. Outcome of halo immobilisation of 104 cases of cervical spine injury. Scot Med J. 2004;49(3):90–2.

27. Garfin SR, Botte MJ, Waters RL, Nickel VL. Complications in the use of the halo fixation device. J Bone Joint Surg Am. 1986;68a(3):320–5.

28. Elliott DM, Sarver JJ. Young investigator award winner: validation of the mouse and rat disc as mechanical models of the human lumbar disc. Spine. 2004;29(7):713–22.

29. Lotz JC, Colliou OK, Chin JR, Duncan NA, Liebenberg E. Compression-induced degeneration of the intervertebral disc: an in vivo mouse model and finite-element study. Spine (Phila Pa 1976). 1998;23(23):2493–506.

30. Simunic DI, Broom ND, Robertson PA. Biomechanical factors influencing nuclear disruption of the intervertebral disc. Spine (Phila Pa 1976). 2001;26(11):1223–30.

31. Stokes IA, Aronsson DD, Spence H, Iatridis JC. Mechanical modulation of intervertebral disc thickness in growing rat tails. J Spinal Disord. 1998;11(3):261–5.

32. Ching CT, Chow DH, Yao FY, Holmes AD. Changes in nuclear composition following cyclic compression of the intervertebral disc in an in vivo rat-tail model. Med Eng Phys. 2004;26(7):587–94.

33. Smith LJ, Fazzalari NL. The elastic fibre network of the human lumbar anulus fibrosus: architecture, mechanical function and potential role in the progression of intervertebral disc degeneration. Eur Spine J. 2009;18(4):439–48.

34. Fu LJ, Chen CS, Xie YZ, Yang JW, Sun XJ, Zhang P. Effect of a new annular incision on biomechanical properties of the intervertebral disc. Orthop Surg. 2016;8(1):68–74.

35. Lotz JC. Load and the spine. How does the goldilocks principle apply? Spine J. 2011;11(1):44–5.

36. Smith EM, Comiskey CM, Carroll AM. A study of bone mineral density in adults with disability. Arch Phys Med Rehabil. 2009;90(7):1127–35.

37. Adams MA, Dolan P. Biomechanics of vertebral compression fractures and clinical application. Arch Orthop Trauma Surg. 2011;131(12):1703–10.

38. Turner CH. Three rules for bone adaptation to mechanical stimuli. Bone. 1998;23(5):399–407.

39. Setton LA, Chen J. Cell mechanics and mechanobiology in the intervertebral disc. Spine (Phila Pa 1976). 2004;29(23):2710–23.

40. Urban JP, Maroudas A. Swelling of the intervertebral disc in vitro. Connect Tissue Res. 1981,9(1).1–10.

41. Maclean JJ, Lee CR, Alini M, Iatridis JC. Anabolic and catabolic mRNA levels of the intervertebral disc vary with the magnitude and frequency of in vivo dynamic compression. J Orthop Res. 2004;22(6):1193–200.

42. MacLean JJ, Lee CR, Alini M, Iatridis JC. The effects of short-term load duration on anabolic and catabolic gene expression in the rat tail intervertebral disc. J Orthop Res. 2005;23(5):1120–7.

43. Walsh AJ, Lotz JC. Biological response of the intervertebral disc to dynamic loading. J Biomech. 2004;37(3):329–37.

44. Wuertz K, Godburn K, MacLean JJ, Barbir A, Donnelly JS, Roughley PJ, Alini M, Iatridis JC. In vivo remodeling of intervertebral discs in response to short- and long-term dynamic compression. J Orthop Res. 2009;27(9):1235–42.

45. Ariga K, Yonenobu K, Nakase T, Hosono N, Okuda S, Meng W, Tamura Y, Yoshikawa H. Mechanical stress-induced apoptosis of endplate chondrocytes in organ-cultured mouse intervertebral discs: an ex vivo study. Spine (Phila Pa 1976). 2003;28(14):1528–33.

46. Lotz JC, Chin JR. Intervertebral disc cell death is dependent on the magnitude and duration of spinal loading. Spine. 2000;25(12):1477–82.

47. Lotz JC, Colliou OK, Chin JR, Duncan NA, Liebenberg E. 1998 Volvo award winner in biomechanical studies - compression-induced degeneration of the intervertebral disc: an in vivo mouse model and finite-element study. Spine. 1998;23(23):2493–506.

48. Choi W, Song S, Chae S, Ko S. Comparison of the extent of degeneration among the normal disc, immobilized disc, and immobilized disc with an endplate fracture. Clin Orthop Surg. 2017;9(2):193–9.

49. Ragab AA, Escarcega AJ, Zdeblick TA. A quantitative analysis of strain at adjacent segments after segmental immobilization of the cervical spine. J Spinal Disord Tech. 2006;19(6):407–10.

6

Open versus arthroscopic Latarjet procedures for the treatment of shoulder instability

Nolan S. Horner[1], Paul A. Moroz[2], Raman Bhullar[3], Anthony Habib[1], Nicole Simunovic[4], Ivan Wong[5], Asheesh Bedi[6] and Olufemi R. Ayeni[1*]

Abstract

Background: The arthroscopic and open Latarjet procedures are both known to successfully treat shoulder instability with high success rates. The objective of this study was to compare the clinical outcomes and positioning of the coracoid graft and screws between the arthroscopic and open Latarjet procedures.

Methods: The electronic databases MEDLINE, EMBASE, and PubMed were searched for relevant studies between database creation and 2018. Only studies directly comparing open and arthroscopic Latarjet procedures were included.

Results: There were 8 included studies, with a total of 580 patients treated arthroscopically and 362 patients treated with an open Latarjet procedure. Several papers found significantly better standardized outcome scores for either the open or arthroscopic procedure but these findings were not consistent across papers. Patients treated with arthroscopic Latarjet procedures had significantly lower initial post-operative pain, however pain scores became equivalent by one month post-operatively. Three of the five included studies found no significant difference in the coracoid graft positioning and two of three included studies found no significant difference in screw divergence angles between the two techniques. Arthroscopic procedures (112.2 min) appear to take, on average, longer than open procedures (93.3 min). However, operative times and complication rates decrease with surgeon experience with the arthroscopic procedure. Overall 3.8% of the patients treated arthroscopically and 6.4% of the patients treated with the open procedure went on to have post-operative complications.

Conclusions: Both open and arthroscopic Latarjet procedures can be used to effectively treat shoulder instability with similarly low rates of complications, recurrent instability and need for revision surgery. Arthroscopic Latarjet procedures are associated with less early post-operative pain but require increased operative time. The evidence does not support there being any significant difference in graft or screw positioning between the two techniques. At this time neither procedure shows clear superiority over the other.

Keywords: Latarjet, Shoulder instability, Arthroscopy, Bone block, Instability, Dislocation

* Correspondence: ayenif@mcmaster.ca
[1]Division of Orthopaedic Surgery, Department of Surgery, McMaster University, 1200 Main St W, Room 4E15, Hamilton, ON L8N 3Z5, Canada
Full list of author information is available at the end of the article

Background

The shoulder is the most commonly dislocated joint and most frequently dislocates anteriorly. The Latarjet is a commonly performed procedure in the treatment of recurrent anterior shoulder instability. This procedure was first characterized in 1954 and modified multiple times since its conception [1]. This procedure classically involves a deltopectoral approach in order to transfer the coracoid process, along with attached soft tissue to the anterior-inferior border of the glenoid. This stabilizes the shoulder through a triple mechanism which uses the conjoint tendon as a sling and the coracoid process as a bony block, while repairing the capsule via fixation to the coracoacromial ligament [2]. That being said, there still exists a number of controversies surrounding the optimal orientation, size and positioning of the graft when preforming the Latarjet procedure [3–5]. For instance, one study found that the Latarjet procedure which involves transfer of the entire horizontal pillar of the coracoid better restored stiffness to the glenohumeral joint in comparison to the Bristow procedure where only the tip of the coracoid is transferred [5]. The Latarjet is a well-established treatment option with good evidence for favourable long term outcomes [6]. Re-dislocation rates following a successful Latarjet procedure are estimated to be 4 to 5% [7].

Advances in technology have recently made an arthroscopic approach to the Latarjet procedure a possibility [8]. Lafosse et al. has proposed that the arthroscopic approach offers advantages such as more accurate bone graft placement, quicker functional recovery, decreased stiffness, and cosmetic benefits [9]. Despite minimal cases of recurrent dislocation in both surgical approaches, theorized disadvantages of the arthroscopic Latarjet include increased cost, longer surgery time, and increased complication rates stemming from challenging graft fixation [10, 11]. This may partially be explained by the arthroscopic Latarjet's complexity and learning curve. Several studies have described a more prolonged learning curve in the arthroscopic Latarjet procedure [10]. However, there currently exist no consensus on whether the arthroscopic or open Latarjet procedure offers overall superior outcomes and/or complication rates.

The purpose of this study is to compare the standardized clinical outcome scores, rates of complication, accuracy of graft and screw positioning and rates of recurrent dislocation between the open and arthroscopic Latarjet procedures by systematically reviewing the literature for comparative studies.

Methods

Search strategy

Three online databases (EMBASE, MEDLINE, and PubMed) were searched by two reviewers (P.M., R.B.) for literature comparing any clinical outcomes or positioning of the graft or screws after arthroscopic and open Latarjet procedures in male and female patients of all ages for the treatment of shoulder instability (Fig. 1). The database search was conducted on March 1, 2018. The inclusion criteria for this search was: (1) Studies comparing outcomes and/or failure rates between open and arthroscopic Latarjet procedures for anterior shoulder instability; (2) Studies comparing the accuracy of the coracoid bone graft or screw positioning; (3) male and female patients of all ages; (4) studies published in English; (5) studies on humans. The exclusion criteria were: (1) any non-surgical treatment studies (e.g. technique articles without outcomes, cadaver studies, review articles, etc.); (2) non-comparative studies.

The following search terms were used: "Latarjet", "Bristow", "Latarjet-Bristow", "Latarjet-patte", "Coracoid" and "Bone block", and "Coracoid" and "Transfer". Both key term and subject heading search methods were used where applicable. A detailed search strategy is presented in Appendix 1: Table 4.

Study screening

Two reviewers (P.M., R.B.) independently screened the titles of the retrieved papers. Any included studies were then screened by abstract. Disagreements at either of these screening stages were resolved by including the papers for full text review. Any disagreements at the full text screening stage were discussed by the reviewers and resolved by a third reviewer (N.H.). A list of references for the papers deemed ineligible at the full text review stage can be found in Appendix 2.

Quality assessment of included studies

A quality assessment of the included studies was completed using the Methodological Index for Non-Randomized Studies (MINORS) Criteria [12]. MINORS is a validated scoring tool for non-randomized studies (e.g. case reports, case series, cohort studies etc.). Each of the 12 items in the MINORS criteria is given a score of 0, 1 or 2 - giving a maximum score of 24 for comparative studies. To the author's knowledge, there is no evidence to categorize the MINORS score. Thus, the MINORS score was categorized apriori as follows: 0–6 to indicate very low quality evidence; 7–10 to indicate low quality of evidence; 10–14 to indicate fair quality of evidence; and > 16 to indicate a good quality of evidence for non-randomized studies.

Data abstraction

Two reviewers (NH, RB) independently abstracted relevant study data from the final pool of included articles and recorded this data in a Microsoft Excel (2013) spreadsheet designed a priori. Demographic information included author, year of publication, sample size, study design, level of evidence, patient demographics (i.e. sex,

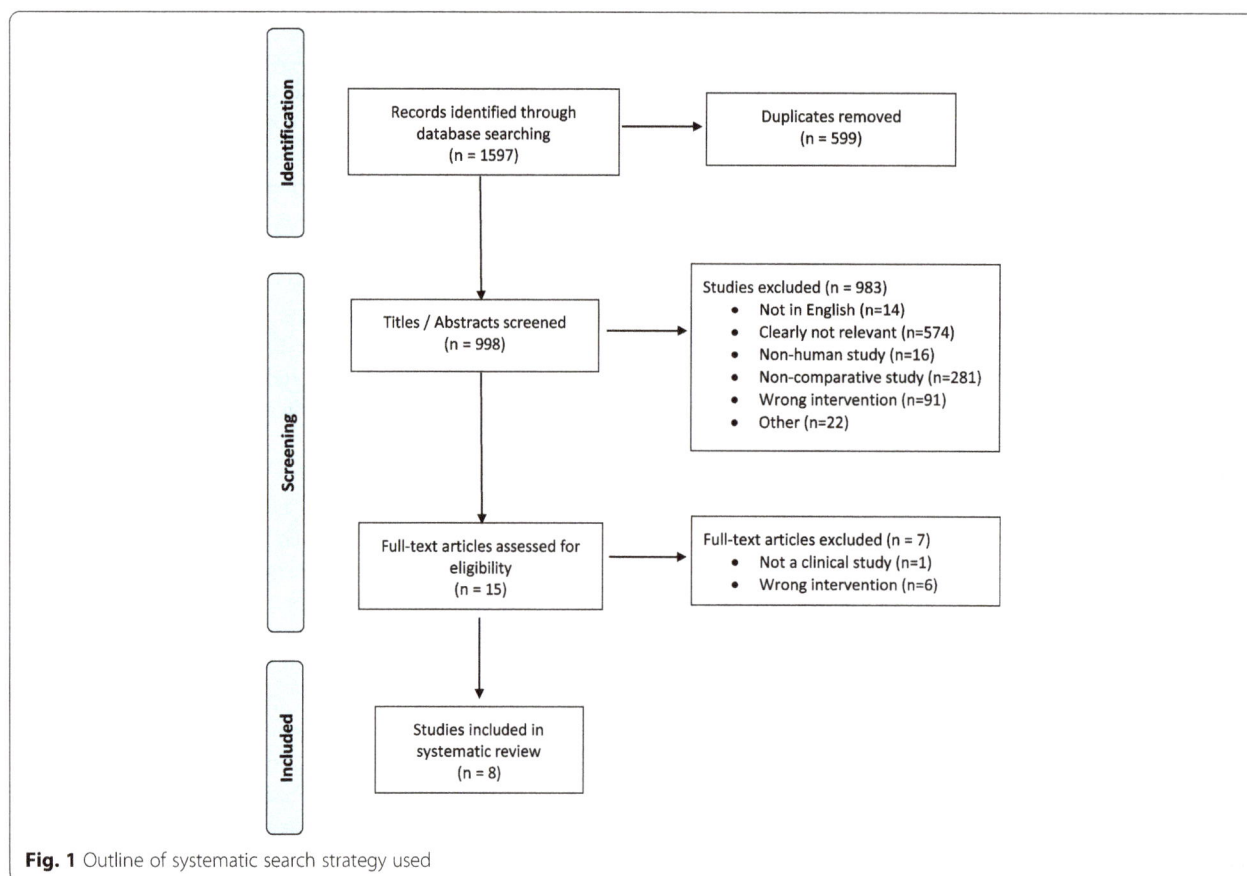

Fig. 1 Outline of systematic search strategy used

age, affected shoulder, follow-up time, % lost to follow-up, etc.) and details of surgery. In addition to demographic information any clinical or information regarding graft or screw positioning was documented. The number of patients requiring further surgery was also abstracted. Finally, any minor or major complications associated with procedures were recorded.

Statistical analysis

Interobserver agreement was assessed at each stage of study screening by calculating a weighted k (kappa). The agreement between the two reviewers assessing the MI-NORS score in duplicate across all studies was calculated using an intraclass correlation coefficient (ICC), which evaluates the consistency of multiple observers measuring the same groups of data. Agreement was categorized a priori as follows: k > 0.61 to indicate substantial agreement, $0.21 < k < 0.60$ to indicate moderate agreement, and $k < 0.20$ to indicate slight agreement. Statistics describing the data collected from the included papers was presented as means, ranges, and measures of variance where appropriate. A meta-analysis was not performed in this study due to the high heterogeneity amongst reported outcomes and the specifics of how the procedure was done.

Results

Study identification and characteristics

Our initial literature search yielded 1597 studies, of which 8 met the inclusion and exclusion criteria for this review (Fig. 1). There was excellent agreement among reviewers at the title (k = 0.76; 95% CI, 0.71 to 0.80), abstract (k = 0.94; 95% CI, 0.90 to 0.98.) and full-text screening (k = 1.0; 95% CI, 1.0 to 1.0) stages. All included studies were published between 2016 and 2018. This included a total of 942 patients, including 580 patients treated arthroscopically and 362 patients treated with an open Latarjet procedure. The mean sample size of the included studies was 117.8 (range 46–390) patients. 81.0% of the patients treated across the studies were male, with a mean age of 27.7 (range 13.6–66) years and mean follow-up 20.6 months. 36.5% of the patients were reported as being lost to follow-up.

Only two studies commented on whether the Latarjet procedures were done as a primary surgery or as a revision surgery after previous shoulder stabilization surgery. Amongst these two studies 98.0% ($n = 100$) of the patients treated arthroscopically and 98.9% ($n = 94$) of the patients treated with an open procedure had not had previous shoulder stabilization surgery. Study demographics are presented in Table 1.

Table 1 Characteristics of included studies

Primary Author, Year	Location	Level of Evidence	Study Design	Inclusion Criteria	Exclusion Criteria	Sample Size – Patients	% Male	Mean age (years)	Follow-up [months]	% Lost to Follow-Up	MINORs score
Cunningham G, 2016 [10]	Switzerland	III	Retrospective comparative cohort	Significant bone loss with indication for Latarjet procedure according to established criteria	Any patient < 16 years of age or with history of previous bone block procedure	Arthroscopic – 28, Open- 36	90.6%	26+/-7.6 (15–45)	6.6+/- 5.9 (1.5–36)	0%	19
Marion B, 2017 [13]	France	II	Prospective comparative cohort	Chronic post-traumatic anterior glenohumoral instability, based on instability severity index score > 3	Not specified	Arthroscopic – 36, Open – 22	77.6%	26.9+/– 7.7	29.8+/–4.4	3.4%	18
Kordasiewicz B, 2017 [16]	Poland	III	Retrospective comparative cohort	All patients undergoing primary shoulder stabilization between 2006 and 2013	Revision cases	Arthroscopic – 62, Open – 48	Not specified	26.9	35.1	8.2%	18
Kordasiewicz B, 2018 [19]	Poland	III	Retrospective comparative cohort	All patients undergoing primary shoulder stabilization between 2006 and 2013	Revision cases	Arthroscopic – 62, Open – 48	Not specified	26.9	36.8	7.6%	18
Metais P, 2016 [15]	France	II	Prospective comparative cohort	Not specified	Not specified	Arthroscopic – 286, Open – 104	Not specified	27.8 (13.6–66.6)	22.7+/–4.1	63.6%	17
Nourissat G, 2016 [14]	France	II	Prospective comparative cohort	Older than 18 years old, experienced at least one shoulder dislocation episode and undergoing anterior bone block surgery	Patients with post-operative complications who required revision surgery	Arthroscopic – 99, Open – 85	Not specified	Not specified	5.5 (1–12)	46.2%	18
Russo A, 2017 [18]	Italy	II	Prospective comparative cohort	Shoulder stabilization with either open or arthroscopic latarjet	Age > 50 years, rotator cuff tears, multidirectional instability, systemic disorders.	Arthroscopic – 25, Open – 21	93.5%	Not specified	Minimum 1-year follow-up	0%	16
Zhu Y, 2017 [17]	China	II	Prospective comparative cohort	1. Diagnosis of recurrent anterior shoulder dislocation 2. Glenoid bone defect greater than 20% on CT 3. Treatment with open Latarjet or arthroscopic Latarjet 4. Agreement to participate in the study 5. Post-op follow up more than 2 years	1. Concomitant musculoskeletal injuries or neurovascular disorders of the ipsilateral shoulder 2. Multi-directional shoulder instability 3. Uncontrolled epilepsy or psychological condition that prevented patients from following post-op rehab	Arthroscopic – 44, Open – 46	75% (68)	30.1	28.8	0%	19

Study quality

There was a total of three (37.5%) level III and five (62.5%) level II studies that met the inclusion criteria (Table 1). The included studies had a mean MINORS score of 17.9 ± 1.0 which indicates a good quality of evidence amongst non-randomized studies (Table 1). There was high agreement (ICC = 0.96 (95% CI, 0.94 to 0.98)) amongst quality assessment scores of included studies using the prespecified criteria.

Outcomes

A summary of the clinical outcomes scores presented in the include studies is presented in Table 2. A variety of scores were used including the visual analog scale (VAS), Western Ontario Shoulder Instability Index (WOSI), Rowe, Walch-Duplay, American Shoulder and Elbow Surgeons Shoulder Score (ASES) and Constant-Murley scores. Both studies that looked at early (< 1 month) post-operative pain found significantly less pain in the arthroscopic group [13, 14]. However one study found no difference in VAS pain scores once patients had reached 30 days post-operatively [14]. One study ($n = 286$ arthroscopic, 104 open, $p < 0.05$) found significantly better post-operative Walch-Duplay scores in the arthroscopic group [15], whereas the other two studies (n = 28 arthroscopic, 36 open, $p > 0.05$; $n = 62$ arthroscopic, 48 open, p > 0.05) reporting post-operative Walch-Duplay scores did not [10, 16]. Interestingly one study ($n = 99$ arthroscopic, 85 open, $p < 0.05$) reported significantly better post-operative WOSI scores in the arthroscopic group [14], whereas another study ($n = 36$ arthroscopic, 22 open, $p = 0.03$) found significantly better WOSI scores in the open group [13]. Similarly, one study (n = 62 arthroscopic, 48 open, p < 0.05) found significantly better Rowe scores in the open group [16], one study ($n = 286$ arthroscopic, 104 open, p < 0.05) found better Rowe scores in the arthroscopic group [14], and one study ($n = 44$ arthroscopic, 46 open, $p = 0.181$) found no significant difference [17]. No studies found significant differences in ASES or Constant-Murley scores.

Five of the included studies reported on radiographic outcomes. Three of the five studies ($n = 126$ arthroscopic, 106 open, $p > 0.05$) found no significant difference in the coracoid graft positioning between the two techniques [13, 18, 19], one study ($n = 25$ arthroscopic, 21 open, $p = 0.025$) found the arthroscopic technique to be significantly more likely to have ideal graft positioning [18], and conversely one study ($n = 44$ arthroscopic, 46 open, $p < 0.001$) found the open procedure to be significantly more likely to have ideal graft positioning [17]. Three of the studies reported on screw divergence angles, two studies ($n = 69$ arthroscopic, 67 open, $p = 0.10$–0.12) found no significant difference between the two techniques [17, 18], and one study ($n = 28$ arthroscopic, 36 open, $p = 0.017$) found the open technique to have significantly less rates of excessively (> 10°) divergent screws [10].

The rates of re-operation, complications, and recurrent instability are shown in Table 3. Overall 3.8% of the patients treated arthroscopically and 6.4% of the patients treated open went on to have post-operative complications. The most common post-operative complications included recurrent instability (arthroscopic – 1.9%, open – 1.4%), graft fracture, failure or non-union (arthroscopic – 1.2%, open – 1.6%) and infection (arthroscopic – 0.9%, open – 1.1%) in both groups.

Table 2 Clinical outcome scores reported in the included studies

Study	Arthroscopic Outcome	Open Outcomes	Significance
Cunningham G, 2016 [10]	Walch Duplay score – 88. Persistant apprehension - 4(5.5%)	Walch Duplay score – 91. Persistant apprehension - 0(0.0%)	Walch Duplay score - no significant difference
Marion B, 2017 [13]	VAS (1 week) - 1.2 +/−1.4 WOSI (2 years) - 372.1+/− 140.9	VAS (1 week) - 2.5+/− 1.4 WOSI (2 years) - 451+/− 158.7	VAS $p = .002$ WOSI $p = 0.03$
Kordasiewicz B, 2017 [16]	Walch - Duplay score - 76.7 Rowe - 78.9 VAS- 1.38 Satisfaction% - 91.9 Residual subjective apprehension - 31%	Walch - Duplay score - 83.9 Rowe - 87.8 VAS- 0.77 Satisfaction% - 96.8 Residual subjective apprehension 28.7%	p < 0.05 for Rowe and Subjective apprehension only. The rest did not reach statistical significance.
Metais P, 2016 [15]	Walch - Duplay score – 92.8. Rowe – 93.4	Walch - Duplay score - 85.9. Rowe – 83.9	Walch-Duplay score $p < 0.0001$ Rowe p < 0.0001
Nourissat G, 2016 [14]	VAS (30 days) - 1.2	VAS (30 days) - 1.6	VAS (30 days) $p = 0.14$ (note significantly lower VAS scores were found in arthroscopic group at earlier follow-ups). WOSI (6 months) - open had significantly better symptoms and sports/recreation/work scores than the arthroscopy group. No significant difference in Lifestyle and Emotion scores.
Zhu Y, 2017 [17]	ASES- 93.3+/− 9.9 Constant Murley Socre - 96.5+/− 3.8 Rowe - 97.1+/− 2.5	ASES- 93.0+/− 5.0 Constant Murley Socre - 95.0+/− 4.1 Rowe - 95.4+/− 5.0	ASES $p = .917$ Constant-Murley $p = .223$ Rowe $p = .181$

Table 3 Complications and reoperation rates reported amongst included studies

Study	Procedure	Number of intra-op complications	Number of post-op complications (including instability)	Number of Revision surgeries	Number of recurrent instability
Cunningham G, 2016 [10]	Open	0%	11%	0%	0%
	Arthroscopic	0%	29%	4%	4%
Marion B, 2017 [13]	Open	0%	0%	0%	0%
	Arthroscopic	0%	6%	8%	3%
Kordasiewicz B, 2017 [16]	Open	13%	13%	8%	6%
	Arthroscopic	8%	10%	13%	5%
Kordasiewicz B, 2018[a] [19]	Open[a]	N/A	N/A	N/A	N/A
	Arthroscopic[a]	N/A	N/A	N/A	N/A
Metais P, 2016 [15]	Open	1%	13%	7%	2%
	Arthroscopic	0%	2%	4%	2%
Nourissat G, 2016 [14]	Open	0%	0%	0%	0%
	Arthroscopic	0%	0%	0%	0%
Russo A, 2017 [18]	Open	N/A	N/A	N/A	N/A
	Arthroscopic	N/A	N/A	N/A	N/A
Zhu Y, 2017 [17]	Open	0%	0%	0%	0%
	Arthroscopic	0%	0%	0%	0%

[a]Kordasiewicz B, 2018 only included hardware complications reported and overlapping patient populations with Kordasiewicz B, 2017, therefore Korasiewicz B, 2018 was not included in any complication calculations

A total of 4.1% of the arthroscopic patients and 3.0% of the open patients required revision surgery. Screw removal (arthroscopic – 1.1%, open – 0.8%) and need for revision due to recurrent instability (arthroscopic – 2.0%, open – 1.4%) were the two most common reasons for revision surgery in both groups. A total of six (1.1%) of the arthroscopic procedures had to be converted to open procedures due to technical difficulties. The average operative time for open procedure was 93.3 min and 112.2 min for arthroscopic procedures. In total 6 (1.1%) patients treated arthroscopically and 7 (2.0%) treated with an open procedure experienced intra-operative complications.

One study which also looked at the learning curve associated with the arthroscopic Latarjet procedure also noted that operative time, rates of complications and need for conversion from arthroscopic to an open procedure due to technically difficulties decreased as surgeons gained experience with the procedure [10].

Discussion

The results of the current study suggest that there is no clear superiority of the open versus arthroscopic approach for Latarjet procedures based on differences in complication rate or recurrence of instability. Several of the papers found superiority for individual standardized outcome scores for either the open or arthroscopic procedure, but these findings were not consistent across papers. Patients being treated with arthroscopic Latarjet procedures have lower reported pain scores in the first couple weeks post-operatively however these scores become equivalent to the open procedures by one month. The average time for the procedure was longer for the arthroscopic procedure compared to the open procedure however no statistical analysis to determine if this was significant was possible due to error of measurements not being reported within the studies. However, the studies did note a significant drop in operative time with the arthroscopic procedure as surgeon experience increased [10]. It should be noted that the studies did not comment on the amount of surgeon experience with each procedure prior to the initiation of the studies, which may have affected results if surgeons were more experienced with one procedure over the other.

Interestingly, the arthroscopic latarjet technique did not show improved positioning of the bone block or of the screws despite the theoretically improved visualization when placing the graft. This is of key importance given the known importance of positioning of the coracoid graft and resulting biomechanical stability of the shoulder [20]. Furthermore, screws that are divergent more than 10 degrees are known to put the suprascapular nerve at risk for injury [21].

We also found that both the arthroscopic and open Latarjet procedures both had relatively low and similar rates of major post-operative complications, recurrent instability and need for revision surgery. Unfortunately, we are unable to comment on whether there was a statistically significant difference in these rates due to the low overall event rate and the low number of studies available on this topic making any meta-analysis underpowered and with large range of variance. It should be noted that not all included Latarjet procedures were primary procedures which may have affected the rate of recurrent instability as rates of failure of the Latarjet procedure may be higher when done as a part of a revision surgery.

Only 1% of the total arthroscopic procedures were converted to open procedures due to technical difficulties. This may, however, be underestimated as it is unclear if all of the studies were reporting this measure. One study did comment on the fact that all of their intra-op conversions to open procedures occurred in their first third of cases with no conversion to open procedures in the remainder of their cases [10]. This suggests that the rates of conversion to open procedures may be very low once surgeons have performed a sufficient number of arthroscopic Latarjet procedures. In fact, several papers in the literature have found performing the Latarjet procedure arthroscopically to have a prolonged learning curve [10, 22].

There exists one previous systematic review on this topic which included 6 of the 8 studies included in this systematic review [23]. The conclusions of Hurley et al. are consistent with the findings of our systematic review which is that both the open and arthroscopic procedures offer significant improvement in clinical outcomes with similar complication rates [23]. However, this systematic review by Hurley et al. does not include all the available literature on the topic [23]. Furthermore, this study quantitatively synthesizes data from multiple studies through a meta-analysis even though multiple studies had retrospective design which generally increases heterogeneity and reduces precision of estimates in a meta-analysis.

This study has numerous strengths including the rigorous methodology which was used in this systematic review. Specifically, a broad search strategy spanning multiple databases was used to ensure that as much of the relevant literature was included as possible. The screening of studies was done in duplicate in order to limit reviewer bias.

The main limitation in this study was the quality of evidence available on the topic. Specifically, there currently exists no randomized studies comparing the arthroscopic and open Latarjet procedures. Furthermore, although only comparative studies were included, no meta-analysis was possible due to the significant heterogeneity in outcomes reported across the studies. Although the outcome measures used

were generally appropriate and validated for this patient population, one study used the constant-Murley score as an outcome which previous authors have found to be a poor outcome measure for shoulder instability [24]. Additionally, the average follow-up of the included studies was less than 2 years and therefore differences in long-term outcomes after arthroscopic and open Latarjet procedures cannot be commented on. This is key as certain outcomes such as the development of osteoarthritis after the Latarjet procedure may only be measurable with longer follow-ups [25]. There was also procedural differences in the study such as screw versus endobutton fixation and open versus a mini-open approach. That being said, the literature on this subject is likely to improve as the arthroscopic Latarjet procedures have only recently been described, and in fact all the included studies in this systematic review were published as recently as 2016. Future large randomized studies comparing the arthroscopic and open procedures will provide further clarity on the possible superiority of one technique over the other as well as the specific indications for each procedure.

Conclusions

Both open and arthroscopic Latarjet procedures can be used to effectively treat shoulder instability with similarly low rates of complications, recurrent instability and need for revision surgery. Arthroscopic Latarjet procedures are associated with less early post-operative pain but require increased operative time. The evidence does not support there being any significant difference in graft or screw positioning between the two techniques. At this time neither procedure shows clear superiority over the other.

Appendix 1

Table 4 Search Strategy

	MEDLINE	EMBASE	PubMED
Search strategy	1. Latarjet.mp. 2. Bristow.mp. 3. Latarjet-bristow.mp. 4. Latarjet-patte.mp. 5. Coracoid.mp. 6. Bone Block.mp. 7. Transfer.mp. 8. 5 and 6 9. 5 and 7 10. 1 or 2 or 3 or 4 or 8 or 9	1. Latarjet.mp. 2. Bristow.mp. 3. Latarjet-bristow.mp. 4. Latarjet-patte.mp. 5 Coracoid.mp. 6. Bone Block.mp. 7. Transfer.mp. 8. 5 and 6 9. 5 and 7 10. 1 or 2 or 3 or 4 or 8 or 9	(Latarjet) OR (Bristow) OR (Latarjet-Bristow) OR (Latarjet-patte) or ((Coracoid) AND ((Bone Block) OR (transfer))
Number of papers retrieved	556	724	317

Appendix 2
References of Studies eliminated at Full Text Screen

1. Bessière C, Trojani C, Carles M, Mehta SS, Boileau P. The open latarjet procedure is more reliable in terms of shoulder stability than arthroscopic bankart repair. *Clin Orthop Relat Res* 2014;472(8):2345–2351.

2. Bokshan SL, DeFroda SF, Owens BD. Comparison of 30-Day Morbidity and Mortality After Arthroscopic Bankart, Open Bankart, and Latarjet-Bristow Procedures: A Review of 2864 Cases. *Orthop J Sports Med* 2017;5(7):2325967117713163.

3. Khan A, Samba A, Pereira B, Canavese F. Anterior dislocation of the shoulder in skeletally immature patients: comparison between non-operative treatment versus open Latarjet's procedure. *Bone Joint J* 2014;96-B(3):354–359.

4. Makhni EC, Lamba N, Swart E, et al. Revision Arthroscopic Repair Versus Latarjet Procedure in Patients With Recurrent Instability After Initial Repair Attempt: A Cost-Effectiveness Model. *Arthroscopy* 2016;32(9):1764–1770.

5. Randelli P, Fossati C, Stoppani C, Evola FR, De Girolamo L. Open Latarjet versus arthroscopic Latarjet: clinical results and cost analysis. *Knee Surgery, Sport Traumatol Arthrosc* 2016;24(2):526–532.

6. Zhang AL, Montgomery SR, Ngo SS, Hame SL, Wang JC, Gamradt SC. Arthroscopic versus open shoulder stabilization: current practice patterns in the United States. *Arthroscopy* 2014;30(4):436–443.

6. Zimmermann SM, Scheyerer MJ, Farshad M, Catanzaro S, Rahm S, Gerber C. Long-Term Restoration of Anterior Shoulder Stability: A Retrospective Analysis of Arthroscopic Bankart Repair Versus Open Latarjet Procedure. *J Bone Joint Surg Am* 2016;98(23):1954–1961.

Abbreviations
ASES: American Shoulder and Elbow Surgeons Shoulder Score; ICC: Intraclass correlation coefficient; MINORS: Methodological Index for Non-Randomized Studies; VAS: Visual analog scale; WOSI: Western Ontario Shoulder Instability Index

Funding
No funding was received for the completion of this project.

Authors' contributions
NH – collected data, analyzed and interpreted data, wrote and edited manuscript. PM – screened studies, collected data, helped with preparation of the manuscript. RB – screened studies, collected data, helped with preparation of the manuscript. AH – Preparation and editing of the manuscript. NS – Statistical analysis, editing and formatting of the manuscript. IW – Content expert, editing of the manuscript. AB – Content expert, editing of the manuscript. OA – Supervised project, concept expert, editing of the manuscript. All authors read and approved the final manuscript.

Author details
[1]Division of Orthopaedic Surgery, Department of Surgery, McMaster University, 1200 Main St W, Room 4E15, Hamilton, ON L8N 3Z5, Canada. [2]Faculty of Medicine, University of British Columbia, Vancouver, BC, Canada. [3]Faculty of Medicine, Royal College of Surgeons in Ireland - Medical University of Bahrain, Manama, Bahrain. [4]Department of Health Research Methods, Evidence and Impact, McMaster University, Hamilton, ON, Canada. [5]Department of Orthopaedic Surgery, Dalhousie University and Nova Scotia Health Authority, Halifax, NS, Canada. [6]MedSport, Department of Orthopaedic Surgery, University of Michigan, Ann Arbor, MI, USA.

References
1. Latarjet M. Treatment of recurrent dislocation of the shoulder. Lyon Chir. 1954;49(8):994–7.
2. Young AA, Maia R, Berhouet J, Walch G. Open Latarjet procedure for management of bone loss in anterior instability of the glenohumeral joint. J Shoulder Elb Surg. 2011;20(2):S61–9. https://doi.org/10.1016/j.jse.2010.07.022.
3. Young AA, Baba M, Neyton L, Godeneche A, Walch G. Coracoid graft dimensions after harvesting for the open Latarjet procedure. J Shoulder Elb Surg. 2013;22(4):485–8. https://doi.org/10.1016/J.JSE.2012.05.036.
4. Boons HW, Giles JW, Elkinson I, Johnson JA, Athwal GS. Classic versus congruent coracoid positioning during the Latarjet procedure: an in vitro biomechanical comparison. Arthrosc J Arthrosc Relat Surg. 2013;29(2):309–16. https://doi.org/10.1016/J.ARTHRO.2012.09.007.
5. Giles JW, Degen RM, Johnson JA, Athwal GS. The Bristow and Latarjet procedures: why these techniques should not be considered synonymous. J Bone Joint Surg Am. 2014;96(16):1340–8. https://doi.org/10.2106/JBJS.M.00627.
6. Mizuno N, Denard PJ, Raiss P, Melis B, Walch G. Long-term results of the Latarjet procedure for anterior instability of the shoulder. J Shoulder Elb Surg. 2014;23(11):1691–9. https://doi.org/10.1016/j.jse.2014.02.015.
7. Hovelius L, Sandström B, Olofsson A, Svensson O, Rahme H. The effect of capsular repair, bone block healing, and position on the results of the Bristow-Latarjet procedure (study III): long-term follow-up in 319 shoulders. J Shoulder Elb Surg. 2012;21(5):647–60. https://doi.org/10.1016/j.jse.2011.03.020.
8. Lafosse L, Lejeune E, Bouchard A, Kakuda C, Gobezie R, Kochhar T. The Arthroscopic Latarjet Procedure for the Treatment of Anterior Shoulder Instability. Arthrosc J Arthrosc Relat Surg. 2007;23(11):1242.e1–1242.e5. https://doi.org/10.1016/j.arthro.2007.06.008.
9. Lafosse L, Boyle S. Arthroscopic Latarjet procedure. J Shoulder Elb Surg. 2010;19(2):2–12. https://doi.org/10.1016/j.jse.2009.12.010.
10. Cunningham G, Benchouk S, Kherad O, Lädermann A. Comparison of arthroscopic and open Latarjet with a learning curve analysis. Knee Surg Sports Traumatol Arthrosc. 2016;24(2):540–5. https://doi.org/10.1007/s00167-015-3910-3.
11. Randelli P, Fossati C, Stoppani C, Evola FR, De Girolamo L. Open Latarjet versus arthroscopic Latarjet: clinical results and cost analysis. Knee Surgery Sport Traumatol Arthrosc. 2016;24(2):526–32. https://doi.org/10.1007/s00167-015-3978-9.
12. Slim K, Nini E, Forestier D, Kwiatkowski F, Panis Y, Chipponi J. Methodological index for non-randomized studies (min- ors): development and validation of a new instrument. ANZ J Surg. 2003;73(9):712–6.
13. Marion B, Klouche S, Deranlot J, Bauer T, Nourissat G, Hardy P. A prospective comparative study of arthroscopic versus mini-open Latarjet procedure with a minimum 2-year follow-up. Arthroscopy. 2017;33(2):269–77. https://doi.org/10.1016/j.arthro.2016.06.046.
14. Nourissat G, Neyton L, Metais P, et al. Functional outcomes after open versus arthroscopic Latarjet procedure: a prospective comparative study. Orthop Traumatol Surg Res. 2016;102(8):S277–9. https://doi.org/10.1016/j.otsr.2016.08.004.
15. Metais P, Clavert P, Barth J, et al. Preliminary clinical outcomes of Latarjet-Patte coracoid transfer by arthroscopy vs. open surgery: prospective multicentre study of 390 cases. Orthop Traumatol Surg Res. 2016;102(8): S271 6. https://doi.org/10.1016/j.otsr.2016.08.003

16. Kordasiewicz B, Małachowski K, Kicinski M, Chaberek S, Pomianowski S. Comparative study of open and arthroscopic coracoid transfer for shoulder anterior instability (Latarjet)-clinical results at short term follow-up. Int Orthop. 2017;41(5):1023–33. https://doi.org/10.1007/s00264-016-3372-3.

17. Zhu Y, Jiang C, Song G. Arthroscopic versus open Latarjet in the treatment of recurrent anterior shoulder dislocation with marked glenoid bone loss: a prospective comparative study. Am J Sports Med. 2017;45(7):1645–53. https://doi.org/10.1177/0363546517693845.

18. Russo A, Grasso A, Arrighi A, Pistorio A, Molfetta L. Accuracy of coracoid bone graft placement: open versus arthroscopic Latarjet. Joints. 2017;5(2): 85–8. https://doi.org/10.1055/s-0037-1603934.

19. Kordasiewicz B, Kicinski M, Małachowski K, Wieczorek J, Chaberek S, Pomianowski S. Comparative study of open and arthroscopic coracoid transfer for shoulder anterior instability (Latarjet)-computed tomography evaluation at a short term follow-up. Part II. Int Orthop. 2018; https://doi.org/10.1007/s00264-017-3739-0.

20. Wellmann M, Petersen W, Zantop T, et al. Open shoulder repair of osseous glenoid defects: biomechanical effectiveness of the Latarjet procedure versus a contoured structural bone graft. Am J Sports Med. 2009;37(1):87–94. https://doi.org/10.1177/0363546508326714.

21. Lädermann A, Denard PJ, Burkhart SS. Injury of the suprascapular nerve during Latarjet procedure: an anatomic study. Arthrosc J Arthrosc Relat Surg. 2012;28(3):316–21. https://doi.org/10.1016/j.arthro.2011.08.307.

22. Castricini R, De Benedetto M, Orlando N, Rocchi M, Zini R, Pirani P. Arthroscopic Latarjet procedure: analysis of the learning curve. Musculoskelet Surg. 2013;97(S1):93–8. https://doi.org/10.1007/s12306-013-0262-3.

23. Hurley ET, Fat DL, Farrington SK, Mullett H. Open versus arthroscopic Latarjet procedure for anterior shoulder instability: a systematic review and meta-analysis. Am J Sports Med. 2018; https://doi.org/10.1177/0363546518759540.

24. Conboy VB, Morris RW, Kiss J, Carr AJ. An evaluation of the constant-Murley shoulder assessment. J Bone Joint Surg Br. 1996;78(2):229–32.

25. Bouju Y, Gadéa F, Stanovici J, Moubarak H, Favard L. Shoulder stabilization by modified Latarjet-Patte procedure: results at a minimum 10 years' follow-up, and role in the prevention of osteoarthritis. Orthop Traumatol Surg Res. 2014;100(4 Suppl):S213–8. https://doi.org/10.1016/j.otsr.2014.03.010.

7

Physical prognostic factors predicting outcome following lumbar discectomy surgery

Alison Rushton[1][*] [iD], Konstantinos Zoulas[2], Andrew Powell[3] and JB Staal[4,5]

Abstract

Background: Success rates for lumbar discectomy are estimated as 78–95% patients at 1–2 years post-surgery, supporting its effectiveness. However, ongoing pain and disability is an issue for some patients, and recurrence contributing to reoperation is reported. It is important to identify prognostic factors predicting outcome to inform decision-making for surgery and rehabilitation following surgery. The objective was to determine whether pre-operative physical factors are associated with post-operative outcomes in adult patients [≥16 years old] undergoing lumbar discectomy or microdiscectomy.

Methods: A systematic review was conducted according to a registered protocol [PROSPERO CRD42015024168]. Key electronic databases were searched [PubMed, CINAHL, EMBASE, MEDLINE, PEDro and ZETOC] using pre-defined terms [e. g. radicular pain] to 31/3/2017; with additional searching of journals, reference lists and unpublished literature. Prospective cohort studies with ≥1-year follow-up, evaluating candidate physical prognostic factors [e.g. leg pain intensity and straight leg raise test], in adult patients undergoing lumbar discectomy/microdiscectomy were included. Two reviewers independently searched information sources, evaluated studies for inclusion, extracted data, and assessed risk of bias [QUIPS]. GRADE determined the overall quality of evidence.

Results: 1189 title and abstracts and 45 full texts were assessed, to include 6 studies; 1 low and 5 high risk of bias. Meta-analysis was not possible [risk of bias, clinical heterogeneity]. A narrative synthesis was performed. There is low level evidence that higher severity of pre-operative leg pain predicts better Core Outcome Measures Index at 12 months and better post-operative leg pain at 2 and 7 years. There is very low level evidence that a lower pre-operative EQ-5D predicts better EQ-5D at 2 years. Low level evidence supports duration of leg pain pre-operatively not being associated with outcome, and very low-quality evidence supports other factors [pre-operative ODI, duration back pain, severity back pain, ipsilateral SLR and forward bend] not being associated with outcome [range of outcome measures used].

Conclusion: An adequately powered low risk of bias prospective observational study is required to further investigate candidate physical prognostic factors owing to existing low/very-low level of evidence.

Keywords: Lumbar discectomy, Microdiscectomy, Back pain, Leg pain, Radiculopathy, Prognostic factors, Prognosis, Systematic review, Narrative analysis

* Correspondence: a.b.rushton@bham.ac.uk; https://www.bham.ac.uk
[1]Centre of Precision Rehabilitation for Spinal Pain [CPR Spine] School of Sport, Exercise and Rehabilitation Sciences, University of Birmingham, Birmingham B15 2TT, UK
Full list of author information is available at the end of the article

Background

Low back pain [LBP] is the leading cause of disability internationally according to the latest Global Burden of Disease study [1]. A key intervention for LBP with radiculopathy is lumbar discectomy surgery. The number of discectomies performed in community hospitals in the United States in 2012 was 184,000 and the cost of these procedures has doubled in the past 10 years to exceed 9 billion dollars in 2012 [2]. In the UK, the number of lumbar discectomies performed increased from 7043 in 2001–2002 to 8478 in 2013–2014 [3].

Systematic reviews support that lumbar discectomy is superior to prolonged non-surgical treatment for short-term pain relief and improvement in function for lumbar radiculopathy [4, 5]. In the most recent synthesis across trials [using a range of outcome measures], surgical success rates have been estimated as 46–75% patients at 6–8 weeks, and 78–95% patients at 1–2 years post-surgery [6], supporting it as an effective procedure for many patients presenting with radiculopathy; but illustrating variability in outcome for patients. Clinical data also suggest ongoing disability is an issue for some patients, with 30–70% patients reported to experience residual pain [7]. Recent studies also suggest that recurrent lumbar disc herniation can occur, contributing to reoperation [14% from latest figures in the UK [8]], and can often lead to worse outcomes for patients [9, 10].

It is therefore important to determine prognostic factors predicting patient outcome following lumbar discectomy. Knowledge of prognostic factors would inform selection of patients for surgery and selection of patients for rehabilitation following surgery. Prognosis is a developing field of research [11], and findings can contribute to the clinical decision making and evaluation of new methods of patient management [12]. Although an increasing number of primary studies investigating prognostic factors for patient outcome following lumbar discectomy have been published, there are only 3 systematic reviews to date that have synthesised and reviewed the existing evidence.

The first systematic review by den Boer [13] investigated potential biopsychosocial factors across 11 prospective studies. They found that lower level of education, lower work satisfaction, longer duration of sick leave, higher severity of pre-operative pain, higher level of passive avoidance coping strategies, and higher level of psychological problems were associated with poor outcome for patients following lumbar discectomy. Outcome was defined as pain, disability or work capacity or their combination. However, risk of bias was not assessed for the included studies, and heterogeneity of outcome measures and candidate predictors limited both analyses and confidence in the review's findings, although a basic rating system of the level of evidence was used. In the second systematic

review, Sabnis and Diwan [14] investigated the timing of lumbar discectomy across 21 prospective and retrospective studies, and randomised controlled trials. They found that long duration of pre-operative leg pain was associated with poor outcome for patients. However, patient outcome was not clearly defined and risk of bias was not assessed for the included studies [an unsupported scoring system was used to assess aspects of quality], which limits confidence in the review's findings, although an early best-evidence rating system was used. In the third systematic review, Schoenfeld and Bono [15] investigated the timing of lumbar discectomy surgery across 11 prospective and retrospective studies. They found that a longer duration of pre-operative symptoms was associated with poor patient outcome and identified 6 months duration of symptoms as the critical point when outcome started to be compromised i.e. symptom duration ≥6 months was associated with poor outcome for patients. A range of outcome measures were employed across studies [Short Form Health Survey [SF36], Oswestry Disability Index [ODI], motor weakness, delayed recovery, Visual Analogue Scale [VAS] pain, Japanese Orthopaedic Association Back Pain Questionnaire [JOABPEQ], psychological disorders, degree of return to activities of daily living, pain/disability score [PDS], failed back surgery syndrome, clinical outcome score, good postoperative outcome score, pain and working capacity]. Along with no assessment of risk of bias for the included studies [an unsupported scoring system was used to assess aspects of quality], the heterogeneity of outcome measures and candidate predictors limited analyses and limits confidence in the findings, although an early best-evidence rating system was used.

There is absence of a PRISMA compliant systematic review of prospective cohort studies with a long-term follow-up to synthesise the data investigating in particular, the physical factors that may be associated with patient outcome following lumbar discectomy which are commonly used as indications for surgery [5]. In addition, although early best-evidence rating systems have been used in previous reviews, none have focused on the key issues for this type of review, for example difference in phases of investigation is very relevant to this field of research to ensure a solid theoretical/conceptual model underpinning studies. Identification of physical prognostic factors, which are utilised for clinician's decision making [16–18], could help inform clinicians which patients are likely to have a more or less favourable outcome. This would allow clinicians to manage their patient's expectations prior to surgery and help their patient's make an informed choice about surgery and alternative management strategies.

Objective

To determine whether pre-operative physical factors are associated with post-operative outcomes in adult patients [≥16 years old] undergoing lumbar discectomy or microdiscectomy.

Methods

This review was guided by a pre-defined and registered protocol [CRD42015024168], and followed method guidelines of the Back Review Group of the Cochrane Collaboration [19], Cochrane Handbook [20] and PRISMA-P [21]. This systematic review is reported in line with the PRISMA statement [22].

Eligibility criteria
Types of studies
Prospective observational studies with a minimum of 1 year follow up. No restriction was placed on publication date.

Participants
Patients [≥16 years old] undergoing first time lumbar discectomy for lumbar disc herniation for irradiating leg pain without a rapid progressive severe motor deficit, cauda equina syndrome or severe comorbid conditions [e.g. arthritis or metabolic bone disease], and with no previous history of other lumbar spine operations.

Interventions
Primary, single-level, standard lumbar open discectomy or microdiscectomy.

Physical prognostic factors
Pre-operative physical prognostic factors including low back and/or leg pain intensity, duration of low back and/or leg pain, lumbar spine range of motion, disability, quality of life, clinical signs of motor deficit, sensory deficit, straight leg raise [SLR] test, crossed SLR test, walking distance.

Outcomes
Outcomes recommended in the evaluation of treatment of spinal disorders [23] were included; specifically disability, physical function, pain intensity and health related quality of life [24, 25].

Exclusion criteria were applied (Table 1).

Information sources
A comprehensive search was performed from inception to 31st March 2017 using key databases:

- CINAHL, EMBASE, MEDLINE, PEDro and ZETOC.
- Hand searches of key journals [Spine, European Spine Journal, The Spine Journal].
- Pubmed
- Screening reference lists by hand in papers that match the eligibility criteria.

Table 1 Criteria for inclusion and exclusion of studies

Inclusion criteria	
Population	16 years or older, male and female
Intervention	Lumbar and lumbosacral standard open discectomy or microdiscectomy Single one level Primary operation with no previous history of other lumbar spine surgery
Prognostic factors	Intensity of back/leg pain Pre-operative duration of back/leg pain Healh related quality of life Range of movement Motor deficit Sensory deficit SLR Walking distance Disability
Study design	Prospective cohort studies ≥1 year follow up
Exclusion criteria	
Population	History of previous back operation Extraspinal cause of low back and/or leg pain Trauma, vertebral fractures, arthritis or metabolic bone disease, scoliosis, spondylolysis, spondlyolisthesis, spinal stenosis or any other notable non-intervertebral disc abnormalities, trauma, rapid progressive motor deficit, cauda equina syndrome
Intervention	Any other lumbar surgical management Lumbar discectomy combined with other surgery
Study design	Studies not published in English language

- Unpublished research: British National Bibliography for Report Literature, Dissertation Abstracts, Index to Scientific and Technical Proceedings, National Technical Information Service, System for Information on Grey Literature.

Search
There was no restriction of the searches to specific languages. The search strategy was developed by one author [KZ] in discussion with a specialist librarian. It was performed independently by two authors [KZ/AP]. A methodological filter for the identification of prognostic studies which has the greatest sensitivity in Medline [26] was adapted for this study and used in combination with a variety of MESH terms and text words. The concepts that were searched included lumbar disc population, with leg pain and/or low back pain presenting symptoms, lumbar discectomy intervention, and studies investigating prognosis as the methodological focus. The Medline OvidSP search is presented in Table 2 as an example.

Study selection
After removing duplicates, screening of the titles and abstracts according to the eligibility criteria (Table 1) was performed independently by 2 authors [KZ/AP] to

Table 2 Example of Medline OvidSP Search Strategy

Searches	Results
1	incidence.sh.
2	follow-up studies.sh.
3	prognos*.tw.
4	predict*.tw.
5	course*.tw.
6	1 or 2 or 3 or 4 or 5
7	Lumbar Vertebrae/ or lumbar.mp.
8	Lumbosacral.mp. [mp = title, abstract, original title, name of substance word, subject heading word, keyword heading word, protocol supplementary concept word, rare disease supplementary word, unique identifier]
9	Intervertebral Disc/ or low back.mp.
10	7 or 8 or 9
11	sciatica.mp. or exp. Sciatica/
12	radicular pain.mp. or Radiculopathy/
13	Intervertebral Disc Degeneration/ or Intervertebral Disc Displacement/ or degenerative disc disease.mp.
14	Low back pain.mp. or Low Back Pain/
15	11 or 12 or 13 or 14
16	Discectomy.mp. or exp. Discectomy/
17	Discectomy.mp. [mp = title, abstract, original title, name of substance word, subject heading word, keyword heading word, protocol supplementary concept word, rare disease supplementary word, unique identifier]
18	Microsurgery/ or microdiscectomy.mp. or Discectomy, Percutaneous/
19	Laminectomy.mp. or Laminectomy/
20	16 or 17 or 18 or 19
21	6 and 10 and 15 and 20

reduce the risk of excluding relevant studies [27]. Full text articles were obtained for the studies that satisfied the inclusion criteria or in any case where eligibility could not be ascertained from the title or abstract. Full text articles were independently screened by 2 authors [KZ/AP]. Discrepancies about inclusion of articles were resolved by discussion and the third author [AR] was planned to resolve any disagreement.

Data collection process
Data were extracted from the studies into standardised forms independently by 2 authors [KZ/AP]. The third author [AR] checked the collected data of the included studies. Investigators were contacted by email to request additional information for missing or unclearly reported data in included studies.

Data items
Data were extracted from each study, including: study population, duration of follow up, prognostic factors, outcome measures and key findings.

Risk of Bias in individual studies
The Quality In Prognostic Studies [QUIPS] tool was used to assess the risk of bias for each individual study.

The QUIPS tool was devised for prognostic factor review questions [28] and has demonstrated acceptable inter-rater reliability [median 83.5%] [29]. It consists of 6 categories-domains of potential biases: study participation, study attrition, prognostic factor measurement, outcome measurement, study confounding, statistical analysis and reporting [29]. Each risk of bias domain was rated independently as 'low', 'moderate' or 'high' according to the responses to prompting items, with all domains weighted equally. Overall classification of risk of bias for individual studies was defined as low risk of bias when all domains were rated as low-moderate risk of bias; and high risk of bias when ≥1 domain was rated as high risk of bias [30]. Risk of bias was rated by two authors [KZ/AP] independently. Discrepancies were resolved by discussion and the third author [AR] was available to resolve any disagreement. Inter-rater agreement was planned to be measured with Cohen's kappa coefficient [31].

Planned method of analysis
According to the protocol and dependent on homogeneity between the included studies, a quantitative analysis was planned. In the situation where a meta-analysis was not justified [owing to high risk of bias and clinical

heterogeneity], a qualitative best evidence synthesis of the results was conducted. This synthesis was based on the risk of bias assessment of the included studies, prognostic factors and the strength of the association with the outcome. Consistency of results across studies was reported to contribute to the overall evidence for an individual candidate prognostic factor. Reporting of multivariable analyses, including odds ratios and 95% Confidence Intervals for dichotomous outcome measures, and βand 95% Confidence Intervals for continuous quantitative outcome measures, and p values were reported where possible. The Grading of Recommendations Assessment, Development and Evaluation [GRADE] method [32] was used to rate the overall quality of evidence for a prognostic factor per outcome [e.g. disability], across studies. The GRADE method criteria have been adapted for prognostic factor research [33]. Huguet et al. [33] modified the GRADE domains including 5 factors that may decrease [phase of investigation, study limitations, inconsistency, indirectness, imprecision and publication bias] and 2 factors that may increase [moderate or large effect size [standardized mean difference 0.5–0.8, or odds ratios 2.5–4.25] [33] and exposure-response gradient] the quality level of evidence. As distinct to GRADE used for assessing intervention studies, study design is not a key feature as longitudinal designs are the only option for prognostic research. Phase of investigation is a distinctive GRADE domain for prognostic research with phase 3 explanatory studies [aiming to understand prognostic pathways] and phase 2 explanatory studies [aiming to confirm independent associations between potential prognostic factor and the outcome measure] providing the highest quality of evidence [33].

Risk of Bias across studies

Visual assessment of potential publication bias with Funnel plots was planned to be performed if > 10 studies with comparable outcome measures were identified.

Results

Study selection

The initial search resulted in 6567 citations. After exclusion of duplicates, 1189 citations were screened by title and abstract. The full texts of 45 studies were retrieved and assessed for eligibility. Eight studies met the eligibility criteria. Figure 1 shows the number of studies at each stage of selection and the main reasons for exclusion. Details of studies excluded at the full text stage are detailed in the Additional file 1: Table S1. Three non-English studies were excluded at the full text stage. Complete agreement was achieved at each stage of the study selection process following the independent assessments of the 2 authors. Of the 8 included studies, 2 acknowledged that

they presented data from the same sample with the later paper by Lewis et al. reporting data at all timepoints [34, 35]. Two further studies appeared to present data from the same sample with the later 2011 article focusing to data on health-related quality of life outcome measures [36, 37]. A request for clarification from the authors did not receive a response. In both cases, data are presented as the same study to ensure appropriate weighting of the evidence in the narrative synthesis. Overall therefore, 6 studies were included reflecting 8 articles.

Study characteristics

The main characteristics of the 6 included studies are presented in Table 3.

Methods

The studies were conducted in four different countries and published between 1979 and 2011. Five studies were published, 1 was unpublished [38] but was presented at a conference and data were acquired after personal communication with the authors. The follow-up period in included studies ranged from 1 to 10 years.

Participants

The total number of participants included across the 6 studies was n = 802 and sample sizes ranged from 82 to 228. Age ranged from 17 to 83 years. After communication with the authors of 3 studies that did not report the age range of the participants [34, 36, 39], it was confirmed that all participants were ≥ 16 years old to enable study inclusion.

Physical prognostic factors

The most common physical prognostic factor that was investigated in 5 studies [34–37, 39–41] was pre-operative duration of leg pain, followed by intensity of pre-operative leg pain investigated in 3 studies [36–38, 41], and pre-operative back pain investigated in 2 studies [36, 37, 41].

Outcome measures

The range of outcome measures included: VAS for pain, ODI, EuroQol-5 Dimension [EQ-5D] score, SF-36, Neurogenic Symptom Score [NSS] and PDS for quality of life, Core Outcome Measures Index [COMI], Clinical Overall Score [COS], MacNab classification of postoperative outcome, satisfaction with treatment and change in leg/back pain.

Risk of Bias within studies

Of the 6 included studies, 1 was assessed as low risk of bias and 5 as high risk of bias (Table 4). Complete agreement in the assessment of risk of bias in all domains was achieved between the 2 authors. The domain 'study attrition' was

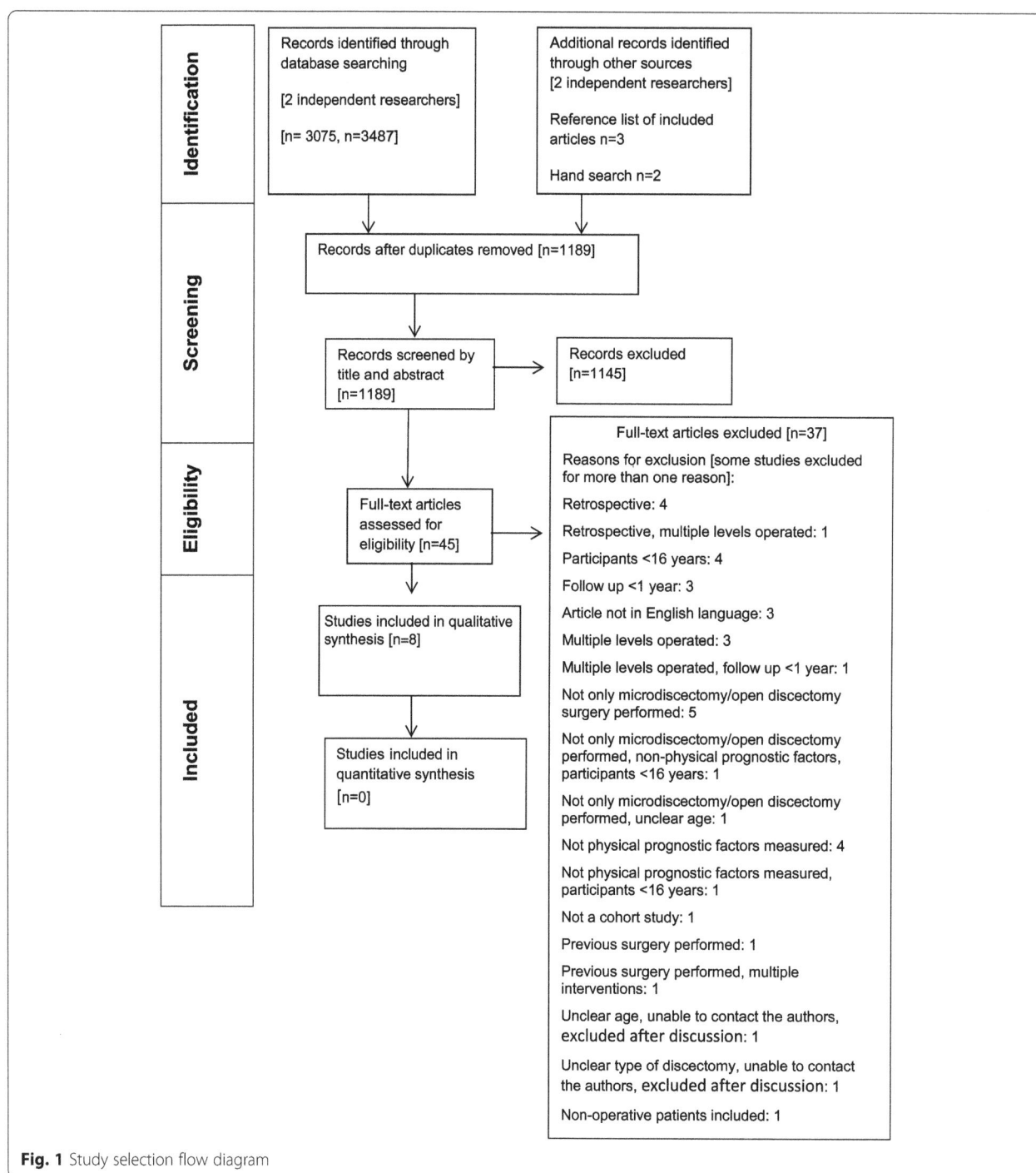

Fig. 1 Study selection flow diagram

rated as high risk of bias in 5 of the studies and only the domain 'outcome' was rated as low risk of bias in all studies. Most studies did not account for all of the important potential confounders in their study design and the risk of selection bias was also high due to incomplete reporting.

Results per physical prognostic factor

Eight different physical prognostic factors were investigated (Table 5). Due to heterogeneity between the included studies [predictors, follow-up timepoints, outcome measures] a meta-analysis was not justified, and a qualitative best evidence synthesis of the results was performed. In particular, there was great diversity in the patient outcomes assessed in the included studies. Using the adapted GRADE method for prognostic research [33] to rate the overall quality of evidence, all included studies were phase 1 predictive modelling or explanatory studies carried out to generate a hypothesis, and

Table 3 Study characteristics

Study	Country	Characteristics of Participants	Follow-up	Physical Prognostic factors	Outcome measures
Divecha et al., 2014	United Kingdom	n = 89 Age: 25–79, mean 48.6 Gender: Male n = 46 [51.7%] Female n = 43 [48.3%]	1 year n = 32 [35%]	• Pre-operative leg pain [% of pain that was radicular, calculated from the Core Outcome Measures Index [COMI]	• COMI score – patient completed assessment through Spine Tango. Includes questions on the severity of leg and back pain. • Definition of outcome unclear for multivariate analyses
Fisher et al., 2004	Canada	n = 82 Age: 17–83, mean 42.2 Gender: Male n = 52 [63.4%] Female n = 30 [36.6%]	1 year n = 71 [87%]	• Pre-operative duration of leg pain in months	• Health Related Quality Of Life [HRQOL] outcome comprising: a. North American Spine Society instruments: Neurogenic Symptom Score and Pain/Disability Score b. Short Form-36 [SF-36] questionnaire
Lewis et al., 1987 (and Weir, 1979)	Canada	n = 100 Age[a]: Mean [SD] 41.7 [1] Gender: Male 75% Female 25%	1 year N = 91 [91%] 5–10 years n = 81 [81%]	• Pre-operative duration of leg pain in months • Ipsilateral straight leg raise (detail of measurement not reported) • Forward bend (detail of measurement tool not reported)	• Relief of back pain • Relief of leg pain • No multivariate analyses
Nygaard et al., 2000	Norway	n = 132 Age[a]: > 18 Gender: Not reported	1 year n = 132 [100%]	• Pre-operative duration of leg pain in months • Pre-operative duration of back pain in months	• Clinical Overall Score, calculated from 40% weighting pain, 20% clinical examination, 20% functional status [Oswestry Disability Index, ODI] and 20% analgesia
Silverplats et al., 2010	Sweden	n = 171 Age[a]: Mean[SD] 39 [11] Gender: Male n = 95 [55.6%] Female n = 76 [44.4%]	2 years n = 154 [90%] Mean[SD] long term 7.3 [1.0] years Range 5.1–9.3 years n = 140 [81%]	• Pre-operative leg pain - recorded with three 0–100 Visual Analogue Scale [VAS] representing 'pain when as worst', 'pain when as least' and 'pain right now'. Mean value of the three scales recorded • Pre-operative back pain - recorded with three 0–100 VAS representing 'pain when as worst', 'pain when as least' and 'pain right now'. Mean value of the three scales recorded • Pre-operative duration of leg pain in months • Pre-operative ODI- self complete questionnaire 0–100	Primary outcomes: • MacNab classification of post-operative outcome [at 2 years] with 4 categories of outcome – excellent, good, fair, poor but unclear how applied as dichotomized outcome in multivariate analyses • Satisfaction with treatment [satisfied, partly, not satisfied, both follow up points] Secondary outcomes: • Change in leg pain [improved, no improvement, worse] • Change in back pain [improved, no improvement, worse]
Silverplats et al., 2011	Sweden	n = 117 Age: 18–66, mean 39 Gender: Male n = 63 [54%] Female n = 54 [46%]	Range 5–8 years 2 years 82% 7 years 76%	• Pre-operative duration of leg pain in months • Pre-operative leg pain [detail of measurement not reported] • Pre-operative back pain [detail of measurement not reported] • Pre-operative EuroQol-5 Dimension [EQ-5D] score for HRQOL self-completion questionnaire 0–100	• Change in EQ- 5D score
Solberg et al., 2005	Norway	n = 228 Age: Mean[SD] 41 [11] Gender: Male n = 114 [63.3%] Female n = 66 [36.7%]	1 year n = 180 [78.9%]	• Pre-operative ODI score - self complete questionnaire 0–100 • Pre-operative duration of leg pain in months • Pre-operative duration of back pain in months • Pre-operative leg pain 0–100 VAS no pain to worst conceivable pain • Pre-operative back pain 0–100 VAS no pain to worst conceivable pain	Primary outcome: • ODI score classified as: a. deterioration [increased ODI] or no deterioration [decreased/unchanged ODI] b. poor [ODI > 39] or good [ODI < 40] Secondary outcomes: • VAS back pain • VAS leg pain

[a] After communication with the authors it was confirmed that all participants were ≥ 16 years old
NOTE: Silverplats et al. 2010 and 2011 reported as two separate rows for clarity of prognostic factors and outcomes

Table 4 Methodological Assessment according to six domains of potential biases [QUIPS][27]

Study [n = 6]	Study Participation	Study Attrition [Follow-up]	Prognostic Factor	Outcome	Confounding Factor	Analysis	Overall Risk of Bias
Divecha et al., 2014	High	High	Moderate	Low	Moderate	Low	High
Fischer et al., 2004	Moderate	High	Moderate	Low	Low	Moderate	High
Lewis et al., 1987 and Weir 1979	High	High	Moderate	Low	High	High	High
Nygaard et al., 2000	High	High	Moderate	Low	High	High	High
Silverplats et al., 2010 and Silverplats et al., 2011	Moderate	Moderate	Low	Low	Low	Low	Low
Solberg et al., 2005	Moderate	High	Low	Low	High	Moderate	High

A study was considered to be of low risk of bias when all domains were rated as low-moderate risk of bias
A study was considered to be of high risk of bias when ≥1 domain[s] were rated as high risk of bias

consequently the quality of evidence was moderate as a starting point (Table 6) [33]. The level of evidence was downgraded in particular for inconsistency, and only upgraded for effect size for 2 prognostic factors.

ODI

The ODI was included in 2 studies [36, 41] as a candidate prognostic factor. There were inconsistencies regarding the association between the ODI and several outcomes. One study [low risk of bias] found no association [leg pain or back pain at 2 or 7 years], while 1 study [high risk of bias] found that higher disability was associated with better patient outcome [ODI at 12 months]. Using GRADE, there is very low level evidence that ODI is not associated with patient outcome.

Duration back pain

Duration of back pain was included in 2 studies [39, 41] as a candidate prognostic factor. Consistent findings from the 2 studies [high risk of bias] found no association with patient outcome [Clinical Overall Score and ODI at 12 months]. Using GRADE, there is very low level evidence that duration of back pain is not associated with patient outcome.

Duration leg pain

Pre-operative duration of leg pain was included in 5 studies [34–39, 41] as a candidate prognostic factor. There were inconsistencies regarding the association between the duration of pre-operative leg pain and numerous outcomes. Three studies [1 low risk of bias and 2 high risk of bias] found no association [leg pain, back pain and ODI at 12 months; leg pain and health-related quality of life at 2 and 7 years] while 2 studies [both high risk of bias] found that shorter pain duration was associated with better patient outcome [Pain Disability Score and Clinical Overall Score at 12 months]. Using GRADE, there is low level evidence that duration of pre-operative leg pain is not associated with patient outcome.

Severity leg pain

Severity of leg pain was included in 3 studies [36–38, 41] as a candidate prognostic factor. There were inconsistencies regarding the association between the severity of leg pain and several outcomes. Two studies [1 low risk of bias and 1 high risk of bias] found no association [health related quality of life at 2 and 7 years; ODI at 12 months], while 2 studies [1 low risk of bias and 1 high risk of bias] found that higher severity of leg pain was associated with better patient outcome [leg pain at 2 and 7 years; Core Outcome Measures Index at 12 months]. Using GRADE, there is low level evidence that higher severity of pre-operative leg pain predicts better Core Outcome Measures Index at 12 months and better post-operative leg pain at 2 and 7 years.

Severity back pain

Severity of back pain was included in 2 studies [36, 37, 41] as a candidate prognostic factor. Consistent findings from the 2 studies [1 low risk of bias and 1 high risk of bias] found no association with patient outcome [ODI at 12 months; back pain and health-related quality of life at 2 and 7 years]. Using GRADE, there is very low level evidence that severity of back pain is not associated with patient outcome.

Health-related quality of life

Health-related quality of life [EQ5D] was included in 1 study [37] as a candidate prognostic factor. The study [low risk of bias] found that low quality of life pre-operatively was associated with better patient outcome [health-related quality of life at 2 years]. Using GRADE, there is very low level evidence that a lower pre-operative EQ-5D predicts better EQ-5D at 2 years.

Straight leg raise and forward bend

Ipsilateral straight leg raise and forward bend were included in 1 study [34] as candidate prognostic factors. The study [high risk of bias] found that ipsilateral straight leg raise and forward bend were not associated

Table 5 Overview of Significant Physical Prognostic Factors: synthesis across included studies [bivariate and multivariable analyses when reported are documented here for consistency - reporting was inconsistent across studies]

Physical prognostic factors	Study and risk of bias	Results	Summary of study findings [based on multivariate analyses; where significant, direction of effect is reported]	gy9	Summary of findings across studies
Oswestry Disability Index [ODI]	Silverplats et al., 2010 LOW risk of bias	Bivariate analyses: • Patients with worse pre-operative ODI scores were more likely to report improvement in leg pain [dichotomized as improvement versus no improvement / worse]. Patients with improved leg pain had pre-operative mean ODI 52 compared to 42 in no improvement/worse group [$p = 0.040$]. • Patients with worse pre-operative ODI scores were more likely to report improvement in back pain [dichotomized as improvement versus no improvement / worse]. Patients with improved back pain had pre-operative mean of 52 compared to 44 in no improvement/worse group [$p = 0.040$]. Multivariable analyses: • ODI was not a significant predictor when using the full model of potential predictors [no measure of association reported] at 2 years or long term follow up.	Pre-operative ODI was not significant as a prognostic factor for leg pain or for back pain at 2 years or long term follow up [mean 7.3 ± 1.0 years].	+ Very low	Using GRADE, there is very low level evidence that ODI is not associated with patient outcome.
	Solberg et al., 2005 HIGH risk of bias	Multivariable analyses: • Using change in ODI score as a dichotomous variable (deterioration or no deterioration of score) in binary stepwise logistic regression analyses, a low pre-operative ODI score was an independent risk factor for 'deterioration' [β [age adjusted] 0.087, $p = 0.011$; β [independent risk factor] – 0.216, $p = 0.013$]. • Using ODI raw score at 12 months as a dichotomous variable ["good" ODI score > 39, or "poor" outcome] pre-operative ODI was not an independent risk factor for a "poor" outcome [no measure of association reported]. Lower ODI score [β = – 0.0442, $p < 0.001$] pre-operatively was a predictor of less improvement in ODI score.	Pre-operative ODI was significant as a prognostic factor for post-operative disability [ODI] at 12 months. *Higher pre-operative ODI predicts better outcome [lower ODI] at 12 months.*		
Duration of back pain	Nygaard et al., 2000 HIGH risk of bias	• Multivariable analyses: Multiple linear regression analysis demonstrated that pre-operative duration of back pain was not predictive of clinical overall score [COS]; coefficient β [Standard error] = – 0.26 [0.16], t test – 1.65, $p = 0.100$.	Pre-operative duration of back pain was not significant as a prognostic factor for COS at 12 months.	+ Very low	Using GRADE, there is very low level evidence that duration of back pain is not associated with patient outcome.
	Solberg et al., 2005 HIGH risk of bias	Multivariable analyses: • Using change in ODI score as a dichotomous outcome variable in binary stepwise logistic regression analyses, duration of back pain was not an independent risk factor for 'deterioration' [β [age adjusted] 0.001, $p = 0.304$]. • Using ODI raw score at 12 months as a dichotomous variable ["good"	Pre-operative duration of back pain was not significant as a prognostic factor for disability [ODI] at 12 months.		

Table 5 Overview of Significant Physical Prognostic Factors: synthesis across included studies [bivariate and multivariable analyses when reported are documented here for consistency - reporting was inconsistent across studies] *(Continued)*

Physical prognostic factors	Study and risk of bias	Results	Summary of study findings [based on multivariate analyses; where significant, direction of effect is reported]	gy9	Summary of findings across studies
		ODI score > 39, or "poor" outcome] in multivariate analyses, duration of back pain was not an independent risk factor for a "poor" outcome [no measure of association reported].			
Duration of leg pain	Fischer et al., 2004 HIGH risk of bias	Multivariable analyses: Patients with longer pre-operative duration of leg pain were more likely to report less improvement in Pain Disability Score [PDS] [$p = 0.026$] after adjustment for gender, age and pre-operative PDS. Mean change PDS 24.4 for duration 0–3 months, 20.0 for duration 3.1–9 months, 13.1 for duration > 9 months [no measures of association reported].	Pre-operative duration of leg pain was significant as a prognostic factor for PDS at 12 months. *Shorter pre-operative duration of leg pain predicts better outcome [lower PDS] at 12 months.*	a	am
	Lewis et al., 1987 and Weir et al., 1979 HIGH risk of bias	Bivariate analyses: • Duration leg pain < 17 months associated with complete relief of back pain in 43/71 cases [61%] at 1 year; 39/65 cases [60%] at 5–10 years. • Duration leg pain ≥17 months associated with complete relief of back pain in 12/19 cases [63%] at 1 year; 9/15 cases [60%] at 5–10 years. • Duration leg pain < 17 months associated with complete relief of leg pain in 54/71 cases [76%] at 1 year; 43/65 cases [66%] at 5–10 years. • Duration leg pain ≥17 months associated with complete relief of leg pain in 12/19 cases [63%] at 1 year; 6/15 cases [40%] at 5–10 years. • Significant association [chi-square of Fisher's exact test] at 1-year follow-up review between duration leg pain and relief of back or leg pain [above]. Shorter duration of leg pain before surgery is associated with relief of leg pain following surgery. Not significant at 5–10 years [results not reported].	Pre-operative duration of leg pain was not significant as a prognostic factor for leg pain and for back pain at 12 months [no multivariable analyses].		
	Nygaard et al., 2000 HIGH risk of bias	Multivariable analyses: • Patients with longer pre-operative duration of leg pain were more likely to report less improvement in COS. Multiple linear regression analysis, coefficient β [Standard error] = 0.98 [0.3], t test 3.23, $p = 0.0016$.	Pre-operative duration of leg pain was significant as a prognostic factor for COS at 12 months. *Shorter pre-operative duration of leg pain predicts better outcome [lower COS] at 12 months.*		
	Silverplats et al., 2010 LOW risk of bias	Bivariate analyses: • Patients with longer pre-operative duration of leg pain were more likely to report improvement in leg pain. Pre-operative short duration [< 6 months] of leg pain predicts good outcome on MacNab [dichotomized outcome] classification [$p = 0.039$] at 2-year follow up and predicts patient satisfaction with treatment [$p = 0.019$] at long term follow-up [mean 7.3 ± 1.0 years].	Pre-operative duration of leg pain was not significant as a prognostic factor for leg pain or health-related quality of life [EQ-5D] at 2 year and long term follow up [mean 7.3 ± 1.0 years].		

Table 5 Overview of Significant Physical Prognostic Factors: synthesis across included studies [bivariate and multivariable analyses when reported are documented here for consistency - reporting was inconsistent across studies] *(Continued)*

Physical prognostic factors	Study and risk of bias	Results	Summary of study findings [based on multivariate analyses; where significant, direction of effect is reported]	gy9	Summary of findings across studies
		Multivariable analyses: • Duration of leg pain was not a significant predictor when using the full model of potential predictors [no measure of association reported].			
	Silverplats et al., 2011 LOW risk of bias	Multivariable analyses: • Duration of leg pain was not a significant predictor for EuroQol-5 Dimension, EQ-5D at 2 years [no measure of association reported].			
	Solberg et al., 2005 HIGH risk of bias	Multivariable analyses: • Duration of leg pain was not an independent risk factor for 'deterioration' [β [age adjusted] 0.008, $p = 0.006$; β [independent risk factor] 0.005, $p = 0.572$]; using change in ODI score as a dichotomous outcome variable (deterioration or no deterioration). • Using ODI raw score at 12 months as a dichotomous outcome variable ["good" ODI score > 39, or "poor" outcome] duration of leg pain was not an independent risk factor for a "poor" outcome [no measure of association reported].	Pre-operative duration of leg pain was not significant as a prognostic factor for disability [ODI] at 12 months.		
Severity leg pain	Divecha et al., 2014 HIGH risk of bias	Bivariate analyses: • Patients with worse pre-operative leg pain were more likely to report improvement in functional outcome. Pearson's correlation coefficient between pre-operative leg pain [%] and Core Outcome Measures Index [COMI] score at 12 months was −0.394 (95% CI -0.653, − 0.053; $p = 0.0256$]. Multivariable analyses: • Patients with higher pre-operative leg pain had significantly lower COMI [$R^2 = 0.155$, $p = 0.03$] at 12 months.	Pre-operative severity of leg pain was significant as a prognostic factor for functional outcome [COMI] at 12 months. *Higher severity pre-operative leg pain predicts better outcome [lower COMI] at 12 months.*	++ Low	Using GRADE, there is low level evidence that higher severity of pre-operative leg pain predicts better Core Outcome Measures Index at 12 months and better post-operative leg pain at 2 and 7 years.
	Silverplats et al., 2010 LOW risk of bias	Bivariate analyses: • Patients with higher pre-operative leg pain were more likely to report improvement in leg pain. Patients with improved leg pain had higher leg pain pre-operatively on VAS [60 versus 47, $p = 0.008$] Multivariable analyses: • For improvement in leg pain the only significant predictor among all potential predictors was pre-operative VAS leg pain ($p = 0.039$). Pre-operative VAS leg pain was also the first and only predictor selected by the stepwise procedure [no measure of association reported].	Pre-operative severity of leg pain was significant as a prognostic factor for leg pain at 2 years and long term follow up [mean 7.3 ± 1.0 years]. Pre-operative severity of leg pain was not significant as a prognostic factor for EQ-5D at 2 years or long term follow up [mean 7.3 ± 1.0 years]. *Higher severity pre-operative leg pain predicts better outcome [lower leg pain] at 2 years and long term follow up [mean 7.3 ± 1.0 years].*		
	Silverplats et al., 2011 LOW risk of bias	Bivariate analyses: Patients with higher pre-operative leg pain were more likely to report improvement in health-related quality of life. Pre-operative VAS leg pain was			

Table 5 Overview of Significant Physical Prognostic Factors: synthesis across included studies [bivariate and multivariable analyses when reported are documented here for consistency - reporting was inconsistent across studies] *(Continued)*

Physical prognostic factors	Study and risk of bias	Results	Summary of study findings [based on multivariate analyses; where significant, direction of effect is reported]	gy9	Summary of findings across studies
		correlated with change in EQ-5D at 2-year follow-up [$r = 0.33$, $p = 0.002$] and at 7-year follow up [$r = 0.23$, $p = 0.04$]. Multivariable analyses: VAS leg pain was not identified as a significant predictor of EQ-5D [no measure of association reported].			
	Solberg et al., 2005 HIGH risk of bias	Bivariate analyses: Patients with higher pre-operative leg pain were more likely to report improvement in disability. Pre-operative VAS leg pain mean [SD; 95%CI] was 63.4 [27.5; 59.3 to 67.4], and at 12 months was 16.8 [21.1; 13.7 to 20.0]. Improvement was 46.5 [33.4, 41.6 to 51.4]. Multivariable analyses: Using change in ODI score as a dichotomous outcome variable, VAS leg pain was not an independent risk factor for 'deterioration' [β [age adjusted] -0.009, $p = 0.481$] at 12 months. Using ODI raw score at 12 months as a dichotomous outcome variable ["good" ODI score > 39, or "poor" outcome] VAS leg pain was not an independent risk factor for a "poor" outcome [no measure of association reported].	Pre-operative severity of leg pain was not significant as a prognostic factor for disability [ODI] at 12 months.		
Severity back pain	Silverplats et al., 2010 LOW risk of bias	Bivariate analyses: Patients with higher pre-operative back pain were more likely to report improvement in back pain. Patients with improved back pain had higher VAS back pain pre-operatively [53 versus 36, $p = 0.001$]. Multivariable analyses: Pre-operative back pain was not a significant predictor when [no measure of association reported] at 2 years or long term follow up [mean 7.3 ± 1.0 years].	Pre-operative severity of back pain was not significant as a prognostic factor for back pain or EQ-5D at 2 years or long term follow up [mean 7.3 ± 1.0 years].	+ Very low	Using GRADE, there is very low level evidence that severity of back pain is not associated with patient outcome.
	Silverplats et al., 2011 LOW risk of bias	Bivariate analyses: Back pain at baseline was not significantly correlated with change in EQ-5D at any follow-up. Multivariable analyses: Back pain was not identified as a significant predictor of EQ-5D at 2 years follow up [no measure of association reported].			
	Solberg et al., 2005 HIGH risk of bias	Bivariate analyses: Baseline VAS back pain (0–100 points) mean [SD; 95%CI] = 51.7 [29.3; 47.4, 56.0]. 12 months 21.3 [22.6; 18.0, 24.6]. Improvement 31.4 [35.6, 25.2–35.6]. VAS back pain pre-operatively not predictive of follow up ODI score at 12 months. Multivariable analyses: VAS back pain was not an	Pre-operative severity of back pain was not significant as a prognostic factor for disability [ODI] at 12 months.		

Table 5 Overview of Significant Physical Prognostic Factors: synthesis across included studies [bivariate and multivariable analyses when reported are documented here for consistency - reporting was inconsistent across studies] *(Continued)*

Physical prognostic factors	Study and risk of bias	Results	Summary of study findings [based on multivariate analyses; where significant, direction of effect is reported]	gy9	Summary of findings across studies
		independent risk factor for 'deterioration' [β–[age adjusted] 0.003, $p = 0.800$]; using change in ODI score as a dichotomous variable [deterioration or no deterioration]. Using ODI raw score at 12 months as a dichotomous variable ["good" ODI score > 39, or "poor" outcome], VAS back pain was not an independent risk factor for a "poor" outcome [no measure of association reported].			
Health-related quality of life [EuroQol-5 Dimension, EQ-5D]	Silverplats et al., 2011 LOW risk of bias	Bivariate analyses: Patients with lower pre-operative EQ-5D were more likely to report improvement in health-related quality of life [EQ-5D]. Pre-operative EQ-5D was correlated with change in EQ-5D at 2-year or 7-year follow-ups [$r = -0.70, p < 0.001$ and $r = -0.71, p < 0.001$]. Multivariable analyses: The only significant predictor of outcome was pre-operative EQ-5D score. The influence of baseline EQ-5D score was estimated [β = − 1.0, 95% CI: − 1.2, − 0.8] at 2 years.	Pre-operative EQ-5D was significant as a prognostic factor for health-related quality of life [EQ-5D] at 2 years. *Lower pre-operative EQ-5D predicts better outcome [lower EQ-5D] at 2 years.*	+ Very low	Using GRADE, there is very low level evidence that a lower pre-operative EQ-5D predicts better EQ-5D at 2 years.
Ipsilateral Straight Leg Raise [SLR]	Lewis et al., 1987 and Weir, 1979 HIGH risk of bias	Bivariate analyses: Positive ipsilateral SLR associated with complete relief of back pain in 47/75 cases [63%] at 1 year; 41/69 cases [59%] at 5–10 years. Negative ipsilateral SLR associated with complete relief of back pain in 9/16 cases [56%] at 1 year; 8/12 cases [67%] at 5–10 years. Positive ipsilateral SLR associated with complete relief of leg pain in 59/75 cases [79%] at 1 year; 42/69 cases [61%] at 5–10 years. Negative ipsilateral SLR associated with complete relief of leg pain in 8/16 cases [50%] at 1 year; 8/12 cases [67%] at 5–10 years. Significant association [chi-square of Fisher's exact test] at 1-year follow-up review between ipsilateral SLR and relief of back or leg pain [above]. Positive ipsilateral SLR before surgery is associated with relief of back and leg pain following surgery. Not significant at 5–10 years [results not reported].	Pre-operative ipsilateral SLR was not significant as a prognostic factor for back pain or leg pain at 5–10 years [no multivariable analyses].	+ Very low	Using GRADE, there is very low level evidence that straight leg raise is not associated with patient outcome.
Forward bend	Lewis et al., 1987 and Weir, 1979 HIGH risk of bias	Bivariate analyses: Forward bend to knee associated with complete relief of back pain in 41/58 cases [71%] at 1 year; 33/50 cases [66%] at 5–10 years. Forward bend to mid tibia or floor associated with complete relief of back pain in 15/33 cases [45%] at 1 year; 16/31 cases [52%] at 5–10 years. Forward bend to knee associated with complete relief of leg pain in	Pre-operative forward flexion was not significant as a prognostic factor for back pain or leg pain at 5–10 years [no multivariable analyses].	+ Very low	Using GRADE, there is very low level evidence that forward bend is not associated with patient outcome.

Table 5 Overview of Significant Physical Prognostic Factors: synthesis across included studies [bivariate and multivariable analyses when reported are documented here for consistency - reporting was inconsistent across studies] *(Continued)*

Physical prognostic factors	Study and risk of bias	Results	Summary of study findings [based on multivariate analyses; where significant, direction of effect is reported]	gy9 Summary of findings across studies
		48/58 cases [83%] at 1 year; 34/50 cases [68%] at 5–10 years. Forward bend to mid tibia or floor associated with complete relief of leg pain in 19/33 cases [58%] at 1 year; 13/31 cases [42%] at 5–10 years. Significant association [chi-square of Fisher's exact test] at 1-year follow-up review between forward bend and relief of back or leg pain [above]. Positive forward bend to knee before surgery is associated with relief of back and leg pain following surgery. Not significant at 5–10 years [results not reported].		

NOTE: Silverplats et al. 2010 and 2011 reported as two separate rows for clarity of prognostic factors and outcomes but combined from 'summary on study findings' column onwards when both studies have reported on a single prognostic factor

with patient outcome [back pain or leg pain at 5–10 years]. Using GRADE, there is very low level evidence that straight leg raise and forward bend are not associated with patient outcome.

Discussion

This is the first systematic review of physical prognostic factors to evaluate their association with patient outcome following lumbar discectomy. Only 6 studies were included, and risk of bias in the included studies was disappointing with only 1 study at low risk of bias. As a consequence, our current understanding of physical prognostic factors is limited.

Based on the strength of association of the prognostic factors investigated and the overall quality of evidence, we know that pre-operative severity of leg pain [low level of evidence] and quality of life [very low level of evidence] are associated with patient outcome. Specifically, higher severity pre-operative leg pain predicts better Core Outcome Measures Index at 12 months and better leg pain at 2 and 7 years; and lower pre-operative EQ-5D predicts better EQ-5D at 2 years. The findings are consistent with den Boer's previous review that found higher severity of pre-operative pain was associated with patient outcome [13]. Greater confidence in low risk of bias studies in situations of inconsistency between study findings contributed to severity of leg pain being identified overall as associated with patient outcome and this may be a limitation of this review. Interestingly, apart from the Core Outcome Measures Index, for both significant factors the prognostic factor and outcome were the same measure, and therefore for both of these factors, the reason they were more likely to report improvement could be due to the fact that

were starting from a higher level of pain or lower level of quality of life initially.

Other potential predictors examined were pre-operative ODI, duration leg pain, duration back pain, severity back pain, ipsilateral SLR and forward bend, and very low quality of evidence found that they were not associated with patient outcome, except for duration of leg pain where the quality of evidence was low. Consistent findings identified that pre-operative duration of back pain and severity of back pain were not associated with patient outcome [clinical overall score and ODI at 12 months; back pain or EQ-5D at 2 or 7 years and ODI at 12 months respectively]. Findings from 1 study [34, 35] identified that pre-operative ipsilateral SLR and forward bend were not associated with patient outcome, although it is difficult to have any confidence in these findings as they were based on bivariate analyses only [Table 5]. Inconsistent findings identified that pre-operative ODI [1 low risk of bias, 1 high risk of bias study] was not associated with patient outcome [leg pain or back pain at 2 and 7 years; ODI at 12 months]. None of these factors had been examined in previous reviews. Inconsistent findings identified that duration leg pain was not associated with patient outcome [Pain Disability Score, ODI, leg pain, back pain and Clinical Overall Score at 12 months; EQ-5D at 2 and 7 years]. This was in contrast to previous reviews that identified pre-operative duration of leg pain as associated with patient outcome [14, 15]. It is however difficult to have confidence in the findings from previous reviews as they themselves were at risk of bias.

In comparison with other systematic reviews [13–15], this review included only prospective cohort studies which are the gold standard design for investigating prognostic factors to enable optimal measurement of

Table 6 Adapted Grading[31] of Recommendations Assessment, Development and Evaluation [GRADE] table for systematic reviews with meta-analysis of prognostic studies for positive outcome across a range of measures

GRADE factor						Factors that may reduce the quality					Factors that may increase the quality		
Prognostic factor [pre-operative measures]	Number of participants	Number of studies	Number of cohorts	Estimated effect size [95% CI]	Phase (design)	Study limitations	Inconsistency	Indirectness	Imprecision	Publication bias	Moderate/large effect size	Dose effect	Overall quality
Oswestry Disability Index [ODI]	399	2	2	Unclear	1	✓	×	✓	×	×	×	×	+ Very low
Duration of back pain	360	2	2	Unclear	1	×	✓	✓	×	×	✓	×	+ Very low
Duration of leg pain	713	5	5	Unclear	1	✓	×	✓	✓	✓	×	×	++ Low
Severity leg pain	488	3	3	Unclear	1	✓	×	✓	✓	✓	×	×	++ Low
Severity back pain	399	2	2	Unclear	1	✓	×	✓	×	×	✓	×	+ Very low
EuroQol-5 Dimension [EQ-5D]	140	1	1	Unclear	1	✓	×	✓	✓	×	×	×	+ Very low
Ipsilateral Straight Leg Raise [SLR]	100	1	1	Unclear	1	×	×	✓	×	×	×	×	+ Very low
Forward bend	100	1	1	Unclear	1	×	×	✓	×	×	×	×	+ Very low

GRADE factors: ✓, no serious limitations; X, serious limitations [or not present for moderate/large effect size]; unclear, unable to rate item based on available information. For overall quality of evidence: +, very low; ++, low; +++, moderate; ++++, high

outcomes and predictors [42]. Our findings illustrate that the current level of evidence is low/very low. An adequately powered low risk of bias prospective observational study that assesses patient outcome at 12 months following surgery is required to further investigate pre-operative severity of leg pain, EQ-5D and duration of leg pain; and those candidate prognostic factors with inconsistent and very low level evidence to date, specifically ODI, duration back pain, severity back pain, ipsilateral SLR and forward bend. Other physical factors worthy of investigation and examined in studies excluded from this review, include pre-operative motor deficit, sensory loss and walking capacity.

Strengths and limitations

This is the first low risk of bias systematic review [self-assessed using AMSTAR 2 [43]] that has synthesised the evidence for physical prognostic factors predicting patient outcome following lumbar discectomy surgery. However, the review is limited by risk of bias across the small number of available studies, and a lack of comparable outcome measures across studies. This lack of comparable outcome measures meant that the definition of outcome taken into the GRADE analysis was broad encompassing a range of domains and outcome measures. The exclusion of 3 non-English studies could be a major limitation of this review as key findings may have been missed; particular as only 6 studies were included. Discussion of this review's findings is limited by the scarce literature in this area and the quality of reporting of individual study results which was inconsistent and poor overall.

Conclusions

Results from this systematic review identified low level evidence that higher severity of pre-operative leg pain predicts better Core Outcome Measures Index at 12 months and better post-operative leg pain at 2 and 7 years. There is very low level evidence that a lower pre-operative EQ-5D predicts better EQ-5D at 2 years. Low level evidence supports duration of leg pain pre-operatively not being associated with outcome, and very low-quality evidence supports other factors [pre-operative ODI, duration back pain, severity back pain, ipsilateral SLR and forward bend] not being associated with outcome [range of outcome measures used]. Research to date is however poor, consisting mostly of high risk of bias studies with inadequate reporting of analyses, not enabling full understanding of the prognostic value of physical factors assessed prior to surgery.

An adequately powered low risk of bias prospective observational study, with clear reporting of multivariable analyses is required to investigate all potential physical factors. Knowledge of the physical prognostic factors is essential to inform clinical decision-making processes regarding selection of patients for surgery and potentially the targeting of patients for rehabilitation following surgery. The results of prospective observational studies can help clinicians to decide which people should receive surgery or rehabilitation. However, a limitation is that a difference in prognosis does not necessarily mean a causal link with the surgery. Therefore, when we understand the prognostic factors we need to investigate them in a randomised controlled trial to investigate predictors of treatment response.

Abbreviations

COMI: Core Outcome Measures Index; COS: Clinical Overall Score; EQ5D: EuroQol-5 Dimension; JOABPEQ: Japanese Orthopaedic Association Back Pain Questionnaire; LBP: Low back pain; NSS: Neurogenic Symptom Score; ODI: Oswestry Disability Index; PDS: Pain disability score; QUIPs: Quality In Prognostic Studies; SF36: Short Form Health Survey; SLR: Straight leg raise; WAS: Visual Analogue Scale

Authors' contributions

AR is Chief Investigator leading protocol development, analyses and dissemination. KZ led on initial drafts of protocol and manuscript; contributing to an MSc award. KZ and AP were the first and second reviewers. AR was the third reviewer. AR and JBS overviewed methodological decisions, data analysis and study quality. All authors contributed to data interpretation, conclusions, and dissemination. All reviewers have read, contributed to, and agreed the final manuscript. AR is the guarantor of the review.

Competing interests

Authors Alison Rushton and J Bart Staal are editorial board members for Musculoskeletal Disorders. The authors declare that they have no competing interests.

Author details

[1]Centre of Precision Rehabilitation for Spinal Pain [CPR Spine] School of Sport, Exercise and Rehabilitation Sciences, University of Birmingham, Birmingham B15 2TT, UK. [2]Polyclinic of Lisieux, Lillebonne, France. [3]ARC Physiotherapy, Saffron Walden, UK. [4]Radboud Institute for Health Sciences, IQ healthcare, Radboud UMC, Nijmegen 6500 HB, The Netherlands. [5]Research group Musculoskeletal Rehabilitation, HAN University of Applied Sciences, Nijmegen, the Netherlands.

References

1. Buchbinder RBF, March LM, et al. Placing the global burden of low back pain in context. Best Pract Res Clin Rheumatol. 2013;27(5):575–89.
2. HCUPnet. Outcomes by 3 laminectomy, excision intervertebral disc. In: National statistics on all stays statistics on specific diagnoses or procedures; 2012.
3. online HES: Procedure and Intervention: 3 character tables. In. Edited by Centre. HaSCI. Accessed 28.7.16 http://www.hesonline.nhs.uk. 2016.
4. Chou R, Baisden J, Carragee EJ, Resnick DK, Shaffer WO, Loeser JD. Surgery for low back pain: a review of the evidence for an American pain society clinical practice guideline. Spine (Phila Pa 1976). 2009;34(10):1094–109.
5. Gibson JNAWG. Surgical interventions for lumbar disc prolapse: updated Cochrane review. Spine. 2007;32(16):1735.
6. Oosterhuis TCL, Maher CG, et al. Rehabilitation after lumbar disc surgery. In: Cochrane Database Syst Rev vol. art. No: CD003007; 2014.
7. Ostelo RWGM, de Vet HC, et al. Economic evaluation of a behavioral-graded activity program compared to physical therapy for patients following lumbar disc surgery. Spine. 2004;29:615–22.
8. Statistics HE. All procedures and interventions 2013/14. In: 3 character All procedures (V33) National Health Service Digital data; 2016.
9. Lebow RL, Adogwa O, Parker SL, Sharma A, Cheng J, McGirt MJ. Asymptomatic same-site recurrent disc herniation after lumbar discectomy: results of a prospective longitudinal study with 2-year serial imaging. Spine. 2011;36(25):2147 51.

10. Parker SL, Mendenhall SK, Godil SS, Sivasubramanian P, Cahill K, Ziewacz J, McGirt MJ. Incidence of low back pain after lumbar discectomy for herniated disc and its effect on patient-reported outcomes. Clin Orthop Relat Res. 2015;473(6):1988–99.

11. Steyerberg EW, Moons KG, van der Windt DA, Hayden JA, Perel P, Schroter S, Riley RD, Hemingway H, Altman DG, Group P. Prognosis research strategy (PROGRESS) 3: prognostic model research. PLoS Med. 2013;10(2):e1001381.

12. Hemingway H, Croft P, Perel P, Hayden JA, Abrams K, Timmis A, Briggs A, Udumyan R, Moons KG, Steyerberg EW, et al. Prognosis research strategy (PROGRESS) 1: a framework for researching clinical outcomes. BMJ. 2013;346:e5595.

13. den Boer JJ, Oostendorp RA, Beems T, Munneke M, Oerlemans M, Evers AW. A systematic review of bio-psychosocial risk factors for an unfavourable outcome after lumbar disc surgery. Eur Spine J. 2006;15(5):527–36.

14. Sabnis AB, Diwan AD. The timing of surgery in lumbar disc prolapse: a systematic review. Indian J Orthop. 2014;48(2):127–35.

15. Schoenfeld AJBM. Does surgical timing influence functional recovery after lumbar discectomy? A systematic review. Clin Orthop Relat Res. 2015;473: 1963–70.

16. Ng LCL, Sell P. Predictive value of the duration of sciatica for lumbar discectomy: a PROSPECTIVE COHORT STUDY. J Bone Joint Surg Br. 2004;86-B(4):546–9.

17. Haugen AJ, Brox JI, Grovle L, Keller A, Natvig B, Soldal D, Grotle M. Prognostic factors for non-success in patients with sciatica and disc herniation. BMC Musculoskelet Disord. 2012;13:183.

18. Lonne G, Solberg TK, Sjaavik K, Nygaard OP. Recovery of muscle strength after microdiscectomy for lumbar disc herniation: a prospective cohort study with 1-year follow-up. Eur Spine J. 2012;21(4):655–9.

19. Furlan A PV, Bombardier C, et al; from the editorial Board of the Cochrane Collaboration Back Review Group: Updated method guidelines for systematic reviews in the Cochrane collaboration back review group. Spine 2009, 34:1929–1941.

20. Higgins JP GS, Eds. : Cochrane handbook for systematic reviews of intervention in., vol. Version 5.1.0: the Cochrane collaboration 2011.

21. Shamseer L, Moher D, Clarke M, Ghersi D, Liberati A, Petticrew M, Shekelle P, Stewart LA, Group P-P. Preferred reporting items for systematic review and meta-analysis protocols (PRISMA-P) 2015: elaboration and explanation. BMJ. 2015;350:g7647.

22. Moher DLA, Tetzlaff J, et al. Preferred reporting items for systematic reviews and meta-analyses: the PRISMA statement. Ann Intern Med. 2009;151(4):264–9.

23. C B. Outcome assessments in the evaluation of treatment of spinal disorders: summary and general recommendations. Spine. 2000;25(24): 3100–3.

24. Solberg T, Johnsen LG, Nygaard ØP, Grotle M. Can we define success criteria for lumbar disc surgery? Estimates for a substantial amount of improvement in core outcome measures. Acta Orthop. 2013;84(2):196–201.

25. Chiarotto A, Deyo RA, Terwee CB, Boers M, Buchbinder R, Corbin TP, Costa LO, Foster NE, Grotle M, Koes BW, Kovacs FM. Core outcome domains for clinical trials in non-specific low back pain. Eur Spine J. 2015;24(6):1127–42.

26. Wilczynski NL, Haynes RB, Hedges T. Developing optimal search strategies for detecting clinically sound prognostic studies in MEDLINE: an analytic survey. BMC Med. 2004;2:23.

27. Edwards P, Clarke M, DiGuiseppi C, Pratap S, Roberts I, Wentz R. Identification of randomized controlled trials in systematic reviews: accuracy and reliability of screening records. Stat Med. 2002;21(11):1635–40.

28. Hayden JA, Cote P, Bombardier C. Evaluation of the quality of prognosis studies in systematic reviews. Ann Intern Med. 2006;144(6):427–37.

29. Hayden JA, van der Windt DA, Cartwright JL, Cote P, Bombardier C. Assessing bias in studies of prognostic factors. Ann Intern Med. 2013;158(4): 280–6.

30. Bruls VEBC, de Bie RA. Prognostic factors of complaints of arm, neck and/or shoulder: a systematic review of prospective cohort studies. Pain. 2015; 156(5):765–88.

31. Landis JR, Koch GG. The measurement of observer agreement for categorical data. Biometrics. 1977;33(1):159–74.

32. Guyatt GH, Oxman AD, Schunemann HJ, Tugwell P, Knottnerus A. GRADE guidelines: a new series of articles in the journal of clinical epidemiology. J Clin Epidemiol. 2011;64(4):380–2.

33. Huguet A, Hayden JA, Stinson J, McGrath PJ, Chambers CT, Tougas ME, Wozney L. Judging the quality of evidence in reviews of prognostic factor research: adapting the GRADE framework. Syst Rev. 2013;2:71.

34. Lewis PJ, Weir BKA, Broad RW, Grace MG. Long-term prospective study of lumbosacral discectomy. J Neurosurg. 1987;67(1):49–53.

35. Weir B. Prospective study of 100 lumboscaral discectomies. J Neurosurg. 1979;50:283–9.

36. Silverplats K, Lind B, Zoega B, Halldin K, Gellerstedt M, Brisby H, Rutberg L. Clinical factors of importance for outcome after lumbar disc herniation surgery: long-term follow-up. Eur Spine J. 2010;19(9):1459–67.

37. Silverplats K, Lind B, Zoega B, Halldin K, Gellerstedt M, Rutberg L, Brisby H. Health-related quality of life in patients with surgically treated lumbar disc herniation: 2- and 7-year follow-up of 117 patients. Acta Orthop. 2011;82(2): 198–203.

38. Divecha MHFB, Verma R. Post-operative outcome following lumbar discectomy: The value of pre-operative radicular pain proportion. In: 8th British Spine Conference 2014. Warwick United Kingdom: European Spine Journal; 2014.

39. Nygaard OPKR, Solberg T. Duration of leg pain as a predictor of outcome after surgery for lumbar disc herniation: a prospective cohort study with 1-year follow-up. J Neurosurg. 2000;92:131–4.

40. Fisher CG, Noonan V, Bishop P, Boyd M, Fairholm D, Wing P, Dvorak M. Outcome evaluation of the operative management of lumbar disc herniation causing sciatica. J Neurosurg. 2004;100(4 SUPPL):317–24.

41. Solberg TØPN, Sjaavik K, Hofoss D. The risk of "getting worse" after lumbar microdiscectomy. Eur Spine J. 2005;

42. Moons KRP, Vergouwe Y, et al. Prognosis and prognostic research: what, why, and how? BMJ. 2009;338(7706):1317–20.

43. Shea BJ, Reeves BC, Wells G, Thuku M, Hamel C, Moran J, Moher D, Tugwell P, Welch V, Kristjansson E, Henry DA. AMSTAR 2: a critical appraisal tool for systematic reviews that include randomised or non-randomised studies of healthcare interventions, or both. BMJ. 2017;358:j4008.

8

The prevalence and associated factors of symptomatic cervical Spondylosis in Chinese adults

Yanwei Lv[1,2,3], Wei Tian[2,3*†], Dafang Chen[1*†], Yajun Liu[3], Lifang Wang[2] and Fangfang Duan[2]

Abstract

Background: Cervical spondylosis adversely affects life quality for its heavy disease burden. The report on the community-based prevalence and associated factors of cervical spondylosis is rare, especially in Chinese population. Whether prevention is needed and how to prevent it is not clear. This study aims to explore its prevalence and related lifestyle factors and provide evidence on prevention of cervical spondylosis.

Methods: A community-based multistage cross-sectional survey of six communities from the Chinese population was conducted. A face-to-face interview was conducted to obtain individual information, and prevalence was calculated. Single-factor analysis and multivariable logistic regressions were used to explore the associated factors in total and subgroup populations.

Results: A total of 3859 adults were analyzed. The prevalence of cervical spondylosis was 13.76%, although it differed significantly among the urban, suburban, and rural populations (13.07%, 15.97%, and 12.25%, respectively). Moreover, it was higher in females than in males (16.51% vs 10.49%). The prevalence among different age groups had an inverted U shape. The highest prevalence was in the age group from 45 to 60 years old. The associated factors differed by subgroups. There were positive associations between engaging in mental work, high housework intensity, and sleep duration of less than 7 h/day with cervical spondylosis. Going to work on foot was a negative factor of cervical spondylosis in the total population. For people aged less than 30 years, keeping the same work posture for 1–2.9 h/day was a special related factor. Exposure to vibration was an associated factor for females aged 45–60 years. Menopause was a special related factor for women.

Conclusions: Prevalence of cervical spondylosis was high in Chinese population. People younger than 60 years were the focus of prevention for cervical spondylosis. Moreover, the characters between male and female and among different age groups were different and required targeted interventions.

Keywords: Cervical spondylosis, Community-based, Cross-sectional study, Prevalence, Associated factors

* Correspondence: tianweijst@vip.163.com; dafangchen@bjmu.edu.cn
†Wei Tian and Dafang Chen contributed equally to this work.
[2]Clinical Epidemiology Research Center, Beijing Jishuitan Hospital, 31#
Xinjiekou Dongjie, West district, Beijing 100035, China
[1]Department of Epidemiology and Biostatistics, Public Health College, Peking
University, 38# Xueyuan Road, Haidian district, Beijing 100191, China
Full list of author information is available at the end of the article

Background

Cervical spondylosis is a chronic degenerative process of the cervical spine. It affects the vertebral bodies and intervertebral disks of the neck and leads to herniated intervertebral disks, osteophytes, and ligament hypertrophy. This may eventually cause compression of the nerve roots and spinal cord [1]. Numbness, weakness, and tingling in the neck and/or arms, pain in the neck and/or arms, neck stiffness, and headaches are the usual symptoms of cervical spondylosis [2]. According to the reports, pain, numbness, and other symptoms were related to depression and insomnia [3, 4]. Although many asymptomatic adults have spondylotic changes according to the imaging examination, cervical spondylosis can cause stenosis of the spinal canal, lateral recess, and foramina and cause clinical symptoms, such as neck pain [5–7]. Neck pain was the most common symptom of cervical spondylosis [8]. The lifetime prevalence of the adult population was 48.5%, and the prevalence of screen-using workers was 55% [9, 10]. According to the global burden of disease study of 2013 [11], in 301 acute and chronic diseases and injuries in 188 countries, neck pain was one of the top 10 causes of years lived with disability. It ranked the fourth globally and the second in China, relatively. Cervical spondylosis not only affects the life quality but also increases the economic burden, since high-cost surgery is a regular treatment method. Therefore, cervical spondylosis might become a public health concern.

Cervical spondylosis is an age-related degeneration and chronic noncommunicable disease. Previous studies showed that age was the main risk factor and a contributor to the incidence of cervical spondylosis. The risk increased with aging [2, 12, 13]. Moreover, several other factors, such as occupational factors, exercises, and so on, exist [14]. In China, the prevalence and related factors were mainly hospital-based studies.However, the community-based prevalence and related factors of cervical spondylosis were rarely reported in Chinese population. With the social development of China and the onset of population aging, a large number of patients with cervical spondylosis

may exist. The lifestyle has changed a lot in Chinese population,but the evidence of whether it needs to be controlled and how to control is lacking.

Therefore, the objective of this study was to report the baseline of the prevalence of cervical spondylosis and its related lifestyle influence factors of Chinese adults and provide evidence on its prevention and management.

Methods

Study participants

The present community-based cross-sectional study was conducted in December 2010. A multistage, stratified sampling method was used to select a representative sample of persons aged 18 years or older and living in Beijing for at least 6 months. The sampling process referred to a previous study [15]. The study protocol was approved by the institutional review board and the ethics committee of the Beijing Jishuitan Hospital, Beijing, China. Written informed consent was obtained from each participant before the data was collected.

Diagnostic criteria

The patients of cervical spondylosis were self-reported doctor-diagnosed. Participants who had been diagnosed in the hospital were the patients. According to the consensus guide, cervical spondylosis was diagnosed by the clinical symptoms, signs and imaging examinations if needed in China. Clinical symptoms and signs were the diagnosis base of cervical spondylosis (Table 1) [16]. According to the clinician judgment, radiography or/and computed tomography or/and magnetic resonance imaging were used for the imaging examinations, and they were mandatory for diagnosing cervical spondylosis.

Data collection

The face-to-face interview was used to collect the information. The information included sociodemographic information, such as place of residence, age, sex, per capita monthly income, education, type of medical insurance, and education level; physical measurement index, including

Table 1 The symptoms and signs of cervical spondylosis

symptoms	signs
Cervical pain aggravated by movement	Poorly localised tenderness
Referred pain (occiput, between the shoulder blades, upper limbs)	Limited range of movement (forward flexion, backward extension, lateral flexion, and rotation to both sides)
Retro-orbital or temporal pain (from C1 to C2)	Minor neurological changes like inverted supinator jerks (unless complicated by myelopathy or radiculopathy)
Cervical stiffness—reversible or irreversible	
Vague numbness, tingling, or weakness in upper limbs	
Dizziness or vertigo	
Poor balance	
Rarely, syncope, triggers migraine, pseudo-angina	

body mass index (BMI, measured as weight in kgdivided by height in m^2) and waist–hip ratio (WHR, the ratio of waist circumference and hip circumference); and lifestyle information containing smoking, drinking, nature of labor (physical-based, mental-based, or mixed), vibration, job posture, working intensity, duration of the same working posture during the day, transportation tools (nonmanpower transportation tool, bicycle, and walking), housework intensity, exercise frequency, exercise intensity, and sleep duration per day. People presently smoking at least one cigarette per day for at least 1 month or having used at least 100 cigarettes during lifetime were defined as smokers. The alcohol drinking group referred to persons whose alcohol consumption was 1000 mL of beer or 100 mL of liquor per week and lasting 1 year or more. Vibration denoted people operating a motor or a similar working environment in which movement was felt as a vibration. Body weight and height were measured by the researchers. A feasibility test of data collection and survey process optimization was done via a pilot study conducted prior to the actual study. A technical training of the investigators was conducted before being sent to interview the participants. Data were doubly entered in parallel using the EpiData 3.1 software (The EpiData Association, Odense, Denmark).

Statistical analysis

Prevalence was reported with a standard error. Area-, age-, and sex-specific prevalences were also reported. Moreover, the prevalence associated with different education levels, BMI, nature of labor, income, drinking, smoking, job posture, transportation tools, sleep duration, vibration, duration of working posture, exercise frequency, exercise intensity, WHR, and menopause of women subgroup was calculated. The single-factor analysis was examined by χ^2 tests or the Kolmogorov–Smirnov test. The multivariate analysis of associated factors was analyzed by the multivariable logistic regression model in the total

population and in gender and age subgroup populations. Only significant variables in the single factor analysis were included in the multivariable model. The variables were selected by stepwise method. All p values were two tailed, not adjusted for multiple tests, and considered significant at $p < 0.05$. All statistical tests were carried out using the SPSS 18.0 software (SPSS Inc., IL, USA).

Results

Participant demographics

The study included 3900 participants, of which 3888 completed the study and 3859 had adequate disease information and were included in the analysis finally. The response rate was 99.7% in total, and 99.6% for males and 99.8% for females. Among the participants, 1820 were males (47.27%) and 2029 were females (52.73%). The mean age was 45.85 ± 16.19 years.

Prevalence of cervical Spondylosis

Among 3859 subjects, 531 were diagnosed with cervical spondylosis, and the prevalence of cervical spondylosis was 13.76% [95% confidence interval (CI): 12.67–14.85%)]. The prevalence of cervical spondylosis in the suburban (15.97%) area was higher than that in the urban and rural areas (13.07% and 12.25%; $p = 0.016$; Fig. 1). The prevalence presented a rising trend with increasing age ($P < 0.001$; Fig. 2). The females had a higher prevalence of cervical spondylosis compared with the males ($P < 0.001$; Fig. 3). Participants with less education had a higher prevalence of cervical spondylosis ($P < 0.001$). The prevalence of cervical spondylosis increased with increasing BMI ($P = 0.001$). A significant difference in the prevalence was found among the three kinds of transportation modes ($P = 0.013$). The sleep duration less than 7 h/day had a higher prevalence compared with those sleeping for no less than 7 h/day ($P < 0.001$). People holding the same working posture for about 1–2.9 h were

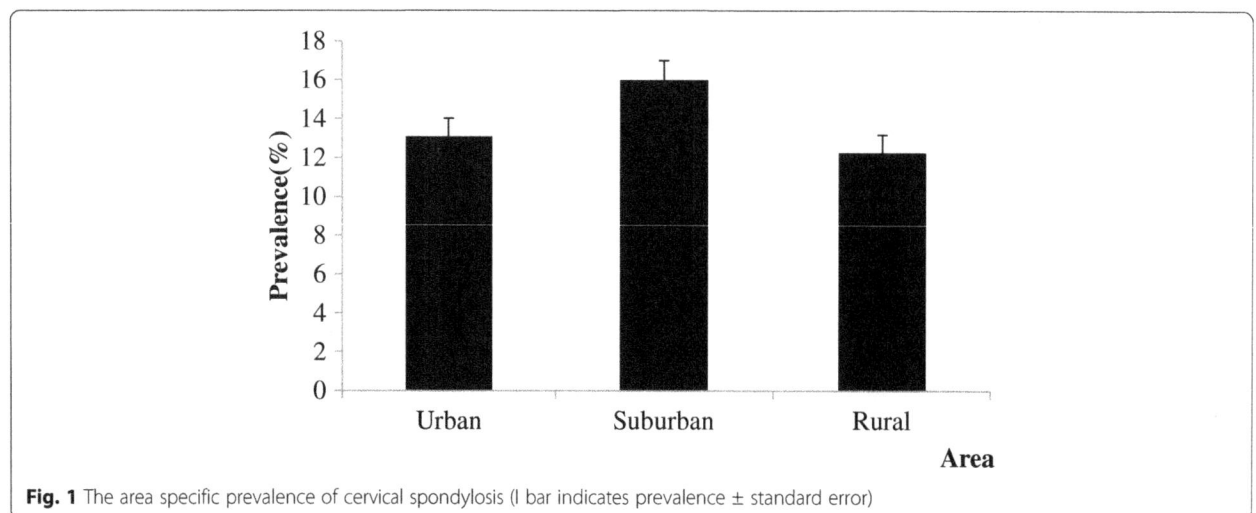

Fig. 1 The area specific prevalence of cervical spondylosis (I bar indicates prevalence ± standard error)

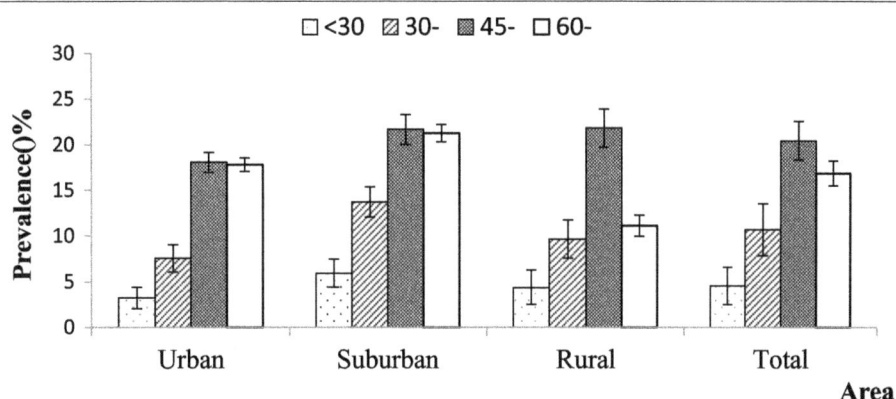

Fig. 2 The age-specific prevalence of cervical spondylosis in different areas (I bar indicates prevalence ± standard error)

more likely to experience cervical spondylosis ($P = 0.015$). The prevalences of higher and lower exercise frequencies groups were both higher than other group ($P < 0.001$). Exercise intensity was related to the prevalence of cervical spondylosis ($P < 0.001$). People whose WHR was central obesity had a higher prevalence compared with the normal people ($P = 0.002$). Menopausal women had a higher prevalence than the nonmenopausal group ($P < 0.001$) (Table 2). Housework intensity was associated with cervical spondylosis (Table 3).

Associated factors for cervical Spondylosis in the Total population

People living in the suburban area, those 30 years or older, females, those engaged in mental work, housework intensity, and those sleeping for less than 7 h/day had a positive association with cervical spondylosis. Going to work on foot was a negative associated factor for cervical

spondylosis; the odds ratio (OR) was 0.690 (95% CI: 0.512–0.929) (Table 4).

Associated Factors for Cervical Spondylosis in the Gender Subgroup

The associated factors for cervical spondylosis were significantly different between men and women. For males, age 30 years or older and having vibration characteristics during their working environment were associated factors for cervical spondylosis. For females, place of residence, age, menopause, mental-based work, housework intensity, and sleeping for less than 7 h/day were associated factors for cervical spondylosis, whereas going to work on foot was a protective associated factor for cervical spondylosis (Table 5).

Associated factors for cervical Spondylosis in the age subgroup

The characteristics of cervical spondylosis differed by age groups. For the people aged less than 30 years, work

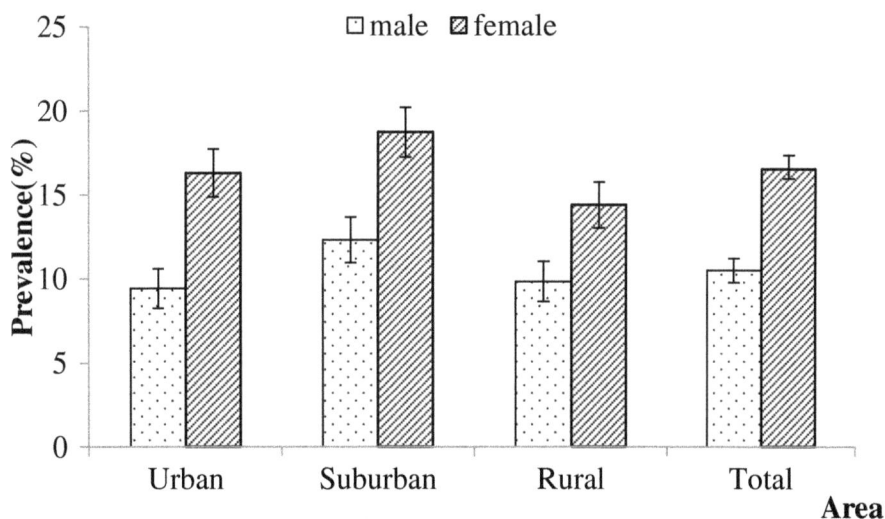

Fig. 3 The sex-specific prevalence of cervical spondylosis in different areas (I bar indicates prevalence ± standard error)

Table 2 Regional and Population-Based Distribution and Characteristics of Cervical spondylosis

	N	n	p	Sp	χ^2	p
Place of residence						
Urban	1293	169	13.07	0.94	8.257	0.016
Suburban	1284	205	15.97	1.02		
Rural	1282	157	12.25	0.92		
Age(years)						
< 30	813	37	4.55	0.73	118.304	< 0.001
30-	1065	114	10.70	0.95		
45-	1199	245	20.43	1.16		
≥ 60	772	130	16.84	1.35		
Sex						
Male	1820	191	10.49	0.72	29.432	< 0.001
Female	2029	335	16.51	0.82		
Education						
Undergraduate or higher	598	60	10.03	1.23	18.503	< 0.001
Junior college	689	75	10.89	1.19		
Senior high school	1121	167	14.90	1.06		
Junior high school or lower	1414	225	15.91	0.97		
BMI(kg/m^2)						
< 18.5	235	15	6.38	1.60	15.559	0.001
18.5-	1912	250	13.08	0.77		
24.0-	1324	201	15.18	0.99		
≥ 28.0	366	59	16.12	2.92		
Nature of labor						
Physical-based	1466	202	13.78	0.90	2.785	0.426
Mental-based	919	140	15.23	1.19		
Mixed	894	114	12.75	1.12		
Per capita monthly income level (¥)						
< 2000	2194	300	13.67	0.73	0.765	0.682
2000-	1400	198	14.14	0.93		
5000-	217	26	12.98	2.21		
Drinking						
Yes	768	115	14.97	1.29	1.191	0.275
No	3091	416	13.46	0.61		
Smoking						
Yes	929	110	11.84	1.06	3.798	0.051
No	2930	421	14.37	0.65		
Job posture						
Sitting	1280	180	14.06	0.97	5.746	0.219
Standing	799	104	13.02	1.19		
Frequently stooping	216	37	17.13	2.57		
Moving	1156	166	14.36	1.03		
Other	405	44	10.86	1.55		

Table 2 Regional and Population-Based Distribution and Characteristics of Cervical spondylosis *(Continued)*

	N	n	p	Sp	χ^2	p
Daily transportation tools						
Non manpower transportation tool	2116	271	12.81	0.73	8.744	0.013
Bicycle	743	127	17.09	1.38		
On foot	992	132	13.31	1.08		
Sleep duration per day (hours/day)						
≥ 7	3002	374	12.46	0.60	28.354	< 0.001
< 7	762	152	19.95	1.45		
Vibration						
Yes	334	50	14.97	2.96	0.451	0.502
No	3525	481	13.65	0.58		
Duration of the same work posture (hr/d)						
< 1	981	124	12.64	1.06	10.440	0.015
1-	987	164	16.62	1.19		
2-	477	69	14.47	1.61		
≥ 3	1411	174	12.33	0.88		
Exercise frequency						
≥ 2 times/week	1107	201	18.16	1.16	35.174	< 0.001
1 time/week	281	41	14.59	2.11		
1 time/2 weeks	77	8	10.39	3.50		
≤ 1 time/month	37	10	27.03	7.40		
No exercise	2336	267	11.43	0.66		
Exercise intensity						
None	2389	272	11.39	0.65	45.389	< 0.001
Mild	759	150	19.76	1.45		
Moderate	158	36	22.78	3.35		
Vigorous	553	73	13.20	1.44		
Waist–hip ratio						
Normal	1602	187	11.67	0.80	9.369	0.002
Central obesity	2243	339	15.11	0.76		
Menopause						
Yes	775	188	24.26	1.54	52.193	< 0.001
No	1145	134	11.70	0.95		

intensity, keeping the same work posture 1–2.9 h/day and the gender were the associated factors for cervical spondylosis. For the group between 30 years and 45 years old, housework intensity was the only associated factor. For 45 and 60 years group, living in the rural area, female gender, engaging in mental work, sleeping less than 7 h/day and vibration exposure in working condition were the associated factors. Going to work on foot was a protective factor for cervical spondylosis. For people aged no less than 60 years, housework intensity, engaging in mental work and mixed work, and daily sleep duration less than 7 h were the associated factors for cervical spondylosis (Table 6).

Discussion

This was an epidemiological study of cervical spondylosis in Chinese population. The prevalence of cervical spondylosis was 13.76%, which was higher than the prevalence of diabetes (9.7%) [17]. According to the data of the population census in 2011, approximately 2.75 million patients suffered from cervical spondylosis in Beijing, a city having a population of 20 million. The prevalence of cervical spondylosis was high not only in the Chinese population but also in other areas of the world. According to a cohort study, the incidence of cervical spondylosis was 13.1% overall, in a total of 47,560 patients [18]. A study in the southwest region of Nigeria found a prevalence of 10.7%

Table 3 The Influence of Working Intensity and Housework Intensity on Cervical spondylosis

	Cervical spondylosis		Not Cervical spondylosis		Kolmogorov-Smirnov Z	P
	meadian	QL	meadian	QL		
Working intensity	5	3	5	3	1.145	0.145
Housework intensity	3	3	3	3	2.918	< 0.001

for cervical spondylosis [19], which was similar to the results of the present study. This indicated that cervical spondylosis was a major public health problem that needed a large-scale intervention.

The prevalence among different age groups had an inverted U shape. The group aged between 45 years and 60 years had the highest prevalence. This might cause absence from work because of the symptoms caused by cervical spondylosis, such as neck pain and so on [20–22]. Therefore, this group needed more preventive measures. Several factors might affect cervical spondylosis. Irrespective of the case–control or longitudinal study, age was an important related factor for cervical spondylosis [23, 24]. These results were consistent with the findings of the present study. Moreover, the present study also revealed

that the strength of association in different age groups was different. Compared with the youngest age group, the adjusted OR was the highest in people aged between 45 and 60 years (OR = 5.303, 95% CI: 3.417–8.229) and second highest in those aged more than 60 years (OR = 4.722, 95% CI: 2.945–7.571). Several reasons might explain this. The first and the most important reason is that the characters might be different in the four age groups (Table 6). For example, for the youngest people aged less than 30 years, work intensity and keeping the same working posture for 1–3 h/day were the associated factors for cervical spondylosis. For people aged 30–45 years, housework intensity was the only associated factor for cervical spondylosis. This result indicated that the prevention measures should be

Table 4 Associated Factors of Cervical spondylosis by Multivariable Logistic Regression

	β	S.E	Wald	P	OR	95% CI	
						lower	upper
Place of residence			7.172	0.028			
Urban					1.000		
Suburban	0.383	0.147	6.809	0.009	1.467	1.100	2.957
Rural	0.302	0.160	3.544	0.060	1.352	0.988	1.851
Age(years)			68.947	< 0.001			
< 30					1.000		
30-	0.845	0.226	13.980	< 0.001	2.327	1.495	3.623
45-	1.668	0.224	55.351	< 0.001	5.303	3.417	8.229
≥ 60	1.552	0.241	41.538	< 0.001	4.722	2.945	7.571
Sex							
Male					1.000		
Female	0.591	0.120	24.146	< 0.001	1.805	1.426	2.285
Nature of labor			10.446	0.005			
Physical-based					1.000		
Mixed	0.207	0.157	1.742	0.187	1.230	0.905	1.671
Mental-based	0.502	0.157	10.260	0.001	1.653	1.215	2.247
Housework intensity	0.086	0.026	10.850	0.001	1.090	1.035	1.147
Modes of daily transportation			6.014	0.049			
Non manpower transportation tool					1.000		
Bicycle	−0.089	0.151	0.348	0.555	0.915	0.681	1.229
On foot	−0.371	0.152	5.966	0.015	0.690	0.512	0.929
Sleep duration per day (<7 h/day)	0.383	0.132	8.410	0.004	1.466	1.132	1.899

Table 5 Epidemiological Characteristics of Cervical spondylosis in Male and Female Populations

	β	Se	Wald	P	OR	95% CI	
						lower	upper
Males							
Age(years)			25.211	< 0.001			
< 30					1.000		
30-	1.027	0.383	7.209	0.007	2.793	1.320	5.911
45-	1.496	0.369	16.401	< 0.001	4.465	2.164	9.210
≥ 60	1.733	0.380	20.749	< 0.001	5.657	2.684	12.923
BMI(kg/m^2)			4.918	0.178			
18.5-					1.000		
< 18.5	−1.676	1.021	2.693	0.101	0.187	0.025	1.385
24-	0.152	0.189	0.649	0.421	1.164	0.804	1.687
≥ 28	0.388	0.299	1.679	0.195	1.474	0.820	2.649
Vibration(yes)	0.471	0.218	4.689	0.030	1.603	1.046	2.450
Females							
Place of residence			4.958	0.084			
Urban					1.000		
Suburban	0.442	0.211	4.389	0.036	1.556	1.029	2.354
Rural	0.413	0.235	3.097	0.078	1.512	0.954	2.397
Age(years)			46.433	< 0.001			
< 30					1.000		
30-	0.654	0.279	5.505	0.019	2.924	1.114	3.323
45-	1.644	0.273	36.222	< 0.001	5.177	3.031	8.843
≥ 60	1.271	0.298	18.135	< 0.001	3.565	2.986	6.399
Menopause(Yes)	0.572	0.217	6.983	0.008	1.772	1.159	2.710
Nature of labor			5.983	0.050			
Physical-based					1.000		
Mixed	0.411	0.225	3.339	0.068	1.508	0.971	2.344
Mental-based	0.522	0.222	5.537	0.019	1.686	1.091	2.605
Housework intensity	0.088	0.038	5.291	0.021	1.092	1.013	1.176
Daily transportation tools			10.013	0.007			
Non manpower transportation tool					1.000		
Bicycle	−0.169	0.211	0.638	0.424	0.845	0.558	1.278
On foot	−0.650	0.207	9.916	0.002	0.522	0.348	0.782
Sleep duration per day (<7 h/day)	0.474	0.187	6.401	0.011	1.606	1.113	2.318

different for different age groups. Second, the occurrence of cervical spondylosis as a chronic disease was the result of the long-term effect of the aforementioned factors. Considering the hysteresis effect, people younger than 60 years were the focus of prevention.

According to the report of Singh S et al., sex showed no significance with cervical spondylosis [23]. Sex was related with cervical spondylosis in this study. In the analysis of gender subgroups, age 30 years or older and vibration exposure in work environment were independent associated factors for cervical spondylosis in males; age 30 years or older, exposure to vibration during their daily work, menopause, those engaged in mental work, housework intensity, and those sleeping for less than 7 h/day were also the associated factors for cervical spondylosis for females, and going to work on foot was a protective factor for cervical spondylosis. The associated factors for females might be related to physiological characteristics and their division of labor.

Work-related factors, such as carrying head loads, were associated with cervical spondylosis [25–27]. For the youngest people aged less than 30 years, work

Table 6 Epidemiological Characteristics of Cervical spondylosis among Different Age Groups

	β	Se	Wald	P	OR	95% CI	
						lower	upper
< 30 years group							
Work intensity	0.329	0.091	13.242	< 0.001	1.390	1.164	1.660
Duration of the same work posture (hours)			9.144	0.027			
< 1					1.000		
1-	2.527	1.049	5.805	0.016	12.522	1.602	97.850
2-	2.169	1.078	4.050	0.044	8.750	1.058	72.346
≥ 3 h	1.629	1.038	2.462	0.117	5.099	0.666	39.013
Gender(Female)	0.917	0.427	4.614	0.032	2.501	1.084	5.771
30-years group							
Housework intensity	0.111	0.052	4.530	0.033	1.117	1.009	1.237
45- years group							
Place of residence			8.023	0.018			
Urban					1.000		
Suburban	0.387	0.239	2.619	0.106	1.473	0.921	2.355
Rural	0.696	0.246	8.020	0.005	2.006	1.239	3.248
Gender(Female)	1.085	0.193	31.782	< 0.001	2.961	2.030	4.318
Nature of labor			7.135	0.028			
Physical-based					1.000		
Mixed	0.067	0.248	0.072	0.788	1.069	0.657	1.739
Mental-based	0.616	0.243	6.439	0.011	1.852	1.151	2.980
Daily transportation tools			6.017	0.049			
Non manpower transportation tool					1.000		
Bicycle	−0.109	0.217	0.252	0.615	0.897	0.586	1.372
On foot	−0.561	0.233	5.793	0.016	0.571	0.361	0.901
Sleep duration per day (<7 h/day)	0.506	0.194	6.771	0.009	1.658	1.133	2.426
Vibration(Yes)	−0.563	0.276	4.156	0.041	0.570	0.332	0.979
≥60 years group							
Nature of labor			7.872	0.020			
Physical-based					1.000		
Mental-based	0.733	0.294	6.237	0.013	2.082	1.171	3.703
Mixed	0.667	0.294	5.153	0.023	2.948	1.095	3.464
Housework intensity	0.136	0.054	6.426	0.011	1.145	1.031	1.272
Sleep duration per day (<7 h/day)	0.518	0.254	4.166	0.041	1.679	1.021	2.760

intensity and keeping the same work posture ranging from 1 to 3 h/day were the associated factors for cervical spondylosis in the present study. Work intensity and the duration of keeping the same work posture were both indicators of neck loading. For this group of people, the cervical spine activity during the appropriate time interval might have some effects, such as turning the head. Occupation, sedentary lifestyle, and unhealthy working posture were the risk factors for cervical spondylosis [28]. For people younger than 30 years, those holding the same work posture for 1–1.9 h and 2–2.9 h had

positive relation with cervical spondylosis, respectively, compared with those who held the same posture for less than 1 h. The present study did not find a significant difference between people holding the same work posture for more than 3 h and those holding the same posture less than 1 h. It might be due to the adaptability of the human body. The present study suggested that the appropriate activity time interval was 1 or less than 1 h.

Occupational low back pain is strongly associated with vibration [29–33]. A positive dose relationship exists between them [34]. The whole-body vibration during daily work was an associated factor of cervical spondylosis in males in this study. Although no report demonstrated the relationship between vibration and cervical spondylosis, occupational factors contributing to the acceleration of spinal degeneration included vehicle driving [35]. Vehicle driving caused vibration. Vibration could cause bone metabolism disorder and bone damage of lumbar vertebra [36]. Therefore, the whole-body vibration was related with the cervical spine. This result could explain why people who traveled by foot had lower prevalence than those who used nonmanpower transportation tool to some degree. Also, going to work on foot gave the body some exercise. Although some exercises had higher risk, some had no risk and others have protective effect [22, 37–41], on foot had positive association on cervical spondylosis in this study.

One study found menopause as an associatedfactor for cervical spondylosis (OR = 1.772, 95% CI: 1.159–2.710). Estrogens can maintain collagens that protect the intervertebral disk [42]. Lou et al. found a relationship between menopause and the degeneration of intervertebral disk [43]. Moreover, the changes in hormone levels during menopause could lead to the degeneration of vertebral endplate, which affected the nutritional distribution of the intervertebral disk, ending in the degeneration of the spine [44]. Females in the perimenopausal period need some health interventions to protect their spine health.

BMI ≥ 28 kg/m^2 had a higher risk for lumbar osteoarthritis in the present study [15]. Obesity was a risk factor for intervertebral disk degeneration and spine disease [15, 46]. Obesity increased the weight of the skeleton and accelerated the intervertebral disk degeneration [47]. Besides, obesity was an inflammatory disorder that could cause the degeneration of intervertebral disk [48]. However, according to a 10-year cohort study [22], no association was found between obesity and degenerative cervical disease. In this study, the prevalence of cervical spondylosis was significantly different in different BMI groups and between normal and central obese groups according to the single-factor analysis. However, obesity and central obesity had no relation to cervical spondylosis in the multivariate analysis. This was probably because the anatomical position of the cervical vertebra was high in the body. It was less influenced by the weight of the body.

Moreover, the negative association between sleeping duration and cervical spondylosis was significant. This was possibly due to biomechanics and emotions. Weight loading was one of the important causes of spinal degeneration [49]. Short hours of sleep per day increased the weight loading time of the spine, thus accelerating its degeneration. Shorter sleep duration per day was associated with emotional stress. Emotional stress was associated with neck pain [50]. Neck pain usually was one of the possible symptoms in the process of cervical spondylosis.

The present study had two limitations. First, the prevalence of cervical spondylosis might have been underestimated because of the definition of cervical spondylosis. In this study, patients with cervical spondylosis were people not only having imaging changes but also having clinical symptoms. Therefore, people even having cervical degeneration imaging changes but no clinical symptoms were excluded. However, according to the current clinical guideline, people having not only imaging changes but also clinical symptoms needed treatment. In addition, if people don't diagnosed in hospital, they were not classified to cervical spondylosis patients.There may be more cervical spondylosis patients in Chinese population. Therefore, the influence of underestimation on policy decisions was less. Second, regarding the evidence level and the relevant strength of the cross-sectional study, a cohort study is needed to provide further evidence of the correlation between the associated factors and cervical spondylosis. However, our findings supplemented the information of cervical spondylosis prevalence in community people which has received little attention from other studies. At the same time, we also reported the prevalence and associated factors in both middle-young and old age group, which was scarcely reported before. Since the middle-young-aged population were the main social labor and should be the focal point for the prevention of cervical spondylosis. Our findings would provide valuable information for the prevention of the disease on lifestyle,especially for middle-young-aged population.

Conclusions

The prevalence of cervical spondylosis was high in Chinese population. People younger than 60 years were the focus of prevention. Moreover, the characters of between male and female and among different age groups were different and required targeted interventions.

Acknowledgements
The Second Hospital of Yanqing arranged the sampled community. The authors thank Tang Xun of Peking University for the design of this study. The authors also thank Xu Xiaochuan, Dr. Wang Yan, Dr. Zhang Guoying, Wang Fei, and Dr. Zhang Lifeng for their support in this survey.

Funding
This study was funded by Chinese National Natural Science Foundation(no:81400923), Beijing Municipal Administration of Hospitals' Youth Programme(no:QML20150405) and Key Project of Chinese National Programs(no:2016YFC0105800 &2016YFC0105801).

Authors' contributions
LVY designed this study and analyzed the data and was a major contributor in writing and revising. TIANW was a major contributor in conception and design and revising. CHEND was a major contributor in conception and design and revising it critically. LIUY made contributions in data collecting and drafting. WANGL contributed in analysis and interpretation of data and

writing. DUAN F made contributions in analysis of data and Writing. All authors read and approved the final manuscript.

Competing interests
The authors declare that they have no competing interests.

Author details
[1]Department of Epidemiology and Biostatistics, Public Health College, Peking University, 38# Xueyuan Road, Haidian district, Beijing 100191, China. [2]Clinical Epidemiology Research Center, Beijing Jishuitan Hospital, 31# Xinjiekou Dongjie, West district, Beijing 100035, China. [3]Department of Spine, Beijing Jishuitan Hospital, 31# Xinjiekou Dongjie, West district, Beijing 100035, China.

References
1. Xiong W, Li F, Guan H. Tetraplegia after thyroidectomy in a patient with cervical spondylosis: a case report and literature review. Medicine (Baltimore). 2015;94:e524.
2. Wang C, Tian F, Zhou Y, He W, Cai Z. The incidence of cervical spondylosis decreases with aging in the elderly, and increases with aging in the young and adult population: a hospital-based clinical analysis. Clin Interv Aging. 2016;11:47–53.
3. Stoffman MR, Roberts MS, King JJ. Cervical spondylotic myelopathy, depression, and anxiety: a cohort analysis of 89 patients. Neurosurgery. 2005;57:307–13. 307-313
4. Paanalahti K, Holm LW, Magnusson C, Carroll L, Nordin M, Skillgate E. The sex-specific interrelationship between spinal pain and psychological distress across time in the general population. Results from the Stockholm public health study. Spine Journal. 2014;14:1928–35.
5. Kelly JC, Groarke PJ, Butler JS, Poynton AR, O'Byrne JM. The natural history and clinical syndromes of degenerative cervical spondylosis. Adv Orthop. 2012;2012:393642.
6. Hartvigsen J, Christensen K, Frederiksen H. Back and neck pain exhibit many common features in old age: a population-based study of 4,486 Danish twins 70-102 years of age. Spine (Phila Pa 1976). 2004;29:576–80.
7. Goode AP, Freburger J, Carey T. Prevalence, practice patterns, and evidence for chronic neck pain. Arthritis Care Res (Hoboken). 2010;62:1594–601.
8. Vogt MT, Cawthon PM, Kang JD, Donaldson WF, Cauley JA, Nevitt MC. Prevalence of symptoms of cervical and lumbar stenosis among participants in the osteoporotic fractures in men study. Spine (Phila Pa 1976). 2006;31:1445–51.
9. Klussmann A, Gebhardt H, Liebers F, Rieger MA. Musculoskeletal symptoms of the upper extremities and the neck: a cross-sectional study on prevalence and symptom-predicting factors at visual display terminal (VDT) workstations. BMC Musculoskelet Disord. 2008;9:96.
10. Fejer R, Kyvik KO, Hartvigsen J. The prevalence of neck pain in the world population: a systematic critical review of the literature. Eur Spine J. 2006;15:834–48.
11. Global, regional, and national incidence, prevalence, and years lived with disability for 301 acute and chronic diseases and injuries in 188 countries, 1990-2013: a systematic analysis for the Global Burden of Disease Study 2013. Lancet. 2015;386:743–800.
12. Nagashima H, Dokai T, Hashiguchi H, Ishii H, Kameyama Y, Katae Y, et al. Clinical features and surgical outcomes of cervical spondylotic myelopathy in patients aged 80 years or older: a multi-center retrospective study. Eur Spine J. 2011;20:240–6.
13. Hadjipavlou AG, Tzermiadianos MN, Bogduk N, Zindrick MR. The pathophysiology of disc degeneration: a critical review. J Bone Joint Surg Br. 2008;90:1261–70.
14. Kepler CK, Hilibrand AS. Management of adjacent segment disease after cervical spinal fusion. Orthop Clin North Am. 2012;43:53–62.
15. Tian W, Lv Y, Liu Y, Xiao B, Han X. The high prevalence of symptomatic degenerative lumbar osteoarthritis in Chinese adults: a population-based study. Spine (Phila Pa 1976). 2014;39:1301–10.
16. Binder AI. Cervical spondylosis and neck pain. BMJ. 2007;334:527–31.
17. Yang W, Lu J, Weng J, Jia W, Ji L, Xiao J, et al. Prevalence of diabetes among men and women in China. N Engl J Med. 2010;362:1090–101.
18. Schairer WW, Carrer A, Lu M, Hu SS. The increased prevalence of cervical spondylosis in patients with adult thoracolumbar spinal deformity. J Spinal Disord Tech. 2014;27:E305–8.
19. Oguntona SA. Cervical spondylosis in south west Nigerian farmers and female traders. Ann Afr Med. 2014;13:61–4.
20. Labbafinejad Y, Imanizade Z, Danesh H. Ergonomic risk factors and their association with lower back and neck pain among pharmaceutical employees in Iran. Workplace Health & Safety. 2016;64:586–95.
21. Andersen LL, Mortensen OS, Hansen JV, Burr H. A prospective cohort study on severe pain as a risk factor for long-term sickness absence in blue- and white-collar workers. Occup Environ Med. 2011;68:590–2.
22. Mesas AE, Gonzalez AD, Mesas CE, de Andrade SM, Magro IS, Del LJ. The association of chronic neck pain, low back pain, and migraine with absenteeism due to health problems in Spanish workers. Spine (Phila Pa 1976). 2014;39:1243–53.
23. Okada E, Matsumoto M, Ichihara D, Chiba K, Toyama Y, Fujiwara H, et al. Aging of the cervical spine in healthy volunteers: a 10-year longitudinal magnetic resonance imaging study. Spine (Phila Pa 1976). 2009;34:706–12.
24. Singh S, Kumar D, Kumar S. Risk factors in cervical spondylosis. J Clin Orthop Trauma. 2014;5:221–6.
25. Yang H, Haldeman S, Nakata A, Choi B, Delp L, Baker D. Work-related risk factors for neck pain in the US working population. Spine (Phila Pa 1976). 2015;40:184–92.
26. Nordander C, Hansson GA, Ohlsson K, Arvidsson I, Balogh I, Stromberg U, et al. Exposure-response relationships for work-related neck and shoulder musculoskeletal disorders--analyses of pooled uniform data sets. Appl Ergon. 2016;55:70–84.
27. Naidoo RN, Haq SA. Occupational use syndromes. Best Pract Res Clin Rheumatol. 2008;22:677–91.
28. Haldeman S, Carroll L, Cassidy JD. Findings from the bone and joint decade 2000 to 2010 task force on neck pain and its associated disorders. J Occup Environ Med. 2010;52:424–7.
29. Shelerud RA. Epidemiology of occupational low back pain. Clin Occup Environ Med. 2006;5:501–28.
30. Murgia N, Dell'Omo M, Gambelunghe A, Folletti I, Muzi G, Abbritti G. Epidemiological evidence of possible musculoskeletal, cardiovascular and neoplastic effects in professional drivers. G Ital Med Lav Ergon. 2012;34:310–3.
31. Murtezani A, Ibraimi Z, Sllamniku S, Osmani T, Sherifi S. Prevalence and risk factors for low back pain in industrial workers. Folia Med (Plovdiv). 2011;53:68–74.
32. Palmer KT, Griffin M, Ntani G, Shambrook J, McNee P, Sampson M, et al. Professional driving and prolapsed lumbar intervertebral disc diagnosed by magnetic resonance imaging: a case-control study. Scand J Work Environ Health. 2012;38:577–81.
33. Milosavljevic S, Bagheri N, Vasiljev RM, McBride DI, Rehn B. Does daily exposure to whole-body vibration and mechanical shock relate to the prevalence of low back and neck pain in a rural workforce? Ann Occup Hyg. 2012;56:10–7.
34. Teschke K, Nicol AM, Davies H, Ju S. Whole body vibrations and back disorders among motor vehicle drivers and heavy equipment operators: a review of the scientific evidence. Occup Hyg; 1999.
35. Magora A. Investigation of the relation between low back pain and occupation. IMS Ind Med Surg. 1970;39:465–71.
36. Chang Q, Wei F, Zhang L, Ju X, Zhu L, Huang C, et al. Effects of vibration in forced posture on biochemical bone metabolism indices, and morphometric and mechanical properties of the lumbar vertebra. PLoS One. 2013;8:e78640.
37. Toueg CW, Mac-Thiong JM, Grimard G, Parent S, Poitras B, Labelle H. Prevalence of spondylolisthesis in a population of gymnasts. Stud Health Technol Inform. 2010;158:132–7.
38. Triantafillou KM, Lauerman W, Kalantar SB. Degenerative disease of the cervical spine and its relationship to athletes. Clin Sports Med. 2012;31:509–20.
39. Chang SK, Tominaga GT, Wong JH, Weldon EJ, Kaan KT. Risk factors for water sports-related cervical spine injuries. J Trauma. 2006;60:1041–6.
40. Rastogi R, Bendore P. Effect of naturopathy treatments and yogic practices on cervical Spondylosis--a case report. Indian J Physiol Pharmacol. 2015;59:442–5.
41. Shakoor MA, Ahmed MS, Kibria G, Khan AA, Mian MA, Hasan SA, et al. Effects of cervical traction and exercise therapy in cervical spondylosis. Bangladesh Med Res Counc Bull. 2002;28:61–9.
42. Calleja-Agius J, Muscat-Baron Y, Brincat MP. Estrogens and the intervertebral disc. Menopause Int. 2009;15:127–30.
43. Lou C, Chen HL, Feng XZ, Xiang GH, Zhu SP, Tian NF, et al. Menopause is associated with lumbar disc degeneration: a review of 4230 intervertebral discs. Climacteric. 2014;17:700–4.
44. Wang YX, Griffith JF. Menopause causes vertebral endplate degeneration and decrease in nutrient diffusion to the intervertebral discs. Med Hypotheses. 2011;77:18–20.
45. Teraguchi M, Yoshimura N, Hashizume H, Muraki S, Yamada H, Minamide A, et al. Prevalence and distribution of intervertebral disc degeneration over the entire spine in a population-based cohort: the Wakayama spine study. Osteoarthr Cartil. 2014;22:104–10.

46. Fanuele JC, Abdu WA, Hanscom B, Weinstein JN. Association between obesity and functional status in patients with spine disease. Spine (Phila Pa 1976). 2002;27:306–12.

47. Ricart W, Lopez J, Mozas J, Pericot A, Sancho MA, Gonzalez N, et al. Body mass index has a greater impact on pregnancy outcomes than gestational hyperglycaemia. Diabetologia. 2005;48:1736–42.

48. Rannou F, Corvol MT, Hudry C, Anract P, Dumontier MF, Tsagris L, et al. Sensitivity of anulus fibrosus cells to interleukin 1 beta. Comparison with articular chondrocytes Spine (Phila Pa 1976). 2000;25:17–23.

49. Inoue N, Espinoza OA. Biomechanics of intervertebral disk degeneration. Orthop Clin North Am. 2011;42:487–99.

50. Cote P, van der Velde G, Cassidy JD, Carroll LJ, Hogg-Johnson S, Holm LW, et al. The burden and determinants of neck pain in workers: results of the bone and joint decade 2000-2010 task force on neck pain and its associated disorders. J Manip Physiol Ther. 2009;32:S70–86.

9

Promoting the use of self-management in novice chiropractors treating individuals with spine pain: the design of a theory-based knowledge translation intervention

Owis Eilayyan[1,2]*, Aliki Thomas[1,2], Marie-Christine Hallé[1,2], Sara Ahmed[1,2], Anthony C. Tibbles[3], Craig Jacobs[3], Silvano Mior[3], Connie Davis[4,5], Roni Evans[6], Michael J. Schneider[7], Fadi Alzoubi[1,2], Jan Barnsley[8], Cynthia R. Long[9] and Andre Bussières[1,2]

Abstract

Background: Clinical practice guidelines generally recommend clinicians use self-management support (SMS) when managing patients with spine pain. However, even within the educational setting, the implementation of SMS remains suboptimal. The objectives of this study were to 1) estimate the organizational readiness for change toward using SMS at the Canadian Memorial Chiropractic College (CMCC), Toronto, Ontario from the perspective of directors and deans, 2) estimate the attitudes and self-reported behaviours towards using evidence-based practice (EBP), and beliefs about pain management among supervisory clinicians and chiropractic interns, 3) identify potential barriers and enablers to using SMS, and 4) design a theory-based tailored Knowledge Translation (KT) intervention to increase the use of SMS.

Methods: Mixed method design. We administered three self-administered questionnaires to assess clinicians' and interns' attitudes and behaviours toward EBP, beliefs about pain management, and practice style. In addition, we conducted 3 focus groups with clinicians and interns based on the Theoretical Domain Framework (TDF) to explore their beliefs about using SMS for patients with spine pain. Data were analysed using deductive thematic analysis by 2 independent assessors. A panel of 7 experts mapped behaviour change techniques to key barriers identified informing the design of a KT intervention.

Results: Participants showed high level of EBP knowledge, positive attitude of EBP, and moderate frequency of EBP use. A number of barrier factors were identified from clinicians ($N = 6$) and interns ($N = 16$) corresponding to 7 TDF domains: *Knowledge; Skills; Environmental context and resources; Emotion; Beliefs about Capabilities; Memory, attention & decision making;* and *Social Influence.* To address these barriers, the expert panel proposed a multifaceted KT intervention composed of a webinar and online educational module on a SMS guided by the Brief Action Planning, clinical vignettes, training workshop, and opinion leader support.

(Continued on next page)

* Correspondence: owis.eilayyan@mail.mcgill.ca
[1]School of Physical and Occupational Therapy, McGill University, 3654 Prom Sir-William-Osler, Montréal, QC H3G 1Y5, Canada
[2]Center for Interdisciplinary Research in Rehabilitation of Greater Montreal (CRIR), Montréal, Canada
Full list of author information is available at the end of the article

(Continued from previous page)

Conclusion: SMS strategies can help maximizing the health care services for patients with spine pain. This may in turn optimize patients' health. The proposed theory-based KT intervention may facilitate the implementation of SMS among clinicians and interns.

Keywords: Spine pain, Self-management, Theory-based intervention, Knowledge translation, Theoretical domain framework, Chiropractic, Brief action planning

Background

Spine pain is very common and is a leading cause of disability worldwide [1–5]. Between 50 and 80% of adults suffer from spine pain during their lives [6, 7], which is associated with a high individual (physical, psychological, emotional) and societal burden [6, 8–16]. In Canada, the estimated direct cost of spine pain ranges from $6 to $12 billion annually [17].

Many people with spine pain consult chiropractors for pain relief [18–20]. Clinical practice guidelines (CPGs) generally recommend offering self-management support (SMS) strategies to individuals with spine pain [21–28] as these help reduce the associated individual and societal burden [29]. SMS strategies are designed to facilitate adoption of healthy lifestyle in people with a range of health issues including spine pain and related co-morbidities (e.g. heart disease, type 2 diabetes, depression) [30–39]. In patients with spine pain, SMS can help decrease levels of pain, disability, and psychological distress [40, 41]. However, the routine adoption of evidence-based practices (EBPs) including the use of CPGs remains suboptimal among care providers including chiropractors [42–45]. Barriers to implementing EBPs among chiropractors include: lack of time, lack of generalizability of guidelines, lack of compensation, time since graduation greater than 10 years, insufficient skills or confidence in using findings from the literature, predefined beliefs and a more narrowed scope of practice [43].

SMS interventions empower the patient to be efficiently involved in their own care by involving them in the decision-making process [46, 47]. SMS strategies also necessitate a close collaboration between clinicians and patients [47–49]. However, a number of barriers to implementing SMS among clinicians have been documented, including: the lack of sufficient knowledge and skills to empower patients or to provide them with useful information, lack of time, and unfavourable patient views about this approach. Inadequate communication between clinicians and patients may also limit the use of SMS [50–53]. In addition, organizational barriers could restrict the use of SMS in clinical settings, such as patient overload, short treatment session, and long waiting lists [53]. Together, these barriers can contribute to reducing the effectiveness of SMS. Given the documented barriers to adoption of EBPs - and SMS in particular - changing clinicians' behaviour is challenging [43, 54].

Knowledge Translation (KT) is an approach used to facilitate' behavioural change in practitioners [55]. It can be used to promote the early use of EBP and CPGs during professional training, which may be more effective than changing existing professional practice to support the long-term use of best evidence [56, 57]. EBP requires the integration of research evidence, clinical expertise and patients' preferences into clinical decision-making [58]. Systematic reviews suggest that, while classroom-based teaching primarily improves EBP knowledge, clinically integrated teaching of EBP may be the most effective approach for improving the knowledge, attitudes, skills and behaviours associated with the use of EBP. Thus, academic programs must first lay down the foundations of EBP over the course of professional training, and then move students along a trajectory of progressive development of EBP competencies [56, 59]. Clinically integrated teaching of EBP delivered in the clinical setting can support deeper reflection on practice through actual patient management [60, 61].

Thus, providing chiropractic interns with the opportunity to routinely use CPGs to inform their clinical decisions should increase the likelihood of uptake and sustained use of EBP in their future practices. These interns will be more likely to become lifelong learners and reflective practitioners who will be equipped to overcome barriers to the use of CPGs - including SMS – and contribute to reducing research-practice gaps [43].

In Canada, the majority of practising chiropractors (58%) are trained at the Canadian Memorial Chiropractic College (CMCC) [62]. While CMCC revised its curriculum to promote the sustainable use of EBP among graduates, structured SMS that allows for patient-centred goals such as the Brief Action Planning (BAP) [63] has not yet been integrated into the curriculum [64]. Consequently, supervisory clinicians and interns do not systematically use SMS with patients across the CMCC outpatient teaching clinics [64].

The objectives of this study were to 1) estimate the organizational readiness for change toward using SMS at the Canadian Memorial Chiropractic College (CMCC), Toronto, Ontario from the perspective of Directors and Deans, 2) estimate the attitudes towards and self-reported use of evidence-based practice (EBP) behaviours, as well as beliefs about pain management among supervisory clinicians and chiropractic interns, 3) identify potential barriers and enablers to using SMS, and 4) design a theory-based tailored Knowledge Translation (KT) intervention to increase the use of SMS.

Conceptual framework

The Theoretical Domain Framework (TDF) has been used across several health disciplines, settings, and conditions to assess barriers to change and guide the development of theory-based interventions [65–69]. The TDF covers the main factors that influence behaviour change in clinical practice: *Knowledge, Skills, Social/Professional Role and Identity, Beliefs about Capabilities, Optimism, Beliefs about Consequences, Reinforcement, Intentions, Goals, Memory/Attention and Decision Processes, Environmental Context and Resources, Social Influences, Emotion,* and *Behavioural Regulation* [70].

Materials
Study design

Mixed-methods sequential transformative design comprising both quantitative and qualitative analyses. Ethical approval was obtained from the Research Ethics Board of McGill University (McGill IRB: A08-E54-16B), and written informed consent was obtained from all participants.

Setting

Five outpatient-teaching clinics of the Canadian Memorial Chiropractic College (CMCC), a major teaching institution in Ontario were approached to participate in the study.

The development of a KT intervention aiming to promote the use of SMS was guided by a systematic approach proposed by French et al. (2012) [69]. The approach includes 4 questions:

1) Who needs to do what, differently? (i.e. identify the evidence-practice gap). For this question, the literature suggests that the use of SMS among clinicians is suboptimal [50–53].
2) Using a theoretical framework (i.e. TDF [70]), which barriers and enablers need to be addressed? and
3) Which intervention components (behaviour change techniques and mode(s) of delivery) could overcome the modifiable barriers and enhance the enablers?

The latter 2 questions were addressed in two separate phases: Phase 1A aimed to 1) explore CMCC organizational readiness to use of EBP and SMS (Quantitative), 2) explore clinicians' and interns' behaviours and attitudes towards the use of EBP and their beliefs about pain management (Quantitative). Phase 1B aimed to identify barriers and enablers to the use of SMS

among a subgroup of clinicians and interns who were representative of CMCC clinicians and interns in terms of age, gender, and years of experience (Qualitative). Results from phase 1 were integrated and used to inform phase 2, where we mapped key barriers to using SMS. Ultimately, the findings served to design KT intervention components to address these barriers.

4) How can behaviour change be measured and understood? This question is beyond the scope of this paper.

Phase 1A targeting objectives 1 and 2: Clinicians' and interns' behaviours and attitudes toward EBP use, and the organizational readiness for change in healthcare settings (Quantitative Data)

Participants Chiropractic interns working within 20 Patient Management Teams (PMTs) and their 20 supervisory clinicians were invited to participate in this phase. Chiropractic interns had to be in their final year at CMCC and working in one of these 20 PMTs. Directors and deans at CMCC (decision makers) were also invited to participate in the study.

Data collection Study instruments

The decision makers at CMCC completed the Organizational Readiness for Implementing Change (ORIC) questionnaire which assesses organizational readiness for change in healthcare settings [71]. Clinicians and interns completed 3 self-administered questionnaires: 1) The Knowledge, Attitude, and Behaviour Questionnaire (KABQ) that assesses knowledge, attitudes, and behaviour toward EBP [72], 2) the Pain Attitudes and Beliefs Scale (PABS) which assesses the strength of 2 treatment orientations of health care practitioners: biomedical and behavioural orientations [73], and 3) the practice style questionnaire to classify clinicians and interns based on their practice [74].

Organizational readiness for implementing change (ORIC) The ORIC is comprised of 12 questions forming 2 domains: change commitment and change efficacy [71]. Each question is rated on 5-point Likert scale (Strongly Disagree – Strongly Agree), scores range 12–60, with higher scores indicating high readiness for change among organization members [71]. The ORIC has good psychometric properties [71].

Knowledge, attitude, and behaviour questionnaire (KABQ) The KABQ is a 33–item validated questionnaire comprised of 4 EBP domains: knowledge, attitudes, behaviours and outcomes/decisions [72]. The 'knowledge' domain includes 8 items each rated on a 7-point Likert scale, with higher scores indicating a higher level of EBP knowledge. The 'attitudes towards EBP' domain contains 14 items rated on a 7-point Likert scale, with higher scores indicating more positive attitudes toward EBP. The "Behaviour towards EBP" domain includes 8 items rated on a 5-point Likert scale, with higher scores indicating a higher frequency of using EBP. Lastly, the "outcomes/decisions" domain includes 3 items rated on a 6-point Likert scale, with lower scores indicating less favourable patient outcomes and poorer clinical evidence-based decision making [72]. This questionnaire has demonstrated good psychometric properties [72].

Pain attitudes and beliefs scale (PABS) The PABS questionnaire assesses the strength of 2 treatment orientations of health care practitioners: biomedical and behavioural orientations [73]. The amended version of the PABS is comprised of 19 items (10 biomedical items and 9 behavioural items) [75]. Each question is rated on a 6-point scale "('Totally disagree' = 1 to 'Totally agree' = 6)", where higher scores on a subscale indicate a stronger treatment orientation [75]. The PABS has acceptable psychometric properties [73, 76].

Practice style questionnaire The practice style questionnaire is used to classify clinicians into 4 categories based on their style of practice: Seekers, Receptives, Traditionalists, and Pragmatists [74]. The questionnaire includes 17 statements about clinicians' practice rated on 5-point Likert scale (Strongly Agree – Strongly Disagree).

Procedure A member of the research team and Director of Clinical Education and Patient Care at CMCC (C.J.) personally introduced the study to the CMCC decision makers ($N = 20$) and at a faculty meeting. Decision makers who agreed to participate in the study completed the ORIC tool online.

We first pilot tested the KABQ, PABS, and practice style questionnaires with one volunteering PMT composed of a supervisory clinician and seven interns. Team member (C.J.) sent these PMT participants an email with a link to the online survey along with a feedback form. Respondents were invited to indicate the length of time needed to complete the questionnaire and any questions or comments they had regarding the clarity of the questionnaires. Feedback received allowed the research team to correct typographical errors and develop an appendix providing additional clarifications for a few questions for which the wording or the meaning appeared to be confusing. C.J. then sent an email to all supervisory clinicians ($N = 20$) and interns ($N = 173$) of the remaining PMTs informing them about the study (e.g., goal, timeline and procedures) and inviting them to dedicate half an hour of their administrative time to complete the

questionnaires in the upcoming week. To avoid coercion, clinicians were invited to complete the same questionnaires at the same time as their interns, but in a different room. All supervisory clinicians and interns received the link to the online surveys and the appendix providing additional clarifications about the surveys via an email sent by C.J. An online consent form preceded the surveys.

Sample size and data analysis Descriptive analysis was conducted for the 4 administered questionnaires using SAS 9.4 [77]. The scores were calculated for each subscale of the KABQ, PABS, and ORIC. For the practice style questionnaire, the frequency of each category was calculated. The associations between demographic variables and the sub-scores/total score of each questionnaire were assessed using simple and multiple linear regression models. The socio-demographic variables included age, gender, education, grade point average (GPA), and clinical experience. B-coefficients were used to assess the association between KABQ and PABS with other factors. All studied factors were considered as categorical variables with the exception of age, which was a continuous variable.

Sample size in multiple regression depends upon the number of studied variables following the rule of thumb of ($N \geq 50 + 8$ m), where m refers to number of studied (predictors) variables [78]. As this study included 5 predictors, a sample size of 106 subjects was needed to run a multiple linear regression with an alpha of 0.05 and 80% power (as a function of medium effect size) [78, 79].

Phase 1B: Barriers and enablers to the use SMS (qualitative)

We conducted three 90-min focus groups with a subset of supervisory chiropractors and interns to identify the key barriers and enablers to the use SMS.

Focus group guide The interview topic guide was developed based on the TDF framework [70] and further informed by our previous work [80–84]. The topic guide included 27 open-ended questions which covered all 14 TDF domains, with on average 2–3 questions per domain. Probing questions were used for further clarification if needed (See Additional file 1). Each focus group took approximately 90 min.

Procedure A member of the research team (C.J.) sent an invitation email to all clinicians and interns at CMCC to participate in a focus group. The email included a link to an online form requesting potential participants' authorization to be contacted by the research team and asking them to provide their name, contact information and a few socio-demographic information. Three focus groups were conducted: one with 6 clinicians, and two with 8 interns each. All focus groups took place in person at CMCC. A research assistant, experienced in conducting qualitative interviews based on the TDF, facilitated the focus groups. All participants completed and signed a consent form prior to the focus groups. Each focus group took approximately 90 min, was audio recorded, anonymized and transcribed verbatim.

Data analysis The analysis in this study followed the same analysis used by the research team previously [68, 82]. The focus group data were coded deductively by 2 independent reviewers (HO & OE). Disagreements were resolved by 2 other team members who have previous experience with using the TDF (AB and FZ). Each transcript was divided into different statements that were coded into relevant TDF domains. Statements were then linked with specific beliefs. A specific belief is defined as "a core statement that captures a common theme from multiple response statements and provides detail about the role of a given domain in influencing practice behaviour" [68, 80]. The specific beliefs were classified into one of 3 categories based on the likelihood that they would 1) increase (facilitator), 2) decrease (barrier), or 3) have no influence on the use of SMS. Similar specific beliefs within each TDF domain were identified and grouped into overarching themes. Three criteria were used concurrently to identify the key barriers: frequency of belief, importance of the belief, and contrasting beliefs.

Sample size The sample size needed for deriving thematic saturation from focus groups cannot be determined in advance. The literature suggests having 2–3 focus groups, a size of 8 participants each to discover most of the themes about the studied area [85]. There was no a priori plan to assess the saturation of focus group data. However, both clinicians and interns indicated almost identical barriers to using SMS.

Phase 2: Intervention design The aim of phase 2 was to review the key barriers identified in phase 1 in order to inform the design of a KT intervention to address these barriers.

Participants Seven research team members with experience using Behaviour Change Techniques (BCTs) and the TDF attended a half-day meeting to consider and propose possible KT intervention components. The team included 3 KT researchers, a researcher in medical education, 2 CMCC faculty members, and 1 patient representative.

Procedure All possible KT intervention components were first selected by a subgroup of 3 team members (AB, AT, OE) after mapping key TDF barriers onto corresponding BCTs (as per Michie et al. [86, 87]). Other team members received the results of this mapping exercise for consideration prior to the group meeting. Findings were reviewed by the team members, and they were asked to brainstorm other possible KT intervention components. Consensus on the selection of KT intervention components and modes of delivery was reached based on the evidence of their effectiveness and the feasibility of implementation.

The selected KT interventions in this study that aimed to promote the use of SMS were guided by Brief Action Planning (BAP) framework [63]. The literature supported the use of the BAP framework to enable the implementation of SMS [63, 88]. The framework was developed based on motivational interviewing, and it was considered an excellent SMS program for busy clinics [63].

Results
Phase 1A— ORIC, KABQ, BAPS and practice style
The data set included 12 decision makers, 14 clinicians, 115 chiropractic interns, with a mean age of 57 ± 6.3 years, 46 ± 12 years and 27 ± 2.4 years, respectively. Twenty-five percent of decision makers, 14% of clinicians, and 46% of interns and were females. The raw data are presented in Additional files 2 & 3.

Results from the ORIC showed that decision makers perceived that members of the CMCC were highly committed (mean = 20.6 ± 3.5) to, and confident about (mean = 29.3 ± 4) implementing SMS for patients with spine pain in CMCC outpatient teaching clinics, Fig. 1 A&B.

Results from the KABQ revealed that both clinicians and interns had high levels of knowledge about EBP (Clinician mean = 29.1 ± 3.7, Intern mean = 28.5 ± 4), positive attitudes towards the use of EBP (Clinician mean = 50.1 ± 6.2, Intern mean = 54.4 ± 5.4) and moderate frequency of using EBP (Clinician mean = 12.9 ± 3.3, Intern mean = 12.8 ± 2.8). The participants reported having favourable patient outcomes and good clinical evidence-based decision-making (Clinician mean = 13.3 ± 2.9, Intern mean = 12.1 ± 2.2). While interns had a significantly stronger behavioural than biomedical treatment orientation, clinicians did not show a significant difference in treatment orientation (Table 1). Lastly, 54% (7/13) of clinicians have a traditional practice style (their intervention decisions are guided by their clinical experience [89]), while 81% (87/108) of interns have a pragmatic practice style (their practice primarily depends on the workload [89]). Neither clinicians nor interns were classified as seekers (their intervention decisions are guided by evidence [89]), Fig. 2.

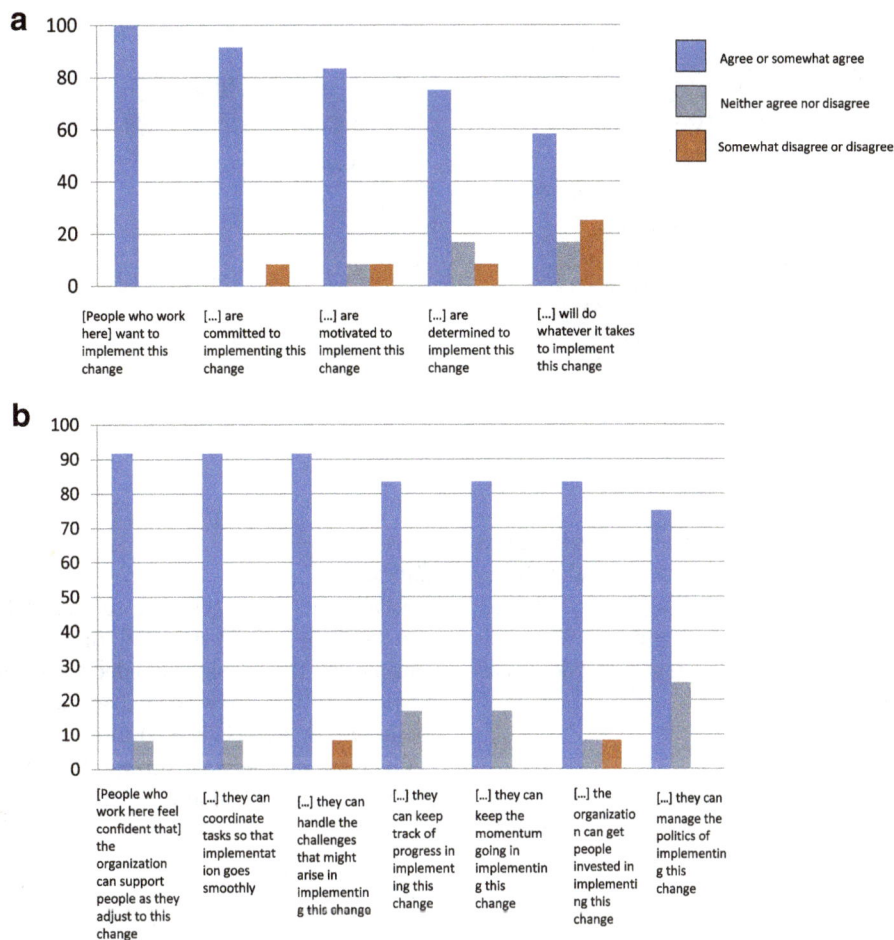

Fig. 1 Response frequency (%) on ORIC. **a** Response frequency (%) on the "Change commitment subscale" of the ORIC, **b** Response frequency (%) on the "Change efficacy (confidence) subscale" of the ORIC. Agree or somewhat agree, Neither agree nor disagree, Somewhat disagree or disagree

The multiple regression models showed that none of the demographic factors appeared to influence the interns' self-reported use of EBP. However, the model revealed that men had significantly higher knowledge of EBP than women ($\beta = 1.74$, $p = 0.043$) and interns who had a previous university degree had more negative attitudes toward EBP ($\beta = 4.3$, $p = 0.035$). Regression analyses were not conducted on the clinician and decision-maker data due to the small sample sizes.

Phase 1B—Focus groups

We conducted one focus group with 6 supervisory clinicians and 2 focus groups with 8 interns each. Clinicians'

and interns' average age was 40.8 ± 6 years and 27 ± 2.8 years, respectively. Almost 33% (2/6) and 44% (7/16) of the clinicians and interns were females, respectively. Clinicians who participated in the focus group had an average of 12.7 ± 4.4 years of clinical experience.

Key themes identified within relevant domains

We identified 720 statements from clinicians representing 38 specific beliefs and 18 themes. For interns, 509 statements were found and represented 56 specific beliefs and 22 themes (Additional files 4, 5, 6 and 7). Four key TDF domains were considered to have a greater likelihood to influence the targeted behaviour among both clinicians and

Table 1 Behavioural and biomedical treatment orientation among supervisory clinicians and interns

Group	Behavioural Treatment Orientation	Biomedical Treatment Orientation	p-value*
Clinicians (N = 13)	34.69 (5.7)	29.31 (7.4)	0.12
Interns (N = 108)	34.96 (4.3)	32.6 (5.9)	0.001

*Dependent t test

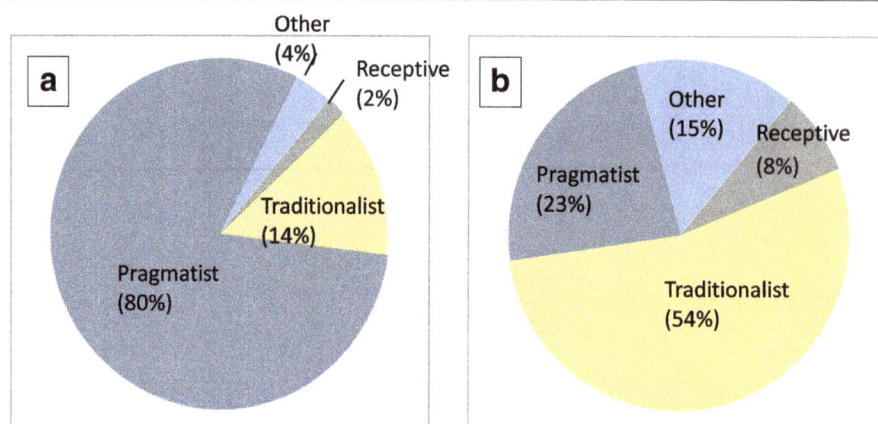

Fig. 2 Interns' and clinicians' practice style trait. **a** Interns' practice style trait, **b** Clinicians' practice style trait

interns: 1) Knowledge; 2) Skills; 3) Environmental context and resources; and 4) Emotion. In addition, another 3 key TDF domains were considered to have a greater influence on the targeted behaviour among only interns: 1) Beliefs about Capabilities; 2) Memory, attention and decision making; and 3) Social Influence.

Key TDF domains (phase 1)
Shared domains by supervisory clinicians and interns
Four key TDF domains were shared by both clinicians and interns: 1) Knowledge; 2) Skills; 3) Environmental context and resources; and 4) Emotions.

Knowledge
Clinicians
Sixteen statements were mapped to the knowledge domain. Three specific beliefs corresponded to the statements forming 2 themes: awareness of SMS and knowledge of SMS. Almost all clinicians stated that they did not attend a specific course on SMS, and that they had acquired a little knowledge of SMS from different courses. In addition, they said that there was a lack of a comprehensive SMS course. Most participants indicated that they were aware of SMS guidelines and evidence.

There were conflicting opinions between clinicians regarding interns' knowledge of SMS: 3 clinicians considered that interns to lack knowledge of SMS, while 2 clinicians considered interns to have adequate knowledge of SMS.

Interns
Fifty-four statements were associated with the knowledge domain. Three specific beliefs corresponded to the statements forming 2 themes: awareness of SMS and knowledge of SMS. Most interns indicated that they were aware of SMS guidelines and evidence, and had enough knowledge of SMS. Few interns stated that formal SMS courses were needed.

Skills
Clinicians
Twelve statements referred to the skills domain. Two specific beliefs corresponded to the statements representing one theme: skills needed to use SMS. Most clinicians stated that they needed to gain the skills required to use SMS, especially communication skills. Also, the clinicians indicated that interns had the skills needed to use SMS, as they had already attended SMS lectures.

Interns
Forty-one statements pertained to the skills domain. These statements formed 3 specific beliefs and one theme: skills needed to use SMS. Almost half of interns stated that they lacked the skills to use SMS efficiently, and indicated that they were not trained on SMS. Furthermore, the interns referred to the need for training courses to gain skills required to use SMS. Few interns mentioned that they lacked the skills to support behavioral change.

Environmental context and resources
Clinicians
Thirty-one clinician statements were mapped on to the environmental context and resources domain. These statements represented 4 specific beliefs and formed 3 themes: 1) lack of time; 2) clinic's characteristics; and 3) patients' characteristics. Most of the clinicians stated that lack of time was a barrier to the use of SMS. Participants reported that the clinic's characteristics (e.g. having rehabilitation equipment and sufficient space, collaborative clinicians, and having interns on placement) could facilitate the use of SMS among clinicians. Furthermore, clinicians indicated that patient's characteristics could restrict the use of SMS, including patient's lack of compliance, resources, or time; patient's priorities; psychological overlay; not accepting the condition;

not trusting the clinicians; and/or language and cultural barriers.

Interns

Seventy statements linked to the environmental context and resources. The statements represented 8 specific beliefs and formed 6 themes: 1) lack of time; 2) clinic's characteristics; 3) patients' characteristics; 4) financial issues; 5) lack of guidelines; and 6) course training. Almost half of interns stated that lack of time was a barrier to the use of SMS. Interns who participated in the focus groups listed the clinic's characteristics that could facilitate the use of SMS: collaborative clinicians, having kinesiology students to refer patients to, and smaller caseload. On the other hand, interns indicated that certain clinic characteristics could restrict the use of SMS: lack of space and equipment, staff shortage, clinician characteristics (unaware of guidelines), lack of communication with peers, and not having enough exposure to different patient conditions. Furthermore, the interns stated that certain patient characteristics could restrict the use of SMS, including: fear avoidance behaviour, lack of patient adherence to SMS, lack of patient motivation to use SMS, and/or patient preference for passive care.

In addition, interns reported 2 additional major barriers: financial considerations and internship requirements. The interns believed that focusing on SMS and active care may result in losing patients who preferred a passive care approach. Interns were also concerned that using SMS would increase the duration of their treatment sessions, thereby causing them to see fewer patients. Regarding internship program requirements, the interns stated that the use of SMS was not a program requirement.

Emotion

Clinicians

Eleven statements were associated with the emotion domain. These statements corresponded to 3 specific beliefs and formed one theme: anxiety about the use of SMS. Although almost all clinicians felt anxious when using SMS with patients who had psychological overlay, almost half of participants felt excited about using SMS. One clinician felt terrified of having self-management guidelines; he thought that this might discourage students from using their clinical judgement.

Interns

Thirty-three statements mapped to the emotion domain. The statements corresponded to 5 specific beliefs and formed one theme: feelings toward the use of SMS. Some interns felt concerned and frustrated when patients did not adhere to SMS or if they had psychological overlay. On the other hand, some interns felt exited and optimistic about the use of SMS. Furthermore, some interns stated that they felt disappointed because of certain clinicians' behaviours, including: prioritizing one treatment over another, non-awareness of the guidelines, and not using SMS.

Key domains identified only for interns

Three additional TDF domains were identified among interns: 1) *Beliefs about Capabilities; 2) Memory, attention and decision making; and 3) Social Influence.*

Beliefs about capabilities

The interns provided 52 statements that were associated with the beliefs about capabilities domain, representing 6 specific beliefs and 2 themes: acceptance and capabilities. Almost all interns stated that they were confident in managing spine pain using SMS, and they had the ability to use SMS. However, most interns indicated that the delivery of SMS was not easy, and the factors that could increase their level of confidence included observing patients benefits from SMS, having experience with SMS, and asking clinicians and colleagues.

Memory, attention & decision making

Twenty-three statements were mapped to the domain of memory, attention & decision-making. The statements represented 5 specific beliefs and formed one theme: decision making on use of SMS. Most of the interns stated that their decisions on SMS varied according to patients' needs. However, some interns mentioned that they did not follow a guideline to guide decisions on the use of SMS; one intern used intuition to decide whether or not to use SMS. Interestingly, one intern decided to not use SMS in order to keep patients coming to the clinic, as the patients preferred passive treatments. Lastly, few interns decided to refer patients with psychological overlay to other healthcare providers.

Social influence

Thirty-four statements were related to the social influence domain. These statements corresponded to 4 specific beliefs and formed one theme: influence of others. Almost half of the interns stated that the clinicians' perception of SMS restricted their use of SMS, while the other half mentioned that clinicians' views facilitated their use of SMS. About half of participants mentioned that they consulted either supervisory clinicians or colleagues on the use of SMS. In addition, interns indicated that patients who preferred passive care could influence their decision to use SMS.

Phase 2 — Final selection of knowledge translation intervention components

Additional file 8 presents the BCTs mapped onto key barriers identified. The research team members considered intervention components to facilitate the use of SMS among clinicians and interns for patients with spine pain, based on current evidence and feasibility of implementation at CMCC clinics. The proposed intervention includes 6 components: 1) supportive handouts summarizing how to use the SMS guided by the BAP; 2) webinar describing the benefits of using SMS and the BAP in particular; 3) an online educational module with professional actors demonstrating the delivery of the BAP by a clinician with a patient; 4) clinical vignettes to apply the BAP using case scenarios; 5) a training workshop to practice and receive feedback when delivering the BAP; and 6) use of an opinion leader. The main roles of the opinion leader are to advise colleagues about SMS practice and ease the delivery of SMS.

Taking into account the teaching institution calendar year and curriculum, the KT intervention will be delivered as follows: clinicians and interns will first be asked to complete the self-study webinar and online educational module. They will then receive practice BAP and feedback from the opinion leaders. Clinicians and interns will also receive supportive materials on motivational interviewing and on how to deliver SMS guiding by BAP. They will also attend one- day training session delivered by a BAP trainer and have more opportunity to practice SMS and get personalised feedback. Further, 2 clinicians agreeing to act as champions (i.e. opinion leaders) will attend a BAP training to become certified in this approach prior to implementation the KT intervention. The main roles of the opinion leaders will be to support other clinicians and interns in using SMS and to provide them with coaching on applying the BAP with patients. Additional file 9 presents the final selection of KT intervention.

Discussion

Organisational support increases the likelihood of clinicians' successful uptake of EBP and CPG recommendations [90, 91]. Decision makers working at CMCC perceived that faculty and supervisory clinicians were highly committed to and confident about implementing SMS for patients with spine pain. Participating clinicians and interns showed positive attitudes toward EBP, and behaviours associated with EBP, which is consistent with the literature [92, 93]. These findings suggest that SMS strategies can be implemented in this environment.

Nonetheless, some barriers corresponding to four TDF domains that restricted both clinicians' and interns' use of SMS: *Knowledge, Skills, Environmental context and resources, and Emotion.* Aadditional barriers corresponding

to three TDF domains that restricted the intern' use of SMS were: *Beliefs about Capabilities; Memory, attention & decision making; and Social Influence.* To address these barriers, a panel of experts mapped BCTs to each barrier and selected the appropriate intervention components.

Both clinicians and interns felt that they needed more training to improve their knowledge and skills on the use of SMS, and they reported that lack of time was a key barrier to using SMS. Interns also indicated that they had a lack of confidence to use SMS. These findings are consistent with the literature showing that clinicians do not have sufficient knowledge and confidence in how to use SMS, and that they lack the appropriate training and competence to use SMS with patients [94, 95]. Furthermore, as the clinicians and interns did not receive intensive training on SMS, they admited sometimes feeling anxious about the use of SMS with complex patients. These findings are supported by the planned change theories, where the knowledge and skills are required to achieve confidece, [96], which may reduce the likelihood of anxiety [97]. In addition, according to these theories the presence of an opinion leader may improve one's confidence regarding behavior change [96].

Not surprisingly, novices starting to develop their clinical judgment skills and working under the supervisory clinicians faced additional challenges in using SMS than clinicians. Interns indicated that they lacked the confidence and knowledge needed to routinely incorporate SMS, did not follow a systematic process to deliver SMS to patients, and had to rely on supervisory clinicians' advice, even though some may not be comfortable or willing to use SMS in their own clinical practice. Together, these findings support the need to target both chiropractic interns and supervisory clinicians with strategies to help them improve their uptake and use of SMS in the clinical teaching environment.

Both clinicians and interns were generally motivated to use SMS in the clinical setting. This might be related to their beliefs about the effectiveness of SMS as well as to the collaborative nature of the relatiosnhips between clinicians and colleagues, and the support from managers. In addition, the interns in this study stated that they would keep delivering SMS if it improved patients' health outcomes. This is consistent with the operant learning theory where the achievements of a behaviour determines the continued use of that behaviour in the future [68].

The expert panel proposed different KT intervention strategies based on BCTs aimed at addressing the key barriers to using SMS among clinicians and interns. The selected KT intervention components formed a multifaceted theory-based intervention, which aims to simultaneously overcome several barriers [98]. The main KT intervention components were selected based on the current evidence [99] and feasibility to be implemented in the chiropractic clinical settings. These include supportive educational material, a webinar, an online educational module, a training workshop, and support by opinion leaders. A high-quality review demonstrated that implementing educational meetings, either alone or combined with other interventions, significantly improved the clinicians' practice in the clinical setting [100]. Furthermore, two high-quality reviews showed that using educational material was effective for improving healthcare providers' practice [101, 102]. Educational material could change clinicians' beliefs, which may result in behaviour change among clinicians toward adherence to EBP [103]. In contrast, three other high-quality reviews showed that educational meetings had mixed effects for improving clinicians' practice [104–107].

Of interest, the literature supported the effectiveness of internet-based learning (e.g. webinar, online module) on clinicians' knowledge [108, 109]; internet-based learning had a larger positive effects than no intervention [109]. However, it had small effect comparing to non-internet learning [109]. Lastly, the literature supports the effectiveness of having an opinion leader, alone or combined with other interventions, to facilitate clinicians' practice behaviour change [110, 111] and promote the adherence to EBP [112]. Interestingly, the availability of an opinion leader was proposed as a factor that made the new intervention implementation quicker [113]. Opinion leader has a small but worthy effect on clinicians behaviour change [114].

Strengths/ limitations

To our knowledge this is the first study aimed at developing a theory-based intervention to support the use of SMS among chiropractors and interns within an educational setting. The KT intervention components in this study were developed based on behavioural change theories using a systematic approach with a panel of experts. This may increase the likelihood of successful use of SMS in the clinical setting. A limitation of this study is that the results cannot be generalized to all chiropractic clinics. While the inclusion of additional clinicians may have resulted in different views, barriers identified are similar to those found on the use of multimodal care by practicing chiropractors when managing neck pain [68].

Conclusion

The key TDF factors that influence the uptake of SMS among clinicians and interns included: *knowledge, skill, environmental context and resources,* and *emotion.* Three additional TDF factors were identified only by interns: *Beliefs about Capabilities; Memory, attention & decision making;* and *Social Influence.* This may optimize the delivery of self-management support in spine pain clinics. The effectiveness of the selected KT intervention component remains to be tested.

Additional files

> **Additional file 1:** "Topic guide for focus groups with chiropractic interns and clinicians". It provides the interview guide for focus group. (DOCX 14 kb)
>
> **Additional file 2:** An Excel sheet that provides the raw data for clinicians and interns (XLSX 99 kb)
>
> **Additional file 3:** An Excel sheet that provides the raw data for decision makers (XLSX 10 kb)
>
> **Additional file 4:** "Thematic analysis based on the TDF – Clinicians". It provides number of clinicians' statements for each TDF domain, TDF specific beliefs and themes. (DOCX 17 kb)
>
> **Additional file 5:** "Thematic analysis based on the TDF – Interns". It provides number of clinicians' statements for each TDF domain, TDF specific beliefs and themes. (DOCX 18 kb)
>
> **Additional file 6:** "Specific Beliefs for each TDF with illustrative quotes – Clinicians". It provides clinicians quotes representing specific TDF domains and beliefs. (DOCX 17 kb)
>
> **Additional file 7:** "Specific Beliefs for each TDF with illustrative quotes – Interns". It provides interns quotes representing specific TDF domains and beliefs. (DOCX 20 kb)
>
> **Additional file 8:** "Mapping behaviour change techniques on key domains, proposed KT interventions and actions". It provides a list of self-management-TDF barriers and the proposed KT interventions. (DOCX 19 kb)
>
> **Additional file 9:** "Final Selection of KT Intervention Components and Related Learning". It provides the final selection of KT intervention for clinicians and interns to promote the use of self-management support in the clinic. (DOCX 14 kb)

Abbreviations

BAP: Brief action planning; BCT: Behavioural change technique; CMCC: Canadian Memorial Chiropractic College; CPGs: Clinical practice guidelines; EBP: Evidence-based practice; IQR: Interquartile range; KABQ: Knowledge, Attitude, and Behaviour Questionnaire; KT: Knowledge translation; ORIC: Organizational Readiness for Implementing Change; PABS: Pain Attitudes and Beliefs Scale; PAM: Patient activation measure; PMT: Patient Management Teams; SMS: Self-management strategy; TDF: Theoretical domain framework

Acknowledgements

We acknowledge CMCC for the support to conduct this research project.

Funding

Canadian Chiropractic Guidelines Initiative. The funding body did not influence the study design, analysis, and results.

Authors' contributions

MCH helped in conducting the focus groups. OE analysed the quantitative and qualitative data under the supervision of AB and AT (principle investigators). OE, AB, AT, CJ, ACT, CD, FA, and JB contributed to the design of Knowledge Translation intervention. All authors: OE, AB, AT, MCH, CJ, ACT, CD, FA, JB, SA, SM, RE, MJS and CL contributed to the preparation of the manuscript. All authors have read and approved the manuscript.

Competing interests

The authors declare that they have no competing interests.

Author details

[1]School of Physical and Occupational Therapy, McGill University, 3654 Prom Sir-William-Osler, Montréal, QC H3G 1Y5, Canada. [2]Center for Interdisciplinary Research in Rehabilitation of Greater Montreal (CRIR), Montréal, Canada. [3]Canadian Memorial Chiropractic College, North York, Canada. [4]University of British Columbia, Vancouver, Canada. [5]Centre for Collaboration, Motivation and Innovation, Vancouver, Canada. [6]University of Minnesota, Minneapolis, USA. [7]University of Pittsburgh, Pittsburgh, USA. [8]University of Toronto, Toronto, Canada. [9]Palmer College Davenport, Davenport, USA.

References

1. Global Burden of Disease Study 2013 Collaborators. Global, regional, and national incidence, prevalence, and years lived with disability for 310 diseases and injuries, 1990–2015: a systematic analysis for the global burden of disease study 2015. Lancet. 2016;388(10053):1545–602.

2. Hartvigsen J, et al. What low back pain is and why we need to pay attention. Lancet. 2018;391(10137):2356–67.

3. Vos T, et al. Years lived with disability (YLDs) for 1160 sequelae of 289 diseases and injuries 1990–2010: a systematic analysis for the global burden of disease study 2010. Lancet. 2012;380(9859):2163–96.

4. Hoy D, et al. Measuring the global burden of low back pain. Best Pract Res Clin Rheumatol. 2010;24(2):155–65.

5. Johannes CB, et al. The prevalence of chronic pain in United States adults: results of an internet-based survey. J Pain. 2010;11(11):1230–9.

6. De Souza L, Frank A. Conservative management of low back pain. Int J Clin Pract. 2001;55(1):21–31.

7. The burden of musculoskeletal conditions at the start of the new millennium. World Health Organ Tech Rep Ser. 2003;919:i–x, 1–218, back cover

8. Andersson GBJ. Epidemiological features of chronic low-back pain. Lancet. 1999;354(9178):581–5.

9. Scheermesser M, et al. A qualitative study on the role of cultural background in patients' perspectives on rehabilitation. BMC Musculoskelet Disord. 2012;13(1):5.

10. Almeida DB, et al. Is preoperative occupation related to long-term pain in patients operated for lumbar disc herniation? Arq Neuropsiquiatr. 2007;65:758–63.

11. Chin KR, et al. Success of lumbar microdiscectomy in patients with Modic changes and low-back pain: a prospective pilot study. J Spinal Disord Tech. 2008;21(2):139–44. https://doi.org/10.1097/BSD.0b013e318093e5dc.

12. Horng Y-S, et al. Predicting health-related quality of life in patients with low back pain. Spine. 2005;30(5):551–5. https://doi.org/10.1097/01.brs.0000154623.20778.f0.

13. Kim T-S, et al. Interrelationships among pain, disability, and psychological factors in young Korean conscripts with lumbar disc herniation. Mil Med. 2006;171(11):1113–6.

14. Mannion AF, et al. A prospective study of the interrelationship between subjective and objective measures of disability before and 2 months after lumbar decompression surgery for disc herniation. Eur Spine J. 2005;14(5):454–65.

15. Di Iorio A, et al. From chronic low back pain to disability, a multifactorial mediated pathway: the InCHIANTI study. Spine (Phila Pa 1976). 2007;32(26):E809–15.

16. Hicks GE, et al. Trunk muscle composition as a predictor of reduced functional capacity in the health, aging and body composition study: the moderating role of back pain. J Gerontol A Biol Sci Med Sci. 2005;60(11):1420–4.

17. Brown A, et al. Costs and Outcomes of Chiropractic Treatment for Low Back Pain. Ottawa: Canadian Coordinating Office for Health Technology Assessment; 2005.

18. Cote P, Cassidy JD, Carroll L. The treatment of neck and low back pain: who seeks care? Who goes where? Med Care. 2001;39(9):956–67.

19. Partner JD. Americans' perceptions of chiropractic. Washington: Gallup, Inc; 2015.

20. Beliveau PJH, et al. The chiropractic profession: a scoping review of utilization rates, reasons for seeking care, patient profiles, and care provided. Chiropr Man Therap. 2017;25(1):35.

21. Stochkendahl MJ, et al. National Clinical Guidelines for non-surgical treatment of patients with recent onset low back pain or lumbar radiculopathy. Eur Spine J. 2018;27(1):60–75.

22. National Guideline C. National Institute for Health and Care Excellence: Clinical Guidelines. In: Low Back Pain and Sciatica in Over 16s: Assessment and Management. London: National Institute for Health and Care Excellence (UK) Copyright (c) NICE; 2016.

23. Qaseem A, et al. Noninvasive treatments for acute, subacute, and chronic low back pain: a clinical practice guideline from the American College of Physicians. Ann Intern Med. 2017;166(7):514–30.

24. Wong JJ, et al. Clinical practice guidelines for the noninvasive management of low back pain: a systematic review by the Ontario protocol for traffic injury management (OPTIMa) collaboration. Eur J Pain. 2017;21(2):201–16.

25. Pierre Côté, et al., Enabling recovery from common traffic injuries: a focus on the injured person; UOIT-CMCC Centre for the study of disability prevention and rehabilitation. 2015.

26. Bryans R, et al. Evidence-based guidelines for the chiropractic treatment of adults with neck pain. J Manip Physiol Ther. 2014;37(1):42–63.

27. Bussieres AE, et al. The Treatment of Neck Pain-Associated Disorders and Whiplash-Associated Disorders: A Clinical Practice Guideline. J Manipulative Physiol Ther. 2016;39(8):523–564.e27.

28. Chou R, et al. Diagnosis and treatment of low back pain: a joint clinical practice guideline from the American College of Physicians and the American pain society. Ann Intern Med. 2007;147(7):478–91.

29. Newman SP. Chronic disease self-management approaches within the complex organisational structure of a health care system. Med J Aust. 2008;189(10 Suppl):S7–8.

30. Hanson R, Gerber K. Coping with chronic pain: a guide to patient self-management. NewYork: Guilford Press; 1990.

31. Turk DC, Meichenbaum D, Genest M. Pain and Behavioral Medicine: A Cognitive-Behavioral Perspective. New York: The Guilford Press; 1983.

32. Bertozzi L, et al. Effect of therapeutic exercise on pain and disability in the management of chronic nonspecific neck pain: systematic review and meta-analysis of randomized trials. Phys Ther. 2013;93(8):1026–36.

33. Von Korff M, et al. Chronic spinal pain and physical-mental comorbidity in the United States: results from the national comorbidity survey replication. Pain. 2005;113(3):331–9.

34. Ritzwoller DP, et al. The association of comorbidities, utilization and costs for patients identified with low back pain. BMC Musculoskelet Disord. 2006;7:72.

35. Hartvigsen J, Natvig B, Ferreira M. Is it all about a pain in the back? Best Pract Res Clin Rheumatol. 2013;27(5):613–23.

36. Sallis R, et al. Strategies for promoting physical activity in clinical practice. Prog Cardiovasc Dis. 2015;57(4):375–86.

37. Marzolini S, et al. Musculoskeletal Comorbidities in Cardiac Patients: Prevalence, Predictors, and Health Services Utilization. Arch Phys Med Rehabil. 2012;93(5):856–62.

38. Bodenheimer T, MacGregor K, Shafiri C. Helping patients manage their chronic conditions. Oakland: California HealthCare Foundation; 2005.

39. Gore M, et al. The burden of chronic low back pain: clinical comorbidities, treatment patterns, and health care costs in usual care settings. Spine (Phila Pa 1976). 2012;37(11):E668–77.

40. Oliveira VC, et al. Effectiveness of self-management of low back pain: systematic review with meta-analysis. Arthritis Care Res (Hoboken). 2012;64(11):1739–48.

41. Newman S, Steed L, Mulligan K. Self-management interventions for chronic illness. Lancet. 2004;364(9444):1523–37.

42. Canadian Chiropractic Resources Databank (CCRD), National Report. A comprehensive inventory of practical information about Canada's licensed chiropractors. Toronto: The Canadian Chiropractic Association; 2011.

43. Bussieres AE, et al. Evidence-based practice, research utilization, and knowledge translation in chiropractic: a scoping review. BMC Complement Altern Med. 2016;16:216.

44. Bussieres AE, et al. Self-reported attitudes, skills and use of evidence-based practice among Canadian doctors of chiropractic: a national survey. J Can Chiropr Assoc. 2015;59(4):332–48.

45. Foster NE, et al. Prevention and treatment of low back pain: evidence, challenges, and promising directions. Lancet. 2018;391(10137):2368-83.

46. Hibbard JH. Moving toward a more patient-centered health care delivery system. Health Aff (Millwood). 2004;(Suppl Variation):Var133–5.

47. Holman H, Lorig K. Patient self-management: a key to effectiveness and efficiency in care of chronic disease. Public Health Rep. 2004;119(3):239–43.

48. Bodenheimer T, et al. Patient self-management of chronic disease in primary care. Jama. 2002;288(19):2469–75.

49. Bodenheimer T, Wagner EH, Grumbach K. Improving primary care for patients with chronic illness. Jama. 2002;288(14):1775–9.

50. May S. Self-management of chronic low back pain and osteoarthritis. Nat Rev Rheumatol. 2010;6(4):199–209.

51. Briggs AM, et al. Consumers' experiences of back pain in rural Western Australia: access to information and services, and self-management behaviours. BMC Health Serv Res. 2012;12:357.

52. Eilayyan O, et al. Developing Theory-Informed Knowledge Translation Strategies to facilitate the Delivery of Low Back Pain Self-management support in Clinical Practice. Quebec: McGill University; 2017.

53. Gordon K, et al. Barriers to self-management of chronic pain in primary care: a qualitative focus group study. Br J Gen Pract. 2017;67(656):e209–17.

54. Straus S, Tetroe J, Graham I. Knowledge translation in health care: moving from evidence to practice. Second ed. Chichester, West Sussex: Wiley; 2013.

55. Curran JA, et al. Knowledge translation research: the science of moving research into policy and practice. J Contin Educ Heal Prof. 2011;31(3):174–80.

56. Thomas A, M. A. Becoming an evidence-based practitioner. In: Law M, MacDermid J, editors. Evidence-based rehabilitation: A guide to practice. 3rd ed. Thorofare, NJ: Slack Incorporated; 2014.

57. Thomas A, Saroyan A, Snider LM. Evidence-based practice behaviours: a comparison amongst occupational therapy students and clinicians. Can J Occup Ther. 2012;79(2):96–107.

58. Dawes M, et al. Sicily statement on evidence-based practice. BMC Med Educ. 2005;5(1):1.

59. Thomas A, Saroyan A, Lajoie SP. Creation of an evidence-based practice reference model in falls prevention: findings from occupational therapy. Disabil Rehabil. 2012;34(4):311–28.

60. Dizon JM, Grimmer-Somers KA, Kumar S. Current evidence on evidence-based practice training in allied health: a systematic review of the literature. Int J Evid Based Healthc. 2012;10(4):347–60.

61. Khan KS, Coomarasamy A. A hierarchy of effective teaching and learning to acquire competence in evidenced-based medicine. BMC Med Educ. 2006;6:59.

62. Blanchette MA, et al. Chiropractors' characteristics associated with their number of workers' compensation patients. J Can Chiropr Assoc. 2015; 59(3):202–15.

63. Gutnick D, et al. Brief action planning to facilitate behavior change and support patient self-management. J Clin Outcomes Manag. 2014;21(1):17–29.

64. Tibbles A, Jacobs C. In: Eilayyan O, Bussieres A, editors. CMCC Curriculum; 2017.

65. McGrady ME, et al. Topical review: theoretical frameworks in pediatric adherence-promotion interventions: research findings and methodological implications. J Pediatr Psychol. 2015;40(8):721–6.

66. Dobson F, et al. Barriers and facilitators to exercise participation in people with hip and/or knee osteoarthritis: synthesis of the literature using behavior change theory. Am J Phys Med Rehabil. 2016;95(5):372–89.

67. Mosavianpour M, et al. Theoretical domains framework to assess barriers to change for planning health care quality interventions: a systematic literature review. J Multidiscip Healthc. 2016;9:303–10.

68. Bussières AE, et al. Fast tracking the design of theory-based KT interventions through a consensus process. Implement Sci. 2015;10(1):18.

69. French S, et al. Developing theory-informed behaviour change interventions to implement evidence into practice: a systematic approach using the theoretical domains framework. Implement Sci. 2012;7.

70. Cane J, O'Connor D, Michie S. Validation of the theoretical domains framework for use in behaviour change and implementation research. Implement Sci. 2012;7:37.

71. Shea CM, et al. Organizational readiness for implementing change: a psychometric assessment of a new measure. Implement Sci. 2014;9:7.

72. Shi Q, et al. A modified evidence-based practice- knowledge, attitudes, behaviour and decisions/outcomes questionnaire is valid across multiple professions involved in pain management. BMC Medical Education. 2014;14(1):263.

73. Bishop A. Pain Attitudes and Beliefs Scale (PABS). J Physiother. 2010;56(4):279.

74. Wyszewianski L, Green LA. Strategies for changing clinicians' practice patterns. A new perspective. J Fam Pract. 2000;49(5):461–4.

75. Houben RM, et al. Health care providers' orientations towards common low back pain predict perceived harmfulness of physical activities and recommendations regarding return to normal activity. Eur J Pain. 2005;9(2):173–83.

76. Mutsaers JH, et al. Psychometric properties of the pain attitudes and beliefs scale for physiotherapists: a systematic review. Man Ther. 2012;17(3):213–8.

77. SAS. SAS® 9.4 Software. 2015 [cited 2016 04–03]; Available from: http://support.sas.com/software/94/index.html. Accessed 3 Apr 2016.

78. Green SB. How many subjects does it take to do a regression analysis. Multivariate Behav Res. 1991;26(3):499–510.

79. Cohen J. Statistical power analysis for the behavioral sciences. Hillsdale, N.J: L. Erlbaum Associates; 1988.

80. Francis JJ, et al. Using theories of behaviour to understand transfusion prescribing in three clinical contexts in two countries: development work for an implementation trial. Implement Sci. 2009;4:70.

81. Francis JJ, et al. Evidence-based selection of theories for designing behaviour change interventions: using methods based on theoretical construct domains to understand clinicians' blood transfusion behaviour. Br J Health Psychol. 2009;14(Pt 4):625–46.

82. Bussieres AE, et al. Identifying factors likely to influence compliance with diagnostic imaging guideline recommendations for spine disorders among chiropractors in North America: a focus group study using the theoretical domains framework. Implement Sci. 2012;7:82.

83. Eldridge S, et al. Internal and external validity of cluster randomised trials: systematic review of recent trials. BMJ. 2008;336(7649):876–80.

84. McCullough AR, et al. Defining the content and delivery of an intervention to change AdhereNce to treatment in BonchiEctasis (CAN-BE): a qualitative approach incorporating the theoretical domains framework, behavioural change techniques and stakeholder expert panels. BMC Health Serv Res. 2015;15(1):342.

85. Guest G, Namey E, McKenna K. How many focus groups are enough? Building an evidence base for nonprobability sample sizes. Field Methods. 2017;29(1):3–22.

86. Michie S, et al. From theory to intervention: mapping theoretically derived Behavioural determinants to behaviour change techniques. Appl Psychol. 2008;57(4):660–80.

87. Michie S, et al. The behavior change technique taxonomy (v1) of 93 hierarchically clustered techniques: building an international consensus for the reporting of behavior change interventions. Ann Behav Med. 2013;46(1):81–95.

88. Lorig KR, et al. Chronic disease self-management program: 2-year health status and health care utilization outcomes. Med Care. 2001;39(11):1217–23.

89. Korner-Bitensky N, et al. Practice style traits: do they help explain practice behaviours of stroke rehabilitation professionals? J Rehabil Med. 2007;39(9):685–92.

90. Paramonczyk A. Barriers to implementing research in clinical practice. Can Nurse. 2005;101(3):12–5.

91. Sandstrom B, et al. Promoting the implementation of evidence-based practice: a literature review focusing on the role of nursing leadership. Worldviews Evid-Based Nurs. 2011;8(4):212–23.

92. Walker BF, et al. Evidence-based practice in chiropractic practice: a survey of chiropractors' knowledge, skills, use of research literature and barriers to the use of research evidence. Complement Ther Med. 2014;22(2):286–95.

93. Alcantara J, Leach MJ. Chiropractic attitudes and utilization of evidence-based practice: the use of the EBASE questionnaire. Explore (NY). 2015;11(5):367–76.

94. Jeffery V, Ervin K. Early intervention in chronic disease--four years on: barriers to implementing self-management strategies. J Allied Health. 2014; 43(1):e1–3.

95. Vallis M. Are Behavioural interventions doomed to fail? Challenges to self-management support in chronic diseases. Can J Diabetes. 2015;39(4):330–4.

96. Straus SE, Tetroe J, Graham ID. Theories and Models of Knowledge to Action. In: Knowledge translation in health care : moving from evidence to practice. Chichester, Hoboken: Wiley-Blackwell/BMJ; 2009.

97. Bandura A. Self-efficacy: toward a unifying theory of behavioral change. Psychol Rev. 1977;84(2):191–215.

98. Straus SE, Tetroe J, Graham ID. The Knowledge-to-Action Cycle. In: Knowledge Translation in Health Care: Moving from Evidence to Practice: Blackwell Publishing Ltd; 2009. p. 59–181.

99. The Canadian Agency for Drugs and Technologies in Health (CADTH). Rx for Change database 2011 [cited 2017 Feb 04]; Available from: https://www.cadth.ca/rx-change.

100. Forsetlund L, et al. Continuing education meetings and workshops: effects on professional practice and health care outcomes. Cochrane Database Syst Rev. 2009;(2):Cd003030.

101. French SD, et al. Interventions for improving the appropriate use of imaging in people with musculoskeletal conditions. Cochrane Database Syst Rev. 2010;(1):Cd006094.

102. Farmer AP, et al. Printed educational materials: effects on professional practice and health care outcomes. Cochrane Database Syst Rev. 2008;3: CD004398.

103. Evans DW, et al. The effectiveness of a posted information package on the beliefs and behavior of musculoskeletal practitioners: the UK chiropractors, osteopaths, and musculoskeletal physiotherapists low back pain ManagemENT (COMPLeMENT) randomized trial. Spine (Phila Pa 1976). 2010; 35(8):858–66.

104. Walsh CM, et al. Virtual reality simulation training for health professions trainees in gastrointestinal endoscopy. Cochrane Database Syst Rev. 2012; (6):Cd008237.

105. Gould DJ, et al. Interventions to improve hand hygiene compliance in patient care. Cochrane Database Syst Rev. 2010;(9):Cd005186.

106. Dwamena F, et al. Interventions for providers to promote a patient-centred approach in clinical consultations. Cochrane Database Syst Rev. 2012;12: Cd003267.

107. Thomas L, et al. Guidelines in professions allied to medicine. Cochrane Database Syst Rev. 2000;(2):Cd000349.
108. Cook DA, et al. Instructional design variations in internet-based learning for health professions education: a systematic review and meta-analysis. Acad Med. 2010;85(5):909–22.
109. Cook DA, et al. Internet-based learning in the health professions: a meta-analysis. Jama. 2008;300(10):1181–96.
110. Elueze IN. Evaluating the effectiveness of knowledge brokering in health research: a systematised review with some bibliometric information. Health Inf Libr J. 2015;32(3):168–81.
111. Flodgren G, et al. Local opinion leaders: effects on professional practice and health care outcomes. Cochrane Database Syst Rev. 2011;(8):Cd000125.
112. Doumit G, et al. Local opinion leaders: effects on professional practice and health care outcomes. Cochrane Database Syst Rev. 2007;(1):Cd000125.
113. Dopson S, Fitzgerald L. Knowledge to Action. Oxford: Oxford University Press; 2005.
114. Straus SE, Tetroe J, Graham ID. The Knowledge-to-Action Cycle. In: Knowledge translation in health care : moving from evidence to practice. Chichester, UK: Wiley-Blackwell/BMJ; 2009. Hoboken, N.J.

10

Efficacy of extracorporeal shock wave therapy for knee tendinopathies and other soft tissue disorders

Chun-De Liao[1,2†], Guo-Min Xie[3†], Jau-Yih Tsauo[1], Hung-Chou Chen[2,4,6] and Tsan-Hon Liou[2,5,6*]

Abstract

Background: Extracorporeal shock-wave therapy (ESWT), which can be divided into radial shock-wave therapy (RaSWT) and focused shock-wave therapy (FoSWT), has been widely used in clinical practice for managing orthopedic conditions. The aim of this study was to determine the clinical efficacy of ESWT for knee soft tissue disorders (KSTDs) and compare the efficacy of different shock-wave types, energy levels, and intervention durations.

Methods: We performed a comprehensive search of online databases and search engines without restrictions on the publication year or language. We selected randomized controlled trials (RCTs) reporting the efficacy of ESWT for KSTDs and included them in a meta-analysis and risk of bias assessment. The pooled effect sizes of ESWT were estimated by computing odds ratios (ORs) with 95% confidence intervals (CIs) for the treatment success rate (TSR) and standardized mean differences (SMDs) with 95% CIs for pain reduction (i.e., the difference in pain relief, which was the change in pain from baseline to the end of RCTs between treatment and control groups) and for restoration of knee range of motion (ROM).

Results: We included 19 RCTs, all of which were of high or medium methodological quality and had a Physiotherapy Evidence Database score of ≥5/10. In general, ESWT had overall significant effects on the TSR (OR: 3.36, 95% CI: 1.84–6.12, $P < 0.0001$), pain reduction (SMD: − 1.49, 95% CI: − 2.11 to − 0.87, $P < 0.00001$), and ROM restoration (SMD: 1.76, 95% CI: 1.43–2.09, $P < 0.00001$). Subgroup analyses revealed that FoSWT and RaSWT applied for a long period (≥1 month) had significant effects on pain reduction, with the corresponding SMDs being − 3.13 (95% CI: − 5.70 to − 0.56; $P = 0.02$) and − 1.80 (95% CI: − 2.52 to − 1.08; $P < 0.00001$), respectively. Low-energy FoSWT may have greater efficacy for the TSR than high-energy FoSWT, whereas the inverse result was observed for RaSWT.

Conclusions: The ESWT exerts an overall effect on the TSR, pain reduction, and ROM restoration in patients with KSTDs. Shock-wave types and application levels have different contributions to treatment efficacy for KSTDs, which must be investigated further for optimizing these treatments in clinical practice.

Keywords: Extracorporeal shock wave therapy, Knee, Musculoskeletal disorders, Physical therapy

* Correspondence: peter_liou@s.tmu.edu.tw
†Chun-De Liao and Guo-Min Xie contributed equally to this work.
²Department of Physical Medicine and Rehabilitation, Shuang Ho Hospital, Taipei Medical University, Taipei, Taiwan
⁵Graduate Institute of Injury Prevention and Control, Taipei Medical University, Taipei, Taiwan
Full list of author information is available at the end of the article

Background

Knee soft tissue disorders (KSTDs) are common problems that develop from sports-induced tendon and ligament injuries in athletes [1], and they originate from overuse conditions or traumatic injuries in nonathletes [2–4]. Overall, knee injuries account for up to 35% of common overuse injuries in sports teams [5]. The most common practical problem caused by knee injury is the pain-induced limitation in sports and related activities, particularly walking or running [2, 6]; this problem further exerts negative effects on not only sports participation but also quality of life [7, 8].

Over the past three decades, extracorporeal shock wave therapy (ESWT) has been widely used in clinical practice for managing musculoskeletal disorders, most of which are tendinopathies and enthesopathies [9–13]. Because of its efficacy in exerting analgesic effects and promoting soft tissue remodeling and repair, ESWT has also been successfully used for treating many other soft tissue disorders that occur after sports injuries and traumatic accidents, such as muscular disorders [14, 15], posttraumatic knee stiffness [16, 17], and ligament injuries [18–21], as well as ligament desmitis in animals [22–24]. In addition, for orthopedic conditions, ESWT serves as a noninvasive alternative to conservative treatment (i.e., steroid injections) or surgery [25, 26]. ESWT provides a mechanical stimulus that is conducted by pulse acoustic waves, and through mechanotransduction, this stimulus is converted into a series of biochemical signals within the targeted tissues, enhancing tissue regeneration [9, 13, 27]. Consequently, the production of proteins, nitric oxide, and specific growth factors causes responses leading to increased neoangiogenesis, tenocyte and fibroblast proliferation, and collagen synthesis, further enhancing tissue catabolism, healing, and remodeling [28–33]. Acoustic cavitation formed in the negative (tensile) phase of the shock wave is the second effect of ESWT; this effect also promotes tissue regeneration by increasing cellular membrane permeability, and it efficiently breaks down calcification deposits (i.e., calculi disintegration) in soft tissues [9, 13, 34]. The aforementioned cascades of biological events support that ESWT can be employed to reduce pain, increase blood flow in ischemic tissues, soften calcified tissues, treat tissue fibrosis, and release adhesions, as well as relieve posttraumatic knee stiffness, thereby improving physical function and performance in sports activities.

On the basis of the delivery pathway for the propagation of acoustic energy through biological tissue, shock wave therapy can be divided into two types: focused shock wave therapy (FoSWT) and radial shock wave therapy (RaSWT) [11, 34, 35]. The differences in the therapeutic effects of FoSWT and RaSWT have been discussed [11, 36–39], and each therapy should be considered an independent modality derived from multiple techniques that generate shock wave pulses [11, 37, 38]. However, it remains unclear whether any difference exists in the therapeutic effects of FoSWT and RaSWT on KSTDs. The intensity at the focal point of the shock wave, which is measured as energy flux density (EFD; mJ/mm^2) per impulse, may influence the therapeutic effects of ESWT [34, 36]. In clinical practice, the EFD levels of ESWT range from 0.001 to 0.5 mJ/mm^2 [36, 37, 40, 41]. Administering ESWT repeatedly and at a very high dosage may increase the risk of treatment failure [42] and increase the onset of adverse events [43, 44]. Thus, it is important to enhance the efficiency of ESWT by determining the differences in the efficacy of various ESWT application levels. The overall pooled effects of different shock-wave types and dosage levels on KSTDs should be further investigated.

Several studies have investigated the efficacy of ESWT for lower limb musculoskeletal conditions or knee tendinopathy through systemic reviews or meta-analyses [45–47]. Nevertheless, two of such studies have selected articles published in a specific language [46, 47]. In addition, other than patellar tendinopathy, most KSTDs have not been included in previous meta-analyses, such as pes anserine tendinopathy [48], fabella syndrome [49, 50], popliteal cyamella [51], iliotibial band friction syndrome [52], infrapatellar fat pad syndrome [53], and posttraumatic tendon and ligament stiffness, which contribute to joint contracture [16, 17]. Restrictions on language in the study inclusion criteria may result in a high risk of bias (i.e., language bias) in research areas such as alternative treatment (e.g., ESWT serves as an alternative to conservative medicine for musculoskeletal conditions) [54]. The aim of the current systematic review and meta-analysis was to determine the efficacy of ESWT in reducing pain and improving functional outcomes in patients with KSTDs at immediate (≤1 month), short-term (>1 month, ≤3 months), medium-term (>3 month, ≤6 months), and long-term (>6 months) follow-up (FU). We also performed subgroup analyses to compare the efficacy of ESWT in reducing pain and improving functional outcomes between different shock-wave types, energy levels (i.e., high and low energy), intervention periods [i.e., short (<1 month) and long (≥1 month)], control group types (i.e., placebo, noninvasive comparison, and invasive comparison), treated populations (i.e., athletes and nonathletes), disease types (i.e., tendinopathy and other KSTDs), and cointervention designs (i.e., monotherapy and cointervention).

Methods

Design

This study was conducted in accordance with the Preferred Reporting Items for Systematic Reviews and Meta-Analysis guidelines [55]. A comprehensive search of online databases and search engines was performed up to June 2018. Original research articles on the clinical efficacy of ESWT for KSDTs were aggregated and coded. To minimize publication and language biases, no limitation was imposed on the publication year or language. Primary sources were MEDLINE, PubMed, the Excerpta Medica dataBASE, the Cochrane Library, the Physiotherapy Evidence Database (PEDro), the China Knowledge Resource Integrated Database, and Google Scholar. Secondary sources were papers cited in the articles retrieved from the aforementioned sources and articles published in journals that were not available in the aforementioned databases. The search was restricted to published or in-press articles reporting human studies. If English titles were not provided in non-English articles, they were translated to English by using translation software (Ginger Software, Inc.). Two researchers (CDL and HCC) independently searched for articles, screened studies, and extracted data in a blinded manner. Any disagreements between the researchers were resolved through consensus, with other research team members (JYT and GMX) acting as arbiters.

Search strategy

We used the following keywords in the Excerpta Medica dataBASE to identify articles reporting studies applying shock wave therapy for KSTDs and associated conditions: ["shock wave therapy" OR "extracorporeal shock wave therapy"] AND [("knee soft tissue disorder" OR "knee musculoskeletal disorder" OR "patella/patellar/patellofemoral") OR ("tendinitis/tendinopathy/peritendinopathy" OR "ligament injury/desmitis" OR "apicitis" OR "apophysitis" OR "enthesopathy" OR "plica" OR "tenosynovitis" OR "synovitis" OR "bursitis" OR "iliotibial band friction syndrome" OR "pes anserine tendinopathy" OR "fabella syndrome" OR "popliteal cyamella" OR "Osgood–Schlatter disease" OR "Jumper's knee")] AND ["Randomized controlled trial" OR "Randomization"]. The detailed search formulas used for each database are presented in Additional file 1.

Study selection

The trial inclusion criteria were (1) randomized controlled trials (RCTs); (2) RCTs in which controls received a placebo through sham shock wave application or underwent noninvasive/invasive treatment (e.g., exercise, injections, or surgery); (3) RCTs involving KSTDs including tendinopathy and other noncartilage soft tissue disorders; (4) trials in which the primary outcomes included pain that was measured using a quantifiable scale (e.g., a visual analog scale [VAS]) and the successful treatment rate that was measured using a ranking scale (e.g., the Roles and Maudsley score [56] or Likert-type scale [57, 58]); (5) trials in which the secondary

outcomes included physical function and disability that were assessed using questionnaires for patient-reported outcomes (e.g., the Victorian Institute of Sport Assessment-Patella questionnaire [59]) or measured using performance-based testing (e.g., the vertical jump test); and (6) trials containing the following application parameters: wave characteristics, EFD, number of shock impulses, number and duration of treatment sessions, and frequency of treatment. Trials reporting one primary or secondary outcome were included if they also fulfilled other inclusion criteria. If more than one primary or secondary outcome measure was reported for pain or function, respectively, we extracted data for the outcomes of pain (e.g., the VAS) and function (e.g., assessment for activities of daily living), which are considered to be of the greatest importance in patients and to be disease specific [60].

The trial exclusion criteria were (1) animal trials; (2) trials with a non-RCT design such as a case report, case series, or prospective trial without a comparison group; and (3) trials using ESWT to treat knee cartilage disorders such as chondromalacia, meniscus injury, and degenerative osteoarthritis.

Data extraction

We developed and refined a data extraction sheet for the included trials [37]. Study characteristics, namely the author name, publication year, study design, participants (i.e., sample size, age, sex, and training status), disease type, symptom onset duration, study group interventions and comparison (including cointerventions), FU duration, outcome measures (including assessment tools), and ESWT application parameters, were extracted according to the standardized data extraction sheet [61]. Information on the side effects of ESWT, loss to FU, author conflict of interest disclosures, and funding sources in each trial was also extracted to assess agenda bias and other potential biases [62]. For all included trials, we also confirmed whether the results of each employed outcome measure which was described in the Methods section being fully reported in the Results section to assess bias that may result from selective outcome reporting [62]. One researcher (CDL) extracted the relevant data from the included trials, and another researcher (HCC) reviewed the extracted data. The reviewers contacted the study authors to confirm any necessary information. Any disagreement between the two researchers was resolved through consensus. A third researcher (THL) was consulted if the disagreement persisted.

Outcome measures

The primary outcomes—pain intensity and the successful treatment rate—were calculated as standardized mean differences (SMDs) and odds ratios (ORs) relative to the placebo or comparison control, respectively. Secondary outcomes—patient-reported and performance-based outcome measures—were also calculated as SMDs relative to the placebo or active control.

Assessment of methodological quality

The PEDro classification scale was used to assess the risk of bias of the included RCTs [63, 64]. The methodological quality of all included trials was independently assessed by two researchers (CDL and HCC) through the PEDro classification scale. Any disagreement between the two researchers was resolved through consensus. A third researcher (THL) was consulted if the disagreement could not be resolved.

The PEDro classification scale is a valid measure of the methodological quality of clinical RCTs [63], as recommended for nonpharmacological studies [65]; all 10 item scores are summed to yield a total score ranging from 0 to 10 points, where a summary score ≥ 6 points typically defines adequate trial quality [66]. On the basis of the PEDro score, the methodological quality of each included RCT was rated as high ($\geq 7/10$), medium (4–6/10), or low ($\leq 3/10$) [67].

Assessment of risk of bias

The same two researchers (CDL and HCC) independently assessed the risk of bias in the included studies by using the Cochrane risk of bias tool [68, 69]. Any difference of opinion was resolved during a consensus meeting; if the difference persisted, a third reviewer (THL) became involved. The following seven bias domains (11 judgement items) related to bias in estimates of intervention effects were assessed [61]: selection bias (i.e., random sequence generation, allocation concealment, and similarity at baseline), performance bias (i.e., blinding of participants and personnel, blinding of therapists or care providers, and avoidance of cointerventions or similar), detection bias (i.e., blinding and timing of outcome assessment); attrition bias (i.e., incomplete outcome data), reporting bias (i.e., selective reporting), agenda bias (i.e., author conflict of interest disclosures), and other sources of potential bias (e.g., unvalidated outcome measures). According to its quality, each included trial was classified to have low, high, or unclear risk of bias [69].

We also examined adverse events, when reported; however, they were not specified a priori. The FU duration was assessed and defined as immediate (≤ 1 month), short term (> 1 month, ≤ 3 months), medium term (> 3 months, ≤ 6 months), and long term (> 6 months).

Statistical analysis

We computed the effect sizes for the primary and secondary outcome measures in each trial by following the Cochrane Handbook for Systematic Reviews [69]. In each trial, the treatment effect of ESWT (i.e., the effect size) on the primary outcome (i.e., pain score) was estimated based on the changes in the score at each FU time point relative to the baseline score [i.e., difference between the mean scores at pretreatment and FU time point], as well as standard deviations (SDs) in each group. If the exact variance of paired differences was not reported, it was imputed by assuming a correlation coefficient of 0.8 between the baseline and FU pain scores [70, 71]. If data were reported as median (range), they were recalculated algebraically from the trial data for imputing the sample mean and SD [72]. In addition, the pooled effect size of ESWT was estimated by calculating the weighted SMD along with 95% CIs by using the inverse variance-weighted method. Using the methodology of a previous study [67], we categorized the magnitude of the SMD in accordance with the following version of Cohen's criteria [73], which was proposed by Hopkins [74]: trivial ($d < 0.20$), small ($0.20 \leq d < 0.60$), medium ($0.60 \leq d < 1.20$), and large ($d \geq 1.20$). The OR along with the corresponding 95% CI was estimated for dichotomous outcomes (i.e., successful treatment rate). For the secondary outcomes of physical mobility and disability, the effect size was calculated as the SMD, thus constituting a combined outcome measure without units.

Statistical heterogeneity was assessed using the I^2 statistic, and a result of $\chi^2 > 50\%$ and $P < 0.05$ was defined as evidence of significant heterogeneity across trials [75]. Fixed- or random-effects models were used depending on the absence or presence of significant heterogeneity ($P > 0.05$ and $P < 0.05$), respectively.

Subgroup analyses were performed according to the shock-wave type (i.e., FoSWT and RaSWT), energy level (i.e., high and low energy), intervention period [i.e., short (< 1 month) and long (≥ 1 month)], (i.e., placebo, noninvasive comparison, and invasive comparison), treated populations (i.e., athletes and nonathletes), disease type (i.e., tendinopathy and other KSTDs), and cointervention design (i.e., monotherapy and cointervention) in the included trials. We used a cutoff EFD value of 0.2 mJ/mm² for high and low energy [40], and an EFD range with the upper limit of 0.2 mJ/mm² or higher was also considered as a high energy level.

Using SPSS statistical software (Version 17.0; IBM, Armonk, NY, USA), we investigated potential publication bias through the visual inspection of a funnel plot [76] and Egger's regression asymmetry test [77]. $P < 0.05$ was considered statistically significant. All analyses were conducted using RevMan 5.3 (The Nordic Cochrane Centre, Copenhagen, Denmark).

We graded the levels of evidence (LoE) for each outcome of interest according to the guideline of evidence synthesis [78] derived from the criteria of van Tulder [79] (Table 1).

Results

Trial selection process

Figure 1 presents a flowchart of the selection process. The final sample for meta-analysis comprised 19 RCTs [16, 17, 48, 51–53, 80–92], totally including 1189 patients [mean (SD) age: 34.7 (9.4) years]. Of all patients, 562 received ESWT and 627 received a placebo or other comparative treatments.

Study characteristics

Table 2 summarizes the demographic data and study characteristics of the included RCTs. All patients in the included RCTs had experienced symptoms for 3 months or longer, except for those in one RCT, except for those in one RCT, who experienced traumatic knee synovitis for 2 months [92]. ESWT was used to treat orthopedic conditions including patellar tendinopathy (eight RCTs) [81–85, 87, 88, 90], pes anserine tendinopathy (two RCTs) [48, 80], anterior cruciate ligament (ACL) injury (two RCTs) [86, 89], traumatic knee synovitis (one RCT) [92], Osgood–Schlatter disease (one RCT) [91], iliotibial band syndrome (one RCT) [52], and infrapatellar fat pad injury (one RCT) [53]. In addition, it was used to treat posttraumatic knee stiffness (two RCTs) [16, 17] and popliteal cyamella (one RCT), which represents gastrocnemius tendinopathy [51].

Among the 19 included RCTs, 6 used ESWT as monotherapy [16, 53, 80, 83, 88, 91], 1 used acupuncture therapy as adjunctive therapy [90], and 12 employed different types of cointerventions that included physiotherapy, acupuncture therapy, exercise training, manual therapy, and pharmacological medication [17, 48, 51, 52, 81, 82, 84–87, 89, 92]. Moreover, 9 RCTs reported an FU duration of 6 or 12 months [51, 52, 80, 82, 84–88], whereas the remaining 10 reported a short-term FU of ≤3 months [16, 17, 48, 53, 81, 83, 89–92].

Regarding the comparative alternatives administered to their control group, 9 RCTs used sham or no ESWT application [17, 48, 51, 81, 83, 84, 87, 89, 92], whereas 12 RCTs with a comparison control design used either noninvasive (conservative treatment [51, 52, 80, 81, 88–91] and specifically prescribed exercise training [51, 86]) or invasive (injection treatment [85] and acupuncture [53, 82]) treatment as ESWT alternatives.

The ESWT parameters and treatment protocols employed are summarized in Table 3. Of the eight RCTs that used FoSWT, five applied high-energy FoSWT [51, 84–87] and three applied low-energy FoSWT [16, 48, 83]. Of the 11 RCTs that used RaSWT, 5 employed high-energy RaSWT [52, 82, 88–90] and 6 employed low-energy RaSWT [17, 53, 80, 81, 91, 92]. Of all 19 RCTs, 18 applied an ESWT protocol comprising three to six treatment sessions over an intervention duration of 2–6 weeks [16, 17, 48, 52, 53, 80–85, 87–92], whereas one used a single ESWT session [86]. During ESWT sessions, local anesthesia was not administered at the treatment site in all included RCTs, except one, in which ESWT was applied immediately after surgery while patients were still under anesthesia [86].

Methodological quality of included RCTs

The methodological quality score of each RCT is listed in Tables 2 and 4. Regarding the cumulative PEDro score, interrater reliability was acceptable and the intraclass correlation coefficient was 0.98 (95% CI: 0.95–0.99,

Table 1 Guidelines of evidence synthesis[a]

Level of evidence	Criteria of judgement
Strong	Provided by consistent[b], statistically significant pooled results in SMD or OR derived from multiple RCTs, including at least two high-quality RCTs[c]
Moderate	Provided by statistically significant results in one high-quality RCT[c] **or** Provided by inconsistent[b], statistically significant pooled results in SMD or OR derived from multiple RCTs, including at least one high-quality RCT[c] **or** Provided by consistent[b], statistically significant pooled results in SMD or OR derived from multiple medium-quality RCTs[c].
Limited	Provided by statistically significant results in one medium-quality RCT[c] **or** Provided by inconsistent[b], statistically significant pooled results in SMD or OR derived from multiple RCTs, including at least one medium-quality RCT[c] **or** Provided by consistent[b], statistically significant pooled results in SMD or OR derived from multiple low-quality RCTs[c]
Very limited	Provided by statistically significant results in one low-quality RCT[c] **or** Provided by inconsistent[b], statistically significant pooled results in SMD or OR derived from multiple low-quality RCTs[c]
Conflicting	Provided by inconsistent[b], statistically non-significant results in SMD or OR derived from multiple RCTs regardless of quality

RCT randomized controlled trial, SMD standard mean difference, OR odds ratio

[a]Established in accordance with the "Best-evidence synthesis" which was adapted by Dorrestijn et al. [78] from the van Tulder's criteria [79]

[b]Pooled results are considered consistent if no statistically significant heterogeneity (I^2, $P > 0.05$) been identified and those are considered inconsistent if statistically significant I^2 ($P < 0.05$) been identified

[c]Methodological quality of a study is rated based on PEDro score as high (≥7/10), medium (4–6/10), and low (≤3/10)

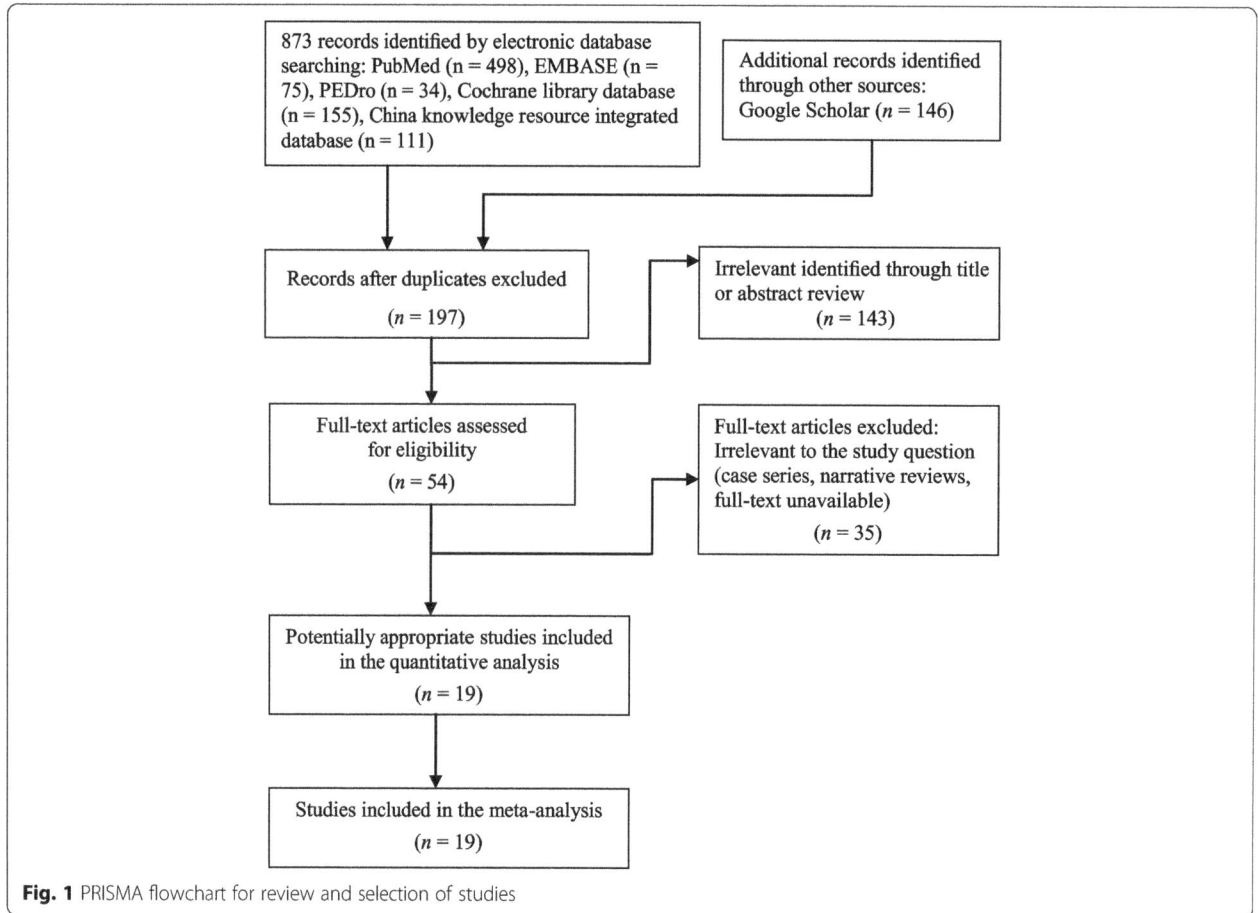

Fig. 1 PRISMA flowchart for review and selection of studies

$P < 0.001$). The methodological quality of all the included RCTs was rated as high or medium, with a median (range) PEDro score of 6 (5–9).

Risk of bias of included RCTs

Figure 2 shows details on each risk of bias item in each included RCT, as judged by the reviewing authors, and Fig. 3 provides an overall summary across the included RCTs. Selection, blinding, and attrition biases were considered to have caused the greatest risks of bias in the included RCTs.

Selection bias

Insufficient information on random sequence generation and allocation concealment led to selection bias in the included RCTs. Less than half of the included RCTs reported the randomization procedure [16, 17, 84–87, 89, 92] and concealed allocation [51, 52, 83, 84, 87] employed.

Performance bias

Difficulty in blinding participants and therapists (or care providers) when administering ESWT interventions with nonplacebo controls were deemed the major sources of performance bias in the included RCTs. The risk of performance bias was considered high in 14 [16, 17, 51–53, 80–82, 85, 88–92] and 16 [16, 17, 51–53, 80–83, 85, 86, 88–92] RCTs because participants and therapists were not blinded, respectively. One RCT applied ESWT immediately after ACL reconstruction surgery under the same anesthesia [86], which enabled masking of the group allocation to the patients while standard postoperative rehabilitation was performed [93]; however, because of the lack of information about whether the patients were blinded for group allocation in this RCT, its risk of bias was considered unclear.

Attrition bias

The assessor was blinded in six RCTs [48, 52, 84–87], and one RCT clearly declared that the assessors were not blinded [16]. However, the remaining 12 RCTs [17, 51, 53, 80–83, 88–92] did not mention blinding of the assessors.

Outcome reporting bias

All RCTs completely reported the results of all outcome measures described in the Methods section, including the pain score, patient-reported functional recovery, and performance-based measured outcomes (Table 2).

Table 2 Summary of included study characteristics

Study author (year) [reference]	Groups	N	Design	Diagnosis	Sex F/M	Age (years) Mean (SD)	Involved side Unilateral/bilateral	Athlete/nonathlete	Duration of symptoms (months) Mean (SD, range)	Cointervention	Follow up time point	Outcome results	Fund or grant§	MQ score*
Chen (2014) [51]	EG: ESWT + MSE	30	RCT, DB	Popliteal cyamella	102/18‡	63.0 (7.4)‡	NR	Nonathlete	10–144‡	None	Baseline	VAS[b,c]; ROM[b,c]	Funded	7/10
	CG 1: USD + MSE	30									Posttest: ≤1, 6 months	Lequesne's index[b,c]		
	CG 2: MSE	30												
	CG 3: Non-ESWT†	30												
Geng (2017) [90]	EG: ESWT + APT	30	RCT	CPT	19/41‡	35.9 (10.2)‡	NR	Nonathlete	4.7 (2.8)‡	None	Baseline	VAS[a,b,c]; PTT[a,b,c]	Funded	6/10
	CG: CT	30									Posttest: 1 month	4-point Likert scale[c]		
Guan (2015) [80]	EG: ESWT	73	RCT	PAT	91/55‡	45.5 (20–80)‡	128/18‡	Nonathlete	12.5 (6–36)‡	None	Baseline	VAS[a,b,c]	NR	6/10
	CG: CT	73									Posttest: 6 months			
Huang (2017) [88]	EG: ESWT	31	RCT	CPT	0/31	22.0 (3.0)	28/3	Athlete	12.0 (6–24)	None	Baseline	VAS[a,b,c]; VISA-p[a,b,c]	Funded	6/10
	CG: CT	30				0/30	21.0 (3.0)	29/1		11.0 (6–20)		Posttest: 1, 3, 12 months	4-point Likert scale[c]		
Jiang (2016) [81]	EG: ESWT	40	RCT	CPT	24/16	35.7 (9.1)	40/0	Nonathlete	4.2 (3.9)	PT	Baseline	VAS[a,b,c]; PJ[b,c]	NR	6/10
	CG: Non-ESWT†	36				21/15	34.4 (10.7)	36/0		4.7 (4.4)	Pain medication	Posttest: ≤1, 2 weeks	KOS-ADLS[a,b,c]		
Khosrawi (2017) [48]	EG: ESWT	20	RCT, SB	PAT	16/4	49.4 (7.8)	NR	Nonathlete	> 3 months‡	STE	Baseline	VAS[a,b,c]; MPQ[a,b,c]	Funded	8/10
	CG: Sham ESWT	20				15/5	50.2 (8.1)				Pain medication	Posttest: ≤1, 2 months			
Liu (2016) [82]	EG: ESWT	50	RCT, SB	CPT	22/28	22.1 (1.5)	50/0	Athlete	4.9 (1.3, 3–6)	APT	Baseline	VAS[a,b,c]; VISA-p[a,b,c]	Funded	6/10
	CG: Iontophoresis	50				23/27	22.2 (1.3)	50/0		5.0 (1.1, 3–6)	Massage	Posttest: ≤1, 3, 6, 12 months	4-point RMS[c]		
Taunton (2003) [83]	EG: ESWT	10	RCT, SB	CPT	5/5	23–52‡	NR	Athlete	> 3 months‡	None	Baseline	VISA-p[a,b,c]	Funded	5/10
	CG: Sham ESWT	10				5/5						Posttest: ≤1, 3 months	Vertical jump test[b,c]		

Table 2 Summary of included study characteristics (Continued)

Study author (year) [reference]	Groups	Age (years) Mean (SD)	Sex F/M	N	Design	Diagnosis	Involved side Unilateral/bilateral	Athlete/ nonathlete	Duration of symptoms (months) Mean (SD, range)	Cointervention	Follow up time point	Outcome results	Fund or grant§	MQ score*
Thijs (2017) [84]	EG: ESWT	30.5 (8.0)	8/14	22	RCT, DB	CPT	NR	Nonathlete	16.3 (18.2, 3–78)	ET exercise	Baseline	VAS^a,b; VISA-p^a,b	NR	9/10
	CG: Sham ESWT	27.3 (5.2)	6/24	30					24.9 (31.6, 3–125)		Posttest: ≤1, 3, 6 months	6-point Likert scale		
Vetrano (2013) [85]	EG: ESWT	26.8 (8.5)	6/17	23	RCT, SB	CPT	23/0	Athlete	17.6 (20.2)	STE	Baseline	VAS^a,b,c; VISA-p^a,b,c	NR	7/10
	CG: PRP	26.9 (9.1)	3/20	23			23/0		18.9 (19.1)		Posttest: 2, 6, 12 months	MBS^a,b,c		
Wang (2014) [86]	EG: ESWT	28.3 (7.4)	5/21	26	RCT, SB	ACL reconstruction	26/0	Nonathlete	21.4 (22.5, 1–72)	PT	Baseline	LFS^a,b,c	Funded	8/10
	CG: Non-ESWT†	27.7 (7.7)	6/21	27			27/0		15.4 (21.9, 1–84)		Posttest: 12, 24 months	IKDC score^a,b		
Weckström (2016) [52]	EG: ESWT	23.7 (2.0)	6/14	11	RCT	ITBS	NR	Nonathlete	60.4 (53.7)	MSE	Baseline	11-point NRS^b;	NR	7/10
	CG: CT	24.2 (2.2)	7/13	13					42.3 (65.1)	STE	Posttest: 1, 2, 12 months	Treadmill test		
Wu (2009) [91]	EG: ESWT	15.9 (11–19)	9/21	30	RCT	OSD	NR	Athlete	3–36	None	Baseline	VAS^a,b,c; MPQ^a,b,c	NR	6/10
	CG: USD	16.5 (14–19)	7/23	30					3–36		Posttest: 0, 3 months	3-point Likert scale^c		
Wu (2016) [89]	EG: ESWT	26.0 (19–38)‡	7/ 55‡	31	RCT	ACL injury	31/0	Nonathlete	3.8 (1–12)‡	PT	Baseline	VAS^a,b,c	NR	6/10
	CG: Non-ESWT†			31			31/0				Posttest: ≤1 month	4-point Likert scale^c		
Yang (2007) [16]	EG: ESWT	34.0 (7.4)	6/22	28	RCT	PTKS	28/0	Nonathlete	6.0 (5.3)	MSE	Baseline	VAS^a,b,c; ROM^a,b,c	NR	5/10
	CG: CPM	33.0 (8.4)	9/20	29			29/0		6.0 (3.3)		Posttest: ≤1 month	4-point Likert scale^c		
Zhang (2016) [92]	EG: ESWT	48.0 (4.6)	10/8	18	RCT, SB	Traumatic synovitis	18/0	Nonathlete	1–2	APT; MSE	Baseline	VAS^a,b,c; ROM^a,b,c;	Funded	6/10
	CG: Non-ESWT†	50.0 (5.8)	11/7	18			18/0		1–2		Posttest: 2, 4, 6 weeks	Swelling^a,b,c, LFS^a,b,c 4-point Likert scale		
Zhang (2017) [17]	EG: ESWT	34.8 (5.6)	7/21	28	RCT	PTKS	28/0	Nonathlete	4.7 (2.3)	PT	Baseline	VAS^a,b,c; ROM^a,b,c;	NR	6/10

Table 2 Summary of included study characteristics (Continued)

Study author (year) [reference]	Groups	Age (years) Mean (SD)	Sex F/M	N	Design	Diagnosis	Involved side Unilateral/bilateral	Athlete/nonathlete	Duration of symptoms (months) Mean (SD, range)	Cointervention	Follow up time point	Outcome results	Fund or grant[§]	MQ score[*]
	CG: Non-ESWT[†]	35.5 (4.9)	9/17	26			26/0		4.3 (2.6)		Posttest: 0 month	HSS[a,b,c]; 4-point Likert scale		
Zhou (2015) [53]	EG: ESWT	25.0 (18–30)[‡]	30/30[‡]	30	RCT	IPFP injury	50/10	Athlete	24 (1–48)[‡]	None	Baseline	VAS[a,b,c];	NR	6/10
	CG: APT			30							Posttest: ≤1 month	4-point Likert scale[c]		
Zwerver (2011) [87]	EG: ESWT	24.2 (5.2)	11/20	31	RCT, DB	CPT	18/13	Athlete	7.3 (3.6)	Sports participation	Baseline	VAS[a,b], VISA-P[a,b];	Funded	9/10
	CG: Sham ESWT	25.7 (4.5)	10/21	31			13/18		8.1 (3.8)	Medical treatment	Posttest: ≤1, 3, 6 months	Knee-loading pain test		

[*] Assessed using the 10-point PEDro classification scale
[†] No application of shock wave treatment
[‡] Value of total sample
[§] Details of the funding information of the studies are presented in Additional file 10: Table S3
[a] Significant improvements in the control group compared with baseline (P < 0.05)
[b] Significant improvements in the experimental group compared with baseline (P < 0.05)
[c] Significant between-group difference for ESWT compared with control (P < 0.05)

MQ methodological quality, EG experimental group, CG control group, ESWT extracorporeal shock wave therapy, RCT randomized controlled trial, DB double blind, VAS visual analog scale, NR not reported, ET eccentric training, VISA-P Victorian Institute of Sport Assessment-Patella, PRP platelet-rich plasma, PTKS posttraumatic knee stiffness, USD ultrasound diathermy, MSE muscular strengthening exercise, APT acupuncture therapy, LPNIR-LI linear polarized near-infrared light irradiation, CT conservative treatment, STE stretching exercise, ITBS iliotibial band syndrome, OSD Osgood–Schlatter disease, CPT chronic patellar tendinopathy, PTT patellar tendon thickness, PT physiotherapy, PAT pes anserine tendinopathy, MPQ McGill pain questionnaire, PI patellar intumesce, KOS-ADLS Knee Outcome Survey-activities of Daily Living Scale, ACL anterior cruciate ligament, LFS Lysholm functional score, MBS Modified Blazina scale, IKDC International Knee Documentation Committee, CPM continuous passive motion, LCSI local corticosteroid injection, HSS Hospital for Special Surgery Knee score, IPFP infrapatellar fat pad, ROM range of mot on

Table 3 Type of wave characteristics, source of stimulation energy, and application parameters

Study author (year) [reference]	Energy generator	Source of energy	Device	Manufacturer	Shock wave treatment protocol					Total treatment sessions	Interval between sessions	Treatment duration (week)
					Application parameters (per session)				Local anesthesia			
					Rate (Hz)	EFD (mJ/mm²)	No. of impulses	TED[a] (mJ/mm²)				
Chen (2014) [51]	Focused	Piezoelectric	Piezowave	Wolf, Germany	1–8	0.03–0.40	2000	60–800	Not used	6	1 week	6
Geng (2017) [90]	Radial	Pneumatic	LGT2500	Longest, China	NR	0.28	2000	560	Not used	4	1 week	4
Guan (2015) [80]	Radial	Pneumatic	DolorClast	EMS, Switzerland	5–7	0.05–0.075	2000–3000	100–225	Not used	3–5	1 week	3–5
Huang (2017) [88]	Radial	Pneumatic	NR	Xiangyu, China	12	0.18–0.31	2000	360–620	NR	5	1 week	5
Jiang (2016) [81]	Radial	NR	NR	NR	2–4	0.10–0.18	2500	100–625	Not used	6	2 days	2
Khosrawi (2017) [48]	Focused	NR	NR	NR	4	0.15	1500	225	Not used	3	1 week	3
Liu (2016) [82]	Radial	Pneumatic	DolorClast	EMS, Switzerland	10	0.21	2000	420	Not used	4	1 week	4
Taunton (2003) [83]	Focused	Electromagnetic	Sonocur	Siemens, USA	NR	0.17	2000	340	Not used	3–5	1 week	3–5
Thijs (2017) [84]	Focused	Piezoelectric	PiezoClast	EMS, Switzerland	1–2	0.20	1000	200	Not used	3	1 week	3
Vetrano (2013) [85]	Focused	Electromagnetic	Modulith SLK	Storz, Switzerland	NR	0.17–0.25	2400	408–600	Not used	3	2–3 days	2
Wang (2014) [86]	Focused	Electrohydraulic	OssaTron	HMT, Switzerland	NR	0.298	1500	447	Used	1		1
Weckström (2016) [52]	Radial	Pneumatic	Masterpuls MP 100	Storz, Switzerland	15	0.10–0.40	4600	460–1840	Not used	3	1 week	3
Wu (2009) [91]	Radial	Pneumatic	ESWO-AJ	EMS, Switzerland	1–15	0.10–0.12	2000	200–240	Not used	36	2 days	12
Wu (2016) [89]	Radial	Pneumatic	MP50	Storz, Switzerland	5–11	0.15–0.32	2000	300–640	Not used	4	5 days	3
Yang (2007) [16]	Focused	Electrohydraulic	HKESWO-AJ II	Wikkon, China	1	0.06–0.11	1000–2000	60–220	Not used	6	4 days	3–4
Zhang (2016) [92]	Radial	Pneumatic	MP100	Storz, Switzerland	10–15	0.08–0.15	2000–3000	300–640	Not used	18	2 days	6
Zhang (2017) [17]	Radial	Pneumatic	HKESWO-AJ II	Wikkon, China	8	0.11	1800–2000	60–220	Not used	8	3 days	4
Zhou (2015) [53]	Radial	Pneumatic	DolorClast	EMS, Switzerland	8–10	0.10–0.18	2000	200–360	Not used	5	4 days	3
Zwerver (2011) [87]	Focused	Piezoelectric	Piezowave	Wolf, Germany	4	0.10–0.58	2000	200–1160	Not used	3	1 week	3

[a]TED = EFD × number of shock wave impulses

EMS Electro Medical Systems, HMT High Medical Technology, DMT Dornier MedTech, EFD energy flux density, TED total energy dose (intensity × number of shock wave impulses), NR not reported

Table 4 Summary of methodological quality based on the PEDro classification scale[c]

Study author (year) [reference]	Overall[a]	Eligibility criteria[b]	1	2	3	4	5	6	7	8	9	10
Chen (2014) [51]	7/10[d]		X	X	X				X	X	X	X
Geng (2017) [90]	6/10	X	X		X				X	X	X	X
Guan (2015) [80]	6/10	X	X		X				X	X	X	X
Huang (2017) [88]	6/10	X	X		X				X	X	X	X
Jiang (2016) [81]	6/10	X	X		X				X	X	X	X
Khosrawi (2017) [48]	8/10	X	X		X	X		X	X	X	X	X
Liu (2016) [82]	6/10	X	X		X				X	X	X	X
Taunton (2003) [83]	5/10[d]	X	X		X	X			X		X	
Thijs (2017) [84]	9/10	X	X	X	X	X		X	X	X	X	X
Vetrano (2013) [85]	7/10	X	X		X			X	X	X	X	X
Wang (2014) [86]	8/10	X	X	X	X			X	X	X	X	X
Weckström (2016) [52]	6/10	X	X	X	X				X		X	X
Wu (2009) [91]	6/10	X	X		X				X	X	X	X
Wu (2016) [89]	6/10	X	X		X				X	X	X	X
Yang (2007) [16]	5/10	X	X		X				X		X	X
Zhang (2016) [92]	6/10	X	X		X				X	X	X	X
Zhang (2017) [17]	6/10	X	X		X				X	X	X	X
Zhou (2015) [53]	6/10	X	X		X				X	X	X	X
Zwerver (2011) [87]	9/10	X	X	X	X	X		X	X	X	X	X

PEDro Physiotherapy Evidence Database
[a]Points of methodological quality are denoted as "*X*" for fulfilled criteria
[b]Not used to calculate the total score
[c]PEDro classification scale: 1 = random allocation, 2 = concealed allocation, 3 = similarity at the baseline, 4 = subject blinding, 5 = therapist blinding, 6 = assessor blinding, 7 = more than 85% follow-up for at least one key outcome, 8 = intention-to-treat analysis, 9 = between-group statistical comparison for at least one key outcome, 10 = point and variability measures for at least one key outcome. Methodological quality: high, ≥7 points; medium, 4–6 points; low, ≤3 points
[d]Score was determined by a third assessor

Agenda bias

Information on funding sources and authors' conflict of interest disclosures is summarized in Table 2 and Additional file 2. Of the 19 included RCTs, nine were funded by one or more funding sources [48, 51, 82, 83, 86–88, 90, 92], whereas the remaining 10 did not report their funding source [16, 17, 52, 53, 80, 81, 84, 85, 89, 91]. Eight RCTs provided conflict of interest disclosures, of which two declared conflicts [83, 87] and the remaining five declared absence of conflicts [48, 51, 84–86] (Additional file 2: Table S2).

Publication bias

Visual inspection of the funnel plots of pain reduction did not reveal substantial asymmetry (Fig. 4). Egger's linear regression test also indicated no evidence of reporting bias among the trials ($t = -2.03$; $P = 0.06$).

Success or improvement rate

In total, 16 RCTs reported categorical data for pain and general outcomes (Table 2) [16, 17, 48, 52, 53, 82–92]. The treatment success rates (TSRs) for pain severity and global outcomes were mostly assessed using a Likert scale [57, 58]

and were reported by nine RCTs [16, 17, 53, 82, 84, 89–92]. In addition, seven RCTs reported the proportions of patients who experienced pain relief and self-reported improved symptoms after ESWT [48, 52, 83, 85–88].

There was moderate evidence from 16 RCTs [16, 17, 48, 52, 53, 82–92] (842 patients) that general ESWT yielded higher TSRs than did the placebo or active control (OR: 3.36, 95% CI: 1.84–6.12, $P < 0.0001$, $I^2 = 60\%$), regardless of the FU duration, shock-wave type, or application level (Fig. 5a and Additional file 3).

Subgroup analysis according to FU duration (Fig. 6a and Additional file 4) revealed moderate evidence from 11 RCTs [16, 17, 48, 52, 53, 83, 84, 87, 89, 90, 92] (518 patients) that at the immediate FU, general ESWT had a higher pooled OR for the TSR than the comparison control (OR: 3.09, 95% CI: 1.43–6.69, $P = 0.004$, $I^2 = 63\%$). General ESWT had no significant effect on the TSR at short-, medium-, and long-term FU assessments. Another subgroup analysis according to shock-wave type (Table 5) showed moderate evidence from 9 RCTs [17, 52, 53, 82, 88–92] (518 patients) that RaSWT had significant effects on the TSR at short-term, medium-term, and long-term FU assessments, with an overall pooled

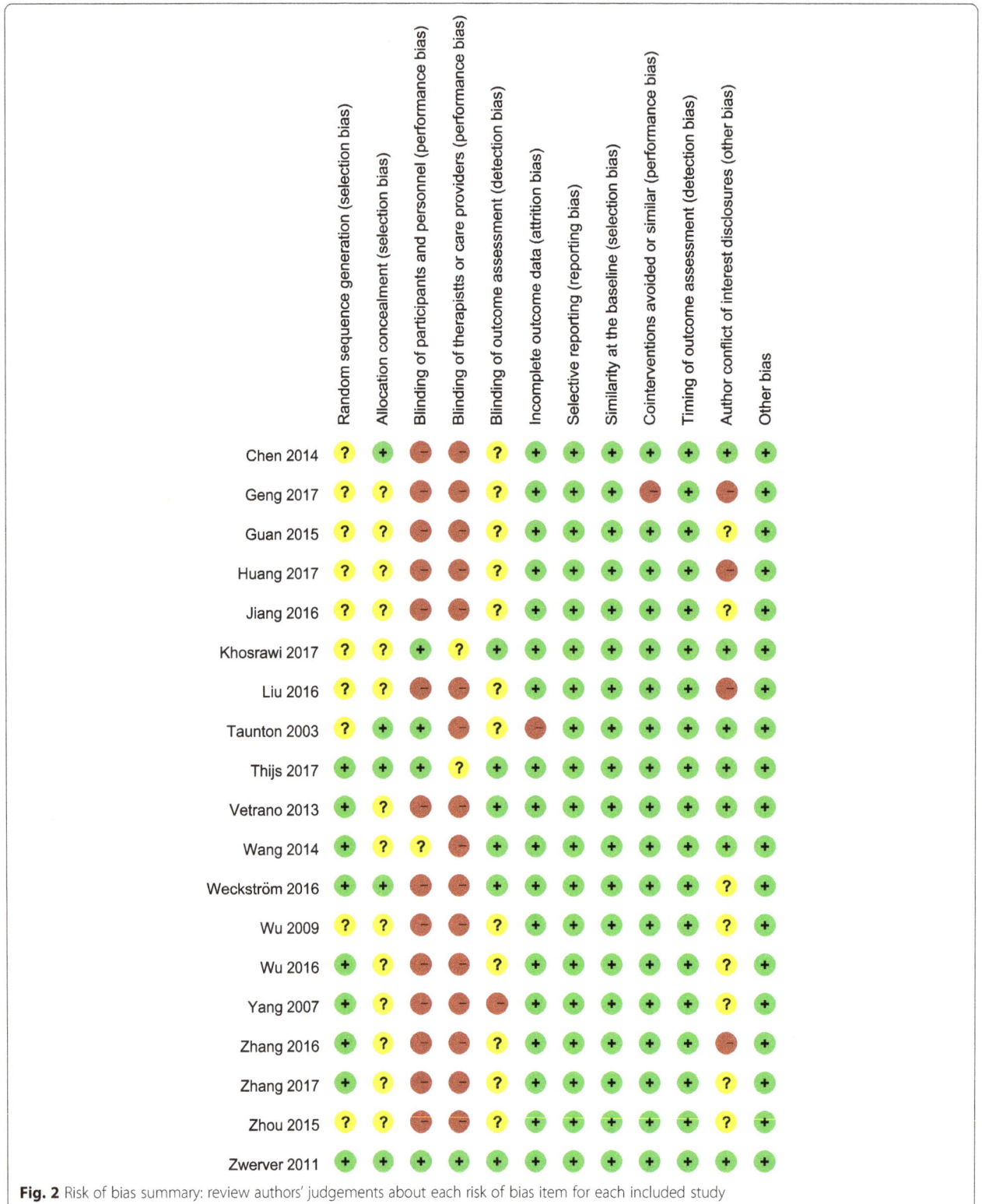

Fig. 2 Risk of bias summary: review authors' judgements about each risk of bias item for each included study

OR of 3.11 ($P = 0.01$, $I^2 = 73\%$), whereas FoSWT had significant effects only at the immediate FU, with an overall pooled OR of 3.28 ($P = 0.001$, $I^2 = 24\%$; LoE, strong; 7 RCTs [16, 48, 83–87], 324 patients).

Subgroup analysis according to shock-wave type, dosage level, and intervention duration (Table 5) revealed moderate evidence that RaSWT administered at high energy (5 RCTs [52, 82, 88–90], 308 patients; OR: 3.98,

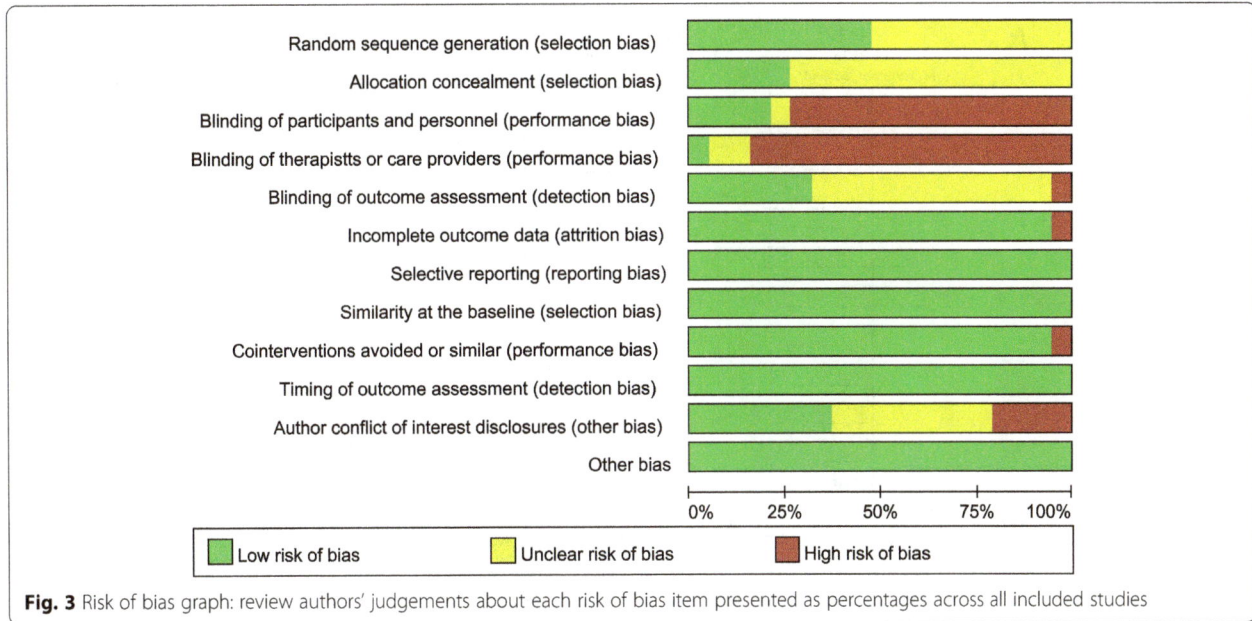

Fig. 3 Risk of bias graph: review authors' judgements about each risk of bias item presented as percentages across all included studies

$P < 0.00001$, $I^2 = 40\%$) and over a long intervention period (6 RCTs [17, 82, 88, 90–92], 375 patients; OR: 5.32, $P < 0.00001$, $I^2 = 0\%$) resulted in a significantly higher TSR than the corresponding control, as indicated by the higher pooled ORs; similar results were noted for FoSWT. Furthermore, low-energy FoSWT also had a higher pooled OR for TSR than its control (3 RCTs [16, 48, 83], 113 patients; OR: 5.32, $P < 0.00001$, $I^2 = 0\%$; LoE, moderate).

Another subgroup analysis according to control intervention showed that FoSWT as well as RaSWT resulted in a higher TSR than did the placebo control (5 RCTs [48, 83, 84, 86, 87], 221 patients; ORs 4.61, $P = 0.0006$, $I^2 = 0\%$; LoE, strong) and noninvasive comparisons (1

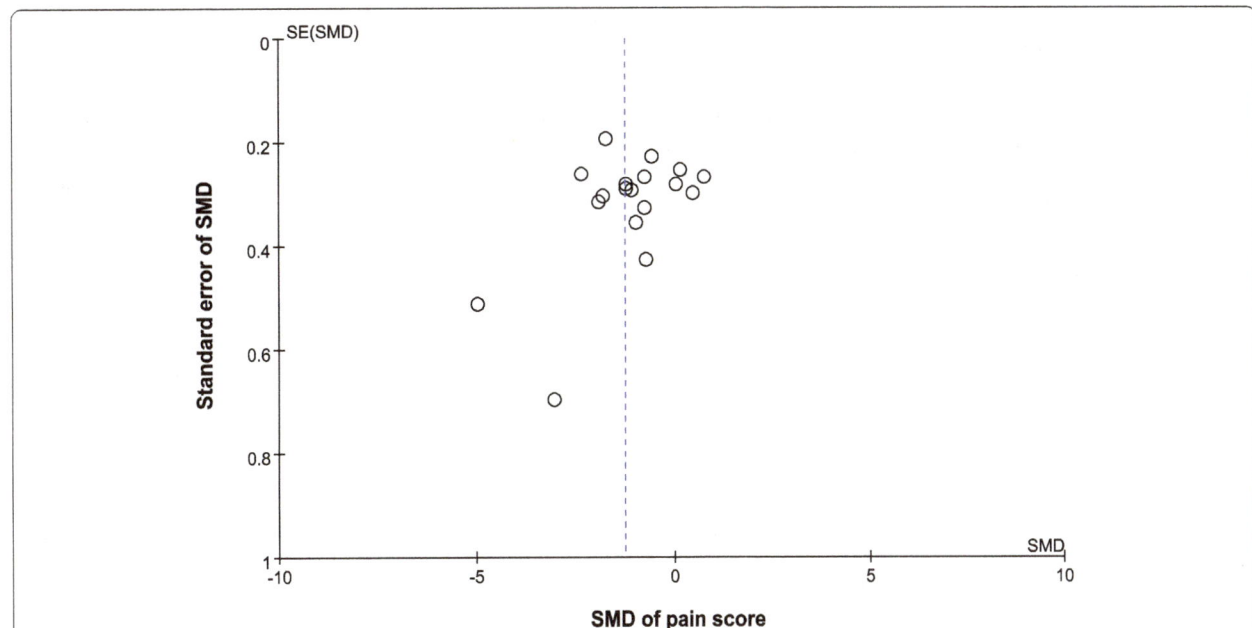

Fig. 4 Funnel plot of standard mean difference (SMD) versus standard error (SE). The SMDs of the pain score are plotted on the x-axis, and the standard error of the SMD is plotted on the y-axis. The vertical dotted line indicates the mean value of the SMDs. Visual inspection of the funnel plot of the SMDs of the pain score did not reveal substantial asymmetry. Egger's linear regression test indicated no evidence of reporting bias among the studies ($t = -2.03$; $P = 0.06$)

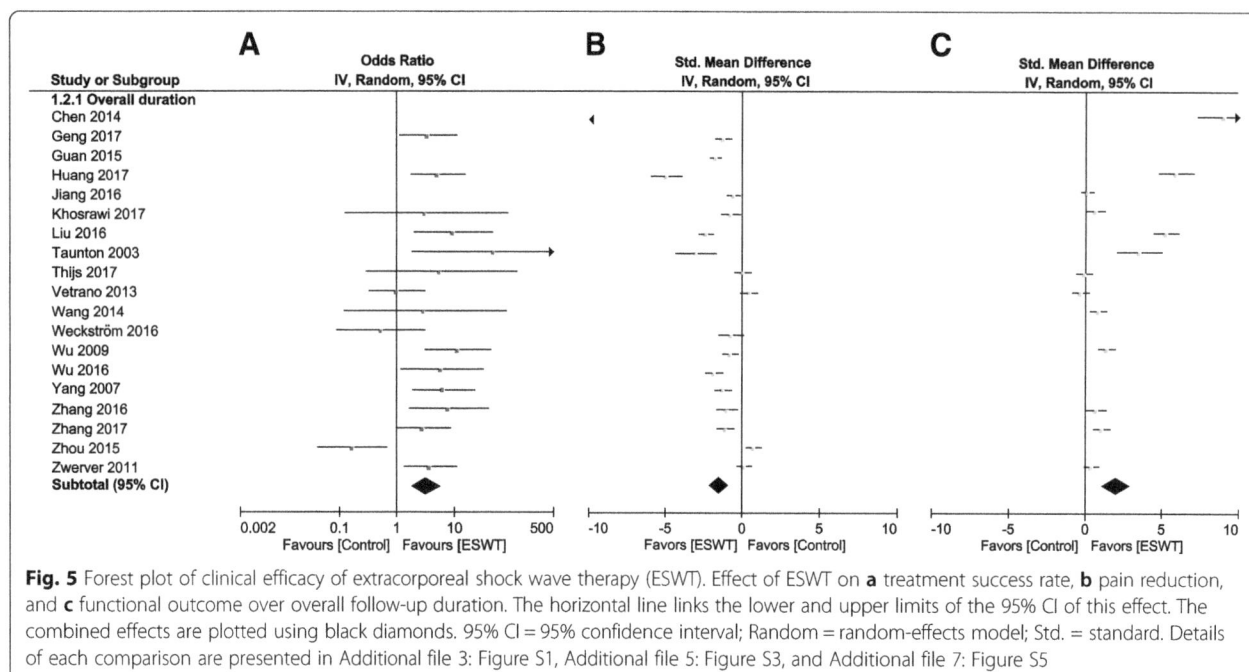

Fig. 5 Forest plot of clinical efficacy of extracorporeal shock wave therapy (ESWT). Effect of ESWT on **a** treatment success rate, **b** pain reduction, and **c** functional outcome over overall follow-up duration. The horizontal line links the lower and upper limits of the 95% CI of this effect. The combined effects are plotted using black diamonds. 95% CI = 95% confidence interval; Random = random-effects model; Std. = standard. Details of each comparison are presented in Additional file 3: Figure S1, Additional file 5: Figure S3, and Additional file 7: Figure S5

RCT [16], 57 patients; ORs 6.40, P = 0.003; LoE, limited; Table 5). No difference was noted in the TSR for pain relief between FoSWT and the invasive comparison control; similar results were obtained for RaSWT.

FoSWT resulted in significantly higher TSRs in both athletes (3 RCTs [83, 85, 87], 124 patients; OR: 2.47, P = 0.02, I^2 = 68%; LoE, moderate) and nonathletes (4 RCTs [16, 48, 84, 86], 200 patients; OR: 5.47, P = 0.001, I^2 = 0%; LoE, strong) than in their control peers (Table 5). However, RaSWT exhibited a significant effect on TSRs in nonathletes alone (5 RCTs [17, 52, 89, 90, 92], 233 patients; OR: 3.22, P = 0.0002, I^2 = 32%; LoE, moderate).

In patients with tendinopathies, both FoSWT and RaSWT exerted significant effects on TSRs, with pooled ORs of 3.62 (P = 0.008, I^2 = 38%; 5 RCTs [48, 83–85, 87], 214 patients; LoE, strong) and 4.67 (P < 0.00001, I^2 = 54%; 5 RCTs [52, 82, 88, 90, 91], 306 patients; LoE, moderate), respectively (Table 5). In patients with other KSTDs, FoSWT employed to treat ACL injury [86] and posttraumatic knee stiffness [16] had a significant effect on the TSRs, with a pooled OR of 5.83 (P = 0.002, I^2 = 0%; LoE, moderate). However, in four RCTs, using RaSWT to treat ACL injury [89], traumatic knee synovitis [92], posttraumatic knee stiffness [17], and infrapatellar fat pad injury [53] did not result in significantly high TSRs (Table 5). Nevertheless, after excluding the RCT with an invasive comparison control [53], RaSWT had a significant effect on TSR among patients with other KSTDs (OR: 4.41, 95% CI: 2.00–9.71, P = 0.0002, I^2 = 0%; LoE, moderate).

When applied with a monotherapy [83] and cointervention [16, 48, 84–87] design, FoSWT exerted a significant effect on TSRs (185 patients, OR: 11.73, P = 0.0002,

I^2 = 0%, LoE, limited and 308 patients, OR: 2.98, P = 0.0005, I^2 = 6%, LoE, strong, respectively; Table 5). However, in the subgroup of RaSWT, only the six RCTs [17, 48, 52, 82, 91, 92] (333 patients) with a cointervention design showed significant effects on TSRs (OR: 4.53, P < 0.00001, I^2 = 48%; LoE, moderate).

Effect on pain reduction
Eighteen RCTs assessed pain severity using the VAS [16, 17, 48, 51–53, 80–85, 87–92]. All pain severity data were transformed into 0–100-mm continuous data. Analysis of transformed pain scores revealed moderate evidence with large effect from 18 RCTs [16, 17, 48, 51–53, 80–85, 87–92] (1084 patients) that pain was significantly ameliorated after ESWT, with an overall pooled SMD of − 1.49 (95% CI: − 2.11 to − 0.87, P < 0.00001, I^2 = 95%) compared with the control group, regardless of the FU duration, shock-wave type, application level, or control intervention type (Fig. 5b and Additional file 5).

Subgroup analysis according to FU duration (Fig. 6b and Additional file 6) indicated moderate evidence with medium effect from 16 RCTs [16, 17, 48, 51–53, 81–84, 87–92] (892 patients) that general ESWT resulted in immediate pain relief, with an SMD of − 1.18 (95% CI: − 1.67 to − 0.68, P < 0.00001, I^2 = 91%), regardless of the shock-wave type, dosage level, or control intervention type. Similar results were obtained for short-term (10 RCTs [48, 52, 82–85, 87, 88, 91, 92], 469 patients; SMD: − 1.07, 95% CI: − 1.84 to − 0.31, P = 0.006, I^2 = 93%; LoE, moderate) and medium-term (6 RCTs [51, 80, 82, 84, 85, 87], 466 patients; SMD: − 1.98, 95% CI: − 3.32 to − 0.64, P = 0.004, I^2 = 97%; LoE, moderate) FUs. Another

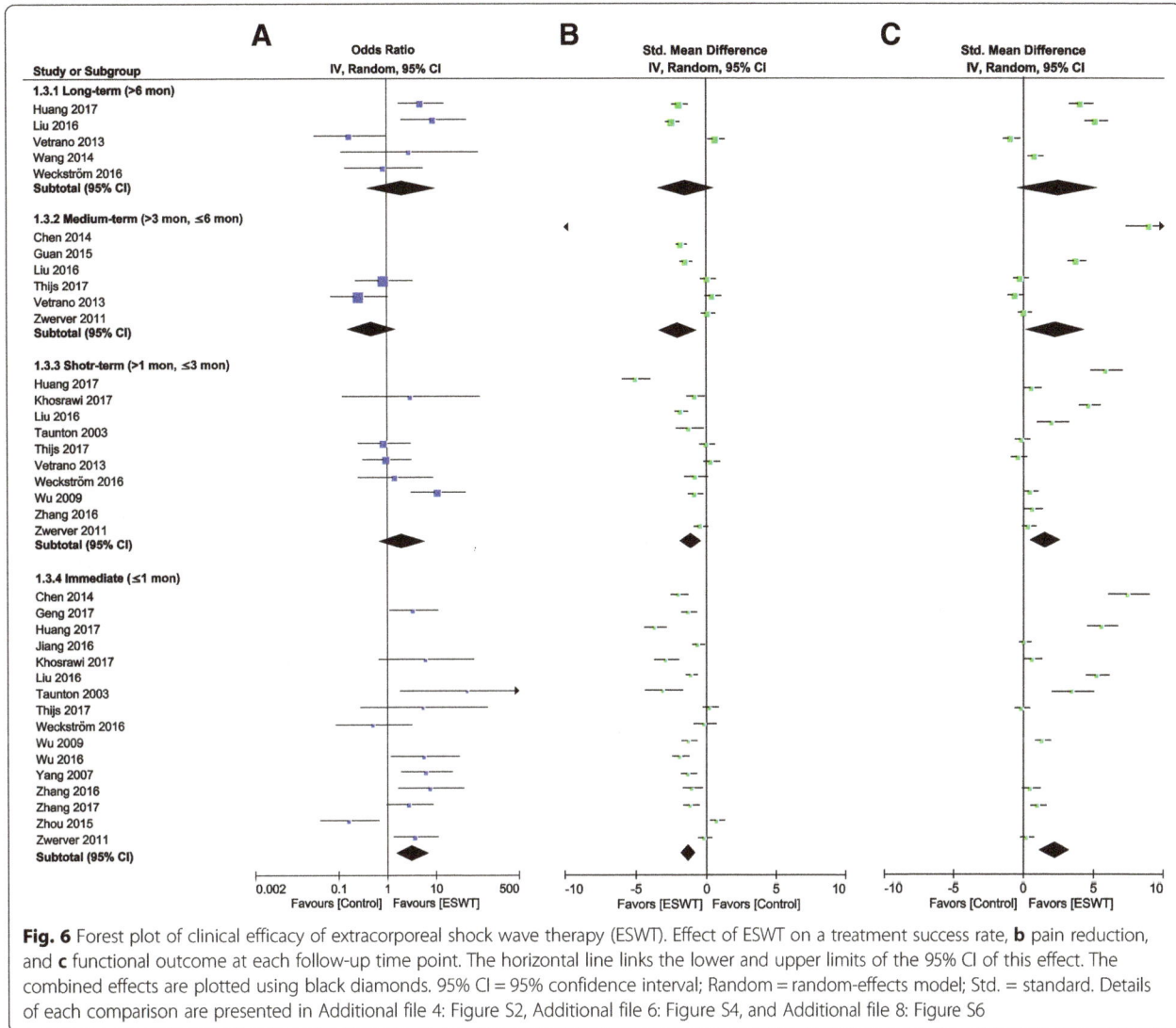

Fig. 6 Forest plot of clinical efficacy of extracorporeal shock wave therapy (ESWT). Effect of ESWT on a treatment success rate, **b** pain reduction, and **c** functional outcome at each follow-up time point. The horizontal line links the lower and upper limits of the 95% CI of this effect. The combined effects are plotted using black diamonds. 95% CI = 95% confidence interval; Random = random-effects model; Std. = standard. Details of each comparison are presented in Additional file 4: Figure S2, Additional file 6: Figure S4, and Additional file 8: Figure S6

subgroup analysis according to shock-wave type (Table 5) revealed that RaSWT had significant effects on pain reduction at each FU, with an overall pooled SMD of −1.36 ($P < 0.0001$, $I^2 = 93\%$; 11 RCTs [17, 52, 53, 80–82, 88–92], 747 patients; LoE, limited). FoSWT also had significant effects on pain reduction at all FU durations except the short-term FU, with an overall pooled SMD of −2.01 ($P = 0.002$, $I^2 = 96\%$; 7 RCTs [16, 48, 51, 83–85, 87], 337 patients; LoE, moderate).

Subgroup analysis according to shock-wave type and application level revealed modrate evidence with large effects that high-energy (4 RCTs [51, 84, 85, 87], 220 patients; SMD: −2.94, 95% CI: −5.05 to −0.82, $P = 0.006$, $I^2 = 97\%$) and low-energy (3 RCTs [16, 48, 83], 117 patients; SMD: −1.47, 95% CI: −2.42 to −0.53, $P = 0.002$, $I^2 = 77\%$) FoSWT as well as long intervention duration (3 RCTs [16, 51, 83], 137 patients; SMD: −3.13, 95% CI: −5.70 to −0.56, $P = 0.02$, $I^2 = 95\%$) exerted significant

effects on pain reduction (Table 5). Similar results were obtained for RaSWT. Neither FoSWT nor RaSWT with an intervention duration of < 1 month exerted a significant effect on pain reduction.

Compared with the placebo control, there were moderate evidences that FoSWT and RaSWT had a significant effect on pain reduction (5 RCTs [48, 51, 83, 84, 87], 234 patients, SMD: −3.22, $P = 0.001$, $I^2 = 97\%$ and 4 RCTs [17, 81, 89, 92], 232 patients, SMD: −1.14, $P < 0.00001$, $I^2 = 56\%$, respectively); similar results were noted in the comparison with the noninvasive controls (Table 5). Compared with the invasive comparison controls, FoSWT and RaSWT did not have a significant effect on pain reduction.

There was moderate evidence with large effect from 4 RCTs [16, 48, 51, 84] (209 patients) that nonathletes experienced significant pain reduction after FoSWT (SMD: −3.61, $P = 0.002$, $I^2 = 97\%$) but athletes did not

Table 5 Summary of subgroup analysis results[a]

Subgroups	Treatment success rate					Pain score reduction					Patient-reported functional improvement				
	Trials (patient), n	OR	(95% CI)	P value	I²(%), LoE[d]	Trials (patient), n	SMD	(95% CI)	P value	I²(%), LoE[d]	Trials (patient), n	SMD	(95% CI)	P value	I²(%), LoE[d]
Follow-up duration															
Focused ESWT															
Overall	7 (324)	3.28	(1.79, 6.02)[b]	0.001	25, S	7 (337)	−2.01	(−3.31, −0.71)[c]	0.002	96, M	7 (333)	1.08	(0.19, 1.97)[c]	0.02	92, M
>6 months	2 (99)	0.33	(0.07, 1.45)[b]	0.14	56, C	1 (46)	0.71	(0.11, 1.31)	0.02	NA, M	2 (99)	−0.01	(−1.66, 1.65)[c]	1.00	94, C
>3 months, ≤6 months	2 (87)	0.49	(0.19, 1.29)[b]	0.15	31, C	4 (220)	−2.74	(−4.85, −0.62)[c]	0.01	97, M	4 (220)	1.81	(−0.14, 3.77)[c]	0.07	97, C
>1 month, ≤3 months	3 (129)	1.02	(0.45, 2.32)[b]	0.96	0, C	5 (220)	−0.31	(−0.78, 0.16)[c]	0.19	65, C	5 (220)	0.42	(−0.17, 1.00)[c]	0.16	76, C
≤1 month	5 (225)	5.53	(2.71, 11.25)[b]	<0.00001	0, S	6 (291)	−1.39	(−2.37, −0.41)[c]	0.005	92, M	5 (234)	2.22	(0.51, 3.92)[c]	0.01	96, M
Radial ESWT															
Overall	9 (518)	3.11	(1.31, 7.38)[c]	0.01	73, M	11 (747)	−1.36	(−2.02, −0.71)[c]	<0.0001	93, L	6 (395)	2.56	(0.92, 4.19)[c]	0.002	97, L
>6 months	3 (185)	4.35	(1.96, 9.63)[b]	0.0003	49, M	2 (165)	−2.13	(−2.52, −1.74)[b]	<0.00001	42, M	2 (165)	4.64	(4.04, 5.25)[b]	<0.00001	68, M
>3 months, ≤6 months	0	NA		NA	NA	2 (246)	−1.59	(−1.88, −1.30)[b]	<0.00001	20, M	1 (100)	3.79	(3.12, 4.45)	<0.00001	NA, L
>1 month, ≤3 months	2 (80)	5.60	(1.97, 15.86)[b]	0.001	69, M	4 (249)	−2.00	(−3.41, −0.58)[c]	0.006	95, L	4 (261)	2.93	(0.48, 5.37)[c]	0.02	98, L
≤1 month	6 (293)	1.88	(0.59, 5.98)[c]	0.28	75, C	10 (601)	−1.07	(−1.67, −0.47)[c]	0.0005	91, L	6 (395)	2.29	(0.73, 3.84)[c]	0.004	97, L
Energy level (EFD)															
Focused ESWT															
≥0.2 mJ/mm²	4 (211)	2.25	(1.08, 4.49)[b]	0.03	8, S	4 (220)	−2.94	(−5.05, −0.82)[c]	0.006	97, M	5 (273)	1.65	(0.21, 3.10)[c]	0.02	96, M
<0.2 mJ/mm²	3 (113)	7.39	(2.52, 21.67)[b]	0.0003	0, M	3 (117)	−1.47	(−2.42, −0.53)[c]	0.002	77, M	2 (60)	1.99	(−0.82, 4.81)[c]	0.17	92, C
Radial ESWT															
≥0.2 mJ/mm²	5 (308)	3.98	(2.18, 7.29)[b]	<0.00001	40, M	5 (311)	−2.17	(−3.23, −1.11)[c]	<0.0001	92, L	2 (165)	5.49	(4.81, 6.17)[b]	<0.00001	0, M
<0.2 mJ/mm²	4 (210)	2.55	(0.43, 15.17)[c]	0.30	86, C	6 (436)	−0.73	(−1.44, −0.02)[c]	0.04	91, L	4 (230)	0.80	(0.19, 1.40)[c]	0.01	79, L
Intervention duration															

Table 5 Summary of subgroup analysis results[a] (Continued)

Subgroups	Treatment success rate					Pain score reduction					Patient-reported functional improvement				
	Trials (patient), n	OR	(95% CI)	P value	I^2 (%), LoE[d]	Trials (patient), n	SMD	(95% CI)	P value	I^2 (%), LoE[d]	Trials (patient), n	SMD	(95% CI)	P value	I^2 (%), LoE[d]
Focused ESWT															
≥1 month	2 (73)	7.89	(2.61, 23.88)[b]	0.0003	0, M	3 (137)	−3.13	(−5.70, −0.56)[c]	0.02	95, M	2 (80)	6.24	(0.86, 11.62)[c]	0.02	95, M
<1 month	5 (251)	1.52	(0.80, 2.87)[b]	0.20	38, C	4 (200)	−0.17	(−0.45, 0.11)[b]	0.23	61, C	5 (253)	0.51	(−0.17, 1.19)[c]	0.14	88, C
Radial ESWT															
≥1 month	6 (375)	5.32	(3.20, 8.83)[b]	< 0.00001	0, M	7 (521)	−1.80	(−2.52, −1.08)[c]	< 0.00001	91, L	5 (315)	1.99	(1.68, 2.30)[c]	< 0.00001	97, L
<1 month	3 (143)	0.78	(0.09, 6.69)[c]	0.82	81, C	4 (226)	−0.58	(−1.64, 0.48)[c]	0.29	93, C	1 (80)	0.11	(−0.33, 0.54)	0.64	NA, C
Control group type															
Focused ESWT															
Placebo	5 (221)	4.61	(1.92, 11.08)[b]	0.0006	0, S	5 (234)	−3.22	(−5.14, −1.31)[c]	0.001	97, M	6 (287)	2.03	(0.70, 3.36)[c]	0.003	95, M
Noninvasive comparison control	1 (57)	6.40	(1.89, 21.68)	0.003	NA, L	2 (117)	−2.07	(−3.73, −0.41)[c]	0.01	92, M	1 (60)	6.98	(5.59, 8.36)	< 0.00001	NA, M
Invasive comparison control	1 (46)	1.00	(0.31, 3.18)	1.0	NA, C	1 (46)	0.36	(−0.22, 0.95)	0.22	NA, C	1 (46)	−0.32	(−0.90, 0.26)	0.28	NA, C
Radial ESWT															
Placebo	3 (152)	4.41	(2.00, 9.71)[b]	0.0002	0, M	4 (232)	−1.14	(−1.42, −0.86)[b]	< 0.00001	56, M	3 (170)	0.70	(0.02, 1.39)[c]	0.04	77, L
Noninvasive comparison control	4 (206)	4.17	(2.23, 7.81)[b]	< 0.00001	61, M	5 (355)	−1.81	(−2.83, −0.80)[c]	0.0005	93, L	2 (125)	3.62	(−0.81, 8.04)[c]	0.11	98, C
Invasive comparison control	2 (160)	1.23	(0.02, 63.55)[c]	0.92	93, C	2 (160)	−0.80	(−3.85, 2.24)[c]	0.61	99, C	1 (100)	5.27	(4.43, 6.12)	< 0.00001	NA, L
Treated populations															
Focused ESWT															
Athlete	3 (124)	2.47	(1.16, 5.27)[b]	0.02	68, M	3 (128)	−0.84	(−2.16, 0.47)[c]	0.21	90, C	3 (128)	0.97	(−0.42, 2.37)[c]	0.17	91, C
Nonathlete	4 (200)	5.47	(1.98, 15.11)[b]	0.001	0, S	4 (209)	−3.61	(−5.86, −1.35)[c]	0.002	97, M	4 (205)	2.35	(0.38, 4.31)[c]	0.02	97, M
Radial ESWT															
Athlete	4 (285)	3.10	(0.50, 19.30)[c]	0.23	87, C	4 (285)	−1.79	(−3.73, 0.15)[c]	0.07	98, C	3 (225)	4.16	(1.09, 7.24)[c]	0.008	98, L
Nonathlete	5 (233)	3.22	(1.75, 5.94)[b]	0.0002	32, M	7 (462)	−1.24	(−1.57, −0.91)[c]	< 0.00001	60, L	3 (170)	0.59	(0.01, 1.18)[c]	0.05	72, L

Table 5 Summary of subgroup analysis results^a (Continued)

Subgroups	Treatment success rate					Pain score reduction					Patient-reported functional improvement				
	Trials (patient), n	OR	(95% CI)	P value	I²(%), LoE^d	Trials (patient), n	SMD	(95% CI)	P value	I²(%), LoE^d	Trials (patient), n	SMD	(95% CI)	P value	I²(%), LoE^d
Treated disease															
Focused ESWT															
Tendinopathy	5 (214)	3.62	(1.28, 5.36)^b	0.008	38, S	6 (280)	−2.29	(−3.84, −0.75)^c	0.004	96, M	6 (280)	1.14	(0.06, 2.21)^c	0.04	94, M
Other KSTDs	2 (110)	5.83	(1.86, 18.26)^b	0.002	0, M	1 (57)	−1.24	(−1.81, −0.67)	<0.0001	NA, L	1 (53)	0.84	(0.27, 1.40)	0.004	NA, M
Radial ESWT															
Tendinopathy	5 (306)	4.67	(2.61, 8.36)^b	< 0.00001	54, M	7 (535)	−1.70	(−2.48, −0.92)^c	<0.0001	93, L	4 (305)	3.47	(0.78, 6.16)^c	0.01	98, L
Other KSTDs	4 (212)	2.13	(0.40, 11.43)^c	0.38	83, C	4 (212)	−0.77	(−1.92, 0.38)^b	0.19	93, C	2 (90)	0.91	(0.47, 1.34)^b	< 0.0001	0, M
Cointervention design															
Focused ESWT															
Monotherapy	1 (16)	45.00	(1.83, 1104.64)	0.0002	NA, L	2 (80)	−5.17	(−6.43, −3.91)^c	<0.0001	98, M	2 (80)	6.24	(0.86, 11.62)^c	0.02	95, M
Cointervention	6 (308)	2.98	(1.61, 5.52)^b	0.0005	6, S	5 (257)	−0.26	(−0.87, 0.35)^c	0.41	83, C	5 (253)	0.29	(−0.12, 0.71)^c	0.17	63, C
Radial ESWT															
Monotherapy	3 (185)	2.18	(0.21, 22.89)^c	0.52	91, C	4 (331)	−1.62	(−3.32, 0.08)^c	0.06	97, C	2 (125)	3.99	(0.31, 7.68)^c	0.03	97, L
Cointervention	6 (333)	3.72	(2.11, 6.57)^b	< 0.00001	33, M	7 (416)	−1.26	(−1.78, −0.75)^c	< 0.00001	82, L	4 (270)	2.11	(0.02, 4.21)^c	0.05	98, L

^a OR odds ratio, I² heterogeneity, LoE level of evidence, SMD standard mean difference, NA not applicable, EFD energy flux density, ESWT extracorporeal shock wave therapy, KSTDs knee soft tissue disorders

^b Fixed-effects model

^c Random-effects model

^d Level of evidence: Strong (S), Moderate (M), Limited (L), Very limited (V), Conflicting (C)

(Table 5). However, after excluding RCTs with a short intervention period [85, 87], we observed a significant effect in athletes (SMD: − 3.03, $P < 0.0001$); similar results were noted for RaSWT.

In patients with tendinopathies, both FoSWT (6 RCTs [48, 51, 83–85, 87], 280 patients) and RaSWT (7 RCTs [52, 80–82, 88, 90, 91], 535 patients) had a significant effect on pain reduction, with pooled SMDs of − 2.29 ($P = 0.004$, $I^2 = 96\%$; LoE, moderate) and − 1.70 ($P < 0.0001$, $I^2 = 93\%$; LoE, limited), respectively (Table 5). In patients with other KSTDs, FoSWT—employed by only one RCT [16] (57 patients) to treat posttraumatic knee stiffness—exerted a significant effect on pain reduction (SMD: − 1.24, $P < 0.0001$; LoE, limited); by contrast, RaSWT—employed by four RCTs to treat ACL injury [89], traumatic knee synovitis [92], posttraumatic knee stiffness [17], and infrapatellar fat pad injury [53] in these patients—did not exert a significant effect (Table 5). Moreover, after excluding an RCT that administered an invasive comparison control [53], we observed that RaSWT had a significant effect on pain reduction in these patients (SMD: − 1.31, 95% CI: − 1.67 to − 0.96, $P < 0.0001$, $I^2 = 53\%$).

There was moderate evidence with large effect from two RCTs [51, 83] (80 patients) that FoSWT employed as monotherapy had a significant effect on pain reduction, with a pooled SMD of − 5.17 ($P < 0.0001$, $I^2 = 98\%$), whereas FoSWT administered with a cointervention, as occurred in five other RCTs [16, 48, 84, 85, 87], did not (Table 5). In contrast to the results for FoSWT, RaSWT employed as monotherapy had no significant effect on pain reduction; however, that with a cointervention, as occurred in seven RCTs [17, 52, 81, 82, 89, 90, 92] (416 patients), did (SMD: − 1.26, $P < 0.00001$, $I^2 = 82\%$; LoE, limited).

Effect on patient-reported functional outcomes

Thirteen RCTs used patient-report questionnaires to evaluate disability, functional mobility, and general outcomes (Table 2) [17, 48, 51, 81–88, 91, 92]. In particular, six RCTs [82–85, 87, 88] used the Victorian Institute of Sport Assessment-Patella questionnaire [59], one [86] used the International Knee Documentation Committee subjective score [94], one [51] used Lequesne's index [95], two [86, 92] used the Lysholm functional score [94], two [48, 91] used the McGill pain questionnaire [96], one [17] used the Hospital for Special Surgery Knee score [97], and one [81] used the Knee Outcome Survey-Activities of Daily Living Scale [98]. Combined analysis revealed moderate evidence with large effect (13 RCTs [17, 48, 51, 81–88, 91, 92], 728 patients; SMD of 2.03 (95% CI: 1.09–2.96, $P < 0.0001$, $I^2 = 96\%$), favoring general ESWT regardless of the FU duration, shock-wave

type, application level, control intervention type, or treated population (Fig. 5c and Additional file 7).

Subgroup analysis according to the FU duration (Fig. 6c and Additional file 8: Figure S6) revealed that general ESWT had an immediate effect on functional outcomes, with an SMD of 2.24 (95% CI: 1.16–3.33, $P < 0.0001$, $I^2 = 97\%$; 11 RCTs [17, 48, 51, 81–84, 87, 88, 91, 92], 629 patients; LoE, moderate), regardless of the shock-wave type, dosage level, or control intervention type. Similar results were observed at short-term (9 RCTs [48, 82–85, 87, 88, 91, 92], 481 patients; SMD: 1.56, 95% CI: 0.46–2.67, $P = 0.006$, $I^2 = 96\%$; LoE, moderate) and medium-term (5 RCTs [51, 82, 84, 85, 87], 320 patients; SMD: 2.28, 95% CI: 0.20–4.35, $P = 0.03$, $I^2 = 98\%$; LoE, moderate) FUs. Another subgroup analysis according to shock-wave type (Table 5) showed limited evidence with large effect from 6 RCTs [17, 81, 82, 88, 91, 92] (395 patients) that RaSWT exerted significant effects on functional recovery at each FU, with an overall pooled SMD of 2.56 ($P = 0.002$, $I^2 = 97\%$). However, FoSWT exerted significant effects only for immediate FUs, with an overall pooled SMD of 1.08 ($P = 0.02$, $I^2 = 92\%$; 7 RCTs [48, 51, 83–87], 333 patients; LoE, moderate).

Subgroup analysis according to shock-wave type and energy level (Table 5) showed moderate evidences with large effects that FoSWT applications with high energy (5 RCTs [51, 84–87], 273 patients; SMD: 1.65, 95% CI: 0.21–3.10, $P = 0.02$, $I^2 = 96\%$) and long intervention duration (2 RCTs [51, 83], 80 patients; SMD: 6.24, 95% CI: 0.86–11.62, $P = 0.02$, $I^2 = 95\%$) had significant effects on pain relief; similar results were noted for RaSWT. Both FoSWT and RaSWT—used by five RCTs [48, 84–87] and one RCT [81], respectively—with a short intervention duration exerted nonsignificant pooled effects on pain reduction.

Compared with the placebo control (six RCTs [48, 51, 83, 84, 86, 87], 287 patients) and noninvasive (one RCT [51], 60 patients) comparisons, moderate evidences with large effects favoring FoSWT (SMD 2.03, $P = 0.003$, $I^2 = 95\%$ and SMD 6.98, $P < 0.00001$, respectively) were observed; no difference was observed between FoSWT and the invasive comparison control, which is in contrast to the results for RaSWT (one RCT [82], 100 patients; SMD 5.27, $P < 0.00001$; LoE, limited; Table 5). In addition, with the placebo control, RaSWT exerted significant effects on function recovery (3 RCTs [17, 81, 92], 170 patients; SMD 0.70, $P = 0.04$; LoE, limited) but not with the noninvasive comparisons.

There was moderate efidence with large effect from four RCTs [48, 51, 84, 86] (205 patients) that FoSWT exerted significant effects on patient-reported functional outcomes in nonathletes (SMD: 2.35, $P = 0.02$, $I^2 = 97\%$) but not athletes (Table 5). However, after RCTs with short intervention duration [85, 87] were excluded,

FoSWT exerted a significant effect in athletes (one RCT [83], 20 patients; SMD: 3.52; $P < 0.00001$; LoE, limited). Athletes (three RCTs [82, 88, 91], 225 patients; SMD: 4.16; $P = 0.008$, $I^2 = 98\%$; LoE, limited), as well as non-athletes (three RCTs [17, 81, 92], 170 patients; SMD: 0.59; $P = 0.05$, $I^2 = 72\%$; LoE, limited), showed significantly improved functional outcomes in response to RaSWT.

For patients with tendinopathies, both FoSWT (six RCTs [48, 51, 83–85, 87], 280 patients) and RaSWT (four RCTs [81, 82, 88, 91], 305 patients) had a significant effect on patient-reported functional outcomes, with pooled SMDs of 1.14 ($P = 0.04$, $I^2 = 94\%$; LoE, moderate) and 3.47 ($P = 0.01$, $I^2 = 98\%$; LoE, limited), respectively (Table 5). Similar results were obtained for patients with other KSTDs receiving FoSWT (one RCT [86], 53 patients; SMD: 0.84, $P = 0.004$; LoE, moderate) or RaSWT (two RCTs [17, 92], 90 patients; SMD: 0.91; $P < 0.0001$, $I^2 = 0\%$; LoE, moderate).

There was moderate evidence with large effect from two RCTs [51, 83] (80 patients) that FoSWT implemented as monotherapy exerted a significant effect on patient-reported functional recovery (SMD: 6.24; $P = 0.02$, $I^2 = 95\%$), whereas FoSWT administered with a cointervention, as occurred in five RCTs [48, 84–87], did not (Table 5). The effect on patient-reported functional recovery was similar in the RCTs that administered RaSWT as a monotherapy (two RCTs [88, 91], 125 patients; SMD: 3.99; $P = 0.03$, $I^2 = 97\%$; LoE, limited) and those with a cointervention design (four RCTs [17, 81, 82, 92], 270 patients; SMD: 2.11, $P = 0.05$, $I^2 = 98\%$; LoE, limited).

Effect on performance-based functional outcomes

Only five RCTs used performance-based tests to evaluate functional recovery: the range of motion (ROM) measurement [16, 17, 51, 92] and the vertical jump test [83]. Four RCTs [16, 17, 51, 92] reported recovery in knee ROM and obtained moderate evidences, favoring FoSWT (two RCTs [16, 51], 117 patients) and RaSWT (two RCTs [17, 92], 90 patients), with consistent significant pooled SMDs of 2.61 (95% CI: 2.11–3.12, $P < 0.00001$, $I^2 = 0\%$) and 1.09 (95% CI: 0.64–1.53, $P < 0.00001$, $I^2 = 0\%$), respectively, regardless of the FU duration (Additional file 9). There was limited evidence with large effect from one RCT [83] (20 patients) that FoSW group exibited a significantly greater height in vertical jump test (SMD: 2.15; $P = 0.0002$, 95% CI: 1.00–3.30) compared with the placebo control group (Additional file 9).

Side effects of ESWT

The adverse events and loss to FU in each included RCT are summarized in Additional file 10. In all included RCTs, no clinically relevant adverse events, side effects,

or severe complications (e.g., hematomas, tendon rupture, and other abnormal musculoskeletal events) were reported after ESWT. Loss to FU in the FoSWT group occurred in four RCTs [51, 84, 85, 87], in which one to seven patients (3.2 to 31.8%) in the ESWT group withdrew from the study due to unknown reasons or reasons unrelated to the intervention. No patient was lost to FU in two FoSWT RCTs [16, 86], whereas the two other RCTs employing FoSWT [48, 83] did not provide information on adherence to shock-wave treatment. Compared with patients in the FoSWT group, no patient receiving RaSWT in 10 RCTs [17, 52, 53, 81, 82, 88–92] dropped out; however, one RCT using RaSWT [80] did not provide information on the number of patients lost to FU.

Discussion

Summarizing the evidence obtained in this meta-analysis

In this meta-analysis, we conducted a comprehensive search to select previous RCTs of the clinical efficacy of ESWT in patients with KSDTs. The results revealed significant moderate evidence of the safety and efficacy of general ESWT in increasing the TSR, reducing pain, enhancing patient-reported functional recovery, and improving performance-based functional outcomes in patients with KSTDs, regardless of the FU duration, shock-wave type, application level, control-intervention type, or treated population. Low-energy FoSWT may have higher efficacy in increasing the TSR and enhancing patient-reported functional outcomes than high-energy FoSWT. The reverse was the case for RaSWT. The intervention duration may have a higher influence on the efficacy of both RaSWT and FoSWT for KSTDs than the energy level.

Superiority of different shock-wave types and application levels

The present study demonstrated the pooled effects of ESWT for KSTDs according to the shock-wave type, energy level in EFD, and intervention duration, in contrast to previous systemic reviews of the efficacy of ESWT for lower-extremity musculoskeletal disorders [36, 45–47, 99]. Previously, van der Worp et al. compared the effects of FoSWT and RaSWT on patellar tendinopathy, and the treatment protocol comprised a low energy level (0.12 mJ/mm^2) and a short intervention period (3 weeks); they found no significant differences in the effects of FoSWT and RaSWT on the TSR and functional recovery at short-term (7 weeks) and medium-term (14 weeks) FU [100]. Król et al. revealed similar results for the effects of FoSWT and RaSWT on pain reduction at 3-, 6-, and 12-week FU time points in patients with elbow tendinopathy [101]. Compared with the aforementioned results, the present study that focused on KSTDs showed inconsistent results; that is, RaSWT exerted significant effects on the TSR and functional recovery at each FU time point, whereas FoSWT exerted significant effects only at immediate FU. Results of the present study may indicate that RaSWT is more likely to result in the highest treatment success or functional recovery than FoSWT. Nevertheless, this study also demonstrated that FoSWT and RaSWT with an application of a short intervention period had no difference in treatment efficacy. The discrepancy between the results of our meta-analysis and the findings of van der Worp [100] may be due to most RCTs included in our meta-analysis used a longer intervention period (> 3 weeks) and a higher EFD (> 0.12 mJ/mm^2) than those used by van der Worp did. These differences in the intervention period and EFD further explain our findings regarding the difference in athletes' responses to FoSWT and RaSWT. Athletes receiving FoSWT were mainly included from RCTs with short intervention periods, and those receiving RaSWT were mostly included from RCTs with long intervention periods. In addition, these differences also explain the difference in the effects of FoSWT on pain reduction and patient-reported functional recovery between RCTs with a monotherapy design and those with a cointervention design.

The influence of shock wave energy or dose on efficacy remains debatable. Previous studies have identified a dose-related effect on the treatment efficacy of ESWT. High-energy ESWT is recommended for treating calcified tendinitis [38, 102–104], whereas a low dose is more likely to result in the highest TSR and pain reduction for plantar fasciitis than medium or high doses [105, 106]. The inconsistency in the results of previous studies may arise from the inconsistent cutoff points set for low- and high-energy ESWT, which were set at 0.08 mJ/mm^2 [102, 103, 105], 0.12 mJ/mm^2 [38, 104, 106], and 0.33 mJ/mm^2 [107] for low-energy ESWT and at 0.12 mJ/mm^2 [38, 104], 0.28 mJ/mm^2 [102, 103, 105, 106], and 0.78 mJ/mm^2 [107] for high-energy ESWT, regardless of treated conditions. In the present study, we used an EFD value of 0.20 mJ/mm^2 as the cutoff for low and high energy levels; the results reveal that compared with high-energy FoSWT, the low-energy FoSWT may exert greater effects on the TSR and functional recovery and may exert similar effects on pain reduction in patients with KSTDs. Contrary to the results of FoSWT, high-energy RaSWT showed significant efficacy for all outcomes, whereas low-energy RaSWT did not. Given that an EFD of < 0.2 mJ/mm^2 has been identified as the optimal energy for FoSWT for tissue regeneration [30, 40, 108–110] and that low-energy RaSWT seems to have limited biological effects on human tendinopathy [33], results in this study may indicate the optimal use of low-energy FoSWT and high-energy RaSWT for enhancing clinical efficacy, particularly for the patients with KSTDs.

The other findings of this meta-analysis are as follows: (i) The intervention period may influence the efficacy of FoSWT or RaSWT. To date, few studies have analyzed various ESWT protocols based on the corresponding intervention periods. This meta-analysis demonstrated that an intervention period of ≥1 month exerted significantly effects on all outcomes favoring ESWT whereas a short intervention period (< 1 month) did not, regardless of ESWT type. This meta-analysis further identified no difference in the efficacy of FoSWT and RaSWT for KSTDs when both therapies were applied with a short intervention period in combination with either high or low EFD. The aforementioned results are supported by the results of previous studies, which showed that RaSWT with a short intervention period (< 1 month) exhibits efficacy similar to that of FoSWT with the same intervention period (< 1 month), regardless of the energy level [100, 101]. (ii) For treating KSTDs, both FoSWT and RaSWT had significant effects on the TSR versus their placebo control or noninvasive comparisons. Furthermore, FoSWT and RaSWT which are noninvasive therapies may be alternatives to such invasive interventions as local corticosteroid injection. However, in this meta-analysis, limited RCTs regarding the efficacy of ESWT versus invasive interventions were available. Thus, we could not obtain conclusive results in favor of ESWT over invasive interventions. Additional RCTs are required to determine the difference in efficacy between ESWT applications and invasive interventions. We further observed that the pooling RCTs with different type of controlled comparisons in the same subgroup may affect the efficacy of ESWT. For example, The subgroup including patients with other KSTDs than tendinopathy exhibited nonsignificant responses to RaSWT in terms of the TSR and pain reduction. The subgroup comprised patients from four RCTs of which only one conducted by Zhou et al. employed RaSWT versus an invasive intervention [53]. After the exclusion of Zhou's study from meta-analyses, the results showed significant effects on the TSR and pain reduction favoring RaSWT, and heterogeneity was improved. (iii) Our meta-analysis indicated that low-energy FoSWT exerted higher effects on the TSR and patient-reported functional recovery than high-energy FoSWT, and the RaSWT showed an inverse case. The shock waves applied in FoSWT and RaSWT have different physical characteristics, and the original source of energy production differs between these therapies. The acoustic wave generated in FoSWT is transmitted into the deep tissue and centrally converges on the targeted tissue, whereas that generated in RaSWT radially penetrates the body [13, 34]. Based on the nature of energy transconduction, the two shock-wave types have different magnitudes of energy (i.e., EFD) at the same tissue depth; in addition, the FoSWT sequentially travels further and has a greater impact on deeper tissues, whereas the RaSWT has superficially maximal energy at its origin [11]. Therefore, it is reasonable that the energy level of RaSWT should be higher than that of FoSWT for producing the same pulse energy at deeper targeted tissues, which may explain the discrepancy in the efficacy of high-energy and low-energy FoSWT and RaSWT for KSTDs in this meta-analysis.

Strengths and limitations

Compared with previous systemic reviews and meta-analyses of the efficacy of ESWT for knee orthopedic conditions [45–47], we included only RCTs to ensure level 1a evidence for therapy [111], and we included non-English trials [16, 17, 53, 80–82, 88–92, 112–115]. We also included RCTs involving soft tissue disorders other than patellar tendinopathy [16, 17, 48, 51–53, 80, 86, 89, 91, 92, 113]. Furthermore, we pooled comprehensive data to distinguish clinical efficacy levels at immediate, short-term, medium-term, and long-term FU, and we compared the clinical efficacy of different ESWT applications, namely different shock-wave types, application levels (i.e., energy in EFD and intervention duration), types of comparison controls, and treated populations (i.e., athletes and nonathletes). We performed comprehensive subgroup analyses to identify differences between different study designs (i.e., comparison types and patient types) and application levels (i.e., shock-wave type, energy level, and intervention duration).

Our meta-analysis has some limitations. First, not all types of KSTDs were included in this meta-analysis. Thus, the results may not be generalizable to other upper or lower limb conditions such as supraspinatus tendinopathy and Achilles' tendinopathy. Second, although the data did not suggest substantial publication bias and suggested a significant effect size for pain reduction, favoring general ESWT, we observed heterogeneity across the included trials. The noted heterogeneity may be due to the varying designs and application protocols of the included RCTs. Third, other application parameters such as the rate of shocks (impulses per second, Hz), number of treatments, and interval between treatments, which may interfere with therapeutic response, were not considered in comparisons in this study [9, 42]. Fourth, most of the 20 RCTs included in this meta-analysis described patient-reported outcomes; only five RCTs reported performance-based functional outcomes including knee ROM [17, 51, 86, 92] and jump height in the vertical jump test [83]. In our meta-analysis, RCTs reporting other performance-based functional outcomes, such as muscle strength, balance, and mobility, were not available. Compared with patient-reported outcome measures, performance-based outcome measures can provide more objective information on physical function in patients with knee disorders [116–118]. Thus, more data on performance-based physical functional outcomes are required to differentiate the efficacy of various ESWT applications. Fifth, in this meta-analysis, high risks of selection, blinding, and performance biases were identified; other potential biases, including agenda bias and biases resulting from cointerventions and loss to FU, were also noted. Because nearly half of the included RCTs reported funding information, and had a cointervention design and because more drop-out events were reported for FoSWT than for RaSWT, the results of this meta-analysis should be interpreted with consideration of the aforementioned potential biases. Finally, other confounding factors, such as age, sex, participation in sports, physical activity level, work type, and rate of return to sports and work, which may have contributed to treatment efficacy, were not considered in the analysis of the TSR.

Conclusions
Findings

This study obtained moderate evidence that general ESWT significantly increases TSR, reduces pain, and improves functional recovery in patients with KSTDs, based on meta-analysis of RCTs with acceptable methodology quality (PEDro score $\geq 5/10$) but high risks of potential selection, blinding, and performance biases. Additionally, this study provided limited to moderate evidence that both FoSWT and RaSWT with long intervention periods are superior to those with short intervention periods, regardless of the energy level. For long intervention periods, ESWTs can be ordered as follows in terms of their pooled effects on overall clinical outcomes for KSTDs: low-energy FoSWT, high-energy RaSWT, and high-energy FoSWT therapy. Furthermore, ESWT can be effectively performed with no severe adverse events other than a few minor side effects [101]. Both shock-wave therapies are worth considering in the treatment of soft tissue disorders, particularly KSTDs.

Implications for clinical practice

Our findings can help clinicians in identifying alternatives to conventional management strategies of KSTDs for determining the optimal treatment strategy.

Cautious application of ESWT for certain KSTDs

The generalizability of our findings is limited to the KSTDs reported in this meta-analysis. In addition, because our meta-analysis did not include sufficient RCTs involving KSTDs such as infrapatellar fat pad injury, traumatic knee synovitis, iliotibial band syndrome, posttraumatic knee stiffness, and gastrocnemius tendinopathy, ESWT should be cautiously applied for treating these KSTDs. Additional RCTs of the treatment effects of ESWT on KSTDs other than patellar tendinopathies are required to demonstrate the clinical efficacy of ESWT.

Additional files

Additional file 1: Table S1. Search formulas for each database. (PDF 272 kb)

Additional file 2: Table S2. Summary of funding information and the declaration of conflict of interest for each included trial. (PDF 262 kb)

Additional file 3: Figure S1. Data and forest plot of clinical efficacy of extracorporeal shock wave therapy for the treatment success rate over the overall follow-up duration. (PDF 86 kb)

Additional file 4: Figure S2. Data and forest plot of clinical efficacy of extracorporeal shock wave therapy for the treatment success rate at each follow-up time point. (PDF 69 kb)

Additional file 5: Figure S3. Data and forest plot of clinical efficacy of extracorporeal shock wave therapy for pain reduction over the overall follow-up duration. (PDF 90 kb)

Additional file 6: Figure S4. Data and forest plot of clinical efficacy of extracorporeal shock wave therapy for pain reduction at each follow-up time point. (PDF 108 kb)

Additional file 7: Figure S5. Data and forest plot of clinical efficacy of extracorporeal shock wave therapy for patient-reported functional outcomes over the overall follow-up duration. (PDF 701 kb)

Additional file 8: Figure S6. Data and forest plot of clinical efficacy of extracorporeal shock wave therapy for patient-reported functional outcomes at each follow-up time point. (PDF 93 kb)

Additional file 9: Figure S7. Data and forest plot of clinical efficacy of extracorporeal shock wave therapy for performance-based functional outcomes over the overall follow-up duration. (PDF 60 kb)

Additional file 10: Table S3. Complications and adverse events in the included trials. (PDF 364 kb)

Abbreviations
ACL: Anterior cruciate ligament; CI: Confidence interval; EFD: Energy flux density; ESWT: Extracorporeal shock wave therapy; FoSWT: Focused shock wave therapy; FU: Follow-up; KSTDs: Knee soft tissue disorders; LoE: Level of evidence; OR: Odds ratio; PEDro: Physiotherapy Evidence Database; RaSWT: Radial shock wave therapy; RCT: Randomized control trial; ROM: Range of motion; SD: Standard deviation; SMD: Standard mean difference; TSR: Treatment success rate; VAS: Visual analog scale

Acknowledgments
The authors thank Ching-Ya Hsieh for her assistance in database search and table editing. This manuscript was edited by Wallace Academic Editing.

Funding
This study received no fund or grant. The authors received no financial support for the research and authorship of this article. The authors certify that they have no affiliations with or financial involvement in any organization or entity with a direct financial interest in the subject matter or materials discussed in this article.

Authors' contributions
CDL, JYT, and HCC conceived and designed the study. CDL, HCC, JYT, and GMX searched and selected relevant studies. CDL, HCC, and THL extracted and interpreted data. CDL, HCC, and THL analyzed the data. CDL and THL wrote the paper. JYT and GMX revised the manuscript. CDL, GMX, JYT, HCC, and THL critically reviewed and approved the final manuscript.

Competing interests
The authors declare that they have no competing interests.

Author details
[1]School and Graduate Institute of Physical Therapy, College of Medicine, National Taiwan University, Taipei, Taiwan. [2]Department of Physical Medicine and Rehabilitation, Shuang Ho Hospital, Taipei Medical University, Taipei, Taiwan. [3]Department of Neurology, Ningbo Medical Center Lihuili Eastern Hospital, Taipei Medical University, Zhejiang, China. [4]Center for Evidence-Based Health Care, Shuang Ho Hospital, Taipei Medical University, Taipei, Taiwan. [5]Graduate Institute of Injury Prevention and Control, Taipei Medical University, Taipei, Taiwan. [6]Department of Physical Medicine and Rehabilitation, School of Medicine, College of Medicine, Taipei Medical University, No. 250 Wu-Hsing Street, Taipei, Taiwan.

References
1. Morelli V, Braxton TM Jr. Meniscal, plica, patellar, and patellofemoral injuries of the knee: updates, controversies and advancements. Prim Care. 2013;40: 357–82.
2. Barr KP. Review of upper and lower extremity musculoskeletal pain problems. Phys Med Rehabil Clin N Am. 2007;18:747–60.
3. Liu SH, Cui ZG, Han XZ, Liu KM, Wang AQ. The therapeutic effect analysis of three kinds of methods for the management of post traumatic knee stiffness. Zhonghua Wai Ke Za Zhi. 2012;50:814–7.
4. Pujol N, Boisrenoult P, Beaufils P. Post-traumatic knee stiffness: surgical techniques. Orthop Traumatol Surg Res. 2015;101:S179–86.
5. Leppänen M, Pasanen K, Kannus P, et al. Epidemiology of overuse injuries in youth team sports: a 3-year prospective study. Int J Sports Med. 2017;38: 847–56.
6. Myklebust G, Bahr R, Nilstad A, Steffen K. Knee function among elite handball and football players 1-6 years after anterior cruciate ligament injury. Scand J Med Sci Sports. 2017;27:545–53.
7. Farrokhi S, Chen YF, Piva SR, Fitzgerald GK, Jeong JH, Kwoh CK. The influence of knee pain location on symptoms, functional status, and knee-related quality of life in older adults with chronic knee pain: data from the osteoarthritis initiative. Clin J Pain. 2016;32:463–70.
8. Weber CD, Horst K, Nguyen AR, et al. Return to sports after multiple trauma: which factors are responsible?-results from a 17-year follow-up. Clin J Sport Med. 2017;27:481–6.
9. Ioppolo F, Rompe JD, Furia JP, Cacchio A. Clinical application of shock wave therapy (SWT) in musculoskeletal disorders. Eur J Phys Rehabil Med. 2014;50: 217–30.
10. Saggini R, Di Stefano A, Saggini A, Bellomo RG. Clinical application of shock wave therapy in musculoskeletal disorders: part I. J Biol Regul Homeost Agents. 2015;29:533–45.
11. van der Worp H, van den Akker-Scheek I, van Schie H, Zwerver J. ESWT for tendinopathy: technology and clinical implications. Knee Surg Sports Traumatol Arthrosc. 2013;21:1451–8.
12. Wang CJ. Extracorporeal shockwave therapy in musculoskeletal disorders. J Orthop Surg Res. 2012;7:11.
13. Loske AM. Extracorporeal Shock Wave Therapy. In: Graham RA, Davison L, Horie Y, editors. Medical and Biomedical Applications of Shock Waves. Cham: Springer International Publishing; 2017. p. 189–250.
14. Kim YW, Chang WH, Kim NY, Kwon JB, Lee SC. Effect of extracorporeal shock wave therapy on hamstring tightness in healthy subjects: a pilot study. Yonsei Med J. 2017;58:644–9.
15. Astur DC, Santos B, de Moraes ER, Arliani GG, Dos Santos PR, Pochini AC. Extracorporeal shockwave TERAPY to treat chronic muscle injury. Acta Ortop Bras. 2015;23:247–50.
16. Yang JH, Zhang PD, Xian XQ, Zhang ZM, Peng XW. Extr acorporeal shock wave therapy for tr aumatic knee joint functional disorder. J Clin Rehabil Tissue Eng Res. 2007;11:5179–82. https://doi.org/10.3321/j.issn:1673-8225. 2007.26.036. Available from: http://www.wanfangdata.com.cn/details/detail. do?_type=perio&id=xdkf200726036
17. Zhang XQ. Observation of curative effect by extracorporeal shock wave combined with rehabilitation training for traumatic knee joint function disorder. China Prac Med. 2017;12:29–31. https://doi.org/10.14163/j.cnki.11-5547/r.2017.11.012. Available from: http://www.wanfangdata.com.cn/details/detail.do?_type=perio&id=zgsyyy201711012
18. Guo HJ. Shock wave therapy for spine on the curative effect observation and rehabilitation guidance of ligament inflammation. China Health Stand Manage. 2014;23:1–2. https://doi.org/10.3969/J.ISSN.1674-9316.2014.23.001. Available from: http://www.wanfangdata.com.cn/details/detail.do?_type=perio&id=zgwsbzgl201423001.

19. Qin JZ, Dong QR, Fan ZY, Li LB. Extracorporeal shock wave therapy for the ankle ligament injuries in athletes:a prospective study. Chinese J Rehabil Med. 2015;30:355–8. https://doi.org/10.3969/j.issn.1001-1242.2015.04.009. Available from: http://www.wanfangdata.com.cn/details/detail.do?_type=perio&id=zgkfyxzz201504009.

20. Romeo P, d'Agostino MC, Lazzerini A, Sansone VC. Extracorporeal shock wave therapy in pillar pain after carpal tunnel release: a preliminary study. Ultrasound Med Biol. 2011;37:1603–8.

21. Du BC, Yang XM, Guan QL, WT T, Pan ZX. Extracorporeal shockwave therapy in anterolateral ankle soft tissue impingement syndrome. Prac J Med Pharm. 2017;34:678–80. https://doi.org/10.14172/j.issn1671-4008.2017.08.003. Available from: http://www.wanfangdata.com.cn/details/detail.do?_type=perio&id=syyyzz201708003

22. Yocom AF, Bass LD. Review of the application and efficacy of extracorporeal shockwave therapy in equine tendon and ligament injuries. Equine Vet Educ. 2017. https://doi.org/10.1111/eve.12780. Available from: https://onlinelibrary.wiley.com/doi/abs/10.1111/eve.12780.

23. Gallagher A, Cross AR, Sepulveda G. The effect of shock wave therapy on patellar ligament desmitis after tibial plateau leveling osteotomy. Vet Surg. 2012;41:482–5.

24. Waguespack RW, Burba DJ, Hubert JD, et al. Effects of extracorporeal shock wave therapy on desmitis of the accessory ligament of the deep digital flexor tendon in the horse. Vet Surg. 2011;40:450–6.

25. Langer PR. Two emerging technologies for achilles tendinopathy and plantar fasciopathy. Clin Podiatr Med Surg. 2015;32:183–93.

26. Smith WB, Melton W, Davies J. Midsubstance tendinopathy, percutaneous techniques (platelet-rich plasma, extracorporeal shock wave therapy, Prolotherapy, radiofrequency ablation). Clin Podiatr Med Surg. 2017;34:161–74.

27. Romeo P, Lavanga V, Pagani D, Sansone V. Extracorporeal shock wave therapy in musculoskeletal disorders: a review. Med Princ Pract. 2014;23:7–13.

28. de Girolamo L, Stanco D, Galliera E, et al. Soft-focused extracorporeal shock waves increase the expression of tendon-specific markers and the release of anti-inflammatory cytokines in an adherent culture model of primary human tendon cells. Ultrasound Med Biol. 2014;40:1204–15.

29. Notarnicola A, Moretti B. The biological effects of extracorporeal shock wave therapy (eswt) on tendon tissue. Muscles Ligaments Tendons J. 2012;2:33–7.

30. Vetrano M, d'Alessandro F, Torrisi MR, Ferretti A, Vulpiani MC, Visco V. Extracorporeal shock wave therapy promotes cell proliferation and collagen synthesis of primary cultured human tenocytes. Knee Surg Sports Traumatol Arthrosc. 2011;19:2159–68.

31. Visco V, Vulpiani MC, Torrisi MR, Ferretti A, Pavan A, Vetrano M. Experimental studies on the biological effects of extracorporeal shock wave therapy on tendon models. A review of the literature. Muscles Ligaments Tendons J. 2014;4:357–61.

32. Wang CJ. An overview of shock wave therapy in musculoskeletal disorders. Chang Gung Med J. 2003;26:220–32.

33. Waugh CM, Morrissey D, Jones E, Riley GP, Langberg H, Screen HR. In vivo biological response to extracorporeal shockwave therapy in human tendinopathy. Eur Cell Mater. 2015;29:268–80.

34. Ogden JA, Toth-Kischkat A, Schultheiss R. Principles of shock wave therapy. Clin Orthop Relat Res. 2001;387:8–17.

35. Cheing GL, Chang H. Extracorporeal shock wave therapy. J Orthop Sports Phys Ther. 2003;33:337–43.

36. Foldager CB, Kearney C, Spector M. Clinical application of extracorporeal shock wave therapy in orthopedics: focused versus unfocused shock waves. Ultrasound Med Biol. 2012;38:1673–80.

37. Schmitz C, Csaszar NB, Milz S, et al. Efficacy and safety of extracorporeal shock wave therapy for orthopedic conditions: a systematic review on studies listed in the PEDro database. Br Med Bull. 2015;116:115–38.

38. Speed C. A systematic review of shockwave therapies in soft tissue conditions: focusing on the evidence. Br J Sports Med. 2014;48:1538–42.

39. Storheim K, Gjersing L, Bolstad K, Risberg MA. Extracorporeal shock wave therapy (ESWT) and radial extracorporeal shock wave therapy (rESWT) in chronic musculoskeletal pain. Tidsskr Nor Laegeforen. 2010;130:2360–4.

40. Rompe JD, Furia J, Weil L, Maffulli N. Shock wave therapy for chronic plantar fasciopathy. Br Med Bull. 2007;81–82:183–208.

41. Speed CA. Extracorporeal shock-wave therapy in the management of chronic soft-tissue conditions. J Bone Joint Surg Br. 2004;86:165–71.

42. Notarnicola A, Maccagnano G, Tafuri S, et al. Prognostic factors of extracorporeal shock wave therapy for tendinopathies. Musculoskelet Surg. 2016;100:53–61.

43. Haake M, Boddeker IR, Decker T, et al. Side-effects of extracorporeal shock wave therapy (ESWT) in the treatment of tennis elbow. Arch Orthop Trauma Surg. 2002;122:222–8.

44. Roerdink RL, Dietvorst M, van der Zwaard B, van der Worp H, Zwerver J. Complications of extracorporeal shockwave therapy in plantar fasciitis: systematic review. Int J Surg. 2017;46:133–45.

45. Korakakis V, Whiteley R, Tzavara A, Malliaropoulos N. The effectiveness of extracorporeal shockwave therapy in common lower limb conditions: a systematic review including quantification of patient-rated pain reduction. Br J Sports Med. 2017;52:387–407.

46. Mani-Babu S, Morrissey D, Waugh C, Screen H, Barton C. The effectiveness of extracorporeal shock wave therapy in lower limb tendinopathy: a systematic review. Am J Sports Med. 2015;43:752–61.

47. van Leeuwen MT, Zwerver J, van den Akker-Scheek I. Extracorporeal shockwave therapy for patellar tendinopathy: a review of the literature. Br J Sports Med. 2009;43:163–8.

48. Khosrawi S, Taheri P, Ketabi M. Investigating the effect of extracorporeal shock wave therapy on reducing chronic pain in patients with pes anserine bursitis: a randomized. Clinical- Controlled Trial Adv Biomed Res. 2017;6:70–4.

49. Seol PH, Ha KW, Kim YH, Kwak HJ, Park SW, Ryu BJ. Effect of radial extracorporeal shock wave therapy in patients with Fabella syndrome. Ann Rehabil Med. 2016;40:1124–8.

50. Driessen A, Balke M, Offerhaus C, et al. The fabella syndrome - a rare cause of posterolateral knee pain: a review of the literature and two case reports. BMC Musculoskelet Disord. 2014;15:100.

51. Chen TW, Lin CW, Lee CL, et al. The efficacy of shock wave therapy in patients with knee osteoarthritis and popliteal cyamella. Kaohsiung J Med Sci. 2014;30:362–70.

52. Weckstrom K, Soderstrom J. Radial extracorporeal shockwave therapy compared with manual therapy in runners with iliotibial band syndrome. J Back Musculoskelet Rehabil. 2016;29:161–70.

53. Zhou K, Li XJ. The comparison of acupuncture and shock wave therapeutics for the injury of infrapatellar fat pad. China J Modern Med. 2015;25:91–4.

54. Song F, Parekh S, Hooper L, et al. Dissemination and publication of research findings: an updated review of related biases. Health Technol Assess. 2010;14:1–193.

55. Moher D, Shamseer L, Clarke M, et al. Preferred reporting items for systematic review and meta-analysis protocols (PRISMA-P) 2015 statement. Syst Rev. 2015;4:1.

56. Roles NC, Maudsley RH. Radial tunnel syndrome: resistant tennis elbow as a nerve entrapment. J Bone Joint Surg Br. 1972;54:499–508.

57. Norman G. Likert scales, levels of measurement and the "laws" of statistics. Adv Health Sci Educ Theory Pract. 2010;15:625–32.

58. Carifio J, Perla RJ. Ten common misunderstandings, misconceptions, persistent myths and urban legends about Likert. J Soc Sci. 2007;3:106–16.

59. Mendonca Lde M, Ocarino JM, Bittencourt NF, Fernandes LM, Verhagen E, Fonseca ST. The accuracy of the VISA-P questionnaire, single-leg decline squat, and tendon pain history to identify patellar tendon abnormalities in adult athletes. J Orthop Sports Phys Ther. 2016;46:673–80.

60. Moher D, Hopewell S, Schulz KF, et al. CONSORT 2010 explanation and elaboration: updated guidelines for reporting parallel group randomised trials. Int J Surg. 2012;10:28–55.

61. Furlan AD, Malmivaara A, Chou R, et al. Updated method guideline for systematic reviews in the Cochrane back and neck group. Spine (Phila pa 1976). 2015;40:1660–73.

62. Higgins JPT, Altman DG, Sterne JAC. Chapter 8: Assessing risk of bias in included studies., in Cochrane handbook for systematic reviews of

interventions version 5.1.0 [updated March 2011]. In: JPT H, Green S, editors. The Cochrane Collaboration; 2011.

63. de Morton NA. The PEDro scale is a valid measure of the methodological quality of clinical trials: a demographic study. Aust J Physiother. 2009;55: 129–33.

64. Maher CG, Sherrington C, Herbert RD, Moseley AM, Elkins M. Reliability of the PEDro scale for rating quality of randomized controlled trials. Phys Ther. 2003;83:713–21.

65. Foley NC, Bhogal SK, Teasell RW, Bureau Y, Speechley MR. Estimates of quality and reliability with the physiotherapy evidence-based database scale to assess the methodology of randomized controlled trials of pharmacological and nonpharmacological interventions. Phys Ther. 2006;86:817–24.

66. For the cumulative PEDro score tirgkswctbaticcwctb, da Costa BR, Cummings GG, et al. PEDro or Cochrane to Assess the Quality of Clinical Trials? A Meta-Epidemiological Study. PLoS ONE. 2015;10:e0132634.

67. Briani RV, Ferreira AS, Pazzinatto MF, Pappas E, De Oliveira SD, Azevedo FM. What interventions can improve quality of life or psychosocial factors of individuals with knee osteoarthritis? A systematic review with meta-analysis of primary outcomes from randomised controlled trials. Br J Sports Med. 2018. https://doi.org/10.1136/bjsports-2017-098099. [Epub ahead of print]

68. Higgins JP, Altman DG, Gotzsche PC, et al. The Cochrane Collaboration's tool for assessing risk of bias in randomised trials. BMJ. 2011;343:d5928.

69. Higgins JPT, Green S. Cochrane Handbook for Systematic Reviews of Interventions Version 5.1.0 [updated March 2011]. In: The Cochrane Collaboration; 2011.

70. Follmann D, Elliott P, Suh I, Cutler J. Variance imputation for overviews of clinical trials with continuous response. J Clin Epidemiol. 1992;45:769–73.

71. Abrams KR, Gillies CL, Lambert PC. Meta-analysis of heterogeneously reported trials assessing change from baseline. Stat Med. 2005;24:3823–44.

72. Wan X, Wang W, Liu J, Tong T. Estimating the sample mean and standard deviation from the sample size, median, range and/or interquartile range. BMC Med Res Methodol. 2014;14:1–21.

73. Cohen J. Statistical power analysis for the behavioral sciences. 2nd ed. Hillsdale: Lawrence Erlbaum Associates; 1988.

74. Hopkins WG. A Scale of Magnitudes for Effect Statistics a new view of statistics 2002 [cited 2018 Jun 04]; Available from: http://sportsci.org/resource/stats/effectmag.html.

75. Bowden J, Tierney JF, Copas AJ, Burdett S. Quantifying, displaying and accounting for heterogeneity in the meta-analysis of RCTs using standard and generalised Q statistics. BMC Med Res Methodol. 2011;11:41–53.

76. Sedgwick P, Marston L. How to read a funnel plot in a meta-analysis. BMJ. 2015;351:1–3.

77. Egger M, Davey Smith G, Schneider M, Minder C. Bias in meta-analysis detected by a simple, graphical test. BMJ. 1997;315:629–34.

78. Dorrestijn O, Stevens M, Winters JC, van der Meer K, Diercks RL. Conservative or surgical treatment for subacromial impingement syndrome? A systematic review. J Shoulder Elb Surg. 2009;18:652–60.

79. van Tulder M, Furlan A, Bombardier C, Bouter L. Updated method guidelines for systematic reviews in the cochrane collaboration back review group. Spine (Phila Pa 1976). 2003;28:1290–9.

80. Guan QL, Pan ZX, Wang ZZ, Wang XH. Long-term treatment effect of radial extracorporeal shock wave therapy for pes anserinus tendinitis. People's Military Surgeon. 2015;58:56–7. Available from: http://www.wanfangdata.com.cn/details/detail.do?_type=perio&id=QKC20152015020400012913

81. Jiang DB, Xu XP, Liu P, Liu HX, Zhu XL, Zhang SW. Effect of shock wave therapy on short-term treatment outcomes of post-traumatic patellofemoral joint arthritis. Chinese J Rehabil. 2016;31:349–51. https://doi.org/10.3969/j.issn.1001-1242.2016.03.021. Available from: http://med.wanfangdata.com.cn/Paper/Detail?id=PeriodicalPaper_zgkfyxzz201603021.

82. Liu YB, Zhang ZH, Zhou JR, Li QH. Effect of shockwave therapy on patellar tendon injury after sport fatigue. Sci Technol Vision. 2016;25:45–6. https://doi.org/10.3969/j.issn.2095-2457.2016.25.031. Available from: http://www.wanfangdata.com.cn/details/detail.do?_type=perio&id=hqsgkj201625031

83. Taunton KM, Taunton JE, Khan KM. Treatment of patellar tendinopathy with extracorporeal shock wave therapy. BC Med J. 2003;45:500–7.

84. Thijs KM, Zwerver J, Backx FJ, et al. Effectiveness of shockwave treatment combined with eccentric training for patellar tendinopathy: a double-blinded randomized study. Clin J Sport Med. 2017;27:89–96.

85. Vetrano M, Castorina A, Vulpiani MC, Baldini R, Pavan A, Ferretti A. Platelet-rich plasma versus focused shock waves in the treatment of jumper's knee in athletes. Am J Sports Med. 2013;41:795–803.

86. Wang CJ, Ko JY, Chou WY, et al. Shockwave therapy improves anterior cruciate ligament reconstruction. J Surg Res. 2014;188:110–8.

87. Zwerver J, Hartgens F, Verhagen E, van der Worp H, van den Akker-Scheek I, Diercks RL. No effect of extracorporeal shockwave therapy on patellar tendinopathy in jumping athletes during the competitive season: a randomized clinical trial. Am J Sports Med. 2011;39:1191–9.

88. Huang YQ, Tang BQ, Lin ZD, Luo YG, Liao CC, Wu JC. Clinical observation of external shock wave in the treatment of chronic peripheral patellar tendonitis in soldiers. China Mod Doct. 2017;55:73–6. Available from: http://www.wanfangdata.com.cn/details/detail.do?_type=perio&id=zwkjzlml-yyws201718021

89. Wu XH, Li YG. Clinical effect of comprehensive therapy in treating cruciate ligament injury of knee joint. Anhui Med J. 2016;37:193–5. https://doi.org/10.3969/j.issn.1000-0399.2016.02.020. Available from: http://www.wanfangdata.com.cn/details/detail.do?_type=perio&id=ahyx201602022

90. Geng JB, Li MG, Peng QJ. Efficacy analysis of needle knife combined extracopreal shock wave therapy in the treatment of patellar tendinitis. World Chinese Med. 2017;12:2172–5. https://doi.org/10.3969/j.issn.1673-7202.2017.09.045. Available from: http://www.wanfangdata.com.cn/details/detail.do?_type=perio&id=sjzyy201709046.

91. Wu D, Lu YF. A therapeutical observation on the treatment of tibial tuberosity osteochondritis treated by radial shock wave. Health Res. 2009;29:27–31. https://doi.org/10.3969/j.issn.1674-6449.2009.01.008. Available from: http://www.wanfangdata.com.cn/details/detail.do?_type=perio&id=jkyj200901008.

92. Zhang Q, Ren YR, Li J, Chen J, Wang L. The clinical observation of shock wave combined with systematic rehabilitation on acute traumatic synovitis in knee joint. J Emerg Tradit Chin Med. 2016;25:1141–3. https://doi.org/10.3969/j.issn.1004-745X.2016.06.063. Available from: http://www.wanfangdata.com.cn/details/detail.do?_type=perio&id=zgzyjz201606064

93. Eshuis R, Lentjes GW, Tegner Y, Wolterbeek N, Veen MR. Dutch translation and cross-cultural adaptation of the Lysholm score and Tegner activity scale for patients with anterior cruciate ligament injuries. J Orthop Sports Phys Ther. 2016;46:976–83.

94. Lequesne M. Indices of severity and disease activity for osteoarthritis. Semin Arthritis Rheum. 1991;20:48–54.

95. Melzack R. The McGill pain questionnaire: major properties and scoring methods. Pain. 1975;1:277–99.

96. Narin S, Unver B, Bakirhan S, Bozan O, Karatosun V. Cross-cultural adaptation, reliability and validity of the Turkish version of the Hospital for Special Surgery (HSS) knee score. Acta Orthop Traumatol Turc. 2014;48:241–8.

97. Bouzubar FF, Aljadi SH, Alotaibi NM, Irrgang JJ. Cross-cultural adaptation and validation of the Arabic version of the knee outcome survey-activities for daily living scale. Disabil Rehabil. 2018;40:1817–28.

98. Boutron I, Guittet L, Estellat C, Moher D, Hrobjartsson A, Ravaud P. Reporting methods of blinding in randomized trials assessing nonpharmacological treatments. PLoS Med. 2007;4:e61.

99. Al-Abbad H, Simon JV. The effectiveness of extracorporeal shock wave therapy on chronic achilles tendinopathy: a systematic review. Foot Ankle Int. 2013;34:33–41.

100. van der Worp H, Zwerver J, Hamstra M, van den Akker-Scheek I, Diercks RL. No difference in effectiveness between focused and radial shockwave therapy for treating patellar tendinopathy: a randomized controlled trial. Knee Surg Sports Traumatol Arthrosc. 2014;22:2026–32.

101. Król P, Franek A, Durmala J, et al. Focused and radial shock wave therapy in the treatment of tennis elbow: a pilot randomised controlled study. J Hum Kinet. 2015;47:127–35.

102. Verstraelen FU, In den Kleef NJ, Jansen L, Morrenhof JW. High-energy versus low-energy extracorporeal shock wave therapy for calcifying tendinitis of the shoulder: which is superior? A meta-analysis. Clin Orthop Relat Res. 2014;472:2816–25.

103. Bannuru RR, Flavin NE, Vaysbrot E, Harvey W, McAlindon T. High-energy extracorporeal shock-wave therapy for treating chronic calcific tendinitis of the shoulder: a systematic review. Ann Intern Med. 2014; 160:542–9.

104. Wu YC, Tsai WC, Tu YK, Yu TY. Comparative effectiveness of non-operative treatments for chronic calcific tendinitis of the shoulder: a systematic review and network meta-analysis of randomized-controlled trials. Arch Phys Med Rehabil. 2017;98:1678–92.

105. Chang KV, Chen SY, Chen WS, Tu YK, Chien KL. Comparative effectiveness of focused shock wave therapy of different intensity levels and radial shock

wave therapy for treating plantar fasciitis: a systematic review and network meta-analysis. Arch Phys Med Rehabil. 2012;93:1259–68.

106. Han Y, Lee JK, Lee BY, Kee HS, Jung KI, Yoon SR. Effectiveness of lower energy density extracorporeal shock wave therapy in the early stage of avascular necrosis of the femoral head. Ann Rehabil Med. 2016;40:871–7.

107. Schofer MD, Hinrichs F, Peterlein CD, Arendt M, Schmitt J. High- versus low-energy extracorporeal shock wave therapy of rotator cuff tendinopathy: a prospective, randomised, controlled study. Acta Orthop Belg. 2009;75:452–8.

108. Zhang X, Yan X, Wang C, Tang T, Chai Y. The dose-effect relationship in extracorporeal shock wave therapy: the optimal parameter for extracorporeal shock wave therapy. J Surg Res. 2014;186:484–92.

109. Leone L, Raffa S, Vetrano M, et al. Extracorporeal shock wave treatment (ESWT) enhances the in vitro-induced differentiation of human tendon-derived stem/progenitor cells (hTSPCs). Oncotarget. 2016;7:6410–23.

110. Tam KF, Cheung WH, Lee KM, Qin L, Leung KS. Delayed stimulatory effect of low-intensity shockwaves on human periosteal cells. Clin Orthop Relat Res. 2005;438:260–5.

111. Howick J, Chalmers I, Glasziou P, et al. "Explanation of the 2011 Oxford Centre for Evidence-Based Medicine (OCEBM) Levels of Evidence (Background Document)". 2011 [cited 2018 31 January]; Available from: http://www.cebm.net/index.aspx?o=5653.

112. Lei MM, Zhang L. Therapeutic effect of extracorporeal shock wave therapy on patellar tendinopathy in National Team Athletes. West China Med J. 2012;27:37–9.

113. Liu HB, Zhang MS, Hu ZQ. Clinical observation of extracorporeal shock wave in the treatment of pes anserinus tendonitis. Chinese J Pain Med. 2010;16:379.

114. Xu H, Liu ST. Therapeutic effect of extracorporeal shock wave on patellar paratendinitis and tendinopathy. J Prac Med Tech. 2010;17:1152–3.

115. Zhang L. Efficacy of extracorporeal shock wave for athletes with patellar tendinopathy. Chinese J Rehabil Med. 2008;23:934–5.

116. Bolink SA, Grimm B, Heyligers IC. Patient-reported outcome measures versus inertial performance-based outcome measures: a prospective study in patients undergoing primary total knee arthroplasty. Knee. 2015;22:618–23.

117. van Hove RP, Brohet RM, van Royen BJ, Nolte PA. High correlation of the Oxford knee score with postoperative pain, but not with performance-based functioning. Knee Surg Sports Traumatol Arthrosc. 2016;24:3369–75.

118. Tolk JJ, Janssen RPA, CAC P, et al. The OARSI core set of performance-based measures for knee osteoarthritis is reliable but not valid and responsive. Knee Surg Sports Traumatol Arthrosc. 2017. https://doi.org/10.1007/s00167-017-4789-y. [Epub ahead of print]

11

Associations among knee muscle strength, structural damage, and pain and mobility in individuals with osteoarthritis and symptomatic meniscal tear

Brittney A. Luc-Harkey[1*], Clare E. Safran-Norton[2], Lisa A. Mandl[3], Jeffrey N. Katz[1] and Elena Losina[1]

Abstract

Background: Sufficient lower extremity muscle strength is necessary for performing functional tasks, and individuals with knee osteoarthritis demonstrate thigh muscle weakness compared to controls. It has been suggested that lower muscle strength is associated with a variety of clinical features including pain, mobility, and functional performance, yet these relationships have not been fully explored in patients with symptomatic meniscal tear in addition to knee osteoarthritis. Our purpose was to evaluate the associations of quadriceps and hamstrings muscle strength with structural damage and clinical features in individuals with knee osteoarthritis and symptomatic meniscal tear.

Methods: We performed a cross-sectional study using baseline data from the Meniscal Tear in Osteoarthritis Research (MeTeOR) trial. We assessed structural damage using Kellgren-Lawrence grade and the magnetic resonance imaging osteoarthritis knee score (MOAKS) for cartilage damage. We used the Knee Injury and Osteoarthritis Outcomes Score (KOOS) to evaluate pain, symptoms, and activities of daily living (ADL), and the Timed Up and Go (TUG) test to assess mobility. We assessed quadriceps and hamstrings strength using a hand-held dynamometer and classified each into quartiles (Q). We used Chi square tests to evaluate the association between strength and structural damage; and separate analysis of covariance models to establish the association between pain, symptoms, ADL and mobility with strength, after adjusting for demographic characteristics (age, sex and BMI) and structural damage.

Results: Two hundred fifty two participants were evaluated. For quadriceps strength, subjects in the strongest quartile scored 14 and 13 points higher on the KOOS Pain and ADL subscales, respectively, and completed the TUG two seconds faster than subjects in the weakest quartile. For hamstrings strength, subjects in the strongest quartile scored 13 and 14 points higher on the KOOS pain and ADL subscales, respectively, and completed the TUG two seconds faster than subjects in the weakest quartile. Strength was not associated with structural damage.

Conclusions: Greater quadriceps and hamstrings muscle strength was associated with less pain, less difficulty completing activities of daily living, and better mobility. These relationships should be evaluated longitudinally.

Keywords: Quadriceps, Hamstrings, Timed up and go, KOOS; activities of daily living

* Correspondence: bharkey@bwh.harvard.edu
[1]Orthopaedic and Arthritis Center for Outcomes Research, Department of Orthopedic Surgery, Brigham and Women's Hospital, 60 Fenwood Road, Suite 5016, Boston, MA 02115, USA
Full list of author information is available at the end of the article

Background

Knee osteoarthritis is a leading cause of functional limitation in older adults [1, 2]. Functional limitation is manifest as reductions in both self-reported difficulty performing activities of daily living and in objectively quantified mobility [3–5]. Identifying modifiable factors that contribute to pain, difficulty performing activities of daily living, and mobility is necessary to inform efficient therapeutic regimens that effectively reduce functional limitation in individuals with knee osteoarthritis.

Performing functional tasks requires sufficient lower extremity muscle strength [6]. Individuals with symptomatic knee osteoarthritis demonstrate deficits in quadriceps and hamstrings strength when compared to healthy matched controls [7–10]. It has been suggested that lower quadriceps and hamstrings strength contribute to a variety of clinical features, including poorer patient-reported function [11, 12], worse physical performance [13–15] and disease progression [16]. The relationship between lower extremity muscle strength and clinical features may be confounded, however by radiographic disease severity [17] in addition to demographic characteristics such as sex [18–20] and body mass index (BMI) [18]. As muscle strength is modifiable, understanding the associations between quadriceps and hamstrings strength and a broad set of clinical features could help to determine efficacious treatment targets.

Previous studies assessing the associations between quadriceps and hamstrings muscle strength and clinical features of knee osteoarthritis have quantified muscle strength using instrumentation only available in research laboratories [13–15, 21, 22], precluding their applicability in the clinical setting. Hand-held dynamometers are small, portable devices that allow for the measurement of muscle strength in clinical settings. Strong, positive associations (i.e., Pearson correlation coefficient range = 0.72–0.85) between the assessment of quadriceps and hamstrings muscle strength using a hand-held dynamometer and an isokinetic dynamometer have been reported [23]. Additionally, hand-held dynamometers demonstrate excellent inter-rater and inter-session reliability [24]. Limited research demonstrates hip abductor strength, assessed using a hand-held dynamometer associates with physical function in patients with knee osteoarthritis [25]. Therefore, our purpose was to evaluate the associations among quadriceps and hamstrings strength measured with a hand-held dynamometer and 1) structural damage quantified via radiograph and MRI, 2) patient-reported pain, symptoms and difficulty performing activities of daily living quantified via the Knee Injury and Osteoarthritis Outcomes Score (KOOS), and 3) performance of mobility tasks quantified via the Timed Up and Go (TUG) test in individuals with symptomatic meniscal tear and osteoarthritis. We

hypothesized that less quadriceps and hamstrings strength is associated with greater structural damage (i.e. radiographic severity and depth and size of cartilage damage), greater patient-reported limitations, and poorer mobility.

Methods

Study design

This cross-sectional study utilized baseline data from the Meniscal Tear in Osteoarthritis Research (MeTeOR) trial (NCT00597012). The MeTeOR trial is a multi-center randomized controlled trial comparing arthroscopic partial meniscectomy plus physical therapy versus physical therapy alone for the treatment of symptomatic meniscal tear. Details of the MeTeOR trial have been published previously [26, 27]. At the time of enrollment, participants underwent a baseline imaging assessment and a testing session that included the assessment of patient-reported outcomes, the Timed Up and Go (TUG) test, quadriceps strength and hamstrings strength. All study procedures were approved by the Partners HealthCare Human Research Committee, and all participants provided written consent prior to participation.

Participants

Participants were recruited into the MeTeOR Trial from seven academic referral centers between June 2008 and August 2011 [26, 27]. Briefly, eligible patients of the participating surgeons across each center were identified, screened for eligibility, and referred to research coordinators if interested in participating. Full trial procedures have been published previously [27]. Participants were 45 years or older, and had an MRI of the knee with evidence of a meniscal tear that extended to the meniscal surface. Included participants had baseline imaging evidence of osteoarthritic changes as determined by either MRI evidence of osteophytes or full-thickness cartilage defect, or plain radiographic evidence of osteophytes or joint space narrowing. Exclusion criteria comprised a chronically locked knee, inflammatory arthritis, injection of corticosteroids or hyaluronic acid agents within the past four weeks, contraindications to surgery or physical therapy, bilateral symptomatic meniscal tears, and prior surgery on the index knee. Participants receiving an injection within the previous 4 weeks were excluded as evidence supports short-term improvement in osteoarthritis symptoms following injections [28], and this could obscure treatment effects [27]. Participants with radiographic Kellgren-Lawrence (K-L) grade 4 were also excluded as total knee arthroplasty is more appropriate than arthroscopic partial meniscectomy in this setting [27]. For this study, we analyzed data from each participant's index knee, which we defined as the knee that prompted the participant to seek care. The MeTeOR

Trial was powered to detect a 10-point difference in the WOMAC function scale at 6 months, which was the principal trial outcomes measure. Adopting a Type I error rate of 5% and power of 80%, the target sample size was set at 340 participants. A total of 351 participants were enrolled into the MeTeOR Trial.

Quadriceps strength

Maximal voluntary isometric quadriceps muscle strength was assessed using a hand-held dynamometer (Fig. 1; MicroFET 2; Hoggan Scientific, LLC, Salt Lake City, UT). Participants were seated on an examination table with their knees flexed to 60° and their feet off the ground. The hand-held dynamometer was positioned on the anterior aspect of the distal tibia, just superior to the malleoli. An inelastic strap was secured around the treatment table under the participant, and was used to maintain the position of the hand-held dynamometer and the knee angle during each testing trial [29, 30]. Participants grasped the examination table with their hands for stabilization, and participants were instructed to extend their knee "as hard as possible" into the hand-held dynamometer. Participants continued to exert force into the hand-held dynamometer for 4 s, and the maximum force across the trial was recorded. Three testing trials were completed, and we normalized the average force (Newtons [N]) across the three trials to body mass (N/kg) [19].

Hamstrings strength

Maximal voluntary isometric hamstrings muscle strength was assessed with participants seated on an examination table with their knees flexed to 60° and their feet off the ground (Fig. 1). The hand-held dynamometer was positioned on the posterior aspect of the lower leg, just superior to the malleoli [29]. An inelastic strap was secured around the waist of the assessor who was seated directly in front of the participant. The strap was used to maintain the position of the hand-held dynamometer and the knee angle during each testing

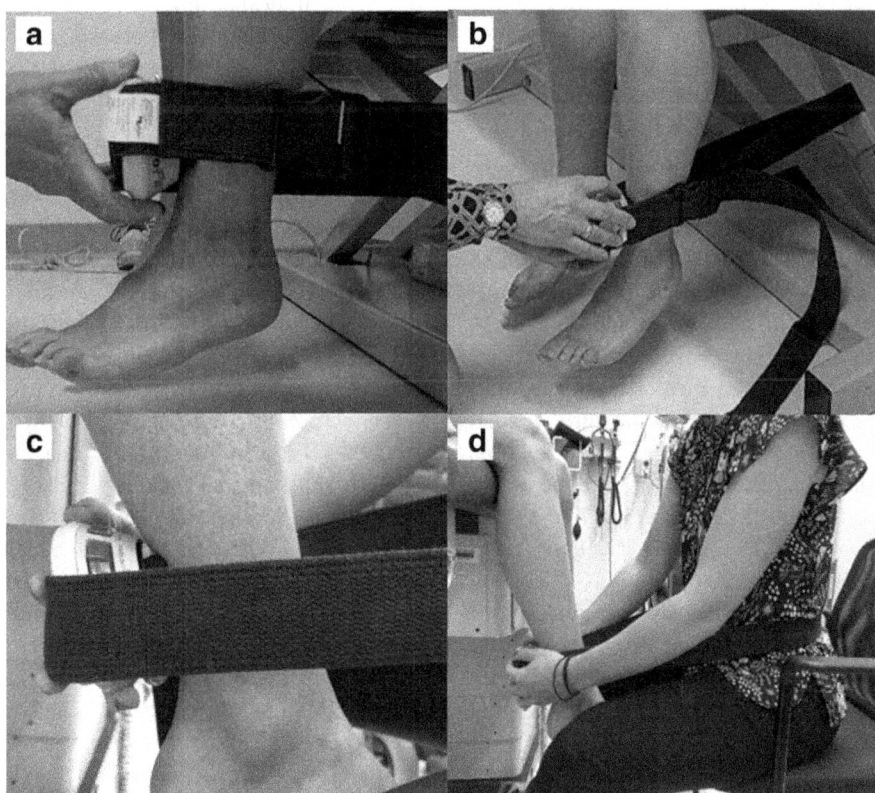

Fig. 1 Muscle Strength Assessment. Legend: For the assessment of quadriceps strength, **a**) the hand-held dynamometer was positioned on the anterior aspect of the distal tibia, just superior to the malleoli, and **b**) participants were seated on an examination table with their knees flexed to 60° and their feet off the ground. An inelastic strap was secured around the treatment table under the participant, and was used to maintain the position of the hand-held dynamometer and the knee angle during each testing trial. For the assessment of hamstring strength, **c**) the hand-held dynamometer was positioned on the posterior aspect of the lower leg, just superior to the malleoli, and **d**) participants were seated on an examination table with their knees flexed to 60° and their feet off the ground. An inelastic strap was secured around the waist of the assessor who was seated directly in front of the participant. The strap was used to maintain the position of the hand-held dynamometer and the knee angle during each testing trial

trial. Participants grasped the examination table with their hands for stabilization, and participants were instructed to flex their knee "as hard as possible" into the hand-held dynamometer. Participants continued to exert force into the hand-held dynamometer for 4 s, and the maximum force across the trial was recorded. Three testing trials were completed, and we normalized the average force (Newtons [N]) across the three trials to body mass (N/kg) [19]. For both quadriceps and hamstrings strength, we categorized the normalized strength values into quartiles (Q) for analysis, with the lowest quartile indicative of the poorest strength.

Structural damage

Structural damage was determined based upon radiographic K-L grade and the size and thickness of cartilage damage on MRI. Radiographic K-L grade was categorized as 0) no radiographic features of osteoarthritis, 1) doubtful joint space narrowing and questionable osteophyte formation, 2) possible joint space narrowing and definite osteophyte formation, and 3) multiple osteophytes and joint space narrowing < 50% [26]. The MRIs were re-read centrally by a single experienced musculoskeletal radiologist, and the size and depth of cartilage damage was classified per the MRI OA Knee Score (MOAKS) criteria. The MOAKS is a semi-quantitative assessment of structural features consistent with knee OA [31]. The MOAKS divides the articular and sub-spinous regions of the knee into 14 sub-regions to quantify the size of cartilage loss (% of surface area in each sub-region) and the depth of cartilage damage (% of full thickness loss in each sub-region). The 14 sub-regions include the patella (medial patella; lateral patella), the femur (medial trochlea; lateral trochlea; medial central femur; lateral central femur; medial posterior femur; lateral posterior femur), and the tibia (anterior medial tibia; middle medial tibia; posterior medial tibia; anterior lateral tibia; middle lateral tibia; posterior lateral tibia) [31]. The size of cartilage damage was categorized as 0) none, 1) < 10%, 2) 10–75%, and 3) > 75%. The depth of cartilage damage was categorized as 0) none, 1) < 10%, 2) 10–75%, and 3) > 75%. All 14 sub-regions were assessed, and we used the maximum score for the size of cartilage damage and for the depth of cartilage damage for analysis [31].

Patient-reported pain and functional status

We assessed baseline patient-reported outcomes using the pain, symptoms and function in activities of daily living (ADL) subscales of the Knee injury and Osteoarthritis Outcomes Score (KOOS) which is a valid and reliable instrument [32]. Within each subscale, scores from each item were summed and divided by the maximum possible score and multiplied by 100 to create a

normalized score ranging from 0 to 100. Lower scores indicate greater pain, greater severity of symptoms, and greater difficulty in performing activities of daily living [32]. A difference of 8 points on each KOOS subscale between quartiles of quadriceps and hamstrings muscle strength represents a clinically meaningful difference in patient reported pain, symptoms and difficulty performing ADL [32].

Mobility

We assessed mobility using the Timed Up and Go (TUG) test [33]. Participants began seated in a chair, and were instructed to rise from the chair without the use of their arms for support, walk 3 m at a self-selected comfortable speed, and return to the seated position. A stopwatch was used to record the time interval from when the participant was instructed to begin the test until s/he returned to the seated position. The TUG test demonstrates excellent test-retest reliability in individuals with knee osteoarthritis [33]. Time to complete the test was recorded in seconds; a longer time to complete the TUG indicates poorer mobility. A difference of 1.14 s on the TUG test between quadriceps and hamstrings strength quartiles represents a clinically meaningful difference in mobility [33].

Statistical analysis

We used means and percentages to describe the sample characteristics. We used separate Chi square tests to determine differences in structural damage (K-L grade and the maximum MOAKS score for size and depth of cartilage damage) across quartiles of quadriceps strength and hamstrings strength. Next, we analyzed the associations between the clinical features (KOOS pain score, KOOS symptoms score, KOOS ADL score, and time to complete the TUG test) and quartiles of quadriceps strength and hamstrings strength using separate analysis of covariance models. We applied a threshold of $P < 0.05$ to determine statistical significance after adjusting for demographic characteristics (age, sex and BMI) and structural damage (K-L grade and the maximum MOAKS score for size and depth of cartilage damage). All analyses were performed using SAS 9.4 statistical software (SAS Institute Inc., Cary, NC).

Results

Sample characteristics

Of the 351 participants who were enrolled into the MeTeOR trial 252 had complete quadriceps and hamstrings strength and clinical features data. Therefore, our sample was comprised of 252 participants. The baseline characteristics for study participants, are presented in Table 1. The mean age for the entire cohort was 58 years (standard deviation [SD] 7; range = 45–87), BMI was

Table 1 Participant characteristics by strength quartile

	Quartile 1 (weakest)	Quartile 2	Quartile 3	Quartile 4 (strongest)	P value
	Quadriceps Strength				
Age	56 (6)	56 (7)	61 (7)	60 (8)	0.889
Sex					0.021
Male	20%	40%	45%	64%	
Female	80%	60%	55%	36%	
BMI	33 (7)	31 (6)	28 (4)	27 (4)	0.061
MOAKS Cartilage Damage Depth Score					0.169
0	27%	41%	20%	36%	
1	22%	22%	24%	25%	
2	44%	29%	41%	34%	
3	7%	8%	15%	5%	
MOAKS Cartilage Damage Size Score					0.011
0	2%	2%	0%	6%	
1	0%	6%	5%	9%	
2	59%	63%	41%	52%	
3	39%	29%	54%	33%	
K-L Grade					0.002
0	12%	13%	9%	5%	
1	12%	27%	12%	33%	
2	39%	49%	39%	39%	
3	37%	11%	39%	23%	
Quadriceps Strength (N/kg)	0.86 (0.28)	1.47 (0.13)	2.02 (0.20)	3.11 (0.57)	< 0.001
KOOS Pain	44 (16)	53 (14)	55 (13)	62 (15)	< 0.001
KOOS Symptoms	43 (15)	47 (15)	43 (15)	47 (13)	0.226
KOOS ADL	53 (19)	60 (17)	67 (14)	72 (16)	< 0.001
TUG Test (s)	12 (5)	10 (4)	9 (3)	9 (2)	0.008
	Hamstrings Strength				
Age	57 (7)	58 (7)	59 (8)	60 (7)	0.627
Sex					0.007
Male	26%	33%	51%	63%	
Female	74%	67%	49%	37%	
BMI	32 (7)	31 (6)	28 (5)	27 (4)	0.081
MOAKS Cartilage Damage Depth Score					0.840
0	35%	30%	30%	28%	
1	21%	16%	29%	28%	
2	36%	43%	33%	35%	
3	8%	11%	8%	8%	
MOAKS Cartilage Damage Size Score					0.544
0	2%	2%	2%	5%	
1	2%	8%	6%	5%	
2	62%	54%	46%	52%	
3	35%	36%	46%	38%	
K-L Grade					0.358

Table 1 Participant characteristics by strength quartile *(Continued)*

	Quartile 1 (weakest)	Quartile 2	Quartile 3	Quartile 4 (strongest)	P value
0	11%	14%	9%	3%	
1	15%	16%	29%	25%	
2	47%	44%	33%	42%	
3	27%	25%	29%	30%	
Hamstrings Strength (N/kg)	0.64 (0.17)	1.10 (0.12)	1.57 (0.15)	2.30(0.41)	< 0.001
KOOS Pain	46 (16)	51 (14)	55 (14)	63 (14)	< 0.001
KOOS Symptoms	44 (15)	45 (16)	44 (15)	47 (14)	0.925
KOOS ADL	55 (18)	60 (18)	66 (16)	74 (14)	< 0.001
TUG Test (s)	12 (5)	10 (3)	9 (3)	9 (2)	0.005

Continuous data presented as mean (standard deviation); categorical data presented percentage; MOAKS = MRI Knee OA Score; KOOS = knee injury and osteoarthritis outcomes score; BMI = body mass index; K-L = Kellgren-Lawrence; N = newtons; ADL = activities of daily living; TUG = Timed Up and Go; p-value corresponds to the difference in each outcome measure across quartiles of muscle strength

30 kg/m^2 (SD 6; range = 19–51), and 57% were female. With respect to structural damage, 9% had K-L Grade 0, 21% had K-L Grade 1, 42% had K-L Grade 2, and 28% had K-L Grade 3. Thirty-one percent received a maximum MOAKS cartilage damage depth score of 0, 23% received a 1, 37% received a 2, and 9% received a 3. Two percent of participants received a maximum MOAKS cartilage damage size score of 0, 5% received a 1, 54% received a 2, and 39% received a 3. The mean scores for the KOOS pain, symptoms and ADL subscales was 54 (SD 16; range = 8–97), 45 (SD 15; range = 10–100) and 64 (SD 18; range = 12–100), respectively, and the mean time to complete the TUG was 10 (SD 4; range = 1–30) seconds. The mean quadriceps strength on the index limb was 1.89 N/kg (SD 0.89; range = 0.18–5.03) and the mean hamstrings strength was 1.39 N/kg (SD 0.66; range = 0.18–3.67).

Quadriceps Strength Associations with Structural Damage, Patient Reported Pain and Functional Status, and Mobility

The distribution of K-L grades significantly differed across quartiles of quadriceps strength (Table 1; $p = 0.002$). The distribution of the maximum MOAKS score for cartilage damage size significantly differed across quartiles of quadriceps strength (Table 1; $p = 0.011$). We did not find that the distribution of the maximum MOAKS score for cartilage damage depth was different across quadriceps strength quartiles (Table 1; $p = 0.169$).

Quadriceps strength was significantly associated with higher KOOS pain scores (mean [SD] Q1 = 44 [16], Q2 = 53 [14], Q3 = 55 [13], Q4 = 62 [15]; $P = 0.001$) and higher KOOS ADL scores (mean [SD] Q1 = 53 [19], Q2 = 60 [17], Q3 = 67 [14], Q4 = 72 [16]; $p = 0.001$). After accounting for age, sex, BMI, and structural damage, the

difference in KOOS pain between the strongest and weakest quartiles was clinically meaningful as KOOS pain scores were on average 14 points higher, indicating less pain, in the strongest quartile of quadriceps strength as compared to the weakest quartile (Fig. 2). Similarly, the difference in KOOS ADL scores between the strongest and weakest quartiles was clinically meaningful as KOOS ADL scores were on average 13 points higher, indicating less difficulty performing activities of daily living, in the strongest quartile of quadriceps strength compared to the weakest quartile of quadriceps strength (Fig. 3). Quadriceps strength was associated with less time to complete the TUG test (mean [SD] Q1 = 12 [5], Q2 = 10 [4], Q3 = 9 [3], Q4 = 9 [2]; $p = 0.009$). After accounting for age, sex, BMI, and structural damage, the difference in the time to

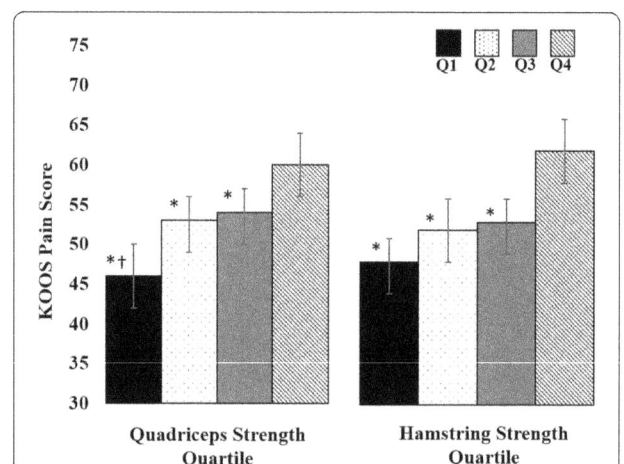

Fig. 2 KOOS Pain Scores by Quartile of Muscle Strength. Legend: Data presented as mean Knee injury and Osteoarthritis Outcomes Score (KOOS) pain scores across each quartile (Q) of muscle strength adjusting for structural damage, age, sex and BMI. * indicates significantly less than quartile 4; † indicates significantly less than quartile 2 and quartile 3

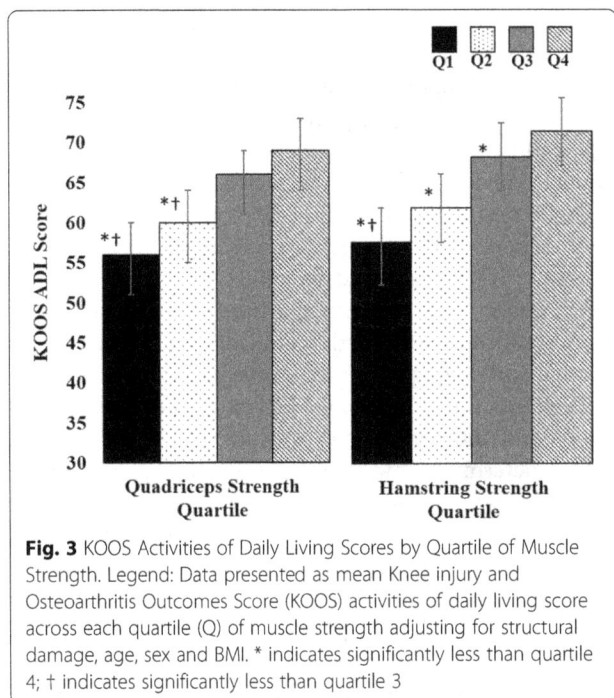

Fig. 3 KOOS Activities of Daily Living Scores by Quartile of Muscle Strength. Legend: Data presented as mean Knee injury and Osteoarthritis Outcomes Score (KOOS) activities of daily living score across each quartile (Q) of muscle strength adjusting for structural damage, age, sex and BMI. * indicates significantly less than quartile 4; † indicates significantly less than quartile 3

complete the TUG test between the strongest and weakest quartiles was clinically meaningful as individuals in the strongest quartile of quadriceps strength completed the TUG test an average of 2 s faster than those in the weakest quartile of quadriceps strength (Fig. 4). We did not find a significant association between quadriceps strength and KOOS symptoms scores (mean [SD] Q1 = 43 [15], Q2 = 47 [15], Q3 = 43 [15], Q4 = 47 [13], $p = 0.226$).

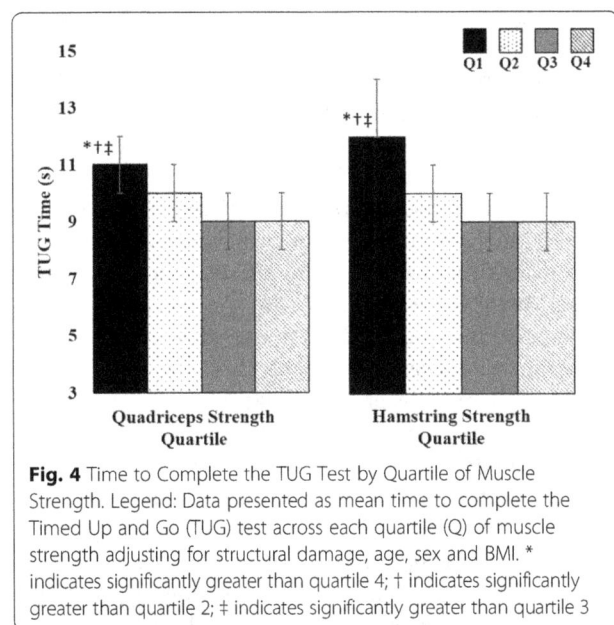

Fig. 4 Time to Complete the TUG Test by Quartile of Muscle Strength. Legend: Data presented as mean time to complete the Timed Up and Go (TUG) test across each quartile (Q) of muscle strength adjusting for structural damage, age, sex and BMI. * indicates significantly greater than quartile 4; † indicates significantly greater than quartile 2; ‡ indicates significantly greater than quartile 3

Hamstrings Strength Associations with Structural Damage, Patient-Reported Pain and Functional Status, and Mobility

We did not find that the distribution of K-L grades differed across quartiles of hamstrings strength (Table 1; $p = 0.36$). We did not find that the distribution of the maximum MOAKS cartilage damage size score differed across quartiles of hamstrings strength (Table 1; $p = 0.54$). We did not find that the distribution of the maximum MOAKS cartilage damage depth score was different across hamstrings strength quartiles (Table 1; $p = 0.84$).

Hamstrings strength was associated with higher KOOS pain (mean [SD] Q1 = 46 [16], Q2 = 51 [14], Q3 = 55 [14], Q4 = 63 [14], $p < 0.001$) and higher KOOS ADL scores (mean [SD] Q1 = 55 [18], Q2 = 60 [18], Q3 = 66 [16], Q4 = 74 [14], $p < 0.001$). After accounting for age, sex, BMI, and structural damage, the differences in KOOS pain and ADL scores between the highest and lowest quartiles were clinically meaningful as KOOS pain scores were on average 13 points higher, indicating less pain, in the strongest quartile of hamstrings strength as compared to the weakest quartile of hamstrings strength (Fig. 2), and KOOS ADL scores were on average 14 points higher, indicating less difficulty performing activities of daily living, in the strongest quartile of hamstrings strength compared to the weakest quartile of hamstrings strength (Fig. 3). Hamstrings strength was associated with less time to complete the TUG test (mean [SD] Q1 = 12 [5], Q2 = 10 [3], Q3 = 9 [3], Q4 = 9 [2], $p = 0.005$). After accounting for age, sex, BMI, and structural damage, the difference in the time to complete the TUG test between the strongest and weakest quartiles was clinically meaningful as individuals in the strongest quartile of hamstrings strength completed the TUG test an average of two seconds faster than those in the weakest quartile of hamstrings strength (Fig. 4). We did not find a significant association between hamstrings strength and KOOS symptoms (mean [SD] Q1 = 44 [15], Q2 = 45 [16], Q3 = 44 [15], Q4 = 47 [14], $p = 0.925$).

Discussion

In this cross-sectional study of individuals with symptomatic meniscal tear and knee osteoarthritis, we observed that greater quadriceps and hamstrings strength were significantly associated with less patient-reported pain and difficulty completing activities of daily living, and better objectively measured mobility after accounting for age, sex, BMI and structural damage. The difference in pain and difficulty performing activities of daily living between the strongest and weakest quartiles of quadriceps and hamstrings strength exceeded the minimal clinically important difference of 8 points for the KOOS [32]. While our cross-sectional results will need to be tested in longitudinal studies, they suggest that increasing quadriceps and hamstrings muscle strength may be beneficial for reducing pain and difficulty performing activities of daily living, and improving mobility in individuals with symptomatic meniscal tear and knee osteoarthritis.

The quadriceps are critical for generating joint actions and attenuating loading during functional tasks such as walking and rising from a chair [6]. In our study, we determined that quadriceps strength was associated with both subjective and objective clinical features of symptomatic knee osteoarthritis. In general, our results agree with previous studies using laboratory-specific instrumentation to quantify quadriceps muscle strength, as greater strength was associated with better functional task performance and less self-reported disability in individuals with knee osteoarthritis [13–15, 21, 22]. Conversely, other studies have determined weak correlation coefficients between lower extremity muscle strength and pain [34, 35]. Contrasting results between our study and previous investigations are likely due to the evaluation of lower extremity muscle strength during a concentric, bilateral leg extension task in one study [35] or the assessment of knee pain using a visual analog scale [34]. We assessed open-chain quadriceps strength using a hand-held device, which allowed us to isolate the quadriceps muscle on the index limb. Our results suggest that quadriceps strength measured in a clinical setting using a hand-held dynamometer is associated with various clinical features that may contribute to functional limitation in individuals with symptomatic meniscal tear and knee osteoarthritis.

Similar to quadriceps strength, we determined that greater hamstrings strength is associated with less pain, less difficulty performing activities of daily living and greater mobility in individuals with symptomatic meniscal tear and knee osteoarthritis. The hamstrings provide dynamic joint stability during walking [6], and greater patient-reported joint stability has been associated with less knee pain [36]. Our results build upon previous work suggesting that hamstrings strength contributes to both subjective [19] and objective [14, 15] clinical features of knee osteoarthritis. Previous studies have determined greater hamstrings strength is associated with less pain and better performance on stair climb and sit to stand assessments [14, 15, 19]. Our results suggest that hamstrings strength contributes to multiple activities of daily living as greater hamstrings strength associated with time to complete the TUG test, which comprises both balance and mobility, and KOOS ADL scores, which assesses the difficulty experienced while completing a variety of daily activities ranging from sitting to ascending and descending stairs. Our results suggest that multiple lower extremity muscles contribute

to clinical features of knee osteoarthritis, and intervention strategies aiming to improve both quadriceps and hamstrings strength may be beneficial.

Classifying our participants into quartiles of quadriceps and hamstrings strength allows us to determine the clinical relevance of quadriceps and hamstrings muscle strength regarding subjective and objective clinical features of knee osteoarthritis. In our cohort, the difference in mean KOOS pain and KOOS ADL scores between the strongest and weakest quartiles of quadriceps and hamstrings muscle strength when adjusted for structural damage and demographic characteristics ranged from 13 to 15 points (Figs. 1 and 2), which represents a clinically meaningful difference in KOOS scores [32]. While we cannot determine how changes in quadriceps and hamstrings muscle strength are associated with changes in clinical features, a previous study has determined that a small reduction in quadriceps and hamstrings muscle strength of approximately 6% was associated with a clinically relevant decline in physical function quantified via the WOMAC [12]. Similarly, individuals in the weakest quartiles of quadriceps and hamstrings muscle strength in our study took on average 2 to 3 s longer to complete the TUG test compared to those in the strongest quartiles, which is greater than the minimum detectible difference of 1.14 s [33]. The TUG test assesses balance and self-selected walking speed, and a greater time to complete the TUG test has been associated with fall risk [37]. Additionally, individuals with slower walking speed are also less likely to meet physical activity guidelines [4]. Individuals with or at risk of developing knee osteoarthritis who take more steps per day have a lower risk of developing functional limitation over 2 years compared to those who take fewer steps per day [3]. Future research is needed to determine how quadriceps and hamstrings muscle strength may contribute to additional features of knee osteoarthritis, such as decreased physical activity, and how improving physical activity may be beneficial for patients with symptomatic meniscal tear and knee OA.

In recent years, multiple clinical trials have demonstrated that arthroscopic partial meniscectomy offers little additional improvement in pain when compared to non-operative interventions for the treatment of symptomatic meniscal tear [26, 38–40]. As the management of symptomatic meniscal tear and knee osteoarthritis transitions to conservative approaches, our results highlight the importance of appropriately strengthening the quadriceps and hamstrings musculature. Previous work demonstrated that a 12-week neuromuscular and strength exercise program consisting of squats, lunges, leg press and hamstring curl exercises improved quadriceps and hamstring muscle strength in patients with meniscal tear [41]. Additionally, high intensity strength training and high velocity power training have been shown to be effective at increasing quadriceps and hamstrings muscle strength in individuals with knee osteoarthritis [42]. Utilizing high intensity strength training and power training may be beneficial for improving lower extremity muscle strength in patients with symptomatic meniscal tear and knee osteoarthritis, and therefore may improve pain and physical function. However, gains in muscle strength following training programs may be limited by underlying deficits in voluntary activation [22, 43]. While improving quadriceps and hamstrings muscle strength is likely beneficial for improving clinical features of knee osteoarthritis, rehabilitation programs may need to treat underlying neural factors (i.e. arthrogenic muscle inhibition) that limit the ability to fully restore muscle strength. Future research is needed to determine the most efficacious therapeutic interventions for improving lower extremity muscle strength in patients with symptomatic meniscal tear and knee osteoarthritis.

While this study improves our understanding of the association between quadriceps and hamstrings muscle strength and subjective and objective clinical features of knee osteoarthritis, there are limitations that should be addressed to inform future research. As our study is cross-sectional in nature, we are unable to determine the causal relationship between quadriceps and hamstrings muscle strength and clinical features of knee osteoarthritis. We also cannot determine how other lower extremity muscles, including the gluteus medius and gluteus maximus, may have contributed to KOOS scores and time to complete the TUG in our study. We limited our inclusion criteria to individuals with mild to moderate knee osteoarthritis based upon K-L grade, therefore it is unknown how our results translate into the larger population of individuals who are at risk of developing knee osteoarthritis or those with end-stage disease. Additionally, we did not determine the presence of bilateral osteoarthritis in this cohort, therefore it remains unknown if the presence of bilateral osteoarthritis may influence our results. We used a hand-held dynamometer to assess quadriceps and hamstrings muscle strength due to its cost-effectiveness, portability and ease of use, rather than an isokinetic dynamometer. However, strong, positive associations (i.e., Pearson correlation coefficient range = 0.72–0.85) between the assessment of quadriceps and hamstrings muscle strength using a hand-held dynamometer and an isokinetic dynamometer have been reported [23]. We also used inelastic straps to stabilize the dynamometer and maintain joint positioning during the assessments, which has been demonstrated to improve the reliability of these measures [30]. We chose to normalized peak force in newtons to body mass to account for differences in body size. The lever arm length was not available in this cohort; therefore, we are unable to determine joint torque. Previous research, however has demonstrated that taking the lever arm length into account for the purpose of normalizing muscle strength does not influence results when compared to normalizing peak force to body mass [19]. Lastly, there are additional factors that may influence quadriceps and hamstrings muscle strength, including neuromuscular activation, muscle co-contraction, and joint range of motion, and we are unable to discern how additional unmeasured factors may contribute to quadriceps and hamstrings muscle strength.

Conclusions

In conclusion, our results demonstrate that quadriceps and hamstrings muscle strength, assessed using a hand-held dynamometer, was associated with subjective and objective clinical features in individuals with symptomatic meniscal tear and knee osteoarthritis. Individuals classified into the strongest quartiles of quadriceps and hamstrings strength reported less pain, less difficulty performing activities of daily living, and demonstrated better mobility than those in the weakest quartiles. The differences in pain and difficulty performing activities of daily living between the strongest and weakest quartiles of muscle strength exceeded the clinically meaningful difference for the KOOS. These results should be confirmed in trials or longitudinal studies, but they suggest that that quadriceps and hamstrings muscle strengthening may be a key component for the non-operative management of symptomatic meniscal tear and knee osteoarthritis.

Abbreviations
ADL: Activities of Daily Living; BMI: Body Mass Index; K-L: Kellgren-Lawrence; KOOS: Knee Injury and Osteoarthritis Outcomes Score; MeTeOR: Meniscal Tear in Osteoarthritis Research; MOAKS: MRI OA Knee Score; N: Newtons; Q: Quartiles; TUG: Timed Up and Go Test

Funding
Research reported in this manuscript was supported by the National Institute of Arthritis and Musculoskeletal and Skin Diseases of the National Institutes of Health under award numbers R01AR055557, K24AR057827, 1P30AR072577 and T32AR055885. The study sponsors had no role in the study design; in the collection, analysis or interpretation of data; in the writing of the manuscript; and in the decision to submit the manuscript for publication.

Authors' contributions
BALH: Conception and design of the study, Analysis and interpretation of data, Drafting of the article, Final approval of the article; CESN: Analysis and interpretation of data, Critical revision of the article for important intellectual content, Final approval of the article; LAM: Analysis and interpretation of data, Critical revision of the article for important intellectual content, Final approval of the article; JNK: Obtaining funding, Conception and design of the study, Analysis and interpretation of data, Critical revision of the article for important intellectual content, Final approval of the article; EL: Obtaining funding, Conception and design of the study, Analysis and interpretation of data, Critical revision of the article for important intellectual content, Final approval of the article.

Competing interests

The authors declare that they have no competing interests.

Author details

[1]Orthopaedic and Arthritis Center for Outcomes Research, Department of Orthopedic Surgery, Brigham and Women's Hospital, 60 Fenwood Road, Suite 5016, Boston, MA 02115, USA. [2]Rehabilitation Services, Brigham and Women's Hospital, Boston, MA, USA. [3]Weill Cornell Medicine, Hospital for Special Surgery, New York, NY, USA.

References

1. Guccione AA, Felson DT, Anderson JJ, Anthony JM, Zhang Y, Wilson PW, et al. The effects of specific medical conditions on the functional limitations of elders in the Framingham study. Am J Public Health. 1994;84(3):351–8.
2. Murray CJ, Richards MA, Newton JN, Fenton KA, Anderson HR, Atkinson C, et al. UK health performance: findings of the global burden of disease study 2010. Lancet. 2013;381(9871):997–1020.
3. White DK, Tudor-Locke C, Zhang Y, Fielding R, LaValley M, Felson DT, et al. Daily walking and the risk of incident functional limitation in knee osteoarthritis: an observational study. Arthritis Care Res (Hoboken). 2014;66(9):1328–36.
4. White DK, Lee J, Song J, Chang RW, Dunlop D. Potential functional benefit from light intensity physical activity in knee osteoarthritis. Am J Prev Med. 2017;53(5):689–96.
5. Dunlop DD, Song J, Lee J, Gilbert AL, Semanik PA, Ehrlich-Jones L, et al. Physical activity minimum threshold predicting improved function in adults with lower-extremity symptoms. Arthritis Care Res (Hoboken). 2017;69(4):475–83.
6. Bennell KL, Wrigley TV, Hunt MA, Lim BW, Hinman RS. Update on the role of muscle in the genesis and management of knee osteoarthritis. Rheum Dis Clin N Am. 2013;39(1):145–76.
7. Hall M, Juhl CB, Lund H, Thorlund JB. Knee extensor muscle strength in middle-aged and older individuals undergoing arthroscopic partial meniscectomy: a systematic review and meta-analysis. Arthritis Care Res (Hoboken). 2015;67(9):1289–96.
8. Thorlund JB, Aagaard P, Roos EM. Thigh muscle strength, functional capacity, and self-reported function in patients at high risk of knee osteoarthritis compared with controls. Arthritis Care Res (Hoboken). 2010;62(9):1244–51.
9. Lewek MD, Rudolph KS, Snyder-Mackler L. Quadriceps femoris muscle weakness and activation failure in patients with symptomatic knee osteoarthritis. J Orthopaed Res. 2004;22(1):110–5.
10. Slemenda C, Brandt KD, Heilman DK, Mazzuca S, Braunstein EM, Katz BP, et al. Quadriceps weakness and osteoarthritis of the knee. Ann Intern Med. 1997;127(2):97–104.
11. Ruhdorfer A, Wirth W, Eckstein F. Longitudinal change in thigh muscle strength prior to and concurrent with minimum clinically important worsening or improvement in knee function: data from the osteoarthritis initiative. Arthritis Rheumatol. 2016;68(4):826–36.
12. Ruhdorfer A, Wirth W, Eckstein F. Relationship between isometric thigh muscle strength and minimum clinically important differences in knee function in osteoarthritis: data from the osteoarthritis initiative. Arthritis Care Res (Hoboken). 2015;67(4):509–18.
13. McAlindon TE, Cooper C, Kirwan JR. Determinants of disability in osteoarthritis of the knee. Ann Rheum Dis. 1993;52(4):258–62.
14. Sharma L, Song J, Hayes K, Pai YC. Physical functioning over three years in knee osteoarthritis: role of psychosocial, local mechanical, and neuromuscular factors. Arthritis Rheum. 2003;48(12):3359–70.
15. Brown K, Kachelman J, Topp R, Quesada PM, Nyland J, Malkani A, et al. Predictors of functional task performance among patients scheduled for total knee arthroplasty. J Strength Cond Res. 2009;23(2):436–43.
16. Culvenor AG, Wirth W, Roth M, Hunter DJ, Eckstein F. Predictive capacity of thigh muscle strength in symptomatic and/or radiographic knee osteoarthritis progression: data from the foundation for the national institutes of health osteoarthritis biomarkers consortium. Am J Phys Med Rehabil. 2016;95(12):931–8.
17. Ruhdorfer A, Wirth W, Hitzl W, Nevitt M, Eckstein F, Investigators O. Association of thigh muscle strength with knee symptoms and radiographic disease stage of osteoarthritis: data from the osteoarthritis initiative. Arthritis Care Res (Hoboken). 2014;66(9):1344–53.
18. Elbaz A, Debbi EM, Segal G, Haim A, Halperin N, Agar G, et al. Sex and body mass index correlate with western Ontario and McMaster universities osteoarthritis index and quality of life scores in knee osteoarthritis. Arch Phys Med Rehabil. 2011;92(10):1618–23.
19. Culvenor AG, Wirth W, Ruhdorfer A, Eckstein F. Thigh muscle strength predicts knee replacement risk independent of radiographic disease and pain in women: data from the osteoarthritis initiative. Arthritis Rheumatol. 2016;68(5):1145–55.
20. Berger MJ, McKenzie CA, Chess DG, Goela A, Doherty TJ. Sex differences in quadriceps strength in OA. Int J Sports Med. 2012;33(11):926–33.
21. Fujita R, Matsui Y, Harada A, Takemura M, Kondo I, Nemoto T, et al. Does the q – h index show a stronger relationship than the h:q ratio in regard to knee pain during daily activities in patients with knee osteoarthritis? J Phys Ther Sci. 2016;28(12):3320–4.
22. Fitzgerald GK, Piva SR, Irrgang JJ, Bouzubar F, Starz TW. Quadriceps activation failure as a moderator of the relationship between quadriceps strength and physical function in individuals with knee osteoarthritis. Arthritis Rheum. 2004;51(1):40–8.
23. Muff G, Dufour S, Meyer A, Severac F, Favret F, Geny B, et al. Comparative assessment of knee extensor and flexor muscle strength measured using a hand-held vs. isokinetic dynamometer. J Phys Ther Sci. 2016;28(9):2445–51.
24. Kim SG, Lee YS. The intra- and inter-rater reliabilities of lower extremity muscle strength assessment of healthy adults using a hand held dynamometer. J Phys Ther Sci. 2015;27(6):1799–801.
25. Tevald MA, Murray A, Luc BA, Lai K, Sohn D, Pietrosimone B. Hip abductor strength in people with knee osteoarthritis: a cross-sectional study of reliability and association with function. Knee. 2016;23(1):57–62.
26. Katz JN, Brophy RH, Chaisson CE, Ld C, Cole BJ, Dahm DL, et al. Surgery versus physical therapy for a meniscal tear and osteoarthritis. N Engl J Med. 2013;368:1675–84.
27. Katz JN, Chaisson CE, Cole B, Guermazi A, Hunter DJ, Jones M, et al. The meteor trial (meniscal tear in osteoarthritis research): rationale and design features. Contemporary clinical trials. 2012;33(6):1189–96.
28. Arroll B, Goodyear-Smith F. Corticosteroid injections for osteoarthritis of the knee: meta-analysis. BMJ. 2004;328(7444):869.
29. Schaubert KL, Bohannon RW. Reliability and validity of three strength measures obtained from community-dwelling elderly persons. J Strength Cond Res. 2005;19(3):717–20.
30. Mentiplay BF, Perraton LG, Bower KJ, Adair B, Pua YH, Williams GP, et al. Assessment of lower limb muscle strength and power using hand-held and fixed dynamometry: a reliability and validity study. PLoS One. 2015;10(10): e0140822.
31. Hunter DJ, Guermazi A, Lo GH, Grainger AJ, Conaghan PG, Boudreau RM, et al. Evolution of semi-quantitative whole joint assessment of knee OA: MOAKS (MRI osteoarthritis knee score). Osteoarthr Cartil. 2011;19(8):990–1002.
32. Roos EM, Lohmander LS. The knee injury and osteoarthritis outcome score (koos): from joint injury to osteoarthritis. Health Qual Life Outcomes. 2003;1:64.
33. Alghadir A, Anwer S, Brismee JM. The reliability and minimal detectable change of timed up and go test in individuals with grade 1-3 knee osteoarthritis. BMC Musculoskelet Disord. 2015;16:174.
34. Steultjens MP, Dekker J, van Baar ME, Oostendorp RA, Bijlsma JW. Muscle strength, pain and disability in patients with osteoarthritis. Clin Rehabil. 2001;15(3):331–41.
35. Reid KF, Price LL, Harvey WF, Driban JB, Hau C, Fielding RA, et al. Muscle power is an independent determinant of pain and quality of life in knee osteoarthritis. Arthritis Rheumatol. 2015;67(12):3166–73.
36. Felson DT, Niu J, McClennan C, Sack B, Aliabadi P, Hunter DJ, et al. Knee buckling: prevalence, risk factors, and associated limitations in function. Ann Intern Med. 2007;147(8):534–40.
37. Shumway-Cook A, Brauer S, Woollacott M. Predicting the probability for falls in community-dwelling older adults using the timed up & go test. Phys Ther. 2000;80(9):896–903.
38. Gauffin H, Tagesson S, Meunier A, Magnusson H, Kvist J. Knee arthroscopic surgery is beneficial to middle-aged patients with meniscal symptoms: a

Associations among knee muscle strength, structural damage, and pain and mobility in individuals...

143

prospective, randomised, single-blinded study. Osteoarthr Cartil. 2014;22(11):1808–16.

39. Yim JH, Seon JK, Song EK, Choi JI, Kim MC, Lee KB, et al. A comparative study of meniscectomy and nonoperative treatment for degenerative horizontal tears of the medial meniscus. Am J Sports Med. 2013;41(7):1565–70.

40. Herrlin SV, Wange PO, Lapidus G, Hallander M, Werner S, Weidenhielm L. Is arthroscopic surgery beneficial in treating non-traumatic, degenerative medial meniscal tears? A five year follow-up. Knee Surg Sports Traumatol Arthrosc. 2013;21(2):358–64.

41. Stensrud S, Risberg MA, Roos EM. Effect of exercise therapy compared with arthroscopic surgery on knee muscle strength and functional performance in middle-aged patients with degenerative meniscus tears: a 3-mo follow-up of a randomized controlled trial. Am J Phys Med Rehabil. 2015;94(6):460.

42. Wallerstein LF, Tricoli V, Barroso R, Rodacki AL, Russo L, Aihara AY, et al. Effects of strength and power training on neuromuscular variables in older adults. J Aging Phys Act. 2012;20(2):171–85.

43. Pietrosimone BG, Saliba SA. Changes in voluntary quadriceps activation predict changes in quadriceps strength after therapeutic exercise in patients with knee osteoarthritis. Knee. 2012;19(6):939–43.

12

Pain coping skills training for African Americans with osteoarthritis study: baseline participant characteristics and comparison to prior studies

Kelli D. Allen[1,2,3*], Liubov Arbeeva[1,2], Crystal W. Cené[2], Cynthia J. Coffman[3,4], Kimberlea F. Grimm[1,2], Erin Haley[5], Francis J. Keefe[6], Caroline T. Nagle[2], Eugene Z. Oddone[3,7], Tamara J. Somers[6], Yashika Watkins[8] and Lisa C. Campbell[5]

Abstract

Background: The Pain Coping Skills Training for African Americans with OsteoaRThritis (STAART) trial is examining the effectiveness of a culturally enhanced pain coping skills training (CST) program for African Americans with osteoarthritis (OA). This disparities-focused trial aimed to reach a population with greater symptom severity and risk factors for poor pain-related outcomes than previous studies. This paper compares characteristics of STAART participants with prior studies of CST or cognitive behavioral therapy (CBT)-informed training in pain coping strategies for OA.

Methods: A literature search identified 10 prior trials of pain CST or CBT-informed pain coping training among individuals with OA. We descriptively compared characteristics of STAART participants with other studies, in 3 domains of the National Institutes of Minority Health and Health Disparities' Research Framework: Sociocultural Environment (e.g., age, education, marital status), Biological Vulnerability and Mechanisms (e.g, pain and function, body mass index), and Health Behaviors and Coping (e.g., pain catastrophizing). Means and standard deviations (SDs) or proportions were calculated for STAART participants and extracted from published manuscripts for comparator studies.

Results: The mean age of STAART participants, 59 years (SD = 10.3), was lower than 9 of 10 comparator studies; the proportion of individuals with some education beyond high school, 75%, was comparable to comparator studies (61–86%); and the proportion of individuals who are married or living with a partner, 42%, was lower than comparator studies (62–66%). Comparator studies had less than about 1/3 African American participants. Mean scores on the Western Ontario and McMaster Universities Osteoarthritis Index pain and function scales were higher (worse) for STAART participants than for other studies, and mean body mass index of STAART participants, 35.2 kg/m^2 (SD = 8.2), was higher than all other studies (30–34 kg/m^2). STAART participants' mean score on the Pain Catastrophizing scale, 19.8 (SD = 12.3), was higher (worse) than other studies reporting this measure (7–17).

(Continued on next page)

---

* Correspondence: kdallen@email.unc.edu
[1]Thurston Arthritis Research Center, University of North Carolina at Chapel Hill, 3300 Thurston Bldg., CB# 7280, Chapel Hill, NC 27599-7280, USA
[2]Department of Medicine, University of North Carolina at Chapel Hill, 125 MacNider Hall CB# 7005, Chapel Hill, NC 27599, USA
Full list of author information is available at the end of the article

(Continued from previous page)

Conclusions: Compared with prior studies with predominantly white samples, STAART participants have worse pain and function and more risk factors for negative pain-related outcomes across several domains. Given STAART participants' high mean pain catastrophizing scores, this sample may particularly benefit from the CST intervention approach.

Keywords: Osteoarthritis, Knee, Hip, Pain coping skills training, Health disparities

Background

African Americans bear a disproportionate burden of chronic pain conditions, including osteoarthritis (OA). Compared with Caucasians, African Americans not only have a higher prevalence of OA, but also more severe pain, functional limitations, and other negative outcomes [1–6]. Because of these well-documented racial differences, the Institute of Medicine has identified interventions to reduce disparities in OA and other musculoskeletal diseases among its top 25 (highest tier) priority topics for comparative effectiveness research [7]. In alignment with this priority, the Pain Coping Skills Training for African Americans with OsteoaRThritis (STAART) study is evaluating the effectiveness of a culturally enhanced pain coping skills training (CST) program for African Americans with OA [8]. There were several factors underlying the choice of a pain CST intervention to address racial disparities in OA-related pain and other outcomes. First, when compared with Caucasians, African Americans with chronic pain conditions report greater levels of pain catastrophizing (i.e., the tendency to focus on and magnify pain sensations and to feel helpless in the face of pain [9–13]), lower perceived ability to cope with and control pain [14], and greater maladaptive coping strategies (i.e., emotion-focused or external coping strategies) [4, 10, 14–16]. These coping-related characteristics have been associated with worse pain, function, and depressive symptoms [17–19]. Second, previous studies indicated that pain coping and other psychological factors are key factors underlying racial differences in OA-related pain [3, 4]. Third, pain CST interventions have been shown to enhance and improve coping strategies, OA-related pain and other outcomes [20–25]. However, there has been very limited study of pain CST interventions among African Americans with OA or other musculoskeletal conditions. This is important because of evidence that behavioral and psychological interventions are most effective when they are adapted to meet the needs and expectations of minority populations [26].

Based on prior studies of racial differences in pain, coping, and social determinants of health [3, 11–16, 27, 28], we expected that baseline characteristics of the STAART study participants, who are all African American, would reflect a worse risk profile than those of participants in prior studies of pain CST or other cognitive behavioral

therapy (CBT)-informed training in pain coping strategies. Therefore, the objective of this analysis was to descriptively compare characteristics of STAART study participants with prior studies of pain CST or CBT-informed pain coping strategies among individuals with OA. In particular, we focused on Individual Level Sociocultural Environment, Biological and Behavioral domains, within the National Institute on Minority Health and Health Disparities (NIMHD) Research Framework [29] as these are of highest relevance to this intervention and population. This Framework also has domains at the Interpersonal Level (e.g., family functioning, patient-clinician relationship), Community Level (e.g. community resources, availability of health services), and Societal Level (e.g., policies and laws); although some items in these domains are also relevant to this intervention and patient group, variables within these domains were not assessed in STAART.

Methods
Overview of STAART study
The STAART study, described in detail previously [8], is a randomized controlled trial of 248 African Americans with symptomatic hip or knee OA. The STAART study enrolled only African Americans (vs inclusion of other racial groups) so that in-depth efforts could be focused on this demographic group with a high risk for poorer OA and pain-related outcomes. STAART participants are equally allocated to pain CST and wait list control groups. The pain CST intervention involved 11 phone-based sessions, delivered approximately weekly and based on previous pain CST programs [20, 22, 23, 25, 30]. Participants in the wait list group received only their usual care for OA, with no study intervention offered until after completion of final follow-up assessments. All measures for these analyses were collected from patients prior to their randomization to treatment conditions. This study was approved by the Institutional Review Boards of the University of North Carolina (UNC), the Durham VA Healthcare System (VA), Duke University Medical Center and East Carolina University.

STAART participants and recruitment methods
Participants were recruited from the UNC Healthcare System and the Durham VA; 124 participants were

enrolled from each site. Study inclusion were 1) Diagnosis of knee or hip OA, verified by self-reported diagnosis from a medical professional, including items based on the American College of Rheumatology clinical criteria for knee or hip OA, 2) Self-report of pain, aching, or stiffness in one or both knees or hips on most days of the week, 3) Patient of the UNC Health Care System or Durham VAMC. Exclusion criteria have been described previously [8] and generally include other pain-related conditions that confound study outcomes or health conditions that would prevent participation in the intervention (e.g., severe hearing loss since this was a phone-based intervention).

Three general methods of recruitment were used. First, potentially eligible patients were identified from UNC and VA medical records, based on OA diagnosis codes; these patients were mailed letters inviting participation, followed by a telephone call. Second, advertisements were posted at study sites and surrounding communities, inviting patients to self-refer to the study. Third, health care providers at study sites could refer patients to the study team directly, with patients' permission, or give study brochures to patients. We used an enhanced informed consent process that included education about the research process, participant bill of rights, and perspectives from African Americans who have participated in research [31].

Measures

The following measures, representing three Individual Level domains from the NIMHD Research Framework, were assessed in-person at baseline by a trained research assistant. Some of these measures are reported for the STAART study sample only (Table 1) because they were not available for any comparator studies, but they represent key constructs related to health disparities and the NIMHD Framework.

Sociodemographics (individual level sociocultural environment domain)

Age Participant age was based on date of birth from the electronic medical record and confirmed through self-report.

Sex Participant sex was based on the electronic medical record and confirmed through self-report.

Ethnicity Participants self-reported whether they were of Hispanic / Latino descent or not.

Education Participants selected from eight options ranging from grade school/junior high to post graduate work or graduate degree. For these analyses we grouped individuals as having "above high school education" or

not, as this was the most common categorization that could be ascertained from comparator studies.

Work status Participants selected from seven options regarding work status, and for these analyses individuals were grouped as either working or not at the time of the study.

Household financial status Participants selected from four options regarding their household's financial situation and were grouped as either "live comfortably" or "meet basic expenses with a little left over for extras" vs. "just meet basic expenses" or "don't even have enough to meet basic expenses."

Marital status Participants selected from five options regarding current marital status and for these analyses were grouped as being married / living with a partner as married or not currently married at the time of the study.

Religiosity This measure was included in STAART because of its cultural relevance in the African American community. The Duke University Religion Index (DUREL) is a five-item measure of religious beliefs and experience [32]. The index consists of 3 subscales, recording the frequency of attendance at religious services (subscale 1; range 1–6), the frequency of private religious activities (subscale 2; range 1–6) and intrinsic religiosity (subscale 3; range 3–15). Higher scores represent more religious activities or religiosity.

Biological vulnerability and mechanisms (individual level biological domain)

Pain and function - Western Ontario and McMaster Universities Osteoarthritis Index (WOMAC) The WOMAC is a measure of lower extremity pain (5 items), stiffness (2 items), and function (17 items) [33, 34]. All items were rated on a Likert scale of 0 (no symptoms) to 4 (extreme symptoms), with a total range of 0–96 and higher scores indicating worse symptoms. Pain and function subscales are also separately reported. Some other studies used the Visual Analog Scale (VAS) version of the WOMAC, which includes the same items but each measured on a 100 mm VAS. For this version, each subscale score ranges from 0 to 100, with higher scores indicating worse symptoms or function. To facilitate comparison of STAART with studies using the WOMAC VAS version, we also transformed pain and function domains to a 0–100 scale, which has been done in prior studies [35, 36].

Arthritis impact measurement scales (AIMS) The AIMS was not collected in the STAART study. However,

Table 1 Characteristics of STAART Participants, Overall and By Site

Characteristic	Total Sample Mean ± SD or N(%)	DVAHCS Mean ± SD or N(%)	UNC Mean ± SD or N(%)
Sociocultural Environment			
Age	59.0 ± 10.3	57.8 ± 10.0	60.2 ± 10.5
Female	122 (49.2%)	26 (21.0%)	96 (77.4%)
Hispanic	7 (2.9%)	2 (1.6%)	5 (4.3%)
Some education above high school	187 (75.4%)	101 (81.5%)	86 (69.4%)
Working	86 (34.7%)	47 (37.9%)	39 (31.5%)
Married or living with partner	103 (41.5%)	63 (50.8%)	40 (32.3%)
Low Perceived Income[a]	83 (33.6%)	39 (31.7%)	44 (35.5%)
Duke University Religion Index			
Attendance at Religious Activities	4.4 ± 1.4	4.1 ± 1.5	4.8 ± 1.2
Private Religious Activities	4.0 ± 1.6	3.8 ± 1.6	4.2 ± 1.5
Intrinsic Religiosity	13.1 ± 2.5	13.1 ± 2.4	13.2 ± 2.6
Biological Vulnerability and Mechanisms			
WOMAC Total[b]	53.0 ± 17.8	56.0 ± 16.6	49.9 ± 18.5
WOMAC Pain	11.0 ± 3.9	11.6 ± 3.8	10.4 ± 3.9
WOMAC Function	37.0 ± 13.2	39.1 ± 12.4	34.9 ± 13.7
PROMIS Pain Interference Score	63.8 ± 6.9	64.0 ± 6.3	63.5 ± 7.5
Short Form-12 - Mental	50.7 ± 11.1	49.8 ± 11.6	51.5 ± 10.7
Short Form-12 - Physical	33.1 ± 9.1	33.1 ± 8.4	33.1 ± 9.7
Duration of Arthritis Symptoms	13.1 ± 10.0	14.6 ± 10.6	11.5 ± 9.1
Number of Self-Reported Comorbidities	8.5 ± 3.9	8.2 ± 3.5	8.8 ± 4.3
Body Mass Index (kg/m^2)	35.2 ± 8.2	33.1 ± 6.5	37.5 ± 9.1
Health Behaviors & Coping Strategies			
CSQ – Total Coping Attempts	93.9 ± 36.6	91.9 ± 39.7	95.8 ± 33.3
CSQ – Diverting Attention	13.9 ± 8.4	12.9 ± 8.6	14.8 ± 8.2
CSQ – Ignoring Sensations	14.1 ± 8.7	15.0 ± 9.6	13.2 ± 7.7
CSQ – Coping Self-Statements	23.6 ± 7.6	23.4 ± 8.2	23.7 ± 6.8
CSQ – Reinterpreting Pain Sensations	8.9 ± 8.4	9.7 ± 8.8	8.1 ± 8.0
CSQ – Praying, Hoping	20.8 ± 8.0	19.8 ± 8.0	21.9 ± 7.9
CSQ – Increasing Behavioral Activities	12.5 ± 7.1	11.0 ± 7.0	14.0 ± 6.9
CSQ – Catastrophizing	11.4 ± 7.6	11.1 ± 7.3	11.7 ± 7.8
Pain Catastrophizing Scale	19.8 ± 12.3	20.4 ± 12.4	19.2 ± 12.1
PHQ-8	6.2 ± 5.3	6.6 ± 5.3	5.7 ± 5.3
Arthritis Self-Efficacy Scale	5.9 ± 2.0	5.6 ± 2.1	6.1 ± 1.8
Self-Efficacy for Pain Communication	78.7 ± 22.0	77.4 ± 22.9	80.1 ± 21.1
Brief Fear of Movement Scale	14.8 (3.5)	14.4 (3.9)	15.2 (3.1)

DVAHCS Durham VA Health Care System, *UNC* University of North Carolina, *WOMAC* Western Ontario and McMaster Universities Osteoarthritis Index, *CSQ* coping strategies questionnaire, *PHQ* patient health questionnaire

[a] Self-report of "just meet basic expenses" or "don't even have enough to meet basic expenses."

[b] Likert scale version of WOMAC

it is a common measure in other OA studies, and therefore we present it for comparator studies when available. Although this does not allow a direct comparison to WOMAC, the AIMS scale provides a general description of the symptom severity of participants in comparator studies. Comparator studies used both the original AIMS, the AIMS2 and the AIMS2 Short Form (AIMS2-SF). The original AIMS includes 45 items across the domains of pain, physical disability and psychological disability [37]; the latter 2 are reported here because of their similarity to

WOMAC domains. Each AIMS domain has a score range of 0–10, with higher scores indicating greater pain or disability. The AIMS2 is an expanded version with 78 items, and the AIMS2-SF has 26 items [38, 39]. AIMS2 domains also have score ranges of 0–10, with higher scores indicating greater pain or disability.

PROMIS pain interference instrument (short form) The PROMIS Pain Interference (Short Form 6a) instrument measures the self-reported consequences of pain across aspects of life including social, cognitive, emotional, physical and recreational activities; this instrument refers to the past 7 days [40] This validated scale has five response options, with scores ranging from one to five; items are summed and re-scaled as a t-score with mean of 50 and standard deviation of 10.

Health-related quality of life (HRQoL) – Short form 12 (SF-12) The Short-Form-12 (SF-12) is a validated measure that covers domains of general health, physical health, work and activity limitations, and emotional health [41]. Physical and Mental Health Composite Scores (PCS & MCS) are computed using the scores of 12 questions and range from 0 to 100, with higher scores indicating better health.

Duration of arthritis symptoms Participants self-reported the number of years they have been experiencing knee and / or hip arthritis symptoms (joint pain, stiffness, or limited movement).

Comorbid illnesses The Self-Administered Comorbidity Questionnaire asks participants to indicate whether or not they have each of 13 physical and psychological health conditions. Participants can also list up to 3 additional conditions. The score range is 0–16 [42].

Body mass index (BMI) BMI was calculated from measured height and weight at baseline.

Health behaviors & coping strategies (individual level behavioral domain)

Coping strategies questionnaire (CSQ) The CSQ is the most commonly used measure of coping among individuals with chronic pain, and its measurement properties have been confirmed in patients with a variety of pain-related conditions [43, 44]. This scale includes 48 items that assess 6 cognitive domains (Catastrophizing, Diverting Attention, Ignoring Sensations, Coping Self-Statements, Reinterpreting Pain Sensations, Praying-Hoping) and 1 behavioral domain (Increasing Behavioral Activities). Each domain includes 6 items, and participants rate the frequency of their use of specific coping strategies on a 7-point Likert

scale from 0 ("Never do that") to 6 ("Always do that"). From the CSQ, we calculated a Coping Attempts Score, which sums all domains other than Catastrophizing. This score was reported because it could be compared to other previous studies [45, 46], and because the factor structure for this score has been replicated in prior research [47–49]. We also separately report scores for the Catastrophizing subscale.

Pain catastrophizing scale (PCS) The PCS is a widely used measure of catastrophic thinking related to pain [50]. This 13-item instrument asks participants to reflect on past painful experiences and to indicate the degree to which they experienced each of the thoughts or feelings when experiencing pain, with each item scored from 0 (not at all) to 4 (all the time). The PCS includes 3 subscales – rumination, magnification, and helplessness. Scores for all items are summed and total scores range from 0 to 52 with a higher score indicating a higher level of catastrophizing.

Depressive symptoms – Patient health questionnaire 8 (PHQ-8) The PHQ-8 is an eight-item survey that consists of items corresponding to depression criteria listed in the *Diagnostic and Statistics Manual Fourth Edition* (DSM-IV) [51]. Each of the eight questions is scored as 0 (not at all) to 3 (nearly every day), so that total scores range from 0 to 24.

Arthritis self efficacy scale This scale includes 8 items asking respondents how certain they are that they can perform specific activities or tasks [52]. Items are scored on a Likert Scale (1 = very uncertain to 10 = very certain); the total score represents a mean of the 8-items, with a range of 1–10. Because of challenges with comparing scores across different versions of this scale, we only included comparator studies that used the 8-item version.

Self-efficacy for pain communication scale – Patient version [53] This 7-item instrument assesses patient's level of confidence in communicating their pain to a "significant other" and receiving understanding and a helpful response. Items are rated on a scale from 10 ("very uncertain") to 100 ("very certain").

Brief fear of movement scale The Brief Fear of Movement Scale is a six item scale for assessing fear of movement in OA [54]. All items are measured on a 4-point scale from "strongly agree" to "strongly disagree." The total score ranges from 6 to 24, with higher scores indicating more fear of movement.

Comparator studies

We aimed to identify prior studies of pain CST and CBT-informed pain coping strategies among individuals with OA (regardless of racial composition), since those are of highest relevance to the STAART study. To identify comparator studies, we performed a literature search (using Pubmed) with search terms of (osteoarthritis) AND (CST OR CBT). We included clinical trials meeting these criteria from any country, resulting in 10 studies. We also compared our identified studies to a recent systematic review of behavioral intervention for OA and found no additional studies to include. For each of study we extracted relevant baseline participant characteristics for comparison to STAART. When participant characteristics were presented only by treatment arm, we contacted authors to request characteristics for the full study sample for simplicity of comparisons. When these were not available we presented characteristics by treatment arm. We compared characteristics between STAART participants and other studies descriptively. Because of the relatively small number of studies and because not all studies assessed all measures of interest, we did not conduct statistical comparisons.

The following are summaries of the studies we identified and included in this comparison. Additional details on participant inclusion criteria and recruitment methods are reported in Additional file 1:

Effectiveness of an Internet-Delivered Exercise and Pain-Coping Skills Training Intervention for Persons With Chronic Knee Pain: A Randomized Trial (Bennell et al., 2017) [45].

- Participants: 148 patients with knee pain.
- Intervention: online educational materials, an interactive, automated 8-module pain CST program (PainCOACH), and seven Skype sessions with a physiotherapist for 12 weeks, focusing on a home exercise program.
- Comparator group: online educational materials only.

Physical Therapist-Delivered Pain Coping Skills Training and Exercise for Knee Osteoarthritis: Randomized Controlled Trial (Bennell et al., 2016) [55, 56].

- Participants: 222 patients with symptomatic knee OA.
- Interventions: pain CST only, exercise only or pain CST/exercise combined. All groups attended 10 individual sessions with a physical therapist for 12 weeks, plus a home program.

Automated Internet-based pain coping skills training to manage osteoarthritis pain: a randomized controlled trial (Rini et al., 2015) [57].

- Participants: 113 participants with hip or knee OA

- Interventions: Internet-based PCST (PainCOACH), eight modules in a self-directed manner at a rate of one per week
- Comparator group: assessment-only control group

Nurse practitioners can effectively deliver pain coping skills training to osteoarthritis patients with chronic pain: A randomized, controlled trial (Broderick et al., 2014) [58].

- Participants: 256 participants with symptomatic knee or hip OA
- Intervention: 10 individual weekly sessions of pain CST
- Comparator group: usual care

Effectiveness of a cognitive-behavioural group intervention for knee osteoarthritis pain: a randomized controlled trial (Helminen et al., 2014) [59].

- Participants: 111 patients with symptomatic knee OA
- Intervention: CBT program for pain management, delivered in 6 weekly group sessions led by both a psychologist and a physiotherapist
- Comparator group: regular general practitioner care only

Cognitive-behavioral treatment for comorbid insomnia and osteoarthritis pain in primary care: the lifestyles randomized controlled trial (Vitiello et al., 2013) [60].

- Participants: 367 individuals with symptomatic OA and insomnia,
- Interventions: CBT for pain and insomnia, CBT for pain or education. CBT interventions were delivered in groups at primary care clinics and consisted of 6 weekly 90-min sessions.
- Comparator group: usual care

Pain coping skills training and lifestyle behavioral weight management in patients with knee osteoarthritis: a randomized controlled study (Somers et al., 2012) [25].

- Participants: 232 individuals with symptomatic knee OA
- Interventions: pain CST plus lifestyle behavioral weight management (BWM), pain CST only, BMW only. Pain CST only and BWM only interventions had 12 weekly 60-min sessions, followed by bi-weekly 60-min sessions for 12 weeks. The BWM only group also had three weekly supervised sessions weekly for the first 12 weeks. The pain CST + BWM group had 12 weekly 120 min sessions, in addition to 3 weekly supervised exercise sessions, followed by bi-weekly 120-min sessions for 12 weeks.
- Comparator group: standard care

Clinical effectiveness of a rehabilitation program integrating exercise, self-management, and active coping strategies for chronic knee pain: a cluster randomized trial (Hurley et al., 2007) [61].

- Participants: 418 individuals with knee pain.
- Interventions: individual rehabilitation, group rehabilitation (8 patients per group). Both individual and group rehabilitation involved 12 sessions (twice weekly for 6 weeks), supervised by a physiotherapist. Content included instruction in pain coping and self-management, as well as an individualized progressive exercise program.
- Comparator group: usual care

Spouse-assisted coping skills training in the management of osteoarthritic knee pain (Keefe et al., 1996) [46].

- Participants: 88 married persons with knee OA
- Interventions: spouse assisted pain CST, conventional pain CST with no spouse involvement arthritis education-spousal support control. Participants in all three interventions met in groups of 4 to 6 patients (or couples) for 10 weekly, 2-h group sessions.

Pain coping skills training in the management of osteoarthritic knee pain: A comparative study (Keefe et al., 1990) [20, 62].

- Participants: 99 patients with knee OA
- Interventions: pain CST, arthritis education. Both interventions met in small groups (6 to 9 patients) for 10 weekly 90-min sessions.
- Comparator: standard care control

Results

At both STAART study sites (UNC, Durham VA), 124 participants were enrolled. At UNC, 381 participants refused and 123 were ineligible; at the Durham VA, 632 participants refused and 77 were ineligible. At UNC, the mean ages for consented, refused, and ineligible patients, respectively, were: 60.2 (standard deviation (SD) = 10.5), 64.0 (SD = 12.9), and 60.1 (SD = 12.7); the proportions of females among those consented, refused, and ineligible, respectively, were: 77, 69 and 70%. At the VA, the mean ages for consented, refused, and ineligible patients, respectively were: 57.8 (SD = 10.0), 59.9 (SD = 11.3), and 61.2 (SD = 11.1); the proportions of females among those consented, refused, and ineligible, respectively, were: 21.0, 11.7 and 18.2%. Characteristics of consented STAART participants, overall and by site, are shown in Table 1. Table 2 compares Sociocultural Environment, Biological Vulnerability and Mechanisms, and Health

Behaviors and Coping variables for STAART participants and comparator studies; this table includes variables for which there was at least one comparator study that included the measure.

Sociocultural environment
Age
The mean age of STAART participants was 59 years (SD = 10.3), with a slightly lower age for VA participants than UNC participants. This mean age was slightly lower than other studies except for Somers et al. [25].

Sex
The proportion of females in the STAART study was 49%, which is lower than in other studies (range: 56–81%); among VA participants, only 21% were female, which reflects the high proportion of males in the VA.

Race and ethnicity
All STAART participants self-identified during screening as being black or African American, per study eligibility requirements. Two other studies included about 1/3 African Americans [25, 57], but the rest 13% or fewer (though several studies did not report information on race). Among STAART participants, 2.9% also self-identified as being of Hispanic or Latino ethnicity. Only Rini et al. reported ethnicity information for the sample, with 11% being of Hispanic or Latino ethnicity [57].

Education
Among STAART participants, 75% reported some education above high school, with the proportion being higher among VA than UNC participants. Proportions of participants with education above high school ranged from 61 to 86% in comparator studies.

Work status
Thirty-four percent of STAART participants reported they were currently working. Proportions of working participants ranged widely among other studies, from 21 to 57%.

Household financial status
Among STAART participants, about 1/3 reported that they could "just meet basic expenses" or "don't have enough to meet basic expenses." We did not identify any comparator studies that measured financial or income status in a manner that could be directly compared with the measure we collected for STAART participants.

Marital status
Forty-two percent of STAART participants were married or living with a partner as married, with a substantially

Table 2 Characteristics of participants in STAART and comparator studies of pain CST and CBT for patients with osteoarthritis

Participant Characteristic	STAART	Bennell et al, 2017 [45]	Bennell et al, 2016 [55]	Rini et al, 2015 [57]	Broderick et al, 2014 [58]	Helminen, 2014 [59]	Vitiello, 2013 [60]	Somers et al, 2012 [25]	Hurley, 2007 [61]	Keefe et al, 1996 [46]	Keefe et al, 1990 [62]
Sociocultural Environment											
Geographic Region	United States (Central North Carolina)	Australia (7 of 8 states)	Australia (Melbourne and Brisbane)	United States (Central North Carolina)	United States (New York, Virginia and North Carolina)	Finland (Kuopio, Eastern Finland)	United States (Washington State)	United States (Central North Carolina)	United Kingdom (Southeast London)	United States (Central North Carolina)	United States (Central North Carolina)
Age[a]	59.0 ± 10.3	61.2 ± 7.1	63.4 ± 8.1	67.6 ± 9.4	67.2 ± 9.5	CBT: 64.5 ± 7.3 Control Group: 62.8 ± 7.2	73.0 ± 8.0	58.0 ± 10.4	Individual Rehab: 66 (50-91) [f] Group Rehab:68 (51-84) Control Group: 67 (51-89)	62.6 ± 10.1	64.0 ± 11.5
Female	49%	56%	60%	81%	77%	69%	78%	79%	70%	61%	72%
Race	100% African American	–	–	70% White 29% African American 2% Other	13% Non-white	–	9% Non-white	38% Non-white	–	–	–
Ethnicity	3% Hispanic/Latino	–	–	11% Hispanic/Latino	–	–	–	–	–	–	–
Education	75% Above High School	75% Above High School	61% Above High School	71% Above High School	72% Above High School	68% Senior High/Vocational School or more	86% Above High School	86% Above High School	–	–	–
Work Status	35% Currently Working	57% Currently Working	51% Currently Working	21% Currently Working	30% Currently Working	21% Currently Working	78% Retired	–	–	–	–
Marital Status	41% Married/Living with Partner	–	–	62% Married/Living with Partner	63% Married/Living with Partner	66% Married/Living with Partner	–	–	–	–	–
Biological Vulnerability & Mechanisms											
WOMAC Total Score[a]	[b]53.0 ± 17.8 [c]53.7 ± 19.1	–	–	–	–	–	–	–	[b]Individual Rehab: 37.5±19.4 Group Rehab: 39.1±19.7 Control Group: 38.6±19.6	–	–
WOMAC Pain Subscale Score[a]	[b]11.0 ± 3.9 [c]55.0 ± 19.4	[b]CST + Exercise: 9.0 ± 2.4 Control: 9.2 ± 2.5	[b]Exercise: 8.6 ± 2.7 CST: 8.7 ± 2.8 CST + Exercise: 9.0 ± 2.8	–	[c]54.8 (17.4)	[c]CBT: 57.6 (53.9 -61.3) [e]Control Group: 56.4 (52.9 -60.0)	–	[c]CST+Weight Management (WM): 47.7 (42.1-55.3) [e] WM: 42.6 (37.7-47.5) CST: 42.8	[b]Individual Rehab: 7.4 ±4.0 Group Rehab: 7.69±4.1 Control Group: 7.7±4.0	–	–

Table 2 Characteristics of participants in STAART and comparator studies of pain CST and CBT for patients with osteoarthritis (*Continued*)

Participant Characteristic	STAART	Bennell et al, 2017 [45]	Bennell et al, 2016 [55]	Rini et al, 2015 [57]	Broderick et al, 2014 [58]	Helminen, 2014 [59]	Vitiello, 2013 [60]	Somers et al, 2012 [25]	Hurley, 2007 [61]	Keefe et al, 1996 [46]	Keefe et al, 1990 [62]
WOMAC Function Subscale Score[a]	[b]37.0 ± 13.2 [c]53.7 ± 19.7	[b] CST + Exercise: 33.1 ± 8.0 Control: 32.5 ± 8.3	[b] Exercise: 34.3 ± 7.2 CST: 35.0 ± 7.4 CST + Exercise: 35.6 ± 7.3	--	[c] 54.6 (17.1)	[c] CBT: 53.0 (48.1 –57.9)[e] Control Group: 48.4 (43.1–53.7)	--	[c]CST+ WM: 47.7 (42.2–53.1)[e] WM: 44.3 (39.5–49.0) CST: 46.2 (41.1–51.3) Control Group: 46.1 (39.7–52.5)	[b]Individual Rehab: 26.4±14.7 Group Rehab: 27.9 ±14.7 Control Group: 27.2±14.6	--	(42.1-53.3) Control Group: 43.4 (37.4-49.5)
Arthritis Impact Measurement Scales 2- Pain Subscale[a]	--	--	--	Internet CST: 4.8 ± 1.7 Control Group: 5.1 ± 1.8	5.1 ± 2.1	--	--	CST+WM: 5.8 (5.3-6.2) WM: 5.3 (4.9-5.7) CST: 5.6 (5.2-6.0) Control Group: 5.5 (4.9-6.1)	--	CST: 5.4 ± 2.1 Spouse Assisted CST: 5.1 ± 1.7 Control Group: 5.2 ± 2.2	CST: 5.4 ± 2.1 Arthritis Education: 5.6 ± 1.9 Control Group: 5.8 ± 1.62
Arthritis Impact Measurement Scales 2 - Physical Function Subscale[a]	--	--	--	Internet CST: 1.7 ± 1.3 Control Group: 1.8 ± 1.0	1.8 ± 1.2	--	--	CST+WM: 1.7 (1.4-1.9) WM: 1.8: (1.1-1.7) CST: 1.6: (1.3-1.8) Control Group: 1.6 (1.2-1.9)	--	CST: 1.8 ± 0.9 Spouse Assisted CST: 1.7 ± 1.1 Control Group: 1.6 ± 0.7	CST: 2.0 ± 1.0 Arthritis Education: 2.1 ± 1.22 Control Group: 1.9 ± 1.2
Years with Arthritis Symptoms[a]	13.1 ± 10.0	CST + Exercise: 15% < 2 years, 51% 2-10 years, 34% >10 years Control: 32% < 2 years, 47% 2-10 years, 20% >10 years	Exercise: 6.0 (3-10)[d] CST: 5.5 (4-10) CST + Exercise: 5.5 (2-10)	--	13.8 ± 9.9	CBT: 8.9 ± 8.7 Control Group: 6.6 ± 4.5	--	--	Individual Rehab: 7 (3-15)[d] Group Rehab: 5 (2.5-11) Control Group: 6 (3-15)	--	--
Number of Comorbidities[a]	8.5 ± 3.9	--	--	1.3 ± 1.1	--	CBT: 5.3 ± 2.8 Control Group: 4.9 ± 3.6	--	--	--	--	--
BMI, kg/m^2 [a]	35.2 ± 8.2	31.4 ± 8.0	31.3 ± 6.1	--	33.4 ± 8.0	CBT: 30.1 ± 6.0 Control Group:	--	CST+ WM: 34.1 (33.0–	Individual Rehab: 30.0 (18–45)[f]	--	--

Table 2 Characteristics of participants in STAART and comparator studies of pain CST and CBT for patients with osteoarthritis (Continued)

Participant Characteristic	STAART	Bennell et al, 2017 [45]	Bennell et al, 2016 [55]	Rini et al, 2015 [57]	Broderick et al, 2014 [58]	Helminen, 2014 [59]	Vitiello, 2013 [60]	Somers et al, 2012 [25]	Hurley, 2007 [61]	Keefe et al, 1996 [46]	Keefe et al, 1990 [62]
	35.2	29.9 ± 6.3						WM: 33.5 (32.4–34.7) CST: 34.4 (33.3–35.5) Control Group: 34.1 (32.8–35.4)	Group Rehab: 30.18 (20–50) Control Group: 30.3 (20–51)		
Health Behaviors and Coping Strategies											
Coping Skills Questionnaire – Total Coping Attempts[a]	93.9 ± 36.6	CST + Exercise: 61.7 ± 24.9 Control: 65.7 ± 24.9	–	–	–	–	–	–	–	CST: 69.2 ± 26.7 Spouse Assisted CST: 67.8 ± 23.2 Control Group: 58.9 ± 22.3	–
Coping Skills Questionnaire – Catastrophizing Subscale[a]	11.4 ± 7.6	–	–	–	7.0 ± 6.4	–	–	CST+WM: 7.4 (5.5–9.3) WM: 6.6 (4.8–8.2) CST: 7.2 (5.5–8.9) Control Group: 6.9 (4.9–8.9)	–	–	–
Pain Catastrophizing Scale[a]	19.8 ± 12.3	CST + Exercise: 8.8 ± 9.2 Control: 10.1 ± 9.6	Exercise: 14.9 ± 8.1 CST: 14.8 ± 9.3 CST+ Exercise: 14.4 ± 9.7	–	–	CBT: 16.9 (13.8–20.0)[e] Control Group: 13.5 (10.7–16.2)	–	–	–	–	–
Arthritis Self-Efficacy Scale[a]	5.9 ± 2.0	–.	–	Internet CST: 6.7 ± 1.8 Control Group: 6.3 ± 2.1	6.0 ± 1.9	–	–	–	–	–	–

CST Coping Skills Training, CBT Cognitive Behavioral Therapy, WOMAC Western Ontario and McMaster Universities Osteoarthritis Index, BMI Body Mass Index
[a]Mean (standard deviation unless otherwise noted); [b]WOMAC Likert scale version; [c]WOMAC Visual Analog Scale or Likert scores transformed to 0-100 scale; [d]Median (Interquartile Range); [e]95% Confidence Intervals; [f]Mean (range)

higher proportion for VA than UNC (51% vs. 32%). In other studies, the proportions of married participants were all higher, ranging from 62 to 66%, though a number of studies did not report marital status. This comparison reflects a potentially greater need or risk for STAART participants.

Religiosity

Among STAART participants, mean scores on the DUREL were relatively high for all domains, including attendance at religious services, private religious activities and intrinsic religiosity. We did not identify any comparator studies that measured this construct.

Biological vulnerability and mechanisms
Pain and function – WOMAC

The mean total WOMAC score (Likert version) among STAART participants was 53.0 (SD = 17.8), which indicates moderate to severe symptoms. WOMAC scores were somewhat worse for the VA group compared to the UNC group. One comparator study reported total WOMAC scores (Likert version) ranging from 38 to 39 [61]; this comparison indicates greater symptom severity among STAART participants. The mean WOMAC pain subscale score (Likert version) among STAART participants was 11.0 (SD = 3.9). Among three comparator studies that reported WOMAC pain scores on the Likert scale, mean values were all lower than for STAART participants (7.7–8.6); this comparison indicates greater pain among STAART participants [45, 55, 61]. When converted to a 0–100 scale, the mean WOMAC pain score among STAART participants was 55.0 (SD = 19.4); this score was worse than [25] or comparable to [59] comparator studies that used the WOMAC VAS version. The mean WOMAC function subscale score (Likert version) among STAART participants was 37.0 (SD = 13.2). Among three comparator studies that reported WOMAC function scores on the Likert scale, mean values were all lower (26–33); this comparison reflects poorer function among STAART participants [45, 55, 61]. When converted to a 0–100 scale, the mean WOMAC function score among STAART participants was 53.7 (SD = 19.7); this score was worse than [25] or comparable to [58, 59] other studies that measured the WOMAC VAS version.

Pain – AIMS

Several studies included AIMS or AIMS2 pain and function scores. Among these, AIMS pain scores ranged from 5.1–5.8 and AIMS2 pain scores ranged from 4.8–5.1; these scores represent modest levels of pain (scale range of 0–10). AIMS function scores ranged from 1.6–2.0 and AIMS2 function scores ranged from 1.7–1.8; these scores represent relatively low levels of functional limitations,

potentially reflecting that these samples were less limited than participants in the STAART study.

Pain interference – PROMIS

Among STAART study participants, the mean score was 63.8 (SD = 6.9). This score indicates that the mean level of pain interference for STAART participants was a little over one standard deviation greater than the average of the general population. We did not identify any comparator studies that included this measure.

HRQoL – SF-12

The mean SF-12 PCS score for STAART participants was 33.1; this is lower than the average score for US men and women aged 60–69 (45.6 and 44.0, respectively), reflecting poorer HRQoL among STAART participants [63]. The mean SF-12 MCS score for STAART participants was 50.1 (SD = 11.1); this is slightly lower than the average score for US men and women aged 60–69 (52.7 and 51.8, respectively), also reflecting somewhat poorer HRQoL among STAART participants [63]. We did not identify any comparator studies that included this measure.

Duration of arthritis symptoms

On average, the self-reported duration of arthritis symptoms was 13.1 years (SD = 10.0), with a longer duration for VA participants than UNC participants. In comparator studies, duration of symptoms ranged from 5 to 14 years, with most having a mean duration lower than the STAART study.

Comorbid illnesses

The mean number of self-reported comorbid illnesses among STAART participants was 8.5 (SD = 3.9). Only two of the comparator studies reported a mean number of comorbidities for participants, and these were lower than in STAART (1.3–5.3), potentially indicating higher risk among our study sample [57, 59]. However, because of different comorbidity measures, the ability to directly to compare studies is limited.

BMI

The mean BMI among STAART participants was 35.2 kg/m^2 (SD = 8.2), which corresponds to Class 2 (moderate risk) obesity; BMI was somewhat lower in the VA group compared to the UNC group. In comparator studies, mean BMI's ranged from 30 to 34 kg/m^2, indicating more risk among STAART participants.

Health behaviors & coping strategies
Pain coping attempts – CSQ

Among STAART participants, the mean Pain Coping Attempts score was 93.9 (SD = 36.6), with slightly higher scores for UNC participants. Two other studies reported this scale [45, 46], with scores ranging from 59 to 69; this indicates that STAART participants were overall engaged in a larger number of coping efforts compared to other studies.

Pain catastrophizing – CSQ

The mean Pain Catastrophizing Scale score was 11.4 (SD = 7.6). This score was higher than two other studies reporting on this scale, in which mean scores ranged from 6.6–7.4 [25, 58]. This comparison suggests greater risk and needs for intervention among STAART participants.

Pain catastrophizing scale

The mean score on the PCS for STAART participants was 19.8 (SD = 12.3). Among three other studies reporting on this scale, mean scores ranged from 7 to 17 [45, 55, 59]. This comparison suggests greater risk and needs for intervention among STAART participants.

Depressive symptoms - PHQ-8

In the STAART study, the mean PHQ-8 score was 6.2 (SD = 5.3), and this was higher for VA participants than UNC participants. This average score indicates low depressive symptoms and is below the cutoff of 10 for depressive disorder [51]. We did not identify comparator studies that used this measure.

Arthritis self efficacy scale

The mean score for STAART participants on this measure was 5.9 (SD = 2.0). Two other studies administered the same version of this scale, and the mean score was similar to STAART participants [57, 58].

Self-efficacy for pain communication scale

The mean score for STAART participants was 78.7 (SD = 22.0); this score indicates a relatively low level of self-efficacy for communicating about pain [64]. We did not identify other comparator studies that used this measure.

Brief fear of movement scale

The mean score for STAART participants was 14.8 (SD = 3.5) on a scale of 6–24, suggesting a relatively high level of fear of movement. None of our comparator studies reported this measure.

Discussion

With a focus on health disparities, the STAART study aimed to reach a patient group with greater OA severity and risk for other negative OA-related outcomes. The study particularly focused on African Americans, who have reported worse OA-related symptoms compared to Caucasians in several studies [2–4, 65, 66]. We also selected recruitment sites that serve many patients with

multiple health challenges and relatively low income levels, since these individuals may be at particular risk for worse OA-related outcomes. Based on descriptions of comparator studies, none had a particular focus on identifying patient populations with greatest risks or needs. We utilized proactive and culturally tailored recruitment methods [8] and were able to meet the study sample size goal within the specified timeline, potentially reflecting a high degree of receptivity to this type of intervention in this patient group. Consented patients were slightly younger than those who declined or were ineligible, but there was a more pronounced gender difference, with the consented group including more females than those who declined or were ineligible. This may be due to greater willingness of women to engage in behavioral and psychological interventions; additional work is needed to understand how to best engage men in these types of programs.

Comparisons to similar studies of pain CST and CBT-informed pain coping strategies demonstrate that STAART participants differ in a number of factors that reflect worse OA severity and greater vulnerability for worsening outcomes, across all three domains we examined within the NIMHD Research Framework:

Sociocultural environment

Based on our review of pain CST and or CBT-informed pain coping studies among patients with OA, STAART is the first to focus exclusively on African Americans. In most comparator studies, proportions of non-white participants were 10% or less, with none greater than about 1/3. This emphasizes the uniqueness and importance of the STAART study in adding to understanding of pain CST interventions among African Americans with OA.

STAART participants also differ from prior studies demographically in other ways that may affect pain-related outcomes and response to a pain CST intervention. Fewer STAART participants are married or living with a partner as married, compared with other studies, likely reflecting the lower rates of marriage among African Americans than Caucasians in general [67]; however, these rates may also partly reflect a lower income status among STAART participants, considering the clinics in which we recruited and the fact that marriage rates decline with lower income. This is an important difference from other studies, since close partners can offer support for pain coping, and being "un-partnered" can place individuals at greater risk for to other health-related or psychosocial stressors [23, 46]. To accommodate both married and single individuals and to reflect that pain communication goes beyond immediate support persons, the intervention encouraged participants to learn skills for communicating about pain with others more broadly, including family members, friends and health care providers. STAART participants, on average, are younger than samples of most prior studies in this area. This is likely due in part to higher risk of OA at younger ages among Veterans, who make up half of the STAART sample [68]. Although younger age is not necessarily a risk factor for worse pain-related outcomes, younger individuals with OA may be more likely to face challenges with continuing employment, particularly in physically demanding occupations. The STAART intervention is telephone-based, with a flexible schedule for calls, which may promote feasibility in working-age participants.

Although we were not able to directly compare financial status of participants across studies due to measurement inconsistency, about 1/3 of STAART participants perceived they "just meet" or "don't even have enough to meet" basic expenses; as noted above, this may be partly reflect the underlying demographic characteristics of the clinics in which we recruited patients. This is important because financial stressors can augment the challenges of coping with chronic illnesses, and therefore individuals with lower income levels may particularly benefit from programs that teach and support coping skills. The telephone-based approach of STAART was also selected because it mitigates financial burdens related to transportation and missing work.

STAART participants reported relatively high levels of religiosity, which is important given the close connections between religiosity and multiple aspects of the pain and pain coping experience [69]. Unfortunately, we did not identify any comparator studies that measured this important construct. We expected that religious values would be important to a substantial proportion of STAART participants, and therefore one aspect of cultural tailoring involved encouraging participants to integrate elements of their spirituality or religious faith into their practice of pain coping when they felt it was important do so [8]. For example, during cognitive restructuring sessions, if participants identified that their faith played an integral role in reframing their pain-related challenges, this was further explored and built upon during the intervention.

Biological vulnerability & mechanisms

Several key variables in this domain also indicate that STAART participants have greater risks and challenges than samples of comparator studies. First, the STAART sample overall had worse OA pain and function than participants in comparator studies. Although we could only make a direct comparison to studies that reported the same version of the WOMAC [45, 55, 61], indirect comparisons to studies using other versions of the WOMAC, as well as the AIMS, suggest STAART participants had worse symptoms [25, 46, 57–59, 62]. The mean total WOMAC score for the STAART sample reflects moderate-to-severe symptoms. We expect this

difference from other studies reflects worse OA symptoms among African Americans than Caucasians, which has been shown in a number of prior studies [2–4].

The STAART sample also had longer symptom duration than most comparator studies [55, 59, 61]. Although it is not clear whether the effectiveness of cognitive behavioral interventions differs based on time since symptom onset, it is an important consideration that overall, this group of patients had been managing their chronic pain for a longer period of time than patients in prior studies of this type. This difference from other studies may partly reflect a younger age of onset of OA among some military personnel and Veterans [68]. BMI was higher in our study than in any of the comparators, including Somers et al. [25], which selected only overweight and obese individuals. This is likely a reflection of higher BMI among African Americans in the US, compared with Caucasians [70]. Although it was difficult to compare comorbidity burden to other studies, STAART participants had a high number of comorbid illnesses (mean of 8.5). This likely reflects the high prevalence of multiple chronic health conditions (e.g. hypertension, diabetes, cardiovascular disease) among African Americans [70], but as noted above, this also may be partly attributable to the general patient populations of the clinics in which we recruited. Little is known about the associations of comorbidity with pain coping in OA, but the challenge of managing multiple health conditions may increase the difficulty of coping with OA-related symptoms.

Health behaviors & coping strategies

STAART participants also differed from prior studies in ways that may indicate greater need for a pain CST intervention. First STAART participants reported higher levels of pain catastrophizing than any other study [25, 45, 46, 55, 58, 59]; prior research has also found higher levels of catastrophizing among African Americans than Caucasians [11–13]. Pain catastrophizing can be improved by CST interventions, which emphasize cognitive restructuring as a strategy to address unhelpful thoughts about pain [20, 22, 24]. Participants in the STAART study also reported more coping attempts than other studies that measured this same construct [45, 46]. This may be due in part to the higher levels of pain experienced by STAART participants compared with prior study samples.

STAART participants reported relatively low levels of Self-Efficacy for Pain Communication. Although none of our comparator studies measured this construct, STAART participants' scores were similar to those of another sample of individuals with OA [64]. Based on prior work by Campbell et al. [71], we expected that many patients would benefit from building skills and confidence in communicating with others about their pain experience;

therefore, a pain communication module was included [8]. Fear of movement scores also were high among STAART participants. Although the STAART CST intervention does not specifically address fear of movement, other modules (e.g. activity pacing, cognitive restructuring) involve related concepts and have potential to reduce pain-related fear of movement. STAART participants had relatively low depressive symptoms, based on the mean PHQ-8 score. Although none of the comparator measures used this same measures, some studies measured depressive symptoms with other measures, including the Beck Depression Inventory, Depression Anxiety Stress Scales, Hospital Anxiety and Depression Scale, and the Geriatric Depression Scale [55, 58–61]; participants in these studies also had scores that indicated normal or low levels of depressive symptoms, similar to the STAART study.

Conclusion

In conclusion, this comparison of STAART participants to prior studies of CST for OA identified differences in a number of key variables related to OA severity and risks for poor pain-related outcomes. In particular, STAART participants have worse OA symptoms, higher BMI, and greater levels of pain catastrophizing compared to other study samples. STAART participants also have a high comorbidity burden, and 1/3 perceive they have relatively low income. These characteristics place STAART participants at greater risk for worse OA related physical and psychological outcomes. However, pain CST programs can improve multiple OA-related outcomes, and STAART participants may gain particular benefit from this intervention approach because of its focus on pain catastrophizing. If results of the STAART study support the effectiveness of pain CST in this group, this will be an important addition to prior literature, given the importance of identifying effective interventions for African Americans, who bear a higher burden of OA.

Abbreviations

AIMS: Arthritis impact measurement scales; AIMS2-SF: AIMS2 Short Form; BMI: Body mass index; BWM: Behavioral weight management; CBT: Cognitive behavioral therapy; CSQ: Coping strategies questionnaire; CST: Coping skills training; DSM-IV: Diagnostic and statistics manual fourth edition; DUREL: Duke University Religion Index; HRQoL: Health-Related Quality of Life; MCS: Mental health composite score; NIMHD: National Institute on Minority Health and Health Disparities; OA: Osteoarthritis; PCS: Pain catastrophizing scale; PCS: Physical health composite score; PCST: Pain coping skills training; PHQ-8: Patient Health Questionnaire 8; SD: Standard deviation; SF-12: Short-Form-12; STAART: Pain Coping Skills Training for African Americans with OsteoaRThritis; UNC: University of North Carolina at Chapel Hill; VA: Durham VA Healthcare System; VAS: Visual analog scale; WOMAC: Western Ontario and McMasters Universities Osteoarthritis Index

Acknowledgements

The study team thanks all of the study participants, without whom this work would not be possible. We thank the following team members for their contributions to the research: Caroline Nagle, Kimberlea Grimm, Ashley Gwyn, Bernadette Benas, Alex Gunn, Leah Schrubbe, Catherine Stanwyck, Erin Haley and Scott Ravyts. The study team also expresses gratitude to the Stakeholder Panel for this project: Ms. Mae Karim, Ms. Sandy Walker, LPN (Chapel Hill Children's Clinic), Mr. Ralph Brown, Yashika Watkins, PhD, MPH (Movement is Life / University of Illinois at Chicago), Teresa J. Brady, PhD (Centers for Disease Control and Prevention), Elaine Hart-Brothers, MD, MPH (Community Health Coalition), and Ms. Laura C. Marrow (Arthritis Foundation). The study team also thanks all of the participants taking part in this research. We thank the authors of the comparator studies included in this manuscript, for their responsiveness regarding their study data: Kim L. Bennell et al., Christine Rini et al., Joan E. Broderick et al., Eeva-Eerika Helminen et al., Michael V. Vitiello et al., and M.V. Hurley et al.

Funding

Research reported in this manuscript was funded through a Patient-Centered Outcomes Research Institute (PCORI) Award (AD-1408-19519). The statements presented in this manuscript are solely the responsibility of the authors and do not necessarily represent the views of the Patient-Centered Outcomes Research Institute (PCORI), its Board of Governors, or Methodology Committee. KDA and LA receive support from National Institute of Arthritis and Musculoskeletal and Skin Diseases Multidisciplinary Clinical Research Center P60 AR062760. KDA and CJC receive support from the Center for Health Services Research in Primary Care, Durham VA Health Care System (CIN 13–410).

Authors' contributions

KDA, LCC, CJC, CWC, FJK, EZO, and TJS contributed to the study design. CJC and LA contributed to plans for and conduct of statistical analyses. LCC, TJS, and EH contributed to the development and administration of the pain coping skills training intervention. All authors contributed to drafting and editing of the manuscript. All authors approved the final manuscript.

Competing interests

The authors declare that they have no competing interests.

Author details

[1]Thurston Arthritis Research Center, University of North Carolina at Chapel Hill, 3300 Thurston Bldg., CB# 7280, Chapel Hill, NC 27599-7280, USA. [2]Department of Medicine, University of North Carolina at Chapel Hill, 125 MacNider Hall CB# 7005, Chapel Hill, NC 27599, USA. [3]Health Services Research and Development Service, Durham VA Medical Center, Durham, NC, USA. [4]Department of Biostatistics and Bioinformatics, Duke University Medical Center, Durham, NC, USA. [5]Department of Psychology, East Carolina University, Greenville, NC, USA. [6]Department of Psychiatry and Behavioral Science, Duke University, Durham, NC, USA. [7]Department of Medicine, Duke University Medical Center, Durham, NC, USA. [8]Institute for Health Research and Policy, University of Illinois at Chicago, Chicago, IL, USA.

References

1. Smith DM, Parmelee PA. Within-day variability of fatigue and pain among African Americans and non-Hispanic whites with osteoarthritis of the knee. Arthritis Care Res (Hoboken). 2016;68(1):115–22.
2. Allen KD. Racial and ethnic disparities in osteoarthritis phenotypes. Curr Opin Rheumatol. 2010;22(5):528–32.
3. Allen KD, Helmick CG, Schwartz TA, DeVellis B, Renner JB, Jordan JM. Racial differences in self-reported pain and function among individuals with radiographic hip and knee osteoarthritis: the Johnston County osteoarthritis project. Osteoarthritis Cartilage. 2009;17(9):1132–6.
4. Allen KD, Oddone EZ, Coffman CJ, Keefe FJ, Lindquist JH, Bosworth HB. Racial differences in osteoarthritis pain and function: potential explanatory factors. Osteoarthritis Cartilage. 2010;18:160–7.
5. Lavernia CJ, Alcerro JC, Rossi MD. Fear in arthroplasty surgery: the role of race. Clin Orthop Relat Res. 2010;468(2):547–54.
6. Vina ER, Ran D, Ashbeck EL, Kwoh CK. Natural history of pain and disability among African-Americans and whites with or at risk for knee osteoarthritis: a longitudinal study. Osteoarthr Cartil. 2018;26(4):471–9.
7. IOM (Institute of Medicine). Initial National Piorities for Comparative Effectiveness Research. Washington DC: The National Academies Press; 2009.

8. Schrubbe LA, Ravyts SG, Benas BC, Campbell LC, Cene CW, Coffman CJ, Gunn AH, Keefe FJ, Nagle CT, Oddone EZ, et al. Pain coping skills training for African Americans with osteoarthritis (STAART): study protocol of a randomized controlled trial. BMC Musculoskelet Disord. 2016;17(1):359.

9. Meints SM, Stout M, Abplanalp S, Hirsh AT. Pain-related rumination, but not magnification or helplessness, mediates race and sex differences in experimental pain. J Pain. 2017;18(3):332–9.

10. Meints SM, Miller MM, Hirsh AT. Differences in pain coping between black and white Americans: a meta-analysis. J Pain. 2016;17(6):642–53.

11. Chibnall JT, Tait RC. Long-term adjustment to work-related low back pain: associations with socio-demographics, claim processes, and post-settlement adjustment. Pain Med. 2009;10(8):1378–88.

12. Edwards RR, Moric M, Husfeldt B, Buvanendran A, Ivankovich O. Ethnic similarities and differences in the chronic pain experience: a comparison of african american, Hispanic, and white patients. Pain Med. 2005;6(1):88–98.

13. Ruehlman LS, Karoly P, Newton C. Comparing the experiential and psychosocial dimensions of chronic pain in african americans and Caucasians: findings from a national community sample. Pain Med. 2005;6(1):49–60.

14. Tan G, Jensen MP, Thornby J, Anderson KO. Ethnicity, control appraisal, coping, and adjustment to chronic pain among black and white Americans. Pain Med. 2005;6(1):18–28.

15. Jones AC, Kwoh CK, Groeneveld PW, Mor M, Geng M, Ibrahim SA. Investigating racial differences in coping with chronic osteoarthritis pain. J Cross Cult Gerontol. 2008;23:339–47.

16. Allen KD, Golightly YM, Olsen MK. Pilot study of pain and coping among patients with osteoarthritis: a daily diary analysis. J Clin Rheumatol. 2006; 12(3):118–23.

17. Somers TJ, Keefe FJ, Pells JJ, Dixon KE, Waters SJ, Riordan PA, Blumenthal JA, McKee DC, Lacaille L, Tucker JM, et al. Pain catastarophizing and pain-related fear in osteoarthritis patients: relationships to pain and disability. J Pain Symptom Manag. 2009;37(5):863–72.

18. Somers TJ, Keefe FJ, Carson JW, Pells JJ, Lacaille L. Pain catastrophizing in borderline morbidly obese and morbidly obese individuals with osteoarthritic knee pain. Pain Res Manag. 2008;13(5):401–6.

19. Allen KD, Coffman CJ, Golightly YM, Stechuchak KM, Keefe FJ. Daily pain variations among patients with hand, hip, and knee osteoarthritis. Osteoarthritis Cartilage. 2009;17(10):1275–82.

20. Keefe FJ, Caldwell D, Williams DA, Gil KM, Mitchell D, Robertson C, Martinez S, Nunley J, Beckham JC, Helms M. Pain coping skills training in the management of osteoarthritic knee pain-II: follow-up results. Behav Ther. 1990;21(4):435–47.

21. Keefe FJ, Caldwell DS. Cognitive behavioral control of arthritis pain. Adv Rheumatol. 1997;81(1):277–90.

22. Keefe FJ, Caldwell DS, Baucom D, Salley A, Robinson E, Timmons K, Beaupre P, Weisberg J, Helms M. Spouse-assisted coping skills training in the management of knee pain in osteoarthritis: long-term followup results. Arthritis Care Res. 1999;12(2):101–11.

23. Keefe FJ, J.A. B, Baucom D, Affleck G, Waugh R, Caldwell DS, Beaupre P, Kashikar-Zuck S, Wright K, Egert J et al: Effects of spouse-assisted coping skills training and exercise training in patients with osteoarthritic knee pain: a randomized controlled study. Pain 2004, 110:539–549.

24. Riddle DL, Keefe FJ, Nay WT, McKee D, Attarian DE, Jensen MP. Pain coping skills training for patients with elevated pain catastrophizing who are scheduled for knee arthroplasty: a quasi-experimental study. Arch Phys Med Rehabil. 2011;92(6):859–65.

25. Somers TJ, Blumenthal JA, Guilak F, Kraus VB, Schmitt DO, Babyak MA, Craighead LW, Caldwell DS, Rice JR, McKee DC, et al. Pain coping skills training and lifestyle behavioral weight management in patients with knee osteoarthritis: a randomized controlled study. Pain. 2012;153(6):1199–209.

26. Miranda J, Bernal G, Lau A, Kohn L, Hwang W-C. State of the science on psychosocial interventions for ethnic minorities. Annu Rev Clin Psychol. 2005;1:113–42.

27. Sullivan MJL, Thorn B, Haythornthwaite JA, Keefe FJ, Martin MI, Bradley LA, Lefebvre JC. Theoretical perspectives on the relation between catastrophizing and pain. Clin J Pain. 2001;17(1):52–64.

28. Allen KD, Bosworth HB, Coffman CJ, Lindquist JH, Sperber N, Weinberger M, Oddone EZ. Racial differences in pain coping efficacy in patients with hip and knee osteoarthritis. In: Annual meeting of the American College of Rheumatology: 2012; Washington, DC; 2012.

29. NIMHD Minority Health and Health Disparities Research Framework. https://www.nimhd.nih.gov/images/research-framework-slide.pdf. Accessed 4 Jan 2018.

30. Campbell LC, Keefe FJ, Scipio C, McKee DC, Edwards CL, Herman SH, Johnson LE, Colvin OM, McBride CM, Donatucci C. Facilitating research participation and improving quality of life for African American prostate cancer survivors and their intimate partners: a pilot study of telephone-based coping skills training. Cancer. 2006;109(2Suppl):414–24.

31. Project I.M.P.A.C.T. – Increase Minority Participation and Awareness of Clinical Trials: http://impact.nmanet.org/wordpress/. Accessed 4 Jan 2018.

32. Koenig HG, Bussing A. The Duke University religion index (DUREL): a five-item measure for use in epidemiological studies. Religions. 2010;1:78–85.

33. Bellamy N. WOMAC: a 20-year experiential review of a patient-centered self-reported health status questionnaire. J Rheumatol. 2002;29(12):2473–6.

34. Bellamy N, Buchanan WW, Goldsmith CH, Campbell J, Stitt LW. Validation study of WOMAC: a health status instrument for measuring clinically important patient relevant outcomes to antirheumatic drug therapy in patients with osteoarthritis of the hip or knee. J Rheumatol. 1988;15:1833–40.

35. Tubach F, Ravaud P, Baron G, Falissard B, Logeart I, Bellamy N, Bombardier C, Felson DT, Hochberg MC, van der Heijde D, et al. Evaluation of clinically relevant states in patient reported outcomes in knee and hip osteoarthritis: the patient acceptable symptom state. Ann Rheum Dis. 2005;64(1):34–7.

36. Quintana JM, Escobar A, Bilbao A, Arostegui I, Lafuente I, Vidaurreta I. Responsiveness and clinically important differences in WOMAC and SF-36 after hip joint replacement. Osteoarthritis Cartilage. 2005;13:1076–83.

37. Meenan RF, Gertman PM, Mason JH. Measuring health status in arthritis. The arthritis impact measurement scales. Arthritis Rheumatism. 1980;32(2):146–52.

38. Meenan RF, Mason JH, Anderson JJ, Guccione AA, Kazis L. AIMS2: the content and properties of a revised and expanded arthritis impact measurement scales health status questionnaire. Arthritis Rheumatism. 1992;35(1):1–10.

39. Ren XS, Kazis L, Meenan RF. Short-form arthritis impact measurement scales 2: tests of reliability and validity among patients with osteoarthritis. Arthritis Care Res. 1999;12(3):163–71.

40. Amtmann D, Cook KF, Jensen MP, Chen WH, Choi S, Revicki D, Cella D, Rothrock N, Keefe F, Callahan L, et al. Development of a PROMIS item bank to measure pain interference. Pain. 2010;150(1):173–82.

41. Ware J Jr, Kosinski M, Keller SD. A 12-item short-form health survey: construction of scales and preliminary tests of reliability and validity. Med Care. 1996;34(3):220–33.

42. Sangha O, Stucki G, Liang MH, Fossel AH, Katz JN. The self-administered comorbidity questionnaire: a new method to assess comorbidity for clinical and health services research. Arthritis Rheumatism. 2003;49(2):156–63.

43. Rosenstiel AK, Keefe FJ. The use of coping strategies in chronic low back pain patients: relationship of patient characteristics and current adjustment. Pain. 1983;17:33–44.

44. Hastie BA, Riley JL, Fillingim RB. Ethnic differences in pain coping: factor structure of the coping strategies questionnaire and coping strategies questionnaire-revised. J Pain. 2004;5(6):304–16.

45. Bennell KL, Nelligan R, Dobson F, Rini C, Keefe F, Kasza J, French S, Bryant C, Dalwood A, Abbott JH, et al. Effectiveness of an internet-delivered exercise and pain-coping skills training intervention for persons with chronic knee pain: a randomized trial. Ann Intern Med. 2017;166(7):453–62.

46. Keefe FJ, Caldwell DS, Baucom D, Salley A, Robinson E, Timmons K, Beaupre P, Weisberg J, Helms M. Spouse-assisted coping skills training in the management of osteoarthritic knee pain. Arthritis Care Res. 1996;9(4):279–91.

47. Keefe FJ, Caldwell DS, Queen K, Gil KM, Martinez S, Crisson JE, Ogden W, Nunley J. Osteoarthritis knee pain: a behavioral analysis. Pain. 1987;28:309–21.

48. Keefe FJ, Caldwell DS, Queen KT, Gil KM, Martinez S, Crisson JE, Ogden W, Nunley J. Pain coping strategies in osteoarthritis patients. J Consult Clin Psychol. 1987;55:208–12.

49. Parker JC, Smarr KL, Buescher KL, Phillips LR, Frank RG, Beck NC, Anderson SK, Walker SE. Pain control and rational thinking. Implications for rheumatoid arthritis. Arthritis Rheum. 1989;32(8):984–90.

50. Sullivan MJL, Bishop SR, Pivik J. The pain catastrophizing scale: development and validation. Psychol Assess. 1995;7:524–32.

51. Kroenke K, Strine TW, Spitzer RL, Williams JB, Berry JT, Mokdad AH. The PHQ-8 as a measure of current depression in the general population. J Affect Disord. 2009;114(1–3):163–73.

52. Brady TJ. Measures of self-efficacy: arthritis self-efficacy scale (ASES), arthritis self-efficacy Scale-8 item (ASES-8), Children's arthritis self-efficacy scale (CASE), chronic disease self-efficacy scale (CDSES), Parent's arthritis self-efficacy scale (PASE), and rheumatoid arthritis self-efficacy scale (RASE). Arthritis Care Res (Hoboken). 2011;63(Suppl 11):S473–85.

53. Porter LS, Keefe FJ, Wellington C, DeWilliams A. Pain communication in the context of osteoarthritis: patient and partner self-efficacy for pain communication and holding back from discussion of pain and arthritis-related outcomes. Clin J Pain. 2008;24(8):662–8.

54. Shelby RA, Somers TJ, Keefe FJ, DeVellis BM, Patterson C, Renner JB, Jordan JM. Brief fear of movement scale for osteoarthritis. Arthritis Care Res. 2012; 64(6):862–71.

55. Bennell KL, Ahamed Y, Jull G, Bryant C, Hunt MA, Forbes AB, Kasza J, Akram M, Metcalf B, Harris A, et al. Physical therapist-delivered pain coping skills training and exercise for knee osteoarthritis: randomized controlled trial. Arthritis Care Res (Hoboken). 2016;68(5):590–602.

56. Bennell KL, Ahamed Y, Bryant C, Jull G, Hunt MA, Kenardy J, Forbes A, Harris A, Nicholas M, Metcalf B, et al. A physiotherapist-delivered integrated exercise and pain coping skills training intervention for individuals with knee osteoarthritis: a randomised controlled trial protocol. BMC Musculoskelet Disord. 2012;13:129.

57. Rini C, Porter LS, Somers TJ, McKee DC, DeVellis RF, Smith M, Winkel G, Ahern DK, Goldman R, Stiller JL, et al. Automated internet-based pain coping skills training to manage osteoarthritis pain: a randomized controlled trial. Pain. 2015;156(5):837–48.

58. Broderick JE, Keefe FJ, Bruckenthal P, Junghaenel DU, Schneider S, Schwartz JE, Kaell AT, Caldwell DS, McKee D, Reed S, et al. Nurse practitioners can effectively deliver pain coping skills training to osteoarthritis patients with chronic pain: a randomized, controlled trial. Pain. 2014;155(9):1743–54.

59. Helminen EE, Sinikallio SH, Valjakka AL, Vaisanen-Rouvali RH, Arokoski JP. Effectiveness of a cognitive-behavioural group intervention for knee osteoarthritis pain: a randomized controlled trial. Clin Rehabil. 2015; 29(9):868–81.

60. Vitiello MV, McCurry SM, Shortreed SM, Balderson BH, Baker LD, Keefe FJ, Rybarczyk BD, Von Korff M. Cognitive-behavioral treatment for comorbid insomnia and osteoarthritis pain in primary care: the lifestyles randomized controlled trial. J Am Geriatr Soc. 2013;61(6):947–56.

61. Hurley MV, Walsh NE, Mitchell HL, Pimm TJ, Patel A, Williamson E, Jones RH, Dieppe P, Reeves BC. Clinical effectiveness of a rehabilitation program integrating exercise, self-management, and active coping strategies for chronic knee pain: a cluster randomized trial. Arthritis Care Res. 2007;57(7):1211–9.

62. Keefe FJ, Caldwell DS, Williams DA, Gil KM, Mitchell D, Robertson C, Martinez S, Nunley J, Beckham JC, Crisson JE, et al. Pain coping skills training in the management of osteoarthritic knee pain: a comparative study. Behav Ther. 1990;21:49–62.

63. Hanmer J, Lawrence WF, Anderson JP, Kaplan RM, Fryback DG. Report of nationally representative values for the noninstitutionalized US adult population for 7 health-related quality-of-life scores. Med Decis Mak. 2006; 26(4):391–400.

64. Porter LS, Keefe FJ, Wellington C, de Williams A. Pain communication in the context of osteoarthritis: patient and partner self-efficacy for pain communication and holding back from discussion of pain and arthritis-related concerns. Clin J Pain. 2008;24(8):662–8.

65. Dillon CF, Rasch EK, Gu Q, Hirsch R. Prevalence of knee osteoarthritis in the United States: arthritis data from the Third National Health and Nutrition Examination Survey 1991-1994. J Rheumatol. 2006;33:2271–9.

66. Jordan JM, Helmick CG, Renner JB, Luta G, Dragomir AD, Woodard J, Fang F, Schwartz TA, Abbate LM, Callahan LF, et al. Prevalence of knee symptoms and radiographic and symptomatic knee osteoarthritis in African Americans and Caucasians: the Johnston County osteoarthritis project. J Rheumatol. 2007;31(4):172–80.

67. Raley RK, Sweeney MM, Wondra D. The growing racial and ethnic divide in U.S. marriage patterns. Futur Child. 2015;25(2):89–109.

68. Cameron KL, Hsiao MS, Owens BD, Burks R, Svoboda SJ. Incidence of physician-diagnosed osteoarthritis among active duty United States military service members. Arthritis Rheum. 2011;63(10):2974–82.

69. Dedeli O, Kaptan G. Spirituality and religion in pain and pain management. Health Psychol Res. 2013;1(3):e29.

70. Cunningham TJ, Croft JB, Liu Y, Lu H, Eke PI, Giles WH. Vital signs: racial disparities in age-specific mortality among blacks or African Americans - United States, 1999-2015. MMWR Morb Mortal Wkly Rep. 2017;66(17):444–56.

71. Campbell LC, Keefe FJ, Scipio C, McKee DC, Edwards CL, Herman SH, Johnson LE, Colvin OM, McBride CM, Donatucci C. Facilitating research participation and improving quality of life for African American prostate cancer survivors and their intimate partners. A pilot study of telephone-based coping skills training. Cancer. 2007;109(2 Suppl):414–24.

13

Diagnosis and treatment of acute Essex-Lopresti injury: focus on terminology

Maurizio Fontana[1], Marco Cavallo[2*], Graziano Bettelli[2] and Roberto Rotini[2]

Abstract

Background: Acute Essex-Lopresti injury is a rare and disabling condition of longitudinal instability of the forearm. When early diagnosed, patients report better outcomes with higher functional recovery. Aim of this study is to focus on the different lesion patterns causing forearm instability, reviewing literature and the cases treated by the Authors and to propose a new terminology for their identification.

Methods: Five patients affected by acute Essex-Lopresti injury have been enrolled for this study. ELI was caused in two patients by bike fall, two cases by road traffic accident and one patient by fall while walking. A literature search was performed using Ovid Medline, Ovid Embase, Scopus and Cochrane Library and the Medical Subject Headings vocabulary. The search was limited to English language literature. 42 articles were evaluated, and finally four papers were considered for the review.

Results: All patients were operated in acute setting with radial head replacement and different combinations of interosseous membrane reconstruction and distal radio-ulnar joint stabilization. Patients were followed for a mean of 15 months: a consistent improvement of clinical results were observed, reporting a mean MEPS of 92 and a mean MMWS of 90.8. One case complained persistent wrist pain associated to DRUJ discrepancy of 3 mm and underwent ulnar shortening osteotomy nine months after surgery, with good results.

Discussion: The clinical studies present in literature reported similar results, highlighting as patients properly diagnosed and treated in acute setting report better results than patients operated after four weeks. In this study, the definitions of "Acute Engaged" and "Undetected at Imminent Evolution" Essex-Lopresti injury are proposed, in order to underline the necessity to carefully investigate the anatomical and radiological features in order to perform an early and proper surgical treatment.

Conclusions: Following the observations, the definitions of "Acute Engaged" and "Undetected at Imminent Evolution" injuries are proposed to distinguish between evident cases and more insidious settings, with necessity of carefully investigate the anatomical and radiological features in order to address patients to an early and proper surgical treatment.

Keywords: Acute Essex-Lopresti injury, Elbow, Wrist, Forearm instability

* Correspondence: marco.cavallo@ior.it
[2]Shoulder and Elbow Unit, IRCCS - Istituto Ortopedico Rizzoli, Via G.C. Pupilli 1, Bologna, Italy
Full list of author information is available at the end of the article

Background

The forearm can be considered as a single articulating unit where the close interdependence of multiple anatomical structures allows forearm rotation, elbow and wrist motion [1, 2]. All of these functions, especially pronation and supination, explain the complex integrated relationship between the bones and soft tissue along the entire length of this anatomical district. The forearm constraints are formed by the Proximal Radio-Ulnar Joint (PRUJ) mainly represented by the Radial Head (RH), the Interosseous Membrane (IOM) particularly in its central and stronger part named Central Band or Interosseous ligament (IOL) [3–5] and Distal Radio-Ulnar joint (DRUJ) represented by the Triangular Fibrocartilage Complex (TFCC) and, when present, by the Distal Oblique Band (DOB). All these anatomic and functional structures can be grouped under the name of the Forearm Unit [6]. In 1951 Peter Essex-Lopresti described the proximal migration of the radius following the surgical excision of. comminuted RH fracture [7]. This longitudinal migration of the radius can generate when a traumatic axial load is transmitted from the wrist to the elbow, causing the combination of DRUJ disruption, rupture of the IOM and RH fracture. After Essex-Lopresti detailed description, this injury pattern gained the eponym of Essex-Lopresti Injury (ELI) [8]. Like other traumatic patterns, this lesion can be classified in the group of unstable fractures of the forearm, characterized by fracture of one or both forearm bones associated with lesion of some forearm main constraints (TFCC, IOM and RH). The lack of at least two constraints can lead to two different acute patterns: a typical ELI or a hidden form, difficult to be detected but still considerably harming the patient's quality of life [9]. The development of these conditions depend from the IOM/TFCC reaction to the energy-related trauma. These lesions are often misdiagnosed in emergency room and not properly treated, leading to a Chronic ELI, a disabling condition extremely difficult to treat with positive outcomes [4, 9–15].

Aim of this work is to focus on the different lesion patterns causing forearm instability, reviewing literature and the cases treated by the Authors and to propose a new terminology for their identification.

Methods

A literature search was performed using Ovid Medline, Ovid Embase, Scopus and Cochrane Library and the Medical Subject Headings vocabulary. The following terms were combined with 'AND' and 'OR': 'essex'; 'lopresti'; 'acute'. A total of 42 articles were The search was limited to English language literature. Papers published before 2018 and clearly reporting clinical results and ELI treatment in acute setting

were considered. A total of 4 articles were finally considered for the review.

For this study all the thirty-two patients affected by ELI who came to the Authors' attention between 2010 and 2016 have been retrospectively reviewed. Adams et al. considered the acute setting within four weeks from trauma, [8] and following this indication five patients have been selected for this study. All patients were males, with mean age of 40 years. The primary injury

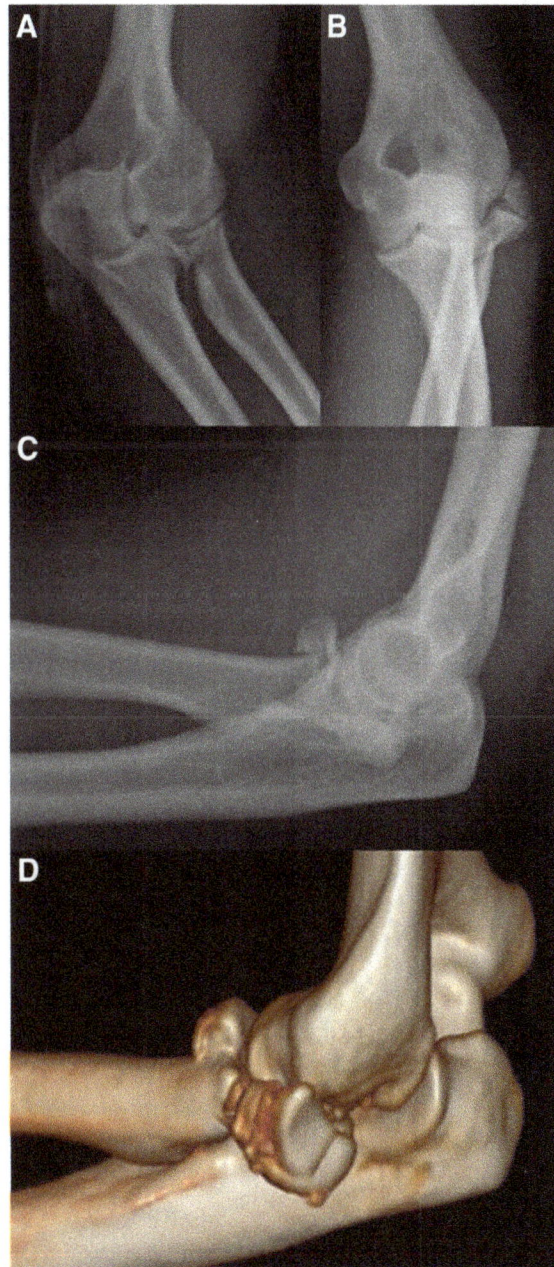

Fig. 1 Clinical case 4, Acute Engaged ELI, pre-operative: elbow. Pre-operative left elbow X-rays (**a**, **b**, **c**) and 3D reconstruction CT scan (**d**) images showing a Mason 3 radial head fracture

causing ELI was by bike fall in two patients, road traffic accident in two cases and fall while walking in one case.

Three cases presented an important proximal longitudinal dislocation of the radius, with the proximal radius engaging into the capitellum (Figs. 1, 2). In one case the RH fracture showed the involvement of radial neck (Mason grade 3) without longitudinal radial proximal dislocation, but in presence of gross instability of elbow and forearm (Fig. 3). In all the cases the lesion was caused by high energy upper limb impact trauma (bike fall, road traffic accident, and so on [16]. Patients' demographics and lesion characteristics are reported in Table 2.

The preliminary evaluation consisted in a clinical complete examination. In particular the investigation of the traumatic mechanism reported by the patient arose the suspect of high energy axial load on the forearm, with possibility of unstable fracture. The clinical examination was performed starting from the elbow stability evaluation (associated lesions of LUCL or MCL), followed by a check of the radial head (tenderness, pronation supination, Xilo Test). The IOM was checked with the "C-Fingers comparative test" [17] (Fig. 4): with this test it is possible to check the tenderness at the level of CB and DOB. In acute cases a vivid painful reaction is

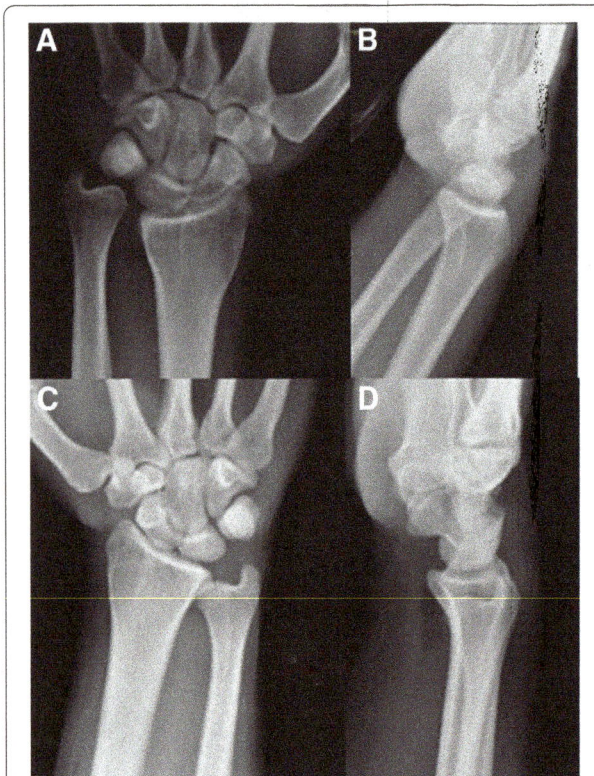

Fig. 3 Clinical case 2: Acute Undetected at Imminent Evolution ELI pattern. Pre-operative X-ray of case n. 2: it is evident the radial head fracture without evident signs of high energy trauma (**a**, **b**). The DRUJ seemed aligned ad regular X-Ray (**c**). Performing the stress test under C-arm view the forearm longitudinal instability was detected (**d**, **e**). The treatment consisted in radial head prosthesis positioning (**g**), IOM plasty and collateral ligaments reconstruction (**f**)

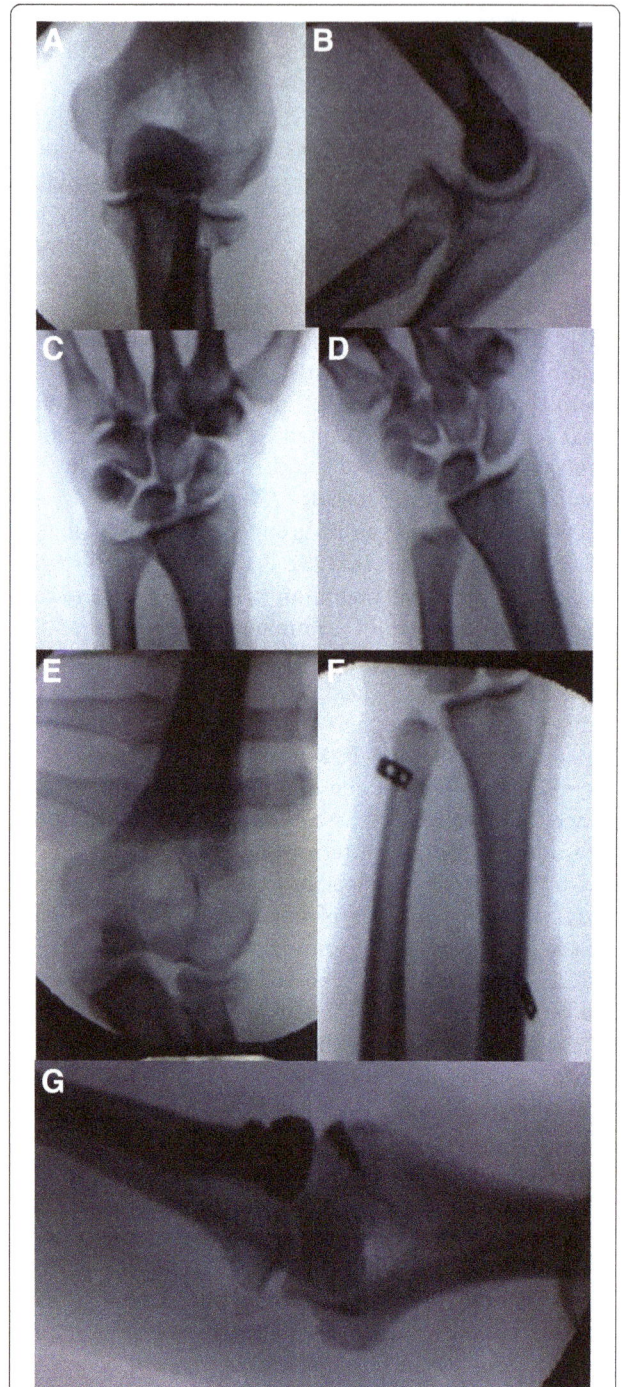

Fig. 2 Clinical case 4, pre-operative: wrist. Pre-operative X-rays of the same patient. The left wrist (**a**, **b**) highlighted a DRUJ lesion, more evident if compared to the right unaffected wrist images (**c**, **d**)

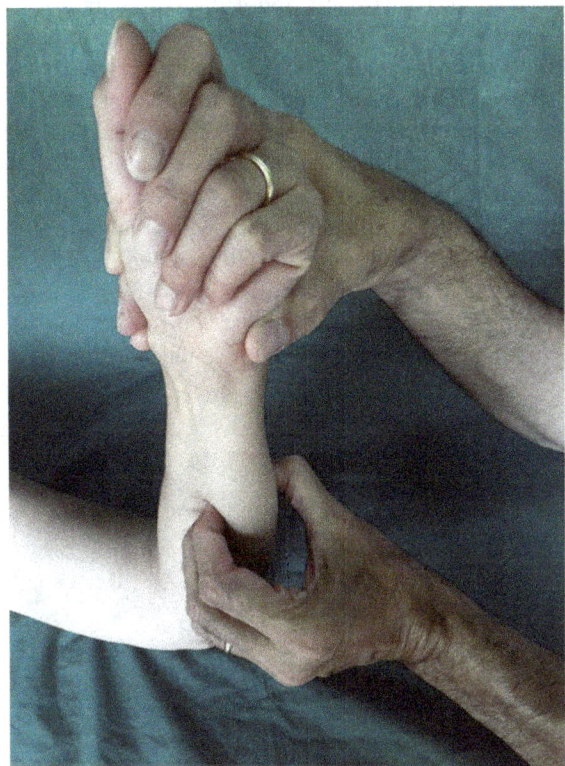

Fig. 4 C-Fingers comparative test. Clinical image of the C-Fingers comparative test: the arm lies on a table, with elbow flexed at 90° and forearm vertical to the floor plane. With the thumb opposite to other fingers (forming the shape of a "C" letter) the surgeon squeezes the forearm space and pushes alternatively in dorsal and palmar direction to feel the muscular-IOM resistance in pronation and supination; the test must be comparative and is generally hindered by muscular hypertrophy and edema

indicative of an IOM laceration. In chronic patients a reduced resistance of one or more segments compared to the counterlateral forearm is suspect for partial or complete IOM tear. The DRUJ was evaluated by the mean of the Tilt test: at the wrist the physician tests the DRUJ with dorsal and volar comparative translation of the ulna in neutral, supination and pronation. Then the potential longitudinal forearm instability was investigated with a comparative wrist X ray, with the detection of a distal radius proximal migration comparing to the counterlateral wrist. An elbow CT scan was performed in all cases to better assess the pathoanathomy of the RH fracture.

Surgery has been performed at a mean of 13 days after trauma. Before the surgical procedure the ELI was confirmed under anesthesia, performing some specific tests to better assess the elbow stability: the ultrasonographic evaluation of the so called "Muscular Hernia Sign" [18] and the axial stress test [19]. A distal radial migration of 3 mm or greater was considered indicative of longitudinal instability [20].

After the confirmation of acute presence of Essex Lopresti syndrome, the surgery was performed with a preliminar positioning of an infraclavear catheter for continuous post operative analgesia. Patients were placed in supine position with a pneumatic tourniquet at the limb's root.

The surgical repair was performed in three steps. Since ELI is a non frequent lesion, not all the three steps were performed in all cases, reflecting the progressive and recent development of knowledge in this pathology.

The first step, performed in all cases, consisted in the positioning of the radial head prosthesis. Using the Kocher interval the implanted prosthesis was unipolar in

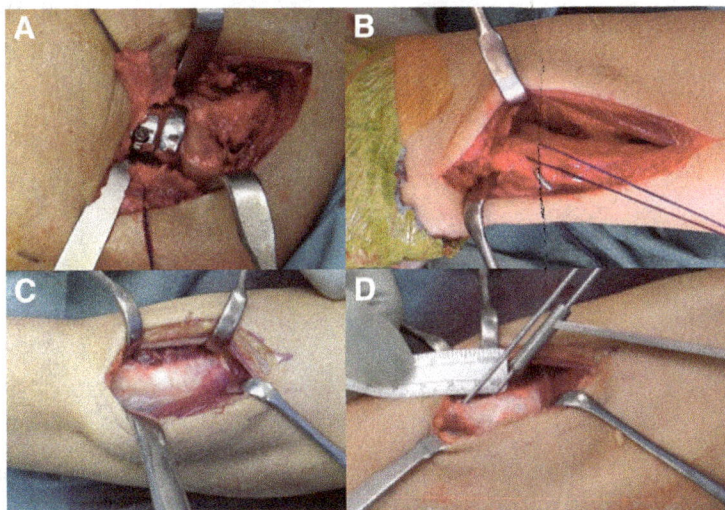

Fig. 5 Surgical images of the procedure, clinical case 3. The radial head prosthesis was firstly positioned (**a**), followed by TFCC reconstruction and DRUJ pinning (**b**). At the level of the maximum radial bow, passing between flexor and extensor muscles, the radial origin of the pronator teres was recognized and isolated (**c**). At intermediate forearm rotation two 1.5 mmm drill were performed (**d**)

three cases and bipolar in two cases, all non cemented with press fit insertion in the radial canal (Fig. 5a).

In patient n.1, only radial head replacement was performed. Patient n.2 was initially underestimated: in emergency room it was classified as isolated Mason 3 radial head fracture and addressed for surgery. It was only under anesthesia and under C-arm view that forearm longitudinal instability was detected. The muscular hernia sign was negative, Axial test positive with a stable DRUJ. The radial head prosthesis was positioned, then IOM and lateral collateral ligaments reconstruction were performed. In Patients n.3 and 4 underwent radial head replacement, TFCC reconstruction, DRUJ pinning and IOM reconstruction. Patient n.5 underwent radial head prosthesis, TFCC reconstruction and DRUJ pinning.

In cases when TFCC reconstruction and DRUJ pinning were performed a dorsal access to the DRUJ was used. The TFCC was re-inserted with a high resistance 0 wire to the ulnar stiloid process with a trans osseous stitch, and the DRUJ was then reduced and fixed by two extra articular Kirschener wires. (Fig. 5b). When a IOM reconstruction was performed (patients n.2,3 and 4) it was used a technique similar to Soubeyrand procedure

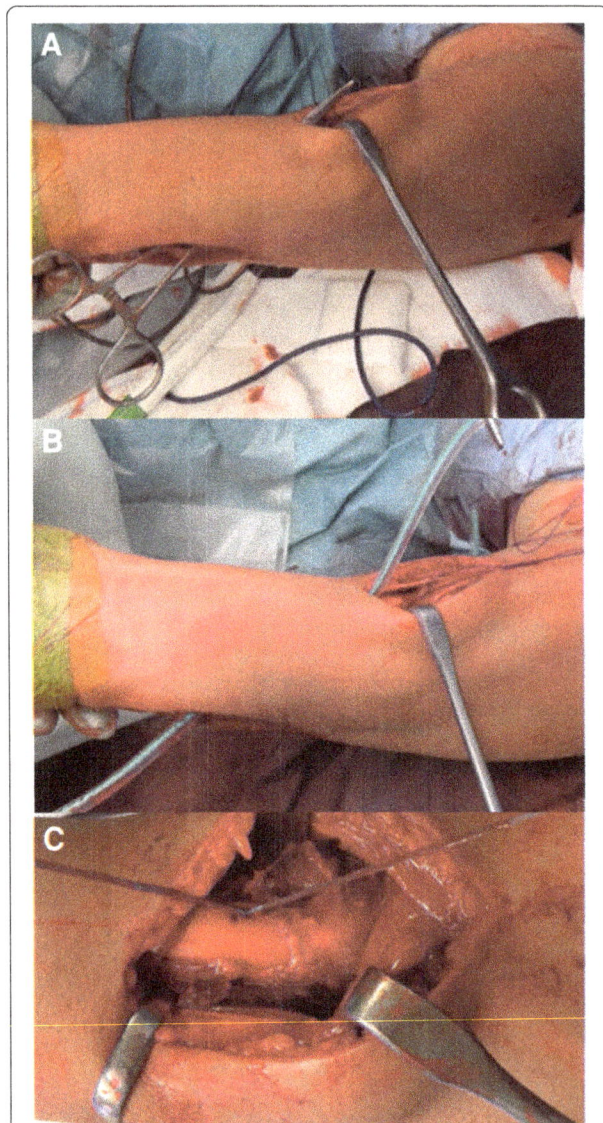

Fig. 6 Surgical images of the procedure clinical case 3. With the help of a smooth tool the path for the stabilizer device was performed, dorsally crossing the forearm bones under the muscular extensor compartment (**a**). The stabilizer device was then put in position with the help of a knee ligament passer (**b**) and finally tensioned (**c**)

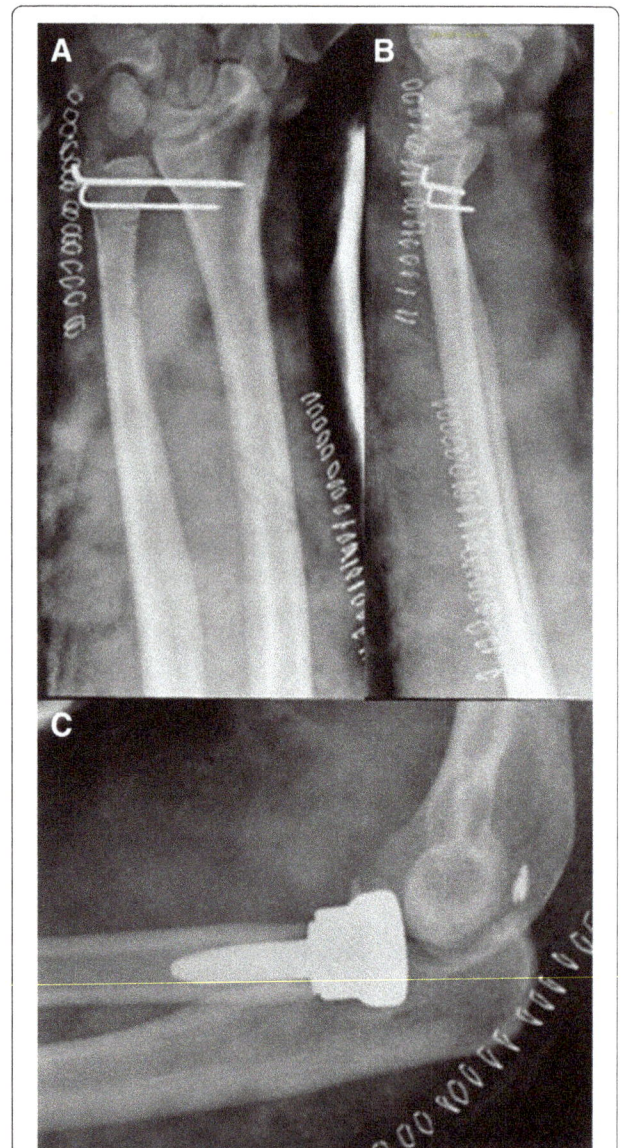

Fig. 7 Post operative X-rays, clinical case 3. Post operative X-rays show the reduced and stabilized DRUJ (**a**, **b**) and the radial head prosthesis (**c**). It is possible to see the radial and ulnar tunnels of the two bundles of the newly reconstructed IOM (**a**)

Table 1 Studies in literature reporting cases of acute Essex-Lopresti injuries

Author	N. of patients operated within 4 weeks	mean follow up, months	MEPS at follow up	MMWS at follow up	mean DRUJ at final FU	Described results
Grassmann et al. [24]	12	59	86.7	88.4	not reported	
Trousdale et al. [15]	5	54	91	80	+ 2.5 mm ulna	
Edwards and Jupiter [10]	5	18	not reported	not reported	+ 2 mm ulna	3 excellent, 1 good, 1 poor
Schnetzke et al. [14]	16	63.6	91.3	81.3	+ 2 mm ulna	

[21] (Figs. 5, 6, 7): at the level of the maximum radial bow and at the opposite part of inner ridge detected under C-arm, a five centimetres incision was performed. Passing between flexor and extensor muscles, the radial origin of the pronator teres was recognized. Keeping the forearm in neutral pronation and supination position, two 1.5 mm drill holes were performed. Other two 1.5 mm drill holes were performed at the level of the distal ulnar neck, with a 20 degrees axis respect to longitudinal forearm axis. As stabilizer device a cadaveric tendon allograft was used in one case (n.4) and a synthetic band (Ultratape, Smith & Nephew,UK) in two cases (patient n.2 and 3). The stabilizer device was then passed, dorsally crossing the forearm bones under the muscular extensor compartment, with the help of a plastic knee ligament passer. Under C-arm view the device was then stretched; pronation supination and radial head pistoning were checked and definitively fixed. Due to LUCL laceration observed, all patients underwent a final LUCL proximal reinsertion and in one case a MCL was proximally reinserted with metallic anchors.

All the patients underwent a post operative cast immobilization for 48 h, followed by progressive passive and active elbow and wrist mobilization. Progressive muscular reinforcement protocol was permitted starting one month after surgery. The DRUJ K wires were surgically removed after 40 days.

All patients of this study have been clinically evaluated at a mean of 17 months of follow up using the Mayo Elbow Performance Score [22] and the Modified Mayo Wrist Score [23]. An X ray investigation has been performed in all cases at final follow up.

Results

Only few reports are present in literature about acute ELI (Table 1): Grassmann et al. [24] identified 12 acute ELI in a group of 295 patients affected by RH fracture. An evident radio-ulnar X-ray discrepancy was found in only five patients, and a partial or complete IOM rupture was diagnosed by MRI in all 12 cases. The authors reported good mid-term results. Trousdale [15] reported a case series of 20 ELI, identifying 5 cases of acute forms: these cases, properly treated, reported good outcome in 4 cases, while the other 15, initially misdiagnosed and treated with RH resection, developed severe pain at distal DRUJ, with good results even after treatment only in 3 cases. In 1987 Edwards and Jupiter [10] reported on 7 patients, 4 operated within one month, with excellent results obtained only in the three cases. The only poor result was experienced by the patient who underwent a RH excision. Duckworth [25] retrospectively reviewed 60 patients affected by RH fracture, identifying 22 patients with radio-ulnar discrepancy. The good short term results (6 months) even after conservative management are to be considered non indicative, since usually patients experience a later worsening and no indication is reported about IOM assessment. The most representative case series have been reported by

Table 2 Patients' demographics and lesion characteristics

Patient n.	Name	age	sex	Injury type	Mason grade	DRUJ discrepancy mm	M hernia sign	Axial test	Essex-Lopresti Injury Type
1	PA	41	M	road traffic accident	3	3	+	+	Acute engaged
2	RM	46	M	bike fall	3	0	−	+	Undetected at Imminent Evolution
3	FDR	33	M	fall while walking	3	7	+	+	Acute engaged
4	CM	42	M	road traffic accident	4	9	+	+	Acute engaged
5	GS	40	M	bike fall	4	6	+	+	Acute engaged

Table 3 Patients intra operative and clinical data set

Patient n.	RH prosthesis	IOM plasty	IOM plasty material	TFCC reinsertion	Reoperation	Final Follow Up time	MEPS at follow up	MMWS	DRUJ at final FU
1	yes	no		no	Ulnar shortening at 9 months	16	83	88	+ 2 mm ulna
2	yes	yes	Ultratape	no	no	15	95	95	+ 0 mm
3	yes	yes	Ultratape	yes	no	15	92	94	+3 mm ulna
4	yes	yes	Allograft	yes	no	25	100	85	+ 2 mm ulna
5	yes	no		yes	no	14	90	92	+ 0 mm

Schnetzke in 2017 [14]: outcome of 16 acute and 15 late ELI were compared. Acute ELI, treated with DRUJ pinning and no IOM reconstruction) showed better clinical and radiological results, with lower rate of reoperations. The authors highlighted how seven patients had a proximalization of more than 2 mm at final follow up, associated with worst outcome: the authors conclude that this observation supports the idea that IOM is not able to heal, and once disrupted the muscle herniation through the laceration prevent its healing [24, 26].

Case n.1 during the post operative rehabilitation protocol complained the onset of persistent wrist pain associated to DRUJ discrepancy of 3 mm (MEPS score 72, MMWS 75), which led to ulnar shortening osteotomy 9 months after the first surgery, with good results at final follow up (MEPS 83, MMWS 88) (as reported in Table 3).

The complete data set is reported in Tables 2 and 3.

Discussion

In 2007 Marc Soubeyrand proposed the "Three Forearm Constraints" concept [27]. The Forearm Unit has to be considered like an association of three main constraints: the PRUJ, the IOM and the DRUJ. Each constraint is essential for stability and movements of the forearm. In case of single constraint damage (distal radius fracture, simple RH fracture, and so on) a pronation-supination decrease occurs, without causing instability (Stage 1). In case of two constraints damage (Stage 2) a partial transversal instability may occur (Criss-Cross lesion, Galeazzi lesion, Monteggia lesions). The disruption of three constraints (Stage 3) causes a longitudinal-transversal instability (Acute). Stage 2 and 3 patterns present an intrinsic instability, and may be grouped under the "Unstable Fractures of the Forearm" definition. In this different conditions, the lack of at least two of the three constraints (TFCC, IOM and RH) can lead to two different patterns. The first is an acute and evident longitudinal instability of the forearm, defined by the authors "Acute Engaged Essex-Lopresti Injury". The second has already been identified by different Authors [7, 9, 10, 15] but still not pointed as specific clinical entity: it shows a more obscure clinical pattern, easy to misdiagnose but still causing instability, defined by Authors "Undetected at Imminent Evolution Acute Essex-Lopresti Injury", observed

also in the two patients reported by Helmerhorst et al. [28]. Usually a correct diagnose is performed in chronic setting, when the symptoms of a longitudinal instability became evident but unfortunately with poor outcome [14]. The clinic extrinsication of one of these two conditions depends

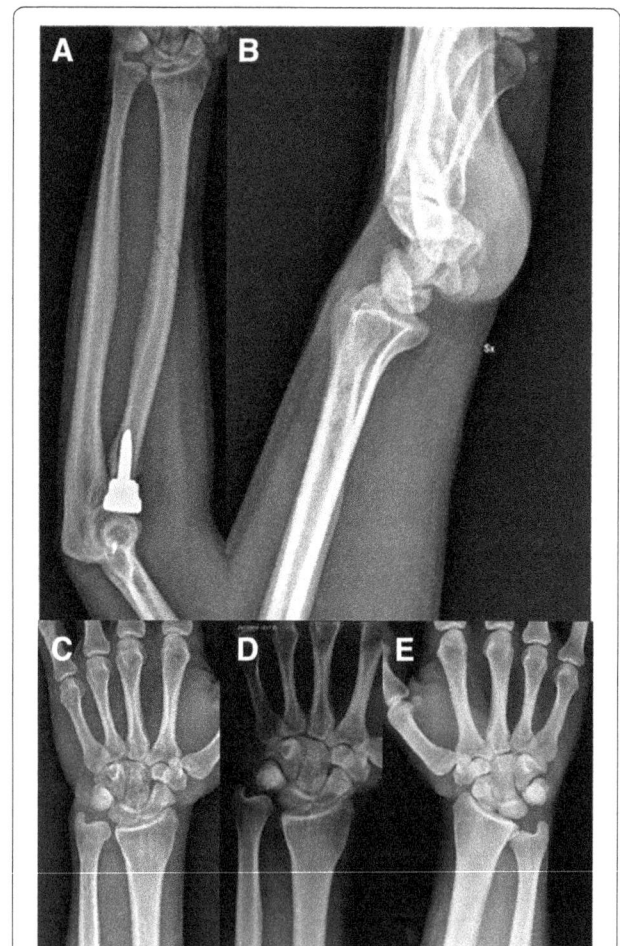

Fig. 8 1 year X-rays, clinical case 3. Follow up X-rays at 1 year of follow up, showing the radial head prosthesis in situ and the whole forearm (**a**). The lateral view shows no dorsal dislocation of the distal ulna (**b**). At the DRUJ a slight recurrence of the ulnar plus is evident (**c**), even if non symptomatic. Nevertheless the improvement preoperative wrist x-ray (**d**) is evident. **e** Image shows the opposite side normal wrist

on the IOM answer to the trauma. In the first case, an immediate proximal translation greater than 5 mm associated with impacted RH fracture into Capitulum Humeri is significative for acute high-henergy complete irreparable IOM and TFCC laceration. Aim of this work was to examine the different lesion patterns that may cause forearm instability, focusing on cases treated by the authors and the few literature reports, in order to better define the different entities.

Among the cases enrolled for this paper, the Authors observed four cases presenting characteristics of Acute Engaged ELI. Unfortunately not all patients received the same treatment: due to the rarity of this condition the knowledge development on anatomopathology and treatment is still ongoing, so it is only in the recent years that it has been properly understood, diagnosed and treated. It is very important to pinpoint how most of the authors indicate that this lesion seems to occur more often than realized up to now, reporting values of around 38% of correct diagnoses performed in excellence centers [8]. Similarly to other series reported in literature, the cases treated with RH implant, IOM reconstruction and TFCC fixation and pinning reported higher scores and better functional outcomes, whereas the patient who underwent the isolated radial head replacement reported worst outcomes, requiring a

shortening ulnar osteotomy to treat the persistent wrist pain. It was noticeable that in this case after the RH replacement a proximal radial migration was barely evident with a DRUJ discrepancy of 3 mm, and the treatment seemed to be sufficient with the experience maturated at that time. A possible explanation is due to a partial IOM/TFCC tear caused by the high-energy trauma, that became complete after repetitive tractions by Biceps Brachii. This condition progressively evolves into a proximal radial migration causing DRUJ instability-discomfort and grip weakness.

These observations lead to the confirmation that there is an elevated possibility to misdiagnose these non evident acute Essex-Lopresti, that in a first step may be considered and treated as simple RH fracture but shortly express the typical symptoms of a forearm instability. Basing on several observation of similar cases, in 2006 in fact Junghbluth et al. introduced the term "missed" Essex-Lopresti [12], characterized by a painful but correctly positioned radial head prosthesis in a context of longitudinal instability of the forearm due to IOM laceration. Patient n.3 (Figs. 2, 5, 6, 7, 8, 9) experienced a progressive worsening of DRUJ discrepancy at follow up compared to post operative control: this may be explained with a slight tension loosening of the IOM and

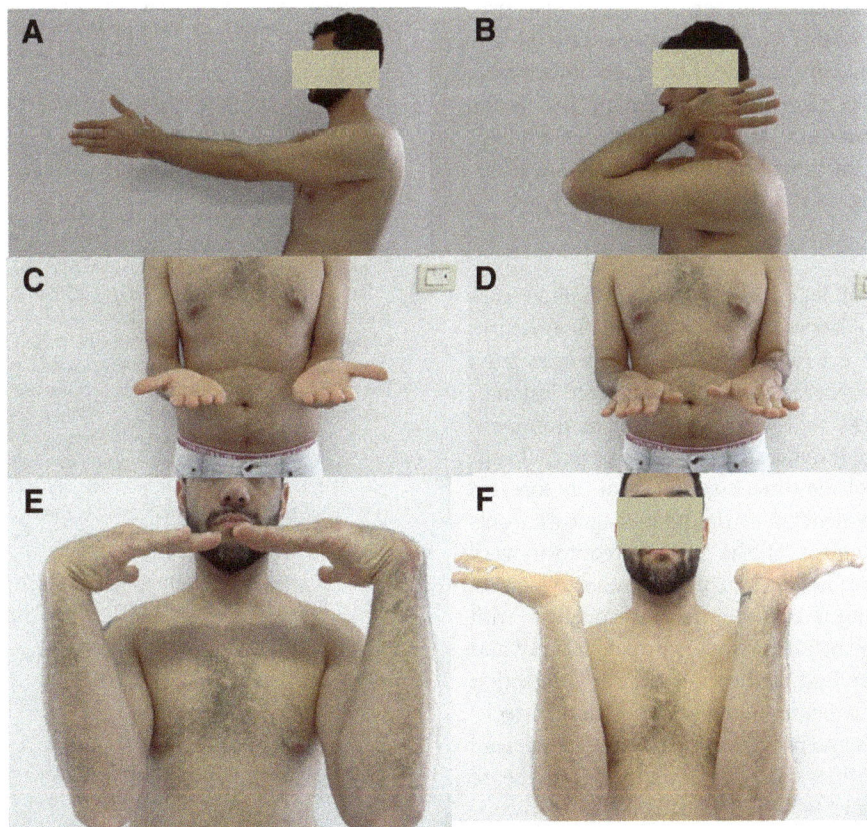

Fig. 9 Clinical follow up, clinical case 3. Follow up clinical aspect at 1 year of follow up, showing a good movement of the elbow (a-d) and the wrist (e, f)

DRUJ reconstruction. At the final follow up this condition was non-symptomatic, supporting the idea that if left untreated the clinical results were prone to deteriorate even more at follow up, as observed in case n.1. These results are consistent with the few reports available in literature (Table 1), with comparable values of MEPS, MMWS and DRUJ discrepancy at follow up. The higher clinical results have been obtained in cases when the IOM have been reconstructed, highlighting the importance of this anatomical structure.

For these reasons it is mandatory to perform an accurate clinical examination to the patient in acute setting, tagging these cases as Undetected at Imminent Evolution ELI and addressing them to a proper and complete treatment. The diagnosis of the acute engaged pattern of ELI is easier to recognize. On the other side, a radial translation inferior to 5 mm associated with Mason 3 radial head fracture, forearm or wrist painful and positive radiological Axial Test is to be considered indicative for an acute IOM laceration, even if not as evident as the acute engaged pattern presentation. Therefore, the diagnosis of Acute Undetected at imminent evolution ELI is difficult, because a proximal radial translation inferior to 3 mm does not lead to an immediate longitudinal instability [29]. Imaging does not give an effective contribution, so the clinical investigation part and the physical examination are fundamental for the correct diagnosis. The main limitation of this study is represented by the low number of cases, mainly because ELI is an uncommon condition. This led to a consequent limitation, that is the different surgical procedure performed and the different approach to ELI. At the same time this reflects the development in the knowledge of this disease over the last years.

Conclusions

From the analysis of literature and the presented case series, ELI can be considered part of the unstable fractures of the forearm, where a radial head fracture is associated to one or more ligament lesions. This is an acute lesion in all cases, that may be evident (Engaged) or at imminent evolution (Undetected) due of the complete or partial rupture of at least two of the three constraints of the forearm unit. The scarce frequency and the poor diagnostic tools make the early diagnosis of the Undetected form very challenging. The comprehension of the lesion dynamics, the accurate anamnesis and clinical investigation with proper tests and the help of a well-conducted X-ray and CT examination may lead to these lesions early detection and treatment with a better outcome. The surgical technique has to follow some progressive steps: the radial head has to be replaced first, then the stability has to be re tested and in case of instability the DRUJ has to be reconstructed along with fixation of the TFCC. The final step should be the IOM reconstruction to give the proper tension to the construct.

Abbreviations
DOB: Distal Oblique Band; DRUJ: Distal Radio-Ulnar joint; ELI: Essex-Lopresti Injury; IOL: Interosseous ligament; IOM: Interosseous Membrane; PRUJ: Proximal Radio-Ulnar Joint; RH: Radial Head; TFCC: Triangular Fibrocartilage Complex

Authors' contributions
MF and RR performed the surgeries, performed the pre operative and post operative clinical examination of the patients and analyzed and interpreted the patient data regarding the forearm instability. MC and GB performed the literature review, collected images, functional scores and were the major contributors in writing the manuscript. All authors read and approved the final manuscript.

Competing interests
The authors declare that they have no competing interests.

Author details
[1]Orthopaedic Department, Infermi Hospital, Viale Stradone 9, 48018 Faenza, Italy. [2]Shoulder and Elbow Unit, IRCCS - Istituto Ortopedico Rizzoli, Via G.C. Pupilli 1, Bologna, Italy.

References
1. Schemitsch EH, Richards R. The effect of malunion on functional outcome after plate fixation of fractures of both bones of the forearm in adults. J Bone Joint Surg Am. 1992;74:1068–78.
2. Stewart RL. Forearm Fractures. in Stannard JP ed, Surgical Treatment of Orthopaedic Trauma. PJ Kregor Ed. Thieme Stuttgard, 2007.
3. Hausmann JT, Vekszler G, Breitenseher M, et al. Mason type-I radial head fractures and interosseous membrane lesions: a prospective study. J Trauma. 2009;66:457–61.
4. Hotchkiss RN. Injuries to the interosseous ligament of the forearm. Hand Clin. 1994;10:391–8.
5. Skahen JR 3rd, Palmer AK, Werner FW, Fortino MD. Reconstruction of the interosseous membrane of the forearm in cadavers. J Hand Surg Am. 1997;22(6):986–94.
6. Adams JE. Forearm instability: anatomy, biomechanics, and treatment options. J Hand Surg Am. 2017;42(1):47–52.
7. Essex Lopresti P. Fractures of the radial head with distal radio–ulnar dislocation: report of two cases. JBJS Br. 1951;33B(2):244–7.
8. Adams JE, Culp RW, Osterman AL. Interosseous membrane reconstruction for the Essex-Lopresti injury. J Hand Surg Am. 2010;35(1):129–36.
9. Green JB, Zelouf DS. Forearm instability. J Hand Surg Am. 2009;34(5):953–61.
10. Edwards GS Jr, Jupiter JB. Radial head fractures with acute distal radioulnar dislocation. Essex-Lopresti revisited. Clin Orthop Relat Res. 1988;234:61–9.
11. Heijink A, Morrey BF, van Riet RP, et al. Delayed treatment of elbow pain and dysfunction following Essex-Lopresti injury with metallic radial head replacement: a case series. J Shoulder Elb Surg. 2010;19:929–36.
12. Jungbluth P, Frangen TM, Arens S, Muhr G, Kälicke T. The undiagnosed Essex-Lopresti injury. J Bone Joint Surg [Br]. 2006;88-B:1629–33.
13. Ruch DS, Chang DS, Koman LA. Reconstruction of longitudinal stability of the forearm after disruption of interosseous ligament and radial head excision (Essex-Lopresti lesion). J South Orthop Assoc. 1999;8(1):47–52.
14. Schnetzke M, Porschke F, Hoppe K, Studier-Fischer S, Gruetzner PA, Guehring T. Outcome of Early and Late Diagnosed Essex-Lopresti Injury. J Bone Joint Surg Am. 2017; 21;99(12):1043–1050.
15. Trousdale RT, Amadio PC, Cooney WP, Morrey BF. Radio-ulnar dissociation. A review of twenty cases. J Bone Joint Surg Am. 1992;74(10):1486–97.
16. Mackey DC, Lui LY, Cawthon PM et al. High-trauma fractures and low bone mineral density in older women and men. JAMA. 2007; 28;298(20):2381–8.
17. Fontana M. Longitudinal Instability of the forearm. In The Elbow, Porcellini G et al. editors, in press.
18. Soubeyrand M, Lafont C, Oberlin C, France W, Maulat I, Degeorges R. The "muscular hernia sign": an original ultrasonographic sign to detect lesion of the forearm's interosseous membrane. SurgRadiolAnat. 2006;28(3):372 8.

19. Davidson PA, Moseley JB, Tullos HS. Radial head fracture. A potentially complex injury. Clin Orthop. 1993;297:224–30.

20. Smith AM, Urbanosky LR, Castle JA, Rushing JT, Ruch DS. Radius pull test: predictor of longitudinal forearm instability. J Bone Joint Surg Am. 2002;84-A(11):1970–6.

21. Soubeyrand M, Oberlin C, Dumontier C, Belkheyar Z, Lafont C, Degeorges R. Ligamentoplasty of the forearm interosseous membrane using the senitindinosus tendon: anatomical study and surgical procedure. Surg Radiol Anat. 2006;28(3):300–7.

22. Broberg MA, Morrey BF. Results of treatment of fracture dislocations of the elbow. Clin Orthop Relat Res. 1987;216:109–19.

23. Cooney WP, Bussey R, Dobyns JH, Linscheid RL. Difficult wrist fractures. Perilunate fracture-dislocations of the wrist. Clin Orthop Relat Res. 1987;214:136–47.

24. Grassmann JP, Hakimi M, Gehrmann SV, et al. The treatment of the acute Essex-Lopresti injury. Bone Joint J. 2014;96-B(10):1385–91.

25. Duckworth AD, Watson BS, Will EM, Petrisor BA, Walmsley PJ, Court-Brown CM, McQueen MM. Radial shortening following a fracture of the proximal radius. Acta Orthop. 2011;82(3):356–9.

26. Loeffler BJ, Green JB, Zelouf DS. Forearm instability. J Hand Surg Am. 2014; 39(1):156–67.

27. Soubeyrand M, Lafont C, De George R, Dumontier C. Pathologie traumatique de la membrane interosseuse de l'avantbras Chir de la Main 2007; 26 : 255–277.

28. Helmerhorst GT, Ring D. Subtle Essex-Lopresti lesions: report of 2 cases. J Hand Surg Am. 2009;34(3):436–8.

29. Wegmann K, Dargel J, Burkhart KJ, Brüggemann GP, Müller LP. The Essex-Lopresti lesion. Strategies Trauma Limb Reconstr. 2012;7(3):131–9.

14

Objective quantification of ligament balancing using VERASENSE in measured resection and modified gap balance total knee arthroplasty

Kyu-Jin Cho[1], Jong-Keun Seon[1], Won-Young Jang[1], Chun-Gon Park[1] and Eun-Kyoo Song[1,2*]

Abstract

Background: Soft tissue balancing which is above all most important factor of total knee arthroplasty, has been performed by subjective methods. Recently objective orthosensor has been developed for compartment pressure measurement. The purpose of this study was: (1) to quantify the compartment pressure of the joint throughout the range of motion during TKA using orthosensor, (2) to determine the usefulness of orthosensor by analyzing correlation between the pressure in both compartment with initial trial and after final implantation, and (3) to evaluate the types and effectiveness of additional ligament balancing procedures to compartment pressure.

Methods: Eighty-four patients underwent total knee arthroplasty (TKA) using VERASENSE Knee System. TKA was performed by measured resection and modified gap balance technique. Compartment pressure was recorded on full extension, 30°, 60°, 90° and full flexion at initial (INI), after each additional procedure, and after final (FIN) implantation. "Balanced" knees were defined as when the compartment pressure difference was less than 15 pounds.

Results: Thirty patients (35.7%) showed balanced knee initially and 79 patients (94.0%) showed balance after final implantation. The proportion of balanced knee after initial bony resection, modified gap balancing TKAs showed significantly higher proportion than measured resection TKAs ($P = 0.004$) On both compartment, the pressure was generally decreased throughout the range of motion. Linear correlation on both compartment showed statistically significant throughout the range on motion, with higher correlation value on the lateral compartment. Total 66 additional ligament balancing procedures were performed.

Conclusion: Using orthosensor, we could obtain 94% quantified balance knee, consequently. And between the techniques, measured resection TKA showed less balanced knee and also required more additional procedures compared to modified gap balancing TKA. Furthermore, with the acquired quantified data during appropriate ligament balancing, the surgeon could eventually reduce the complications associated with soft tissue imbalance in the future.

Keywords: Total knee arthroplasty, Orthosensor, Measured-resection, Gap-balance, Ligament balancing

* Correspondence: eksong@chonnam.ac.kr
[1]Center for Joint Disease, Chonnam National University Hwasun Hospital, 160, Ilsim-Ri, Hwasun-Eup, Hwasun-Gun, Jeonnam 519-809, South Korea
[2]Department of Orthopaedic Surgery, Chonnam National University Hwasun Hospital, 160 Ilsim-Ri, Hwasun-gun, Jeonnam 519-809, South Korea

Background

A successful outcome in total knee arthroplasty depends on various surgical factors including precise bone resection, correct alignment of the components, femoral and tibial rotation, and above all adequate soft tissue balancing [1–3]. Technological advances over the past few years have facilitated accurate alignment and rotation in the surgical field via three-dimensionally guided bone resection such as navigation or ROBODOC systems [4, 5]. However, adequate soft tissue balancing still remains a challenge for many surgeons, especially younger surgeons who lack surgical experience. Further, experienced surgeons traditionally obtain soft tissue balance using their own subjective "feeling" rather than a scientific perspective [6–9]. The soft tissue balancing "feeling" is affected by factors such as surgical experience, patient's BMI, gender, generalized laxity, degree of joint contracture and even the surgeon's daily condition [10, 11].

Despite the excellent long-term clinical results of TKA, with reported survival greater than 95% at 15 years [12, 13], a few patients experience failure. Many factors contributing to dysfunction and pain have been reported [14]. Especially, revision arthroplasty due to instability has been estimated in more than 20% each year, which may be due to inappropriate ligament balancing [15]. Soft tissue balancing of the knee during total knee arthroplasty is a significant factor for postoperative patient satisfaction and implant longevity [16]. Unfortunately, until recently, soft tissue balancing, which can lead to catastrophic failure of the implant, has been determined only by surgeon's judgement with subjective feeling.

Combining the need for objective soft tissue balancing and advanced technology, VERASENSE Knee System (OrthoSensor Inc., Dania Beach, FL) has been introduced, recently. VERASENSE is an orthosensor that enables surgeons to quantify ligament balance based on real-time, evidence-based data during primary and revision TKA (Fig. 1). This disposable device delivers wireless data to an intra-operative monitor to facilitate informed decision-making regarding implant position and soft-tissue releases to improve balance and stability through a full range of motion.

The purpose of this study was: (1) to quantify the compartment pressure of the joint throughout the range of motion during TKA using orthosensor, (2) to determine the usefulness of orthosensor by analyzing correlation between the pressure in both compartment with initial trial and after final implantation, and (3) to evaluate the types and effectiveness of additional ligament balancing procedures to compartment pressure.

Methods

Patient demographic data

Between July 2017 and March 2018, 84 patients (84 knees) who showed varus deformed osteoarthritic knees underwent unilateral posterior cruciate ligament-retaining (CR) or -sacrificing (PS) primary total knee arthroplasty using VERASENSE Knee System (OrthoSensor Inc., Dania Beach, FL) in our hospital. The surgical procedure was approved by our institutional review board (IRB) of Chonnam National University Hwasun Hospital, and written informed consent was obtained from all patients. All patients were implanted with the same total knee system (NexGen™, Zimmer, Inc., Warsaw, IN, USA). Bone resection was performed by either measured resection technique using ROBODOC® system or modified gap balancing technique. Among 84 knees, measured resection

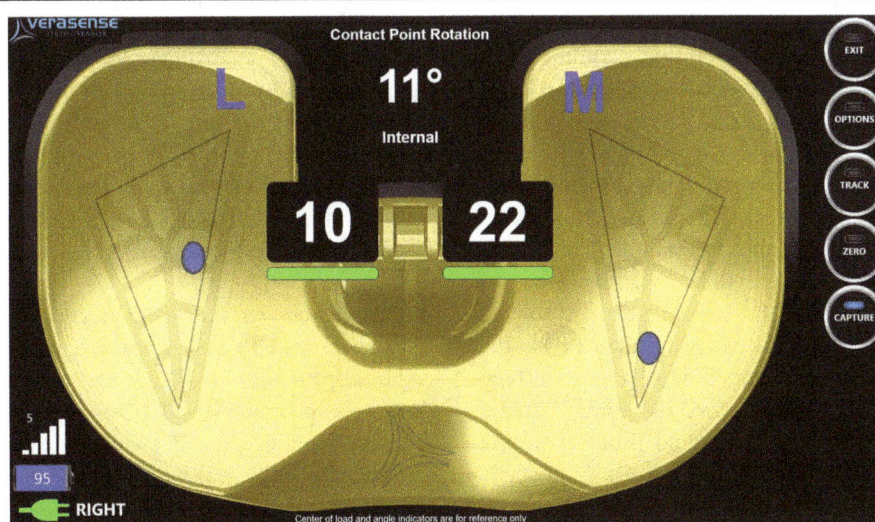

Fig. 1 Quantification of medial and lateral compartment pressure using VERASENSE

TKA was performed in 34 patients (17 CR implants and 17 PS implants) and modified gap balancing TKA was performed in 50 patients (all PS implants). Patients were consisted of 11 men and 73 women ranging in age from 51 to 83 years (mean age: 69.6 years old) at the time of surgery. There were 46 left knees and 38 right knees. The mean mechanical axis was 10.5° varus (range 0.5 to 26.7°). The CR implant was used in 17 patients with mean 9.2° varus deformity (range 0.7 to 19.5°) and the PS implant was used in 67 patients with mean 10.8° varus deformity (range 0.5 to 26.7°). Patients younger than 50 years, those who underwent revision TKA, or previous ligamentous reconstruction, osteotomy, or any other procedures, were excluded from the study.

Preoperatively, all patients underwent standard antero-posterior, lateral radiographic examination, Merchant & Lauren's view, Rosenberg view and standing extremity tele-oroentgenography for evaluation of mechanical alignment. Further, we obtained the preoperative valgus and varus stress views to evaluate the ligament laxity of the knee pre-operatively, and helical computed tomography (CT) to pre-pare ROBODOC® planning for measured resection TKA. All the surgical procedures were carried out by a senior au-thor (EKS) using either ROBODOC® (Curexo Technology Corp, Fremont, CA, USA)-assisted TKA or conventional TKA using modified gap balancing technique.

Surgical procedure and VERASENSE application
Bone resection (measure resection and modified gap balance technique)
All knees were exposed with a standard midline incision with medial parapatellar arthrotomy, and the patella was everted laterally. In ROBODOC®-assisted TKA, the pa-tient's leg was rigidly connected to the robot and bony landmarks of both femur and tibia were registered using a probe. After the registration was successfully accom-plished, bone resection was automatically conducted by ROBODOC® according to preoperative planning using ORTHODOC system with measured resection tech-nique. In the coronal plane, distal femur and proximal tibia cutting were used to cut perpendicular to the mechanical axis, with 7° of posterior slope to the mech-anical axis of the tibia in the sagittal plane. Femoral rota-tional alignment was planned perpendicular to the trans-epicondylar axis and the tibial rotational axis was planned parallel to that of the femur [17]. In conven-tional TKA, after exposing the knee joint, bone resection was performed by tibia first modified gap balance tech-nique. Tibial preparation was carried out using extrame-dullary cutting guide with proximal tibial resection perpendicular to the mechanical axis with 7° posterior slope. Tibial component rotation was aligned to the line connecting the posterior cruciate ligament insertion site and the medial edge to medial 1/3 of the tibial

tuberosity. Distal femoral preparation was carried out by intramedullary rod guide with 5° of valgus, and femoral rotation was determined according to the balanced flexion gap [18].

Intraoperative compartment pressure evaluation using VERASENSE
The VERASENSE Knee System (OrthoSensor Inc., Dania Beach, FL) is a wireless and disposable articular loading quantification device, which is inserted in the tibial com-ponent tray during the surgery. The sensor allows quan-tification of the intraoperative real-time loading data in both medial and lateral compartments of the knee via the full range of movement (Fig. 2).

Once the bony resection was carried out either with the ROBODOC®-assisted measured resection or modi-fied gap balance technique, initially femoral and tibial trial components were implanted and the VERASENSE sensor was inserted into the tibial component tray for initial (INI) quantitative assessment of compartment pressure. After reducing the patella and closing the cap-sule with one or two towel clips, a gentle range of mo-tion was performed by the surgeon. The surgeon held the leg in a neutral position and monitored the medial and lateral loading forces from full extension to full flexion. In order to observe additional details, we divided the range of motion into 5 categories and recorded com-partment pressure in: full extension, 30°, 60°, 90° and full flexion. Less than differential loading of 15 pounds be-tween the medial and lateral compartments, was consid-ered as adequately "balanced" according to previous studies [19]. After initial ligament balance assessment, if the joint showed imbalance (loading difference > 15 pounds), additional soft tissue releases (s) or bony resec-tion were performed and recorded. After each additional ligament balancing procedure, the VERASENSE was inserted in the tibial tray and compartment pressure was re-measured. The orthosensor was routinely re-zeroed before the insertion to minimize the error due to plastic deformation of the sensor. Resultingly, the compartment pressures were recorded initially right after the bone re-section (INI), after each additional procedure, and after the final implantation of the real femoral and tibial com-ponents with the bone cement (FIN).

Additional ligament balancing procedures
In "unbalanced" knees, various ligament balancing pro-cedures were performed. For soft tissue balancing proce-dures, we generally used "pie-crusting" (PC) technique with an 18-guage needle while releasing the ligaments [20]. Medial collateral ligament (MCL) release using the PC technique was most frequently used in soft tissue re-leases, followed by sub-periosteal superficial MCL re-lease using a narrow curved chisel, lateral collateral

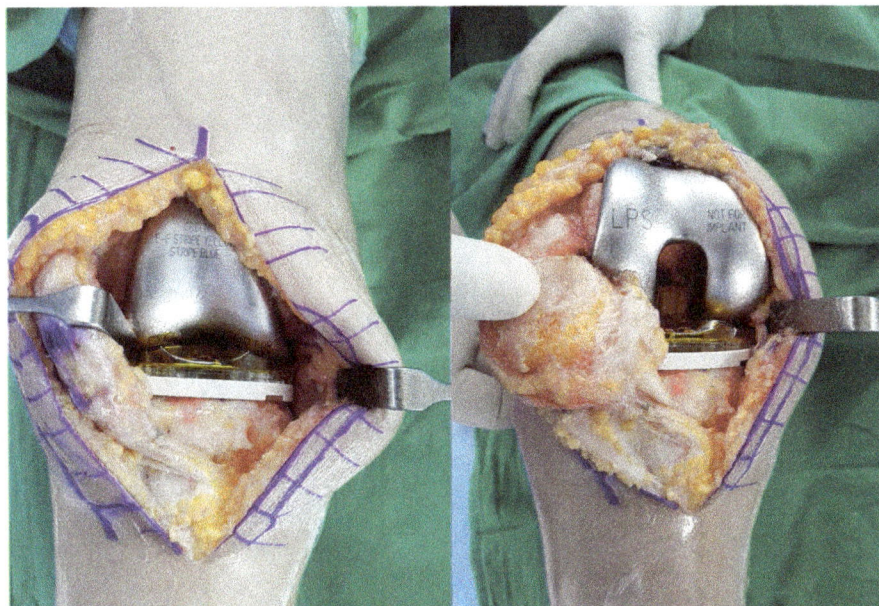

Fig. 2 VERASENSE inserted in the tibial tray in extension and flexion

ligament (LCL) release using PC technique, and iliotibial band (ITB) release. When the joint was too tight to balance by soft-tissue release alone or in valgus-aligned knee after the initial procedure, additional bony resection was performed. Varus or additional proximal tibial recut was mostly performed followed by varus or additional distal femur recut, additional osteophyte removal on medial compartment and posterior tibial slope resection.

Postoperative radiologic evaluation

For radiologic evaluation, standard anteroposterior, lateral and standing extremity teleoreontgenography were used to evaluate the postoperative alignment. Mechanical axis, femorotibial angle (FTA), and posterior slope of the tibia (PTS) were measured from the postoperative radiograph. Also to evaluate the adequate positioning of the implants, coronal and sagittal inclination of femoral and tibial components (α, β, γ, δ) were measured using anteroposterior and lateral radiographs. To determine the intra-observer variation, the radiographic measurement was repeated by the author (observer A) after 1 week. To determine the inter-observer variation, the measurements were performed by 3 experts: the author (observer A), another knee orthopedic surgeon (observer B), and a radiologist (observer C).

Statistical analysis

Means, standard deviations and frequencies were calculated, and paired t-tests were used to evaluate the continuous variables and chi-square test was used for categorical variables. Multiple regression analyses were made to evaluate the intraoperative effectiveness of additional procedures on compartment pressure. Linear correlation analysis was performed to evaluate the relationship between the initial and final pressure differences in both compartments. For radiographic measurement, intra-observer consistency between the two sets of measurements obtained by observer A and inter-observer consistency between the three sets of measurements obtained by observers A, B, and C, were analyzed using Pearson's correlation coefficient and the intra-class correlation coefficient (ICC). ICC > 0.75 was regarded as excellent, ICC 0.40–0.75 was fair to good, and ICC < 0.40 was poor (20). A P value less than 0.05 was considered statistically significant and all statistical analyses were performed using SPSS 24.0 (SPSS, Chicago, IL). Finally, a power analysis was conducted to estimate the required number of the study. The power was set at 80% or higher with $p < 0.05$, and at least 64 knees were required for the study.

Results

Absolute mediolateral compartment pressure difference determined initially (INI) and finally (FIN) were recorded and are shown in Fig. 3. Throughout the range of motion, the measured resection group showed higher initial pressure difference than the modified gap balancing group. Upon initial trial and final measurement after implantation, the proportion of the knees according to the compartment pressure (sum of medial and lateral compartment pressure) is shown in Fig. 4. After final implantation, 95% of the patients showed total compartment pressure less than 200 lbf.

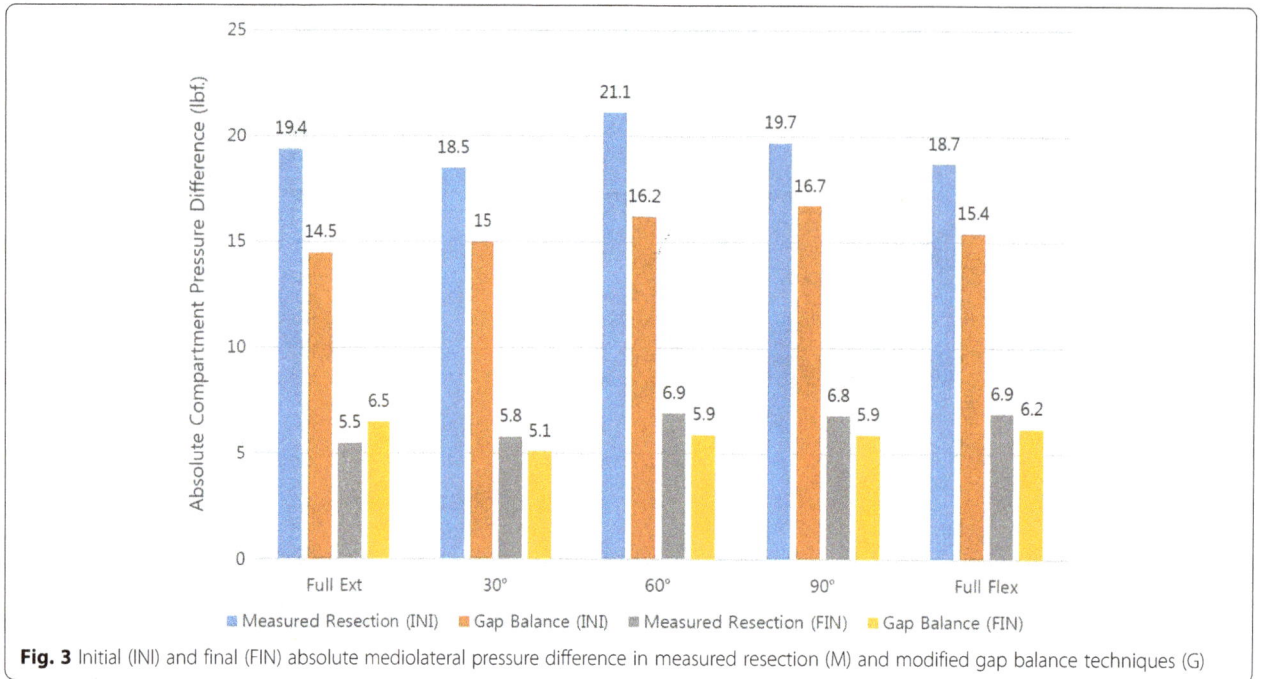

Fig. 3 Initial (INI) and final (FIN) absolute mediolateral pressure difference in measured resection (M) and modified gap balance techniques (G)

Overall (T), measured resection TKAs (M) and modified gap balancing TKAs (G) initial (INI) and final (FIN) compartment pressure on medial and lateral side are shown in Fig. 5. In both medial lateral compartments, the pressure was generally decreased throughout the ROM in both TKA methods. In the medial compartment, the overall final compartment pressure (FIN) was significantly decreased compared with initial pressure (INI) throughout all range of motion ($p < 0.05$), and in the lateral compartment, the overall final compartment pressure was also decreased throughout the ROM especially during 30° flexion and full flexion ($p < 0.05$)

(Table 1). According to TKA methods, both TKA techniques showed significant decrease in the medial compartment at the final measurement, although the lateral compartment did not show significant decrease in both technique (Table 2).

Linear correlation in the medial and lateral compartments was both statistically significant throughout the range of motion, with higher correlation in the lateral compartment. Medial compartment coefficients of determination were as follows: full extension ($R^2 = 0.12$; $P = 0.01$), 30° flexion ($R^2 = 0.084$; $P = 0.007$), 60° flexion ($R^2 = 0.078$; $P = 0.010$), 90° flexion ($R^2 = 0.071$; $P = 0.014$),

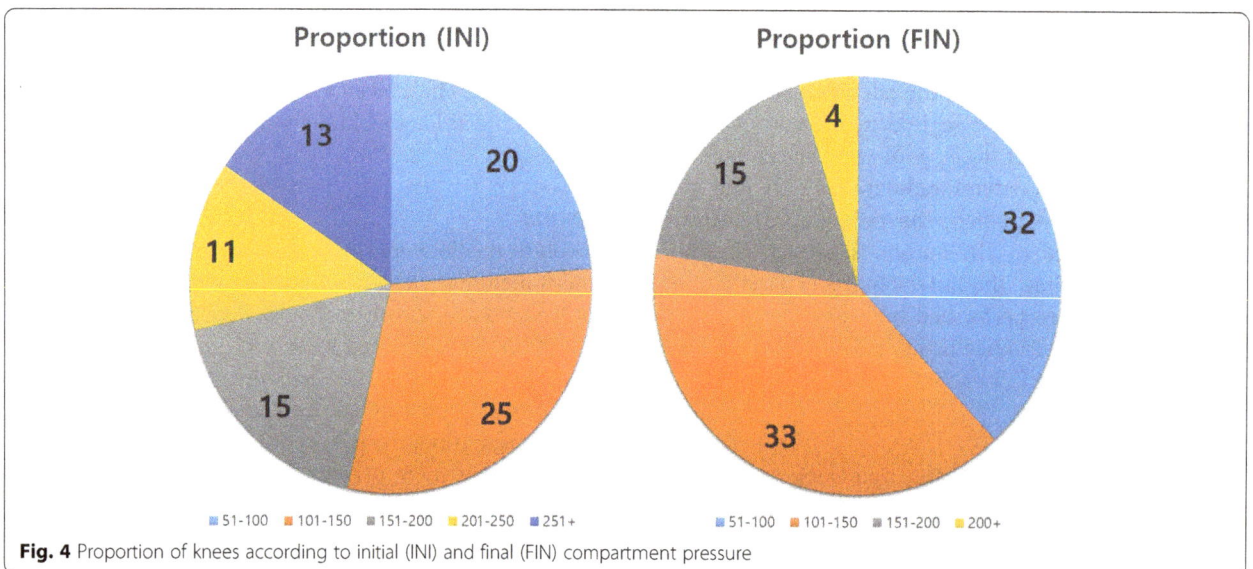

Fig. 4 Proportion of knees according to initial (INI) and final (FIN) compartment pressure

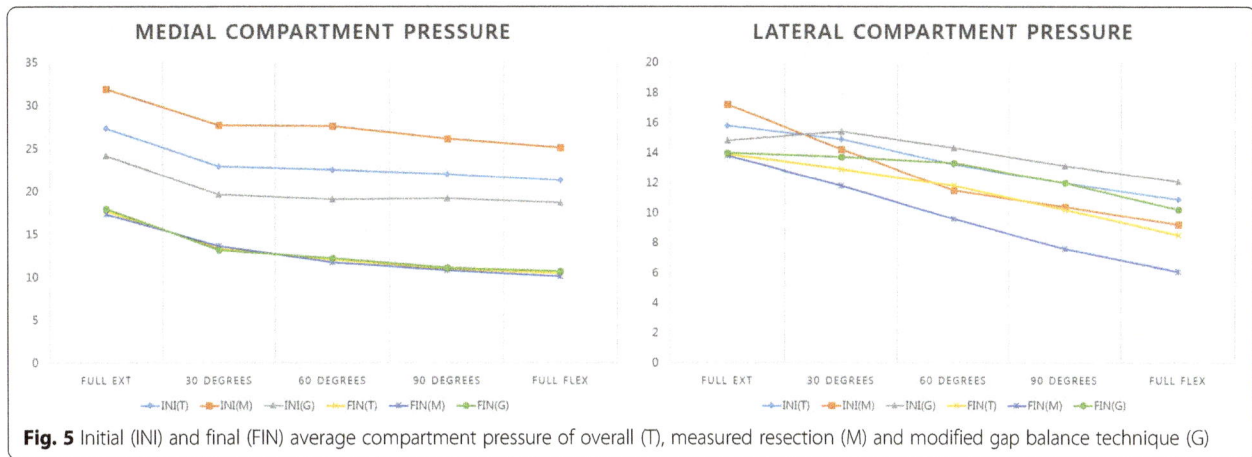

Fig. 5 Initial (INI) and final (FIN) average compartment pressure of overall (T), measured resection (M) and modified gap balance technique (G)

and full flexion ($R^2 = 0.107$; $P = 0.002$). Lateral compartment coefficients of determination were as follows: full extension ($R^2 = 0.306$; $P = 0.000$), 30° flexion ($R^2 = 0.366$; $P = 0.000$), 60° flexion ($R^2 = 0.358$; $P = 0.000$), 90° flexion ($R^2 = 0.376$; $P = 0.000$), full flexion ($R^2 = 0.422$; $P = 0.000$) (Fig. 6).

Thirty patients (35.7%) showed "balanced" knee without a need for additional ligament balancing upon initial measurement and 54 patients showed "imbalance" knee who underwent additional procedures. Among 30 balanced knees, 6 were measured resection TKAs and 24 were modified gap balancing TKAs. After initial bone resection, modified gap balancing TKAs showed significantly higher proportion of "balanced" knees than measured resection TKAs (24 of 50 TKAs vs. 6 of 34 TKAs) ($P = 0.004$). Upon final pressure measurement after ligament balancing and component implantation, 79 patients (94.0%) showed a "balanced" joint with medial and lateral pressure difference less than 15 pounds

Table 1 Overall Comparison of Initial (INI) and Final (FIN) Compartment Pressure

	Initial (lbf.)	Final (lbf.)	P-value[a]
Medial compartment			
Full Extension	27.3 ± 25.8	17.7 ± 7.8	0.001
30°	22.9 ± 25.0	13.3 ± 5.6	0.000
60°	22.5 ± 24.2	12.0 ± 6.3	0.000
90°	22.0 ± 25.7	11.0 ± 6.8	0.000
Full Flexion	21.3 ± 21.5	10.5 ± 7.9	0.000
Lateral compartment			
Full Extension	15.8 ± 11.7	13.9 ± 6.3	0.082
30°	14.9 ± 11.3	12.9 ± 5.6	0.046
60°	13.2 ± 11.3	11.8 ± 6.0	0.174
90°	12.0 ± 11.4	10.2 ± 6.5	0.074
Full Flexion	10.9 ± 11.7	8.5 ± 6.6	0.017

[a]Paired-t test. The p values of < 0.05 was considered significant

Table 2 Initial (INI) and Final (FIN) Compartment Pressure Classified by TKA technique: Measured Resection (M) vs. Modified Gap Balance (G) technique

	Initial (lbf.)	Final (lbf.)	P-value
Medial (G)			
Full Extension	24.1 ± 18.7	18.0 ± 8.6	0.023
30°	19.6 ± 19.0	13.1 ± 5.1	0.025
60°	19.1 ± 18.4	12.2 ± 5.6	0.009
90°	19.2 ± 20.0	11.1 ± 5.9	0.006
Full Flexion	18.7 ± 19.5	10.7 ± 7.5	0.002
Lateral (G)			
Full Extension	14.8 ± 9.8	14.0 ± 6.7	0.510
30°	15.4 ± 11.1	13.6 ± 5.8	0.190
60°	14.3 ± 11.3	13.3 ± 6.2	0.400
90°	13.1 ± 11.9	12.0 ± 9.6	0.365
Full Flexion	12.1 ± 12.6	10.2 ± 6.6	0.129
Medial (M)			
Full Extension	31.9 ± 33.5	17.3 ± 6.3	0.009
30°	27.7 ± 31.5	13.6 ± 6.2	0.008
60°	27.6 ± 30.4	11.7 ± 7.2	0.003
90°	26.1 ± 31.3	10.8 ± 8.1	0.006
Full Flexion	25.1 ± 30.4	10.1 ± 8.6	0.005
Lateral (M)			
Full Extension	17.2 ± 14.0	13.8 ± 5.9	0.075
30°	14.2 ± 11.8	11.8 ± 5.2	0.129
60°	11.5 ± 11.3	9.6 ± 5.0	0.286
90°	10.4 ± 10.5	7.6 ± 5.3	0.105
Full Flexion	9.2 ± 10.2	6.1 ± 5.8	0.061

[a]Paired-t test. The p values of < 0.05 was considered significant
[b]M Measured resection, [c]G Modified gap balance

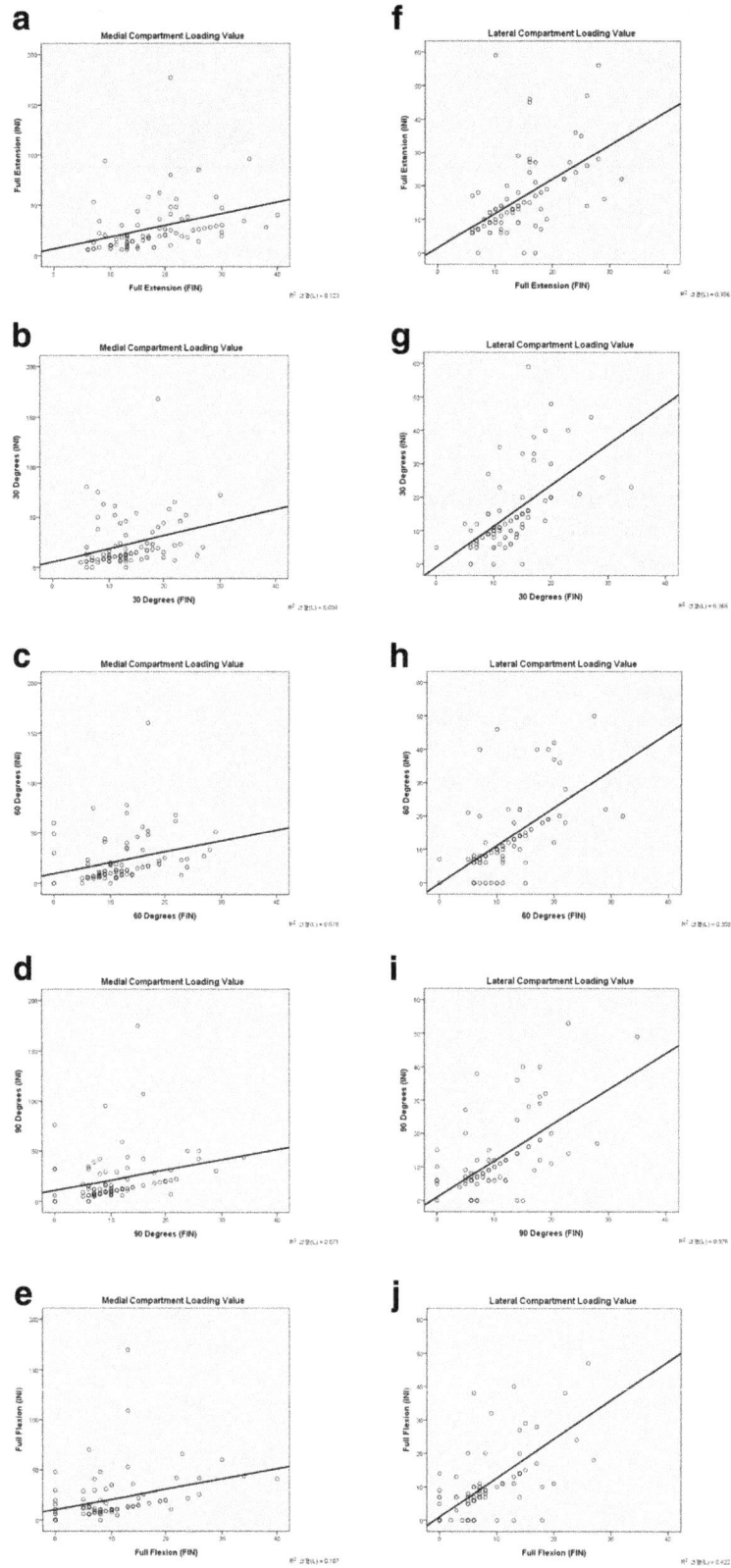

Fig. 6 a-j Linear correlation between initial (INI) and final (FIN) compartment pressure

throughout the full range of motion. Compared with the initial "balanced" knee (35.7%), there was significant improvement following ligament balancing at the final implantation (94.0%) ($P < 0.05$).

For 54 imbalanced knee, total 66 additional ligament balancing procedures (including soft tissue release (s) and bony resection) were carried out: 38 procedures for 28 measured resection TKAs and 28 procedures for 26 modified gap-balancing TKAs. Nine distal femur recuts (varus and neutral resection), 14 proximal tibia recuts (varus and neutral resection), 4 osteophyte removals, and 1 tibia posterior slope recut constituted additional bony procedures; and 26 medical collateral ligament (MCL) releases using pie-crusting (PC) method, 5 sub-periosteal superficial MCL releases, 5 iliotibial band (ITB) releases using PC method, 2 lateral collateral ligament (LCL) releases using PC method were performed for additional soft tissue releases.

The change of compartment pressure due to each additional procedure has been evaluated individually throughout the range of motion, and statistically significant procedures analyzed by regression analysis at each motion, are shown in Table 3. Results of regression analysis of the additional procedures were calculated based on the contributing beta values for each procedure by subtracting the post-procedure compartment pressure from pre-procedure compartment pressure. A positive value indicates improvement in joint pressure, and negative value indicates increased joint pressure while the absolute value indicates effectiveness of the joint pressure improvement. The effect of LCL release using PC method and tibia posterior slope resection procedures could not be analyzed due to lack of cases. However, the loading has been calculated to identify the effect of additional procedures on the compartment pressure throughout the range of motion. On average, bony resection showed relatively higher beta values compared with soft tissue releases. Distal femur recut showed a statistically significant effect on full extension and 90° flexion; proximal tibia recut showed significant effect on full extension; MCL release with PC technique showed effect throughout the range of motion but only significant in full extension; and release of suferficial MCL showed small but significant effect throughout the full range of motion.

On postoperative radiograph, average mechanical axis (MA) was 1.8° varus with 4.7° valgus femorotibial angle (FTA) and 6.2° posterior tibial slope (PTS). According to implant radiologic measurements, femoral and tibial components were also adequate positioned overall (Table 4). And the radiologic measurements showed excellent intra-observer consistency and inter-observer consistency across the 3 observers (Table 5).

Discussion

The most important implication of the study is that, not only measured resection TKA but also modified gap balancing TKA using subjective "feeling" of ligament balancing, can be inaccurate or can show variable results despite abundant experience. Objective quantification using real-time orthosensor improved the soft tissue balance in both TKA techniques.

Until now, most of the studies about kinematics of knee joint have been based on biomechanical models or cadaveric studies [21–23]. Unfortunately, these studies have limitations in understanding the dynamics of the real knee joint. It is difficult to extrapolate the findings from cadaveric studies to living human body due to bias associated with factors such as postmortem contracture and tissue atrophy. Furthermore, in the biomechanical model studies, data application was a demanding procedure, because data are generally acquired from limited specimens.

Further, according to previous studies, although TKAs were carried out in conventional methods with soft tissue balancing intraoperatively, the potential imbalance remains due to subjective ligament balancing. It resulted in a variety of postoperative complications such as instability, stiffness, loosening, etc., which resulted in a significant proportion of TKA failures and revision surgeries [24, 25].

Therefore, we used the VERASENSE system to ensure adequate ligament balancing objectively via quantification

Table 3 Regression analysis of Additional Ligament Balancing Procedures on the joint

	Full Extension	30°	60°	90°	Full Flexion
Distal femur recut	23.8[a]	43.1	40.7	19.1[a]	16.8
Proximal tibia recut	15.0[a]	19.6	42.0	42.6	29.2
Osteophyte removal	12.1	−6.4	4.8	3.6	7.6
MCL[b] PC[c]	16.6[a]	27.0	32.9	34.0	34.0
Sub-periosteal superficial MCL release	9.8[a]	3.1[a]	7.6[a]	− 2.6[a]	7.2[a]
ITB[d]	22.7	−9.6	15.2	2.6[a]	2.5[a]

[a]Multiple regression analysis. The p values of < 0.05 was considered significant
[b]MCL Medial collateral ligament, [c]PC Pie-crusting technique, [d]ITB Iliotibial band

Table 4 Postoperative Radiologic Measurement of the Implant

	α (°)	β (°)	γ (°)	δ (°)
Average	95.2	89.5	2.8	86.4
SD[t]	2.6	2.2	1.9	2.3

α Coronal medial inclination of femoral component, β Coronal medial inclination of tibial component, γ Sagittal inclination of femoral component, δ Sagittal inclination of tibial component, [t]SD Standard Deviation

of the joint intraoperatively, which would reduce the postoperative complications in long-term follow-up.

The initial (INI) and final (FIN) absolute pressure difference between medial and lateral compartments was higher in measured resection TKAs compared with gap balancing technique TKAs. As the femur resection was conducted according to the soft tissue balance in the modified gap balance technique, the quantification results were obtained as expected. But the difference was relatively higher than expected in spite of modified gap technique bone resection. Theoretically, modified gap balance bone resection should not show pressure difference between medial and lateral compartments because the bone resection was already based on patient's ligament balance. In previous studies, the superiority of measured resection and gap balancing technique was still disputed. A few studies reported better outcomes with the gap balancing technique TKAs, whereas other reports showed no significant difference between the techniques in long-term clinical outcomes [3, 26, 27].

The overall initial (INI) and final (FIN) average compartment pressure showed a significant decrease throughout the range of motion in the medial compartment ($p < 0.05$). In the lateral compartment, the overall final loading values were significantly decreased under 30° flexion and full flexion ($p < 0.05$). Correlation analysis suggested that both medial and lateral compartments showed a significant relationship between initial (INI) and final (FIN) pressure throughout the range of motion. Our study indicated that variability of pressure between the initial (INI) and final (FIN) measurements

was equal in both compartments, which facilitated surgical prediction of similar loading measurements with both VERASENSE system and final implanted components. Consequently, the surgeon could expect the same measured compartment pressure with the final implanted components.

Another important implication of the study was that only 30 patients (35.7%), constituting only 1/3 of the patients showed initially "balanced" knee after measured resection or gap balancing TKA. In spite of the abundant experience of the surgeon (EKS) in total knee arthroplasty for more than 30 years, subjective human "feeling" is variable and inaccurate. Fortunately, after additional ligament balancing procedures, a total of 79 patients (94.0%) completed the "balanced" TKA procedure, with load difference lower than 15 lbs. In a previous report of TKAs with a load difference lower than 15 lbs., better shorter-term clinical outcomes were observed compared with "unbalanced" knees with a difference greater than 15 lbs. [19], which underscored the significance of the objective quantification orthosensor, for adequate and satisfactory results. As mentioned before, the subjective and inaccurate procedures associated with traditional ligament balancing [28] have been elucidated through the study.

Excluding the 30 patients who were initially "balanced", 54 patients underwent additional ligament balancing procedure. A total of 66 additional procedures were performed, which accounted for an average of 1.2 procedures per patient. According to our study, generally measured resection TKA patients underwent more additional ligament balancing procedures than modified gap balance TKA patients, 1.36 per person and 1.1 per person, respectively. Bony resection showed higher changes in joint loading, especially distal femur recut was effective in full extension to mid-flexion, and proximal tibia recut was effective during the mid-flexion. These results were similar to previous qualitative studies. For example, Mihalko et al. [29] demonstrated that distal femur

Table 5 Comparison of intra-observer and inter-observer consistency in Radiologic measurements

Observer	A-A		A-B		A-C		B-C	
	ICC[¥]	P-value[a]	ICC	P-value	ICC	P-value	ICC	P-value
MA[b]	0.934	0.005	0.862	0.014	0.871	0.009	0.864	0.015
FTA[c]	0.944	0.004	0.877	0.008	0.854	0.012	0.869	0.010
PTS[d]	0.962	0.005	0.812	0.018	0.828	0.022	0.836	0.015
α	0.952	0.002	0.834	0.012	0.852	0.011	0.847	0.007
β	0.961	0.001	0.882	0.010	0.904	0.005	0.891	0.009
γ	0.918	0.010	0.807	0.024	0.833	0.019	0.829	0.022
δ	0.933	0.005	0.856	0.010	0.872	0.009	0.886	0.005

[a]Pearson's-correlation test. The p values of < 0.05 was considered significant
[b]MA Mechanical Axis, [c]FTA FemoroTibial Angle, [d]PTS Posterior Tibial Slope, α Coronal medial inclination of femoral component, β Coronal medial inclination of tibial component, γ Sagittal inclination of femoral component, δ Sagittal inclination of tibial component, [¥]ICC Intra-class Correlation Coefficient

resection was effective for mid-flexion contractures. Ahn et al. [30] demonstrated the effectiveness of proximal tibia varus resection on severe varus deformities. Among soft tissue release (s), MCL release with PC technique was most frequently used and was also most effective through flexion, which also was similar to many previous studies using MCL release as an important procedure during total knee arthroplasty in varus deformity [31–33]. Although superficial MCL has been known to have a lesser effect in flexion stability [34], our study showed that sub-periosteal superficial MCL release showed small but significant effect on joint loading throughout the range of motion. Postoperative radiographic alignment of patients including mechanical axis, femorotibial angle, posterior slope, and implant positions were within satisfactory range.

However, this study also has a few limitations. First, the group only consisted of 84 patients, and a larger group may have yielded more generalized analyses of the knee joint. Fortunately, our study findings were similar to those reported previously in published studies. Second, we used only a single implant system in all patients. Other implant systems showed different loading values due to differences in implant design. Also, the PCL release being a strong influence on flexion ligament balancing, using two types of implant (CR and PS type) may have produced some bias during interpretation of the data. Third, although the pressure was quantified and presented as digited results on the screen, the measurement was done by a single surgeon, suggesting possible bias. Fourth, we did not compare the long-term clinical and radiological outcomes between objectively balanced TKAs and traditionally subjectively balanced TKAs.

Conclusion

By objective quantification using orthosensor, we observed significant decrease in both medial and lateral compartments pressure after TKA, and could obtain 94% balanced knee, consequently. And between the techniques, measured resection TKA showed less balanced knee in the initial pressure measurement and also required more additional procedures compared to modified gap balancing TKA. But also, we suggest that regardless of TKA surgical methods, additional procedures could be needed for adequate "patient-specific" ligament balancing. Furthermore, with the consistent data of the orthosensor acquired during appropriate ligament balancing, the surgeon could eventually reduce the complications associated with soft tissue imbalance in the future.

Abbreviations

CR: Cruciate-retaining; CT: Computed tomography; FIN: Final; FTA: Femorotibial angle; ICC: Intra-class correlation coefficient; INI: Initial; ITB: Iliotibial band; LCL: Lateral collateral ligament; ma: Mechanical axis; MCL: Medical collateral ligament; PC: Pie-crusting technique; PS: Posterior-sacrificing; PTS: Posterior tibial slope; TKA: Total knee arthroplasty

Authors' contributions
KJC analyzed the results of the statistics and draft the manuscript. JKS participated in its design and statistical analysis. WYJ collected patients' data and categorized. CGP carried out statistical analysis. EKS conceived and designed the study. All authors have read and approved the manuscript.

Competing interests
On behalf of all authors, the corresponding author states that there is no competing of interest.

References

1. Lustig S, Bruderer J, Servien E, Neyret P. The bone cuts and ligament balance in total knee arthroplasty: the third way using computer assisted surgery. Knee. 2009;16(2):91.
2. Hananouchi T, Yamamoto K, AndoW FK, Ohzono K. The intraoperative gap difference (flexion gap minus extension gap) is altered by insertion of the trial femoral component. Knee. 2012;19:601–5.
3. Matsumoto T, Muratsu H, Kawakami Y, Takayama K, Ishida K, Matsushita T, et al. Soft-tissue balancing in total knee arthroplasty: cruciate-retaining versus posterior-stabilised, and measured-resection versus gap technique. Int Orthop. 2014;38(3):531–7.
4. Siddiqi A, Hardaker WM, Eachempati KK, Sheth NP. Advances in computer-aided technology for total knee arthroplasty. Orthopedics. 2017;40(6):338–52.
5. Liow MH, Xia Z, Wong MK, Tay KJ, Yeo SJ, Chin PL. Robot-assisted total knee arthroplasty accurately restores the joint line and mechanical axis. A prospective randomised study. J Arthroplast. 2014;29(12):2373–7.
6. Nagai K, Muratsu H, Takeoka Y, Tsubosaka M, Kuroda R, Matsumoto T. The influence of joint distraction force on the soft-tissue balance using modified gap-balancing technique in posterior-stabilized total knee arthroplasty. J Arthroplast. 2017;32(10):2995–9.
7. Lee SY, Lim HC, Jang KM, Bae JH. What factors are associated with femoral component internal rotation in TKA using the gap balancing technique? Clin Orthop Relat Res. 2017;475(8):1999–2010.
8. Ferreira MC, Franciozi CES, Kubota MS, Priore RD, Ingham SJM, Abdalla RJ. Is the use of spreaders an accurate method for ligament balancing? J Arthroplast. 2017;32(7):2262–7.
9. Kim SH, Lim JW, Jung HJ, Lee HJ. Influence of soft tissue balancing and distal femoral resection on flexion contracture in navigated total knee arthroplasty. Knee Surg Sports Traumatol Arthrosc. 2017;25(11):3501–7.
10. Heesterbeek PJC, Haffner N, Wymenga AB, Stifter J, Ritschl P. Patient-related factors influence stiffness of the soft tissue complex during intraoperative gap balancing in cruciate-retaining total knee arthroplasty. Knee Surg Sports Traumatol Arthrosc. 2017;25(9):2760–8.
11. Wyss TF, Schuster AJ, Münger P, Pfluger D, Wehrli U. Does total knee joint replacement with the soft tissue balancing surgical technique maintain the natural joint line? Arch Orthop Trauma Surg. 2006;126(7):480–6.
12. Ranawat CS, Flynn WF Jr, Saddler S, Hansraj KK, Maynard MJ. Long-term results of the total condylar knee arthroplasty. A 15-year survivorship study. Clin Orthop Relat Res. 1993;286:94–102.
13. Ranawat CS, Flynn WF Jr, Saddler S, Hansraj KK, Maynard MJ. Long-term results followup of anatomic graduated components posterior cruciate-retaining total knee replacement. Clin Orthop Relat Res. 1993;388:51–7.
14. Fehring TK, Odum S, Griffin WL, Mason JB, Nadaud M. Early failures in total knee arthroplasty. Clin Orthop Relat Res. 2001;392:315–8.
15. Mulhall KJ, Ghomrawi HM, Scully S, Callaghan JJ, Saleh KJ. Current etiologies and modes of failure in total knee arthroplasty revision. Clin Orthop Relat Res. 2006;446:45–50.
16. Mihalko WM, Saleh KJ, Krackow KA, Whiteside LA. Soft-tissue balancing during total knee arthroplasty in the varus knee. J Am Acad Orthop Surg. 2009;17(12):766–74.
17. Yim JH, Song EK, Khan MS, Sun ZH, Seon JK. A comparison of classical and anatomical total knee alignment methods in robotic total knee arthroplasty: classical and anatomical knee alignment methods in TKA. J Arthroplast. 2013;28(6):932–7.
18. Oh CS, Song EK, Seon JK, Ahn YS. The effect of flexion balance on functional outcomes in cruciate-retaining total knee arthroplasty. Arch Orthop Trauma Surg. 2015;135(3):401–6.
19. Gustake KA, Golladay GJ, Roche MW, et al. A new method for defining balance: promising short-term clinical outcomes of sensor-guided TKA. J Arthroplast. 2014;29:955–60.

20. Bellemans J, Vandenneucker H, Van Lauwe J, et al. New surgical technique for medial collateral ligament balancing. J Arthroplast. 2010;25(7):1151–6.

21. Onishi Y, Hino K, Watanabe S, Watamori K, Kutsuna T, Miura H. The influence of tibial resection on the PCL in PCL-retaining total knee arthroplasty: a clinical and cadaveric study. J Orthop Sci. 2016;21(6):798–803.

22. Wada K, Hamada D, Tamaki S, Higashino K, Fukui Y, Sairyo K. Influence of medial collateral ligament release for internal rotation of tibia in posterior-stabilized total knee arthroplasty: a cadaveric study. J Arthroplast. 2017;32(1):270–3.

23. Shoifi Abubakar M, Nakamura S, Kuriyama S, Ito H, Ishikawa M, Furu M, et al. Influence of posterior cruciate ligament tension on knee kinematics and kinetics. J Knee Surg. 2016;29(8):684–9.

24. Postler A, Lützner C, Beyer F, Tille E, Lützner J. Analysis of total knee arthroplasty revision causes. BMC Musculoskelet Disord. 2018;19(1):55–60.

25. Naudie DD, Ammeen DJ, Engh GA, Rorabeck CH. Wear and osteolysis around total knee arthroplasty. J Am Acad Orthop Surg. 2007;15(1):53–64.

26. Churchill JL, Khlopas A, Sultan AA, Harwin SF, Mont MA. Gap-balancing versus measured resection technique in total knee arthroplasty: a comparison study. J Knee Surg. 2018;31(1):13–6.

27. Teeter MG, Perry KI, Yuan X, Howard JL, Lanting BA. Contact kinematic differences between gap balanced vs measured resection techniques for single radius posterior-stabilized total knee arthroplasty. J Arthroplasty. 2017; 32(6):1834–8.

28. Elmallah RK, Mistry JB, Cherian JJ, Chughtai M, Bhave A, Roche MW, et al. Can we really "feel" a balanced total knee arthroplasty? J Arthroplast. 2016; 31(9 Suppl):102–5.

29. Mihalko WM, Whiteside LA. Bone resection and ligament treatment for flexion contracture in knee arthroplasty. Clin Orthop Relat Res. 2003; 406(1):141–7.

30. Ahn JH, Back YW. Comparative study of two techniques for ligament balancing in total knee arthroplasty for severe varus knee: medial soft tissue release vs. bony resection of proximal medial tibia. Knee Surg Relat Res. 2013;25(1):13–8.

31. Ha CW, Park YB, Lee CH, Awe SI, Park YG. Selective medial release technique using the pie-crusting method for medial tightness during primary total knee arthroplasty. Knee Surg Sports Traumatol Arthrosc. 2015;23(6):1816–23.

32. Koh IJ, Kwak DS, Kim TK, Park IJ, In Y. How effective is multiple needle puncturing for medial soft tissue balancing during total knee arthroplasty? A cadaveric study. J Arthroplast. 2014;29(12):2478–83.

33. Bellemans J. Multiple needle puncturing: balancing the varus knee. Orthopedics. 2011;34(9):e510–2.

34. Whiteside LA. Soft tissue balancing: the knee. J Arthroplast. 2002;17(4 Suppl 1):23–7.

15

The prevalence of low back pain in the emergency department: a descriptive study set in the Charles V. Keating Emergency and Trauma Centre, Halifax, Nova Scotia, Canada

Jordan Edwards[1,3]* (iD), Jill Hayden[1], Mark Asbridge[1] and Kirk Magee[2]

Abstract

Background: While low back pain is a common presenting complaint in the emergency department, current estimates from Canada are limited. Furthermore, existing estimates do not clearly define low back pain. As such, our main objective was to estimate prevalence rates of low back pain in a large Nova Scotian emergency department using various definitions, and to describe characteristics of individuals included in these groups. An additional objective was to explore trends in low back pain prevalence in our emergency department over time.

Methods: We conducted a cross sectional analysis using six years of administrative data from our local emergency setting. We first calculated the prevalence and patient characteristics for individuals presenting with any complaint of back pain, and for groups diagnosed with different types of low back pain. We explored prevalence over time by analyzing presentation trends by month, day of the week and hour of the day.

Results: The prevalence of patients presenting to the emergency department with a complaint of back pain was 3. 17%. Individuals diagnosed with non-specific/mechanical low back pain with no potential nerve root involvement made up 60.8% of all back pain presentations. Persons diagnosed with non-specific/mechanical low back pain with potential nerve root involvement made up 6.7% of presentation and the low back pain attributed to secondary factors accounted for 9.9% of back pain presentations. We found a linear increase in presentations for low back pain over the study period.

Conclusion: This is the first multi-year analysis assessing the prevalence of low back pain in a Canadian emergency department. Back pain is a common presenting complaint in our local emergency department, with most of these persons receiving a diagnosis of non-specific/mechanical low back pain with no potential nerve root involvement. Future research should concentrate on understanding the management of low back pain in this setting, to ensure this is the proper setting to manage this common condition.

Keywords: Low back pain, Emergency setting, Prevalence estimate, Policy decision maker

* Correspondence: jr860374@dal.ca
[1]Department of Community Health & Epidemiology, Dalhousie University, Halifax, NS, Canada
[3]Department of Epidemiology & Biostatistics, Schulich School of Medicine & Dentistry, Western University, London, ON, Canada
Full list of author information is available at the end of the article

Background

Low back pain is one of the most common forms of musculoskeletal pain, prompting individuals to seek medical care [1, 2]. In 2002, low back pain was the fifth most common reason for all office based physician visits in the US [3]. A systematic review conducted by Dagenais et al., 2008 analyzed the total costs of low back pain to society and estimated that in the US the total costs - direct (medical and nonmedical), indirect costs, and intangible costs of low back pain - are between 84.1 billion and 624.8 billion US dollars annually [4].

Most individuals will develop low back pain at some point in their life, as the lifetime prevalence is between 49 and 90% [5]. It is currently accepted that the management of low back pain should begin in the primary care setting [6], and over half of visits for low back pain are to primary care physicians [5]. Nevertheless, a recent systematic review on the prevalence of low back pain in emergency settings [7] suggests that low back pain is a common presenting complaint to this setting (pooled prevalence estimate 4.3%). Results from the same systematic review [7] indicated that there are a number of gaps in the literature, particularly a lack of clear and detailed definitions of low back pain. Additionally, the review identified a need for studies comparing prevalence results from multiple definitions of low back pain and research conducted in Canada [7].

In this study, we addressed these gaps in the literature by conducting a cross sectional analysis, involving secondary use of data from a large emergency department in Nova Scotia, Canada. Our objectives were to estimate the prevalence of low back pain among patients presenting to the emergency department, using different definitions of low back pain, and to describe the characteristics of patients diagnosed with these distinct definitions of low back pain. Our secondary objective was to assess trends in low back pain prevalence in this emergency department over time.

Methods

Design and data sources

We conducted a cross-sectional analysis of emergency department administrative data collected between the 15th of July 2009 and the 15th of July 2015. All patients presenting to the emergency department were captured in the database.

Emergency department setting

This study was conducted at the Charles V. Keating Emergency and Trauma Centre (QEII emergency department) in Halifax, Nova Scotia, Canada. It is a tertiary care teaching hospital and the largest emergency department in Atlantic Canada with approximately 71,000 patient presentations each year [8].

Data collection

We collected data from the administrative database EDIS (Emergency Department Information System), which is the central information database used in the QEII emergency department. The database contains over one million patient records and offers access to these records in real time. The database is constantly updated with information about patients as they progress through the emergency department. EDIS is currently endorsed by the Canadian Association of Emergency Physicians, L'Association des Médecins d'Urgence du Quebec, the National Emergency Nurses Affiliation, the Canadian Paediatric Society and the Society of Rural Physicians of Canada [9].

We collected data on individuals as they passed through the emergency department. We collected data on patients' presenting complaint codes, presenting level of pain, Canadian Triage and Acuity Scale (CTAS) scores and individuals' time of arrival. Presenting complaints were captured using the EDIS presenting complaint list. Description of the CTAS scores can be found online in Additional file 1.

We gathered data on patient characteristics age, sex and whether patients currently had a primary care provider. Information on primary care providers was captured as a check box when individuals present to the emergency department. We also captured patients emergency department diagnosis using both ICD-9 and ICD-10 codes, as the QEII emergency department switched from the use of ICD-9 codes to ICD-10 codes between July 2012 and Feb 2013.

We collected data on patients' length of stay in the emergency department, whether patients were admitted to hospital following the visit and the details of the type of emergency department visit (e.g. referred to the emergency department or transferred from another health facility). We also captured whether patients had repeat visits to the emergency department, who was responsible for payment in the emergency department (e.g. department of health or workers' compensation) and whether the patient received any imaging services (x-ray, CT, MRI). A list of the characteristics captured can be found in Additional file 2.

Study population

We defined our eligible population as all adults presenting to the emergency department, excluding patients' deceased on arrival. Adults were defined as individuals over the age of 16 (the minimum age of intake in our emergency setting). We included patients who arrived to the emergency department independently or by emergency health services (ambulance or helicopter). The eligible population made up the denominator in our prevalence estimate. This included the total number of emergency department visits [10, 11] and the total number of individual patients presenting to the emergency department [12] over the study period.

The prevalence of low back pain in the emergency department: a descriptive study set...

183

Low back pain definitions

We first explored patient presentations and patient characteristics for individuals presenting with a triage complaint of "back pain" or "traumatic back/spine injury". These codes were used to capture individuals potentially diagnosed with serious or non-serious low back pain. From this population, we defined three clinically relevant low back pain patient groups based on patient's emergency department discharge diagnostic ICD codes: 1. low back pain with no potential nerve root involvement, 2. low back pain with potential nerve root involvement and 3. low back pain with attributed to trauma or other secondary factors (see Additional file 3, Fig. 1). ICD diagnoses included in each group was determined by consultation of previous studies [13, 14] and consensus with three independent researchers, which included an emergency physician and a back pain content expert. In the case of disagreement, discussion between the three reviewers was used to reach consensus.

1) *Non-specific/mechanical low back pain with no potential nerve root involvement* was defined as low back pain not attributed to an identifiable specific pathology [2]. Non-specific low back pain is described as pain, muscle tension, or stiffness localized below the lower edge of the chest and above the upper thigh [15]. For example, we included patients assigned ICD codes 724.5 "back pain" and 847.2 "low back strain" in this group (Additional file 3). A more specific definition of low back pain with no potential nerve root involvement, excluding ambiguous codes (e.g. 715.90 "osteoarthritis"), was used for sensitivity analysis (Table 1).

2) *Non-specific/mechanical low back pain with potential nerve root involvement* was defined as low back pain that included neurological signs and symptoms. This included patients with low back

pain including irritation/compression of a lumbar nerve root). For example, we included patients assigned ICD codes 724.3 "sciatica" and 729.2 "radiculopathy" in this group (Additional file 3).

3) *Low back pain attributed to secondary factors* defined patients presenting with low back pain who are diagnosed with another etiology, for which low back pain may be a symptom, and often requiring different and sometimes urgent care. For example, we included patients assigned ICD codes of 441.9 "aortic aneurysm" and 577.0 "pancreatitis" in this group (Additional file 3).

Individuals presenting with a low back pain complaint, but not meeting the above definitions, were classified as 'other' and further classified for completeness based on independent researcher judgment. These groups were defined as *likely non-specific low back pain with comorbidity* (patients presenting with low back pain, but ultimately diagnosed with an etiology unlikely to have back pain as a symptom; consensus judgement that diagnosis was likely to be a co-morbid condition), or *Non-lumbar back pain* (thoracic or cervical non-specific pain syndromes). Remaining patients with other diagnostic codes were classified as 'unsure'.

Analysis

We calculated the crude prevalence rates for all patients presenting with a complaint of low back pain, and for each of our defined low back pain groups. We performed a sensitivity analysis for the definition of non-specific/mechanical low back pain with no potential nerve root involvement by eliminating ambiguous ICD codes (see Table 1).

We described patient characteristics for each of our defined categories of low back pain. Frequencies and percentages were used to describe categorical variables.

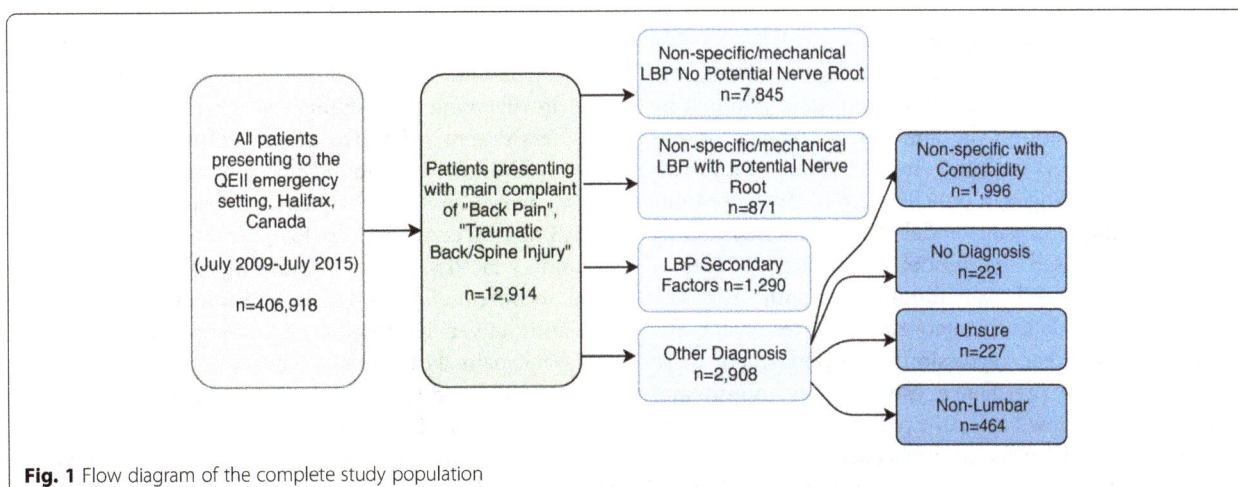

Fig. 1 Flow diagram of the complete study population

Table 1 ICD-9/10 coding for a definition of low back pain that is representative of the literature

Description	ICD-9 Code
Myalgia	729.1
Muscle spasm	728.85
Mechanical Low Back Pain	724.2
Recurrent Low Back Pain	724.2
Back Pain	724.5
Chronic Back Pain	724.5
Pain-Back nyd	724.5
Muscle Spasm Back	724.8
Musculoskeletal Pain	729.1
Other msk	729.9
Chronic Pain (misc)	780.9
Pain nyd (Misc)	780.9
Lumbosacral Strain	846.0
Sprain Sacroiliac Int/Ligament	846.1
Low Back Strain	847.2
Other Sprain/ Strain Trunk	848.8
Description	ICD-10 Code
Myalgia	M79.1
Back Pain	M54.5
Muscle Strain	M62.6
Superficial inj Low Back / Pelvis uncomplicated	S30.80
Ow lower back / pelvis, uncomplicated	S31.0

Continuous variables were described as means and standard deviations, or medians and inter-quartile ranges. Data was tested for normal distribution using the Shapiro-Wilk test. Means were used for variables with results that were normally distributed and medians were used for non-normally distributed data. Krustal-Wallis analysis of non-parametric data was used with a Bonferroni adjustment to test for significant differences between patient characteristics for separate definitions of low back pain. Significance was set at $p = < 0.05$.

Trends in low back pain prevalence over time were assessed using the available six-years of data grouped by month of presentation. The analysis of trend examines the low frequency variation in the data along with non-stationary changes in prevalence [16]. We fitted our data with a random walk model looking for seasonality by month. We used this model as we expect random presentations for back pain month to month [17]. The trend fitting our data was smoothed and tested for linearity using a linear regression. We performed these analyses for both prevalence estimates by month and presentations for low back pain per month. This allowed us to determine the trend in prevalence of low back pain with and without the influence of total presentations to

the emergency setting. Due to partial data in the months of July 2009 and July 2015, we excluded these two months from the time series analysis.

We analyzed presentations by hour of the day and day of the week. We used density plots to explore presentations during separate hours of the day and days of the week and unpaired t-tests to test for significant differences between individuals presenting during work hours (Mon-Fri, 9 AM-5 PM) and non-work hours.

Significance was set at $p = 0.05$ level for all comparative analyses. Analyses were conducted using STATA IC 13.1.

Results

There were a total of 406,918 presentations to the QEII emergency department during our six-year study period, of which 12,914 or 3.17% of individuals presented with a primary complaint of back pain, including "Back Pain" (12,706 presentations) and "Traumatic Back/Spine Injury" (208 presentations). The majority of patients (60.8%) presenting with back pain received a diagnostic code compatible with low back pain no potential nerve root involvement (overall prevalence of 1.93%). Individuals receiving a diagnostic code compatible with low back pain with potential nerve root involvement made up 6.7% of all back pain presentations (overall prevalence 0.22%); the low back pain attributed to secondary factors group accounted for 9.9% of all back pain presentations (overall prevalence 0.32%) (Fig. 1).

Characteristics of patients presenting to the emergency department with a complaint of back pain are described in Table 2. The median age of individuals was 45 (IQR: 30–60), and females made up 53.4% of the population. Patients spent a median length of 3.13 h (IQR: 1.93–5.1) in the emergency department and 34.7% of individuals presenting with back pain received x-rays.

We compared patient characteristics between the three definitions of low back pain: low back pain no potential of nerve root involvement, low back pain with potential nerve root involvement and low back pain attributed to secondary factors (Table 3). We found that individuals with low back pain with no potential nerve root involvement had significantly higher CTAS scores (i.e. "less urgent") than the other definitions of low back pain. Additionally, we found that low back pain with potential nerve root involvement had significantly higher CTAS scores compared to low back pain attributed to secondary factors. We also found that the low back pain with no potential nerve root involvement group had significantly lower age (median 43), compared to both the low back pain with potential nerve root irritation (median 46) and the low back pain attributed to secondary factors (median 58) groups. Furthermore, individuals with low back pain with no potential nerve root involvement were significantly less likely to be admitted to the

Table 2 Patient characteristics of individuals presenting with a complaint of low back pain

Characteristic	Presenting complaint of LBP n = 12,914
Age, years (Median, IQR)	45 (30,60)
Female sex (#,%)	6897 (53.4)
CTAS (median, IQR))	4 (3–4)
Primary Care Provider (#,%)	12,211 (94.5)
Type of ED visit (#,%)	
Direct to Consult	310 (2.4)
Referral from GP	30 (0.2)
Return Visit	36 (0.3)
Missing	2247 (17.4)
Other (Emergency presentation)	10,291 (79.7)
X ray (#,%)	4478 (34.7)
CT (#,%)	968 (7.5)
MRI (#,%)	15 (0.12)
Hospital admission [#(%)]	878 (6.8)
Length of stay, hrs (Median, IQR)	3.13 (1.93–5.1)
Responsibility for payment (#,%)	
Department of Health, NS	10,680 (82.7)
Worker's Compensation Board, NS	852 (6.6)
Other	1078 (8.3)
Missing	304 (2.4)

Note: *LBP* low back pain, *ED* Emergency Department, *HRS* hours, *CTAS* Canadian Triage and Acuity Scale, *IQR* Inter Quartile Range, *GP* General Practitioner, *NS* Nova Scotia

hospital. Results of our Krustal-Wallis analysis are presented in Table 4.

Our sensitivity analysis, which was used to test the robustness of our definition of low back pain with no potential nerve root involvement (eliminating ambiguous codes), resulted in an insignificant difference in prevalence (1.89%) compared to our non-specific low back pain estimate of (1.93%). Furthermore, we found no significant difference in age, sex or CTAS scores between both groups.

In our analysis of prevalence estimates over time, we found that peak hours for presentations for back pain were between 9 AM and 11 AM (Fig. 2). Our results indicate that significantly more individuals presented during non-work hours, 61.8%, compared to work hours (Fig. 3). Also, more persons presented on Mondays (16.6%) compared to all other days of the week (Fig. 4).

Our time series analysis showed that trends in the prevalence of low back pain in the emergency department remained stable over the six years of our study. The monthly prevalence of back pain ranged from 2.73 to 4.09%. There was no linear trend identified in the data; the linear regression resulted in a slope of − 0.001 and an R^2 value of 0.06 (Fig. 5a).

Trend analysis for patient presentations for low back pain revealed a steady increase in patient presentations over the six years of data. The trend in presentations per month ranged from 135 to 230. The linear regression resulted in a slope of 0.42 with a R^2 value of 0.78 (Fig. 5b).

Discussion

Our multi-year study provides evidence that a substantial number of individuals, just over 3 %, present to the QEII emergency department with a complaint of low back pain. We found large variation in prevalence estimates for different definitions of low back pain. Most individuals presenting with back pain were diagnosed with low back pain with no potential nerve root involvement (overall prevalence 1.93%), while individuals with low back pain with potential nerve root involvement had an overall prevalence of 0.22% and individuals with low back pain attributed to secondary factors had an overall prevalence of 0.32%. These estimates are useful as they allow for comparison with other research in the field and they provide context for future prevalence estimates.

Our prevalence estimate for individuals presenting with back pain, 3.17%, is lower than what was observed in a meta-analysis of 16 prevalence studies of low back pain in the emergency department (4.3%) [7]. This difference may be due to the fact that the review included a broad spectrum of emergency settings, which may have different healthcare funding structures and access, and which may serve different patient populations.

Our results are comparable to other studies conducted in similar settings using similar back pain definitions of low back pain with no potential nerve root involvement and low back pain with potential nerve root involvement. For example, a study conducted in Canada [18], and one conducted in the US [13] reported prevalence estimates of 2.2%, and 2.3%, respectively, compared to our prevalence estimate of 2.15% (1.93% low back pain with no potential nerve root involvement and 0.32% low back pain with potential nerve root involvement).

To provide perspective, a study conducted in the US [19], which analyzed top presenting complaints, found that back pain (including neck pain), ranked as being the fifth most common presenting complaint in the emergency department [19]. Another recent analysis of Canadian emergency department visits, performed by the Canadian Institute of Health Information (CIHI), indicated that back pain is the sixth most common reason for an emergency department visit [20].

Studies using only ICD codes to quantify low back pain may be underrepresenting the burden of low back pain in emergency settings. Most studies in this field define prevalence for low back pain with and without a potential of nerve root involvement; however, other studies have not described prevalence of

Table 3 Patient characteristics of individuals presenting with a complaint of low back pain and diagnosed with various definitions of low back pain

Characteristic	Non-specific/mechanical LBP with No Potential Nerve Root Involvement $n = 7845$	Non-specific/mechanical LBP with Potential Nerve Root Involvement $n = 871$	LBP Attributed to Secondary Factors $n = 1290$
Age, years (Median, IQR)	43 (29,57)	46 (36,57)	58 (38,76)
Female sex (#,%)	4133 (52.7)	476 (54.6)	737 (57.1)
CTAS (median, IQR))	4 (3–4)	4 (3–4)	3 (3–3)
Primary Care Provider (#,%)	7411 (94.5)	825 (94.7)	1233 (95.6)
Type of ED visit (#,%)			
Direct to Consult	54 (0.7)	19 (2.2)	142 (11.0)
Referral from GP	12 (0.2)	2 (0.2)	5 (0.4)
Return Visit	19 (0.2)	6 (0.7)	5 (0.4)
Missing	1315 (16.8)	149 (17.1)	227 (17.6)
Other (Emergency presentation)	6445 (82.1)	695 (79.8)	911 (70.6)
Hospital admission [#(%)]	120 (1.5)	39 (4.5)	410 (31.9)
Length of stay, hrs (Median, IQR)	2.8 (1.8–4.4)	2.9 (1.7–4.9)	5.5 (3.5–9.2)
Responsibility for payment (#,%)			
Department of Health, NS	6364 (81.1)	751 (86.2)	1124 (87.1)
Worker's Compensation Board, NS	31 (0.4)	47 (5.4)	28 (2.2)
Other	1292 (16.5)	55 (6.3)	95 (7.4)
Missing	158 (2.0)	18 (2.1)	43 (3.3)

Note: *LBP* low back pain, *ED* Emergency Department, *HRS* hours, *CTAS* Canadian Triage and Acuity Scale, *IQR* Inter Quartile Range, *GP* General Practitioner, *NS* Nova Scotia

the low back pain attributed to secondary factors [7]. Including this group in prevalence estimates is important as it captures a clinically relevant population requiring serious intervention and significant resources. Future research should capture this population to increase the homogeneity of the literature and our understanding of the impact of the low back pain attributed to secondary factors group in various emergency settings.

This is one of the first studies to describe the prevalence and patient characteristics for groups of low back pain patients defined using discharge diagnostic codes. Results indicate that the severity of patients increases as our definitions progress from low back pain with no potential nerve root involvement to low back pain with potential nerve root involvement to low back pain attributed to secondary factors. This was reflected in our analysis of CTAS scores, which decreased with

Table 4 Results of Krustal-Wallis analysis used to test for significant differences between patient characteristics for separate definitions of low back pain ("non-specific/mechanical low back pain with no potential nerve root involvement", "non-specific/mechanical low back pain with potential nerve root irritation" and "low back pain attributed to secondary factors")

Characteristics	No Potential Nerve - Potential Nerve	No Potential Nerve - Secondary	Potential Nerve - Secondary
Age	<	<	<
	$p < 0.001$	$p < 0.001$	$p < 0.001$
Sex (More Females)	No difference	<	No difference
	$p = 0.279$	$p < 0.001$	$p = 0.416$
Length of stay	No difference	<	<
	$p = 0.514$	$p < 0.001$	$p < 0.001$
CTAS (Higher = less severe)	>	>	>
	$p < 0.005$	$p < 0.001$	$p < 0.001$
Hospital admissions	<	<	<
	$p < 0.001$	$p < 0.001$	$p < 0.001$

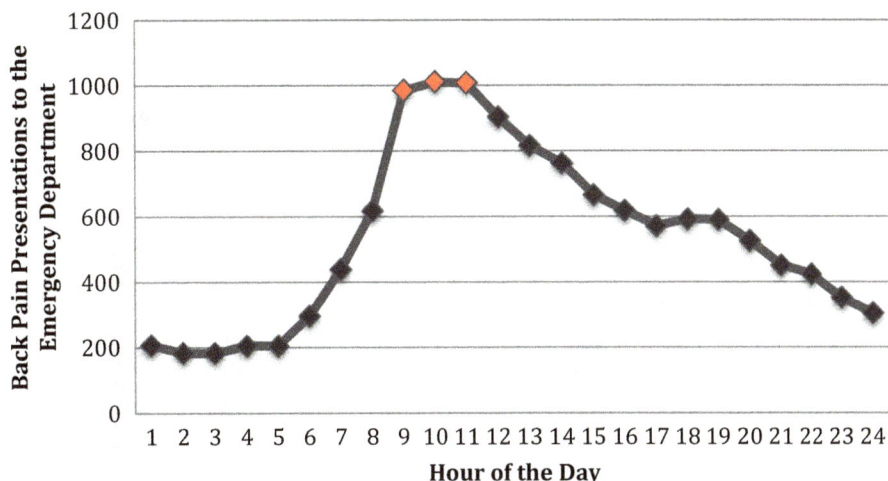

Fig. 2 Patient presentations for back pain by the hour of the day. The analysis includes data from all days of the week. Peak hours of presentation were between 9 and 11 AM

increasing severity of each definition of low back pain. This finding was both statistically and clinically significant. The findings strengthen our confidence and understanding of the severity of each of our definitions of low back pain, as they relate to the amount and urgency of care required for persons presenting with low back pain. We additionally found that for increasingly severe definitions of low back pain, length of stay increases, hospital admissions increase and so does median age of patients. We found that 27.4% of individuals diagnosed with low back pain with no potential nerve root involvement received x-rays. This result is similar to an analysis performed in the US [13], which found 30.5% of individuals received x-rays for back-related presentations to the emergency department. As we were not able to determine whether the x-rays were warranted,

further analysis is required, and could be done by examining the prevalence of individuals presenting with a complaint of back pain along with red flag symptoms.

Our exploration of trends in low back pain presentations to the emergency department over time found that the prevalence of low back pain has remained relatively stable over the six years of the study period. However, there has been a steady increase in the number of presentations for low back pain over the past six years. This indicates that the emergency department has had a relative increase in total patient presentations, including back pain, over the past six years. The increase in emergency department and back pain patients may be due to changes in primary care availability, an increase in population or a decrease in population health. Further research is needed to understand this result, in addition to a broader

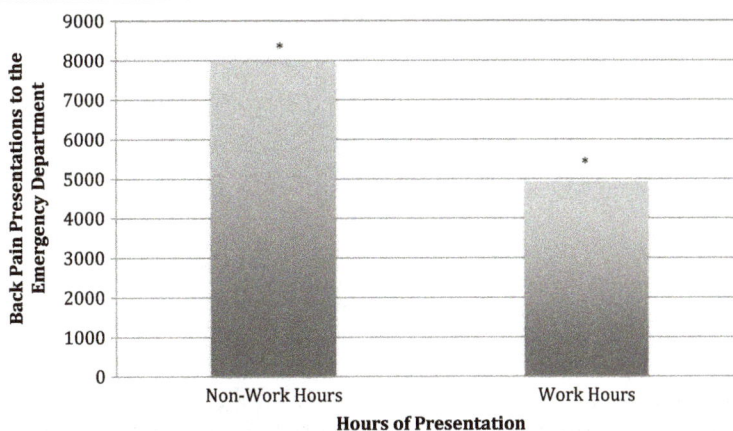

Fig. 3 Patients presenting with low back pain during typical work hours, defined as 9 am to 5 pm Monday to Friday (38.2%) and non-work hours (61.8%) ($p < 0.05$)

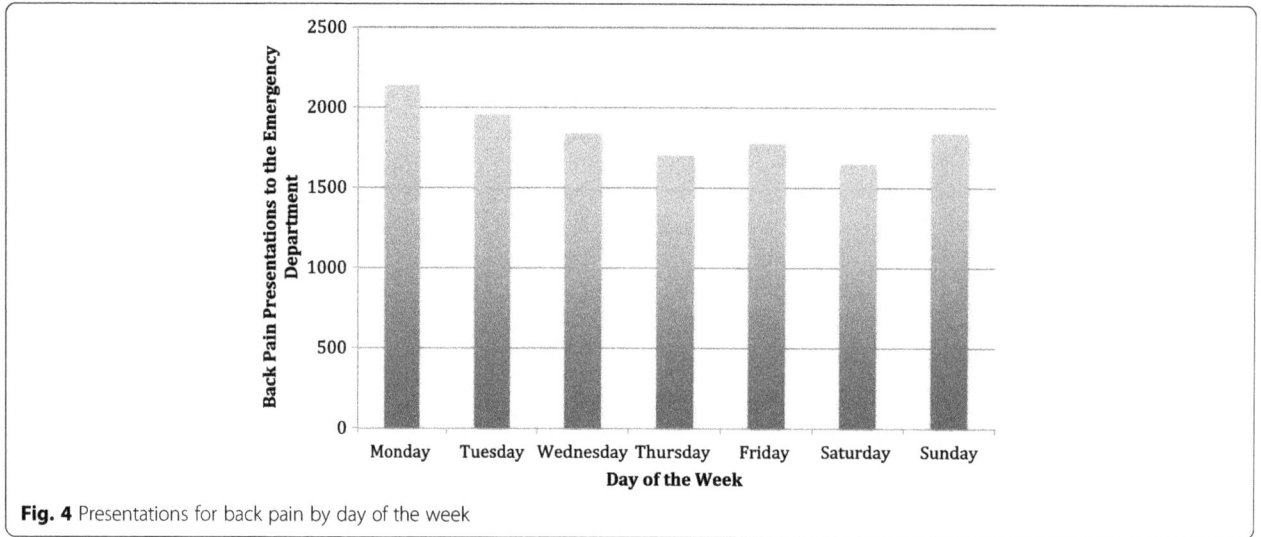

Fig. 4 Presentations for back pain by day of the week

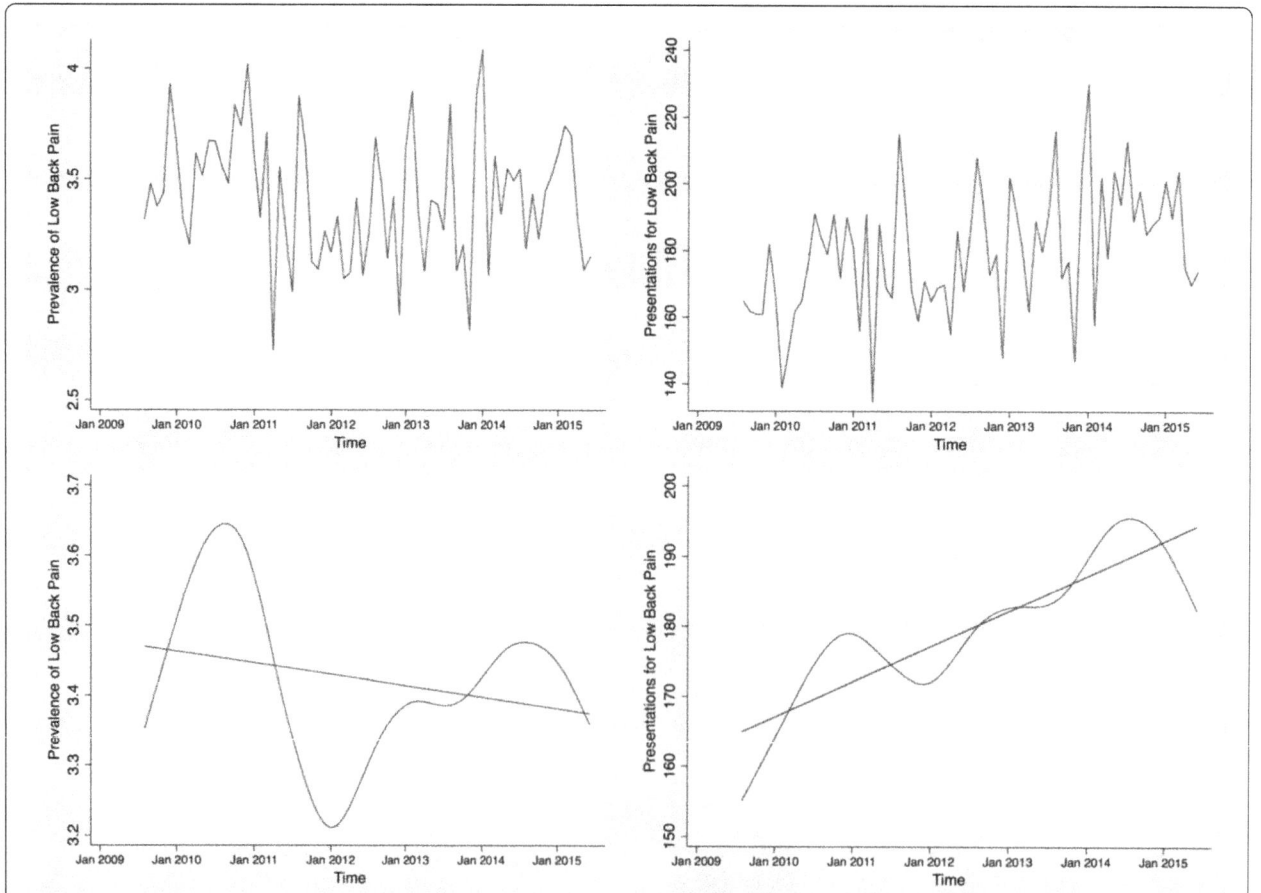

Fig. 5 Prevalence and absolute number of presentations of persons with a complaint of "back pain" or "traumatic back/spine injury" between July 2009 and July 2015 grouped by month. The top panels display raw data and the bottom panels report the smoothed trend analysis with a linear regression. For our estimates of prevalence, the linear regression resulted in a slope of − 0.001 and an R^2 value of 0.060. For our estimates of presentations, the linear regression resulted in a slope of 0.419 and an R^2 value of 0.787

exploration of the use of emergency settings to treat low back pain. A comparison between the treatment of low back pain in emergency settings and primary care settings would be useful to contextualize our findings, and provide insight into whether we should expect increases in presentations of low pain in emergency settings going forward.

Strengths and limitations

A strength of this study was the use of a sensitivity analysis to explore the robustness of our definition of low back pain with no potential nerve root involvement. As we found insignificant differences between the two definitions (prevalence, patient characteristics), we can be confident in the robustness of our definition.

Our use of specific definitions of low back pain will benefit future research exploring the economic impact of back pain. As our separate definitions represent various levels of severity and intervention, they additionally represent different levels of economic impact. Our use of these definitions will provide a better picture of the economic burden of back pain in the emergency department.

We may be underestimating our prevalence estimate of low back pain, as we limited our study population to patients presenting with back pain. Because we used EDIS presenting complaint data to define our study population, our study does not include individuals who did not present with a complaint of back pain, however, left the emergency department with a diagnosis compatible with low back pain.

The accuracy of the presenting and diagnostic codes used in the emergency department administrative data (EDIS) is currently unknown. There may be differences between patient charts and what is recorded in the administrative dataset. The confidence in our results could be improved by performing a validity and reliability study on the EDIS database by comparing results from the database to patient charts [6].

Finally, the results of our study may not be generalizable to other parts of Canada, due to provincial differences in the population of patients seeking care for low back pain in the emergency department; for example socioeconomic status and the availability of emergency health services, as well as the structure of the health care system in Nova Scotia. We recommend that future research address this issue by analyzing prevalence in other emergency settings in Canada, including rural settings.

Conclusions

Back pain is a common presenting complaint to emergency departments. Most individuals presenting with back pain are diagnosed with low back pain with no potential of nerve root involvement; however, we found that some individuals who present with back pain are discharged with other diagnoses. Moving forward,

grouping patients using specific diagnostic codes would help us to better understand the prevalence of low back pain and its economic impact on the emergency department. Canadian research on the topic should include rural settings, where back pain is unexplored. In our local setting, future research should examine the increasing trend in presentations of low back pain and the impact of primary care service access on the prevalence of low back pain in the emergency department. We should also concentrate on understanding the management of low back pain in this setting, to ensure this is the proper setting and approach to manage this common condition.

Abbreviations
CIHI: Canadian Institute of Health Information; CTAS: Canadian Triage and Acuity Scale; EDIS: Emergency Department Information System; ICD: International Classification of Disease; US: United States

Acknowledgements
To Rachel Ogilvie, Andrea Smith, and David Urquhart thank you for all the incredible support and guidance on this work.

Funding
Funding for this study was kindly provided by the Maritime SPOR Support Unit Graduate Scholarship (JE). The larger project was supported by a QEII Foundation TRIC Grant. The funding body did not play a role in study design, analysis, interpretation of the data, or the writing of the manuscript.

Authors contributions
JE and JH conceived the study, designed the study and obtained research funding. MA and KM contributed to the study design and study objectives. JE cleaned and analyzed the data. JE and JH drafted the manuscript and all authors contributed to its revision. JE takes responsibility for the paper as a whole. All authors read and approved the final manuscript.

Competing interest
The authors declare that they have no competing interests.

Author details
[1]Department of Community Health & Epidemiology, Dalhousie University, Halifax, NS, Canada. [2]Department of Emergency Medicine, Charles V. Keating Emergency & Trauma Centre, Halifax, NS, Canada. [3]Department of Epidemiology & Biostatistics, Schulich School of Medicine & Dentistry, Western University, London, ON, Canada.

References
1. Bell JA, Burnett A. Exercise for the primary, secondary and tertiary prevention of low back pain in the workplace: a systematic review. J Occup Rehabil. 2009;19(1):8–24.
2. Walker BF. The prevalence of low back pain: a systematic review of the literature from 1966 to 1998. J Spinal Disord Tech. 2000;13(3):205–17.
3. Deyo RA, Mirza SK, Martin BI. Back pain prevalence and visit rates: estimates from US national surveys, 2002. Spine. 2006;31(23):2724–7.
4. Dagenais S, Caro J, Haldeman S. A systematic review of low back pain cost of illness studies in the United States and internationally. Spine. 2008;8(1):8–20.
5. Scott N, Moga C, Harstall C. Managing low back pain in the primary care setting: the know-do gap. Pain Research and Management. 2010;15(6):392–400.
6. Koes BW, van Tulder M, Lin CW, Macedo LG, McAuley J, Maher C. An updated overview of clinical guidelines for the management of non-specific low back pain in primary care. Eur Spine J. 2010;19(12):2075–94.
7. Edwards J, Hayden J, Asbridge M, Gregoire B, Magee K. Prevalence of low back pain in emergency settings: a systematic review and meta-analysis. BMC Musculoskelet Disord. 2017;18(1):143.

8. Highlights: Charles V. Keating Emergency and Trauma Centre, QEII Health Sciences Centre, Capital Health. Available: https://www.google.com/url?sa=t&rct=j&q=&esrc=s&source=web&cd=1&cad=rja&uact=8&ved=2ahUKEwip-emO7_vcAhWLmOAKHQuDDGkQFjAAegQIBRAC&url=https%3A%2F%2F www.cdha.nshealth.ca%2Fsystem%2Ffiles%2Fsites%2F5153%2Fdocuments% 2Fcharles-v-keating-emergency-amp-trauma-centre.pdf&usg=AOvVaw0c42 JiaHOq_DJBAjzH5E6X.

9. Canadian Association of Emergency Physicians 2015. Canadian Association of Emergency Physicians. Available: https://caep.ca/resources/cedis/.

10. Silman AJ, Jayson MI, Papageorgiou AC, Croft PR. Hospital referrals for low back pain: more coherence needed. J R Soc Med. 2000;93(3):135–7.

11. Niska R, Bhuiya F. Xu J. National hospital ambulatory medical care survey: 2007 emergency department summary. Natl Health Stat Report. 2010;26(26):1–31.

12. Colman, Ronald, and Karen Hayward. Cost of chronic disease in Nova Scotia. GPI Atlantic 2002. Available: https://www.google.com/url?sa=t&rct=j&q= &esrc=s&source=web&cd=1&cad=rja&uact=8&ved=2ahUKEwiViZWO8PvcAh VHNd8KHS_ZCEoQFjAAegQIABAC&url=https%3A%2F%2Fnovascotia. ca%2Fdhw%2Fpublications%2Fcost_chronic_X_6c9Biyg3.

13. Friedman BW, Chilstrom M, Bijur PE, Gallagher EJ. Diagnostic testing and treatment of low back pain in US emergency departments. A national perspective. Spine. 2010;35(24):E1406.

14. Chou R, Qaseem A, Snow V, Casey D, Cross JT, Shekelle P, Owens DK. Diagnosis and treatment of low back pain: a joint clinical practice guideline from the American College of Physicians and the American pain society. Ann Intern Med. 2007;147(7):478–91.

15. Von Korff M, Saunders K. The course of back pain in primary care. Spine. 1996;21(24):2833–7.

16. Cleveland RB, Cleveland WS, McRae JE, Terpenning ISTL. A seasonal-trend decomposition procedure based on loess. J Off Stat. 1990;6(1):3–73.

17. Nau R. Notes on the random walk model: Fuqua School of Business; 2014.

18. Thiruganasambandamoorthy V, Turko E, Ansell D, Vaidyanathan A, Wells GA, Stiell IG. Risk factors for serious underlying pathology in adult emergency department nontraumatic low back pain patients. The Journal of emergency medicine. 2014;47(1):1–1.

19. Kocher KE, Meurer WJ, Fazel R, Scott PA, Krumholz HM, Nallamothu BK. National trends in use of computed tomography in the emergency department. Ann Emerg Med. 2011;58(5):452–62.

20. Canadian Institute for Health Information, A Snapshot of Health Care in Canada as Demonstrated by Top 10 Lists, 2011 (Ottawa, Ont.: CIHI, 2012). Available: https://www.google.com/url?sa=t&rct=j&q=&esrc=s&source= web&cd=2&cad=rja&uact=8&ved=2ahUKEwjVwdWm8PvcAhUDNd8KHX3-DEIQFjABegQICRAC&url=https%3A%2F%2Fsecure.cihi.ca%2Ffree_ products%2FTop10ReportEN-Web.pdf&usg=AOvVaw1nGxRUYceOK-- 1pwiVWO_q.

16

Congenital limb deficiency in Japan: a cross-sectional nationwide survey on its epidemiology

Hiroshi Mano[1†], Sayaka Fujiwara[1†], Kazuyuki Takamura[3], Hiroshi Kitoh[4], Shinichiro Takayama[5], Tsutomu Ogata[6], Shuji Hashimoto[7] and Nobuhiko Haga[1,2*]

Abstract

Background: Congenital limb deficiency is a rare and intractable disease, which impairs both function and appearance of the limbs. To establish adequate medical care, it is necessary to reveal the actual conditions and problems associated with this disease. However, there have been no extensive epidemiological surveys in Japan addressing this disease. This is the first nationwide epidemiological survey of congenital limb deficiency in this country.

Methods: With the cooperation of epidemiology experts, we performed a two-stage nationwide survey to estimate the number of patients with congenital limb deficiency and reveal basic patient features. We targeted orthopaedic surgery, paediatric, and plastic surgery departments. Hospitals were categorized according to the institution type and the number of hospital beds; hospitals were randomly selected from these categories. We selected 2283 departments from a total 7825 departments throughout Japan. In this study, we defined congenital limb deficiency as partial or total absence of the limbs, proximal to the proximal interphalangeal joint of the fingers/lesser toes or interphalangeal joint of the thumb/great toe. We distributed the first survey querying the number of initial patient visits from January 2014 to December 2015. Targets of the second survey were departments that reported one or more initial patient visits in the first survey.

Results: In the first survey, 1767 departments responded (response rate: 77.4%). Among them, 161 departments reported one or more initial patient visits. We conducted the second survey among these 161 departments, of which 96 departments responded (response rate: 59.6%). The estimated number of initial visits by patients with congenital limb deficiency was 417 (95% confidence interval: 339–495) per year in 2014 and 2015. The estimated prevalence of congenital limb deficiency in Japan was 4.15 (95% confidence interval: 3.37–4.93) per 10,000 live births. The sex ratio was 1.40. Upper limbs were more affected than lower limbs.

Conclusions: We revealed the estimated number of initial patient visits per year and birth prevalence of congenital limb deficiency in Japan. Our results will contribute to establishing the disease concept and grades of severity of congenital limb deficiency.

Keywords: Congenital limb deficiency, Epidemiology, Cross-sectional study, Nationwide survey, Birth prevalence

* Correspondence: hagan-reh@h.u-tokyo.ac.jp
†Hiroshi Mano and Sayaka Fujiwara contributed equally to this work.
[1]Department of Rehabilitation Medicine, The University of Tokyo Hospital, Tokyo, Japan
[2]Department of Rehabilitation Medicine, Graduate School of Medicine, The University of Tokyo, Tokyo, Japan
Full list of author information is available at the end of the article

Background

In developed countries, paediatric limb deficiencies are primarily congenital, and result from various causes and phenotypes. Causal factors include environmental insults, such as owing to chemicals and pharmaceuticals, and chromosomal or genetic defects. Thalidomide, warfarin, valproic acid, and phenytoin are well known as causal drugs of limb deficiencies [1]. Some genetic factors associated with hypoplastic limb defects and split hand/split foot malformation have been identified [2]. The prevalence of congenital limb deficiencies is reportedly 4.91 per 10,000 live births in South America (1967–1992) [3], 5.5 per 10,000 total births in Alberta, Canada (1980–2012) [4], and 6.9 per 10,000 total births in Northern Netherlands (1991–2010) [5]. According to the International Clearinghouse for Birth Defects Monitoring Systems (ICBDMS), the prevalence of congenital limb deficiency in Japan is reportedly 3.81 per 10,000 total births (2007–2011) [6]. Although some breakdown has been reported (transverse: 0.29; pre axial: 0.90; post axial: 0.25; intercalary: 1.04; mixed: 0.90; unspecified: 0.43 per 10,000 total births), distinctions between upper or lower limbs, laterality, and other details (e.g., level of transverse deficiency) have not been demonstrated. In addition, it seems difficult to make precise diagnoses at birth in some patients. Regarding anomalies of the upper limbs in the Japanese population, Ogino et al. reported incidences and details such as affected side, associated anomalies, and family history [7]; however, these anomalies consisted mostly of deformities without limb deficiency or reduction such as trigger finger, polydactyly, camptodactyly and clasped thumb, and the situation for deficiency only was uncertain.

Congenital limb deficiency is a rare and intractable disease, and these patients require consecutive care from birth, through the stages of growth, and up to adulthood. However, in Japan, medical care and education systems have been inadequate for affected children. In considering therapeutic approaches, it is necessary to include both the function and appearance of the defect. Treatment approaches vary according to the type of deficiency. For example, children with congenital unilateral transverse upper limb deficiencies are often prescribed prostheses [8]. For radial deficiency, surgeries such as wrist centralization on the ulna and reconstruction of the thumb are the treatment choices [9]. In proximal focal femoral deficiency, surgeries including amputation or rotationplasty may be considered to optimise prosthetic fitting and function [10]. There is debate regarding which surgical approach to choose in certain situations. For example, for Jones type 1a tibial deficiency, one surgical approach is tibial centralization surgery (Brown's procedure), to reconstruct the function of the knee-joint [11]. Another procedure is knee disarticulation to fit a prosthesis [12]. Regarding fibular dysplasia, one approach is foot reconstruction followed by limb-lengthening surgery, to preserve the affected limb; another is Syme's amputation procedure, followed by a prosthetic fitting [13, 14].

In Japan, nationwide epidemiological surveys have been performed in patients with various intractable diseases [15] such as familial Mediterranean fever [16], Moyamoya disease [17, 18], Churg–Strauss syndrome [19], adult Still's syndrome [20], Sjögren's syndrome [21], paediatric acquired demyelinating syndrome [22], and pancreatitis [23, 24]; however, congenital limb deficiency has not been studied in detail. To provide better evidence-based medical care, it is necessary to establish the concept of congenital limb deficiency and its grades of severity. In this study, we aimed to clarify the actual condition of congenital limb deficiency in Japan.

Methods

With the cooperation of the Research Committee on the Epidemiology of Intractable Diseases of Japan, we conducted a two-stage postal survey according to the *Nationwide Epidemiological Survey Manual of Patients with Intractable Diseases* (2nd edition 2006, Ministry of Health, Labour and Welfare of Japan).

This nationwide survey consisted of a first survey, in which the number of patients was estimated, and a second survey, in which basic clinical features were investigated. To achieve a high response rate, it was important to use a simple questionnaire. We confined the first survey to only a query of the number of patients who completed an initial visit. In the second survey, we requested the ages, symptoms, diagnostic details, associated anomalies, family histories of patients, and the previous hospitals and referral to other hospitals as the minimum of demographic and clinical information.

A list of all hospitals in Japan was obtained from the Research Committee on the Epidemiology of Intractable Diseases of Japan. The departments of orthopaedic surgery, paediatrics, and plastic surgery were extracted and subjected to stratified random sampling. Hospitals were categorized according to the institution type and number of hospital beds. Departments were randomly selected from these hospital categories; sampling rates were determined as approximately 5, 10, 20, 40, 80, and 100% for the stratum of general hospitals with 20–99 beds, 100–199 beds, 200–299 beds, 300–399 beds, 400–499 beds, and 500 or more beds, respectively. As the departments that most commonly treat patients with congenital limb deficiency, departments belonging to "the Japanese Association of Children's Hospitals and Related Institutions" and "Rehabilitation Centers for Children with Physical Disabilities" were classified as "special stratum", and all of these were selected for the survey.

Other departments that could not be classified under any of the three departments above (i.e., hospitals in which medical care was provided by a specially associated group of multi-departments) were classified as "other special stratum," and were selected for the survey.

From this selection, 2283 departments (995 orthopaedic surgery departments, 812 paediatric departments, 472 plastic surgery departments), and four special departments were selected from a total of 7825 departments throughout Japan. In May 2016, we distributed the first survey querying the number of initial patient visits from January 2014 to December 2015. In this study, we defined congenital limb deficiency as partial or total absence of the limbs, proximal to the proximal interphalangeal joint of the fingers/lesser toes or interphalangeal joint of the thumb/great toe. We focused on deficiencies that cause relatively severe impairment and disability, for which treatment approaches have been discussed; therefore, we excluded deficits of the middle and distal phalanges. Polydactyly, syndactyly, and malformation or shortening of the limbs without deficit were also excluded from this study.

The targets of the second survey were departments that reported one or more initial patient visits in the first survey. In September 2016, we distributed the second survey querying patient details. In the second survey, patients who were ineligible, those who were not eligible because of their diagnosis or the time of their initial visit, and duplicate patients who were reported by two or more departments, were determined. Patients were identified as duplicated if their information (age, sex, diagnosis, and referral) was consistent among two or more departments. For duplicate patients, we included the data of their latest initial visit at the most recent, to obtain a more precise diagnosis and more detailed information. If a patient had visited more than one hospital during a short time, it is reasonable to think that the first institution saw the necessity for a more precise diagnosis or specialized medical treatment, such as a surgical procedure or prosthesis, and consulted a specialized department and that the most recent institution provided them with medical care. We identified the department for the date of the most recent initial visit as the actual institution that provided medical treatment at that time.

Statistics

The method used to estimate the number of patients is as follows [25, 26]:

Let n be the number of all departments, and n_i be the number of departments with a number of targeted patients i ($i = 0, 1, ...$). Let N be the number of responding departments and N_i be the number of responding departments with a number of patients i ($i = 0, 1, ...$). N and N_i were obtained from the survey, and $\{N_i\}$ followed a multi-hypergeometric distribution under the assumption of random response and under the condition that N is fixed.

Let a be the total number of patients; note that $a = \Sigma$ $i*n_i$. The estimate of a was calculated as.

$$a^\wedge = \sum i * N_i * n/N.$$

The approximate 95% confidence intervals for a were calculated as.

$$(a^\wedge - 1.96\, s, a^\wedge + 1.96\, s),$$

where s is an estimate of standard error of $a^\wedge$ and is given to be.

$$s = \sqrt{\frac{\sum i^2 * \frac{N_i}{N} - \left(\sum i * \frac{N_i}{N}\right)^2}{n-1} * n^3 \left(\frac{1}{N} - \frac{1}{n}\right)}.$$

The number of patients in some strata was estimated using the above method. Let k be the number of strata, $a_1^\wedge, a_2^\wedge, ..., a_k^\wedge$ be the estimated numbers of patients in some strata, and $s_1, s_2, ..., s_k$ be their standard errors. The approximate confidence intervals for the sum of the number of patients in the strata were calculated as.

$$(a.^\wedge - 1.96\, s., a.^\wedge + 1.96\, s.),$$

where $a. = a_1^\wedge + a_2^\wedge + ... + a_k^\wedge$ and $s = \sqrt{s_1^2 + s_2^2 + ... + s_k^2}$.

Using the results of the first survey, the number of patients and 95% confidence intervals were estimated using the above procedure. Additionally, we corrected these using the ineligibility rate and duplication rate from the second survey. To obtain the final estimates and confidence intervals, we multiplied their values in the first survey by "1 – ineligibility rate" and "1 – duplication rate", respectively.

Statistical analysis was performed using JMP® Pro 13.0.0 (SAS Institute Japan) and $p < 0.05$ was considered significant.

Results
Estimation of the number of patients

Table 1 summarizes the results of the first survey and shows the corrected number of patients with the results of the second survey. Of 2283 departments selected from the 7825 departments in Japan, 1767 responded to the first questionnaire concerning the number of patients with initial visits who had congenital limb deficiency: the response rate for the first survey was 77.4%. Details of the number of all, surveyed, and responding departments are shown in Additional file 1. Among them, 161 departments reported one or more patients

Table 1 Number of total, surveyed, and responded departments, and estimated number of patients

Strata	Total Number of Departments	Number of Surveyed Departments	Sampling rate (%)	Number of Responded Departments	Response Rate (%)	Estimated Number of Patients	95% Confidence Interval		
First Survey									
Orthopedic surgery									
University hospital	133	133	100.0	120	90.2	104	87	–	121
General hospital									
≧500 beds	201	201	100.0	155	77.1	25	16	–	33
400–499 beds	213	170	79.8	135	79.4	0	0	–	0
300–399 beds	343	137	39.9	104	75.9	7	0	–	14
200–299 beds	391	79	20.2	59	74.7	0	0	–	0
100–199 beds	1006	100	9.9	75	75.0	40	0	–	96
≦99 beds	1950	96	4.9	64	66.7	0	0	–	0
Special stratum	79	79	100.0	65	82.3	290	230	–	351
Subtotal	4316	995	23.1	777	78.1	466	381	–	551
Pediatrics									
University hospital	125	125	100.0	106	84.8	24	18	–	29
General hospital									
≧500 beds	189	189	100.0	152	80.4	25	18	–	31
400–499 beds	193	154	79.8	128	83.1	8	3	–	12
300–399 beds	302	121	40.1	93	76.9	97	0	–	230
200–299 beds	297	60	20.2	51	85.0	12	0	–	26
100–199 beds	486	48	9.9	33	68.8	0	0	–	0
≦99 beds	786	39	5.0	29	74.4	0	0	–	0
Special stratum	76	76	100.0	50	65.8	15	6	–	25
Subtotal	2454	812	33.1	642	79.1	180	47	–	314
Plastic surgery									
University hospital	89	89	100.0	68	76.4	47	35	–	60
General hospital									
≧500 beds	157	157	100.0	107	68.2	129	6	–	252
400–499 beds	125	100	80.0	75	75.0	30	10	–	50
300–399 beds	127	52	40.9	38	73.1	7	0	–	14

Table 1 Number of total, surveyed, and responded departments, and estimated number of patients *(Continued)*

Strata	Total Number of Departments	Number of Surveyed Departments	Sampling rate (%)	Number of Responded Departments	Response Rate (%)	Estimated Number of Patients	95% Confidence Interval	
200–299 beds	126	25	19.8	20	80.0	0	0 – 0	
100–199 beds	186	19	10.2	13	68.4	0	0 – 0	
≦99 beds	222	11	5.0	8	72.7	0	0 – 0	
Special stratum	19	19	100.0	15	78.9	46	28 – 63	
Subtotal	1051	472	44.9	344	72.9	259	132 – 385	
Other special stratum	4	4	100.0	4	100.0	179	179 – 179	
Total	7825	2283	29.2	1767	77.4	1084	881 – 1287	
Total (per year)						542	441 – 643	
Second Survey								
Total (per year) [a]						417	339 – 495	
Total (per 10,000 live births) [b]						4.15	3.37 – 4.93	

[a]The estimated number of patients and 95% confidence interval was corrected with ineligible rate and duplication rate
[b]We estimated with the assumption that the number of live birth was 1.005million

with an initial visit. We then conducted the second survey among these 161 departments. Ninety-six departments responded to the second questionnaire concerning demographic and clinical information; the response rate for the second survey was 59.6%. Of these 96 departments, whereas a total number of 534 patients had an initial visit in the first survey, 491 patients with initial visits were recorded in the second survey. This difference of 43 patients was considered to represent ineligible patients and those excluded by the target departments. Some departments reported the reasons for exclusion as follows: intermixing of patients whose initial visit did not fall within the target period or did not fit the diagnosis (e.g., patients with acquired limb defects) in the first survey. Of the 491 patients, we excluded 38 ineligible patients and 42 duplicated patients; finally, 411 patients were eligible for inclusion in the analysis of demographic and clinical information. Of the 38 ineligible patients, 27 did not fall within the target period and 11 did not fit the diagnosis (4 patients had deficits of only the middle and/or distal phalanx, 4 had brachydactyly without deficits, 2 had constriction band without deficits, and 1 patient had polydactyly). The ineligibility rate was 15.2% and the duplication rate was 9.3%.

We estimated that the number of initial visits of patients with congenital limb deficiency between 2014 and 2015 was 417 per year, (95% confidence interval 339–495). Considering that at the initial visit, most patients were aged 0 years, and that the number of live births in Japan was 1.004 million in 2014 and 1.006 in 2015, we estimated the prevalence of congenital limb deficiency with the assumption that the number of live births was 1.005 million (average of 2014 and 2015). The estimated prevalence was 4.15 (95% confidence interval 3.37–4.93) per 10,000 live births.

Sex ratio

Among 411 patients reported in the second survey, there were 240 males and 171 females; the sex ratio was 1.40. Assuming an equal sex ratio (50% male, 50% female), a chi-square test yielded $\chi^2 = 11.58$, and $p = 0.0007$. This result suggests that males have a significantly higher prevalence of congenital limb deficiency than females.

Age

Table 2 summarizes the age of patients at their initial visit. Congenital limb deficiencies develop during the foetal stage, or before birth. The age reflects the patients' access to medical care. It is necessary to consider that in cases of duplication, we included data for the date of the most recent initial visit to a department. A total 276 (67.2%) patients visited the hospital at age 0 years. The number of patients with initial visits decreased with advancing age.

Affected limbs

Among 411 patients reported in the second survey, 275 (66.9%) had one affected limb, 83 (20.2%) had two, 23 (5.6%) had three, and 30 (7.3%) had four affected limbs. There were 275 patients (66.9%) with only the upper

Table 2 Patient age at the initial visit

Age	Number of Patients	%
0	276	67.2
1	39	9.5
2	22	5.4
3	18	4.4
4	9	2.2
5	10	2.4
6	6	1.5
7	5	1.2
8	4	1.0
9	3	0.7
10	2	0.5
≥11	12	2.9
Unknown	5	1.2
Total	411	100

limbs affected, 75 (18.2%) with only lower limbs affected, and 61 (14.8%) with both upper and lower limbs affected.

The 411 patients had a total of 630 affected limbs among them. Four limbs had different classifications of deficiency (a total of 634 limb deficiencies) and all four affected limbs had coexisting proximal femoral focal deficiency and fibular dysplasia. Affected limbs were as follows: 218 (34.6%) were right upper limbs, 224 (35.6%) were left upper limbs, 105 (16.7%) were right lower limbs, and 83 (13.2%) were left lower limbs.

Classification of limb deficiency

Table 3 summarizes the classification of limb deficiency. For upper limbs deficiencies, transverse deficiency was the most prevalent (45.5%), followed by longitudinal deficiency(31.2%). For lower limbs deficiency, longitudinal deficiency was the most prevalent (37.0%), followed by transverse deficiency(31.8%). For longitudinal deficiency, whereas there was not much difference between tibial deficiency (33 limbs) and fibular deficiency (37 limbs) in the lower limbs, radial deficiency (110 limbs) was more prevalent than ulnar deficiency (27 limbs) in the upper limbs. For transverse deficiency, both upper limbs and lower limbs had similar tendencies in that distal deficiency comprised a large proportion and proximal deficiency was less frequent. The prevalence rates of intercalary, central, and other finger column deficiency were similar for both upper and lower limbs.

Associated anomalies

Coexisting disorders with relatively high prevalence (over 1%), were cardiac anomaly, vertebral anomaly, renal anomaly, anal atresia, hypospadias, cleft lip/palate and developmental disorders (autism spectrum syndrome or attention deficit hyperactivity disorder) (10.2, 3.6, 2.4, 2.4, 2.2, 1.2, and 1.0% respectively). Eleven patients had chromosomal abnormality: 3 had 17p-related

Table 3 Classification of congenital limb deficiency

	Upper limbs			Lower Limbs			Total	
		Number of deficiencies	%		Number of deficiencies	%	Number of deficiencies	%
Longitudinal	Radial deficiency	110	24.9	Tibial deficiency	33	17.2		
	Ulnar deficiency	27	6.1	Fibular deficiency	37	19.3		
	Not classifiable	1	0.2	Not classifiable	1	0.5		
	Subtotal	138	31.2	Subtotal	71	37.0	209	33.0
Transverse	Shoulder, Upper arm, Elbow	16	3.6	Hip, Thigh, Knee	2	1.0		
	Forearm, Wrist	41	9.3	Lower leg, Ankle	4	2.1		
	Hand	141	31.9	Foot	54	28.1		
	Unknown	3	0.7	Unknown	1	0.5		
	Subtotal	201	45.5	Subtotal	61	31.8	262	41.3
Intercalary	Phocomelia	5	1.1	Proximal femoral focal deficiency	7	3.6		
	Subtotal	5	1.1	Subtotal	7	3.6	12	1.9
Central	Split hand	75	17.0	Split foot	32	16.7		
	Subtotal	75	17.0	Subtotal	32	16.7	107	16.9
Other finger column deficiency		23	5.2		21	10.9	44	6.9
Total		442	100		192	100	634	100

abnormalities (duplication, microduplication and deletion), 4 had trisomy 21, 1 had trisomy 18, 1 had 48 XXXX, and 2 patients unspecified chromosomal abnormalities. Seventeen patients were diagnosed with or suspected of having the following specific syndromes, associations or sequences: 5 patients had VATER association, 4 had Poland syndrome (1 patient concomitantly had Moebius syndrome), 2 had Cornelia de Lange syndrome, and 1 each, had Apert syndrome, CHARGE syndrome, FATCO syndrome, KOSAKI syndrome, Leri-Weill syndrome, Nager syndrome, Silver-Russell syndrome, facioauriculovertebral sequence, and autosomal dominant epidermolysis bullosa dystrophica (we excluded amniotic bands syndrome). Approximately 66.4% of patients had no coexisting disorders.

Family history

Seventeen (4.1%) patients had a family history of congenital limb deficiency, and 165 (40.1%) had no such history. The family histories of 229 (55.7%) patients were unknown. The extent of family history was left to the discretion of each department.

Table 4 shows the details of 17 patients with a positive family history of congenital limb deficiency. The breakdown of these 17 patients was as follows: 9 with split hand deformity; 3 with ulnar deficiency; 2 each with upper limb transverse deficiency, split foot, and tibial deficiency; and 1 each with radial deficiency, lower limb transverse deficiency, and other finger column deficiency. Four patients had multiple types of deficiencies: 1 each with split hand and foot, split hand and tibial deficiency, ulnar deficiency and split foot, and ulnar deficiency and tibial deficiency. Most columns in the questionnaire requiring information about the limb deficiency of family members were left blank; therefore, we could not identify whether the type of deficiencies were the same for these patients.

Discussion

This is the first study providing the detailed epidemiology of congenital limb deficiency in Japan. We achieved a higher response rate (77.4%) for the first survey than the 34–74% of similar studies conducted in Japan [16–24]. This may reflect an interest in limb deficiency by orthopaedic surgeons, paediatricians, and plastic surgeons. The estimated prevalence of congenital limb deficiency in Japan of the present study was similar to that of previous studies in other countries [3–5].

Table 4 Details of patients with a positive family history of congenital limb deficiency

Child	Deficiency of the limb	Associated anomaly	Relation of the relative	Limb anomaly of the relative
1	split hand of right upper limb	none	sibling	(not reported)
2	split hand of right upper limb	none	sibling	(not reported)
3	split hand of right upper limb	none	sibling	(not reported)
4	split hand of right upper limb	none	sibling	(not reported)
5	split hand of both upper limbs and split foot of both lower limbs	none	sibling	(not reported)
6	radial deficiency of left upper limb	Fanconi's anemia	sibling	(not reported)
7	ulnar deficiency of right upper limb	none	sibling	(not reported)
8	transverse deficiency at the level of hand of right upper limb	none	sibling	(not reported)
9	split hand of right upper limb	none	mother	anomalies of radius and ulna
10	split hand of right upper limb	none	father	split hand
11	split hand of both upper limbs	none	father	split hand
12	split hand of left upper limb and tibial deficiency of both lower limbs	none	granduncle	split hand
13	split foot of right lower limb	none	someone other than sibling	(not reported)
14	ulnar deficiency of both upper limbs and split foot of both lower limbs	Leri-Weill syndrome	mother	Madelung deformity, and Leri-Weill syndrome
15	ulnar deficiency of both upper limbs and tibial deficiency of both lower limbs	none	mother and grandmother	upper limb anomaly
16	transverse deficiency at the level of hand of right upper limb	none	relative on the mother's side	toe defect
17	transverse deficiency at the level of foot of both lower limbs	none	father and grandfather on the father's side	anomaly of fifth finger

Whereas the duplication rate in this study seemed reasonable, the ineligibility rate seemed somewhat high. Similar surveys have reported low duplication rates, and the ineligibility rates varied by disease (2.3–13.2%) [17, 18, 20, 21]. One possible reason for the high ineligibility rate in this study was the inconsistent responses by some departments regarding the number of patients who had completed an initial visit and the total number of patients. In similar surveys in Japan, the number of patients and the number of initial patient visits, or only the number of patients were usually requested. In this study, to achieve a high response rate, we only queried the number of initial patient visits, which might have confused respondents.

The prevalence value was also similar to that reported in Japan by ICBDMS [6]; however the classification of congenital limb deficiency was different, especially for intercalary deficiency. In this study, intercalary deficiency included phocomelia and proximal femoral focal deficiency. In the ICBDMS report, a definition of "intercalary" was not available and the "limb reduction defects" did not include "central reduction." These differences in definitions may have influenced the results of our survey. Our results were more similar to those of a study in the Northern Netherlands that reported fewer number of intercalary reduction defects than transverse, longitudinal, and central reduction defects [5].

The sex ratio was 1.40 in this study, which is similar to a study in Alberta, Canada, including 434 male and 344 female patients [4].

For most patients, the initial visit to the most recent institution was made at age 0 years, and the number of initial patient visits decreased with advancing age. Most congenital limb deficiencies are noted at birth, even if they are not diagnosed in detail; however, therapeutic interventions are rarely required in the neonatal period. No radical surgeries or therapies are normally carried out. It is recommended that the first fitting of prostheses commence at about age 6–9 months in children with limb deficiencies [27]; however, prosthetic therapy often begins later in Japan. In particular, prostheses for children with congenital upper limb deficiencies have not been sufficiently prescribed [28]. In our study, we assumed that there were patients who were untreated or were only followed-up without therapy and that some of them visited a specialized hospital for surgeries or prosthetic therapy or sought a second opinion during childhood or later in life.

Upper limbs were more affected than lower limbs in the present study. Previous studies showed the same tendency [4, 5]. Commonly associated anomalies in our survey were cardiac anomaly, vertebral anomaly, renal anomaly, anal atresia, hypospadias, and cleft lip/palate. The study in the Northern Netherlands also indicated cardiovascular anomalies and urinary tract anomalies as anomalies that are frequently present with reduction defects [5]. The specific syndromes, associations, or sequences diagnosed or suspected in more than one patient were already known to be associated with congenital limb deficiency. Considering the data thus far, we feel certain about the validity of the present results.

Seventeen (4.1%) patients had a family history of congenital limb deficiency; however, the family history of 229 (55.7%) patients was unknown. Possible reasons for the substantial number of patients with unknown family histories include the following:

(1) The respondent may have completed the survey in detail, but the family history was truly unknown.

(2) Although respondents reported that there was no family history, the extent was insufficient (e.g., only parents were known to have no limb deficiency, but this information for grandparents was unknown), and the respondent thought it was inadequate to consider as not-existence.

(3) The respondents were too busy to complete the survey in detail.

If patients with "unknown" family histories were excluded, the prevalence of patients with a family history of congenital limb deficiency was 9.3%. It seems reasonable that the prevalence was estimated at 4–10% in this study. Most patients with a family history were those with split hand (a portion of these patients were associated with split foot or tibial deficiency). We speculate that split hand might have a stronger relationship with genetic factors than other limb deficiencies, such as transverse deficiency, of which constriction band is one cause. This is consistent with a study that identified the genetic factor associated with split hand/foot malformation and Gollop-Wolfgang complex (association with split hand and tibial deficiency) among Japanese patients [29]; this is also in keeping with the fact that most split hand/foot malformation, including Gollop-Wolfgang complex, present an autosomal dominant pattern of inheritance [2]. Another speculation is that patients with split hand procreate more frequently than those with other limb deficiencies; further study of this relationship is warranted.

The present survey was cross-sectional and involved analyses of demographics, and clinical information such as prevalence and classification. To promote the development of therapeutic approaches and social support of patients with congenital limb deficiency, further surveys based on the results of this study are required. A longitudinal survey is expected to reveal the actual conditions and challenges throughout life among these patients, such as education, employment, marriage, and reproduction.

Limitations

Although the response rate for the first survey was high (77.4%), the ineligibility rate (15.2%) in the second survey seemed somewhat high. The main reason for exclusion was that the time of the initial visit did not correspond with the target period. In addition, there were some patients who did not fit the appropriate definition of congenital limb deficiency used in this study (defined as partial or total absence of the limbs proximal to the proximal interphalangeal joint of fingers/lesser toes or interphalangeal joint of the thumb/great toe). The disease concept of congenital limb deficiency has not been established in Japan. The estimates number in the present study may have been overestimated or underestimated, or may have changed in accordance with the definition used for this disease.

Conclusions

We estimated the prevalence of congenital limb deficiency in Japan to be 4.15 (95% confidence interval 3.37–4.93) per 10,000 live births. Upper limbs were more affected than lower limbs. For upper limbs, transverse deficiency was the most prevalent, followed by longitudinal deficiency. For lower limbs, longitudinal deficiency was the most prevalent, followed by transverse deficiency. We also revealed information of the sex ratio, age at initial visit, associated anomalies, and family history. Although we believe that our results will contribute to establishing the disease concept and grades of severity of this disease, further surveys, especially longitudinal ones, will be needed to promote the development of therapeutic approaches and social support for patients with congenital limb deficiency.

Acknowledgements
We acknowledged the Ministry of Health, Labour, and Welfare for supporting this work. We are grateful to the occupational therapist, Satoko Noguchi for her contribution to clerical work.

Funding
This work was supported by research grants on Rare and Intractable Diseases of the Ministry of Health, Labour and Welfare of Japan [grant number H26-Nanchitou(Nan)-Ippan-089 and H27-Nanchitou(Nan)-Ippan-036], and by JSPS KAKENHI Grant Number 18K17890. The funder had no role in study design, data collection and analysis, decision to publish, or preparation of the manuscript.

Authors' contributions
The questionnaire of the survey was prepared by SF, KT, HK, ST, TO and NH. Epidemiological advice and ascertainment were provided by SH. The dispatch and receipt of questionnaire were performed by HM, SF, and NH. The analysis was performed by HM. The paper was written by HM and SF with equal contribution. All authors read and approved the final manuscript.

Competing interests
The authors declare that they have no competing interests.

Author details
[1]Department of Rehabilitation Medicine, The University of Tokyo Hospital, Tokyo, Japan. [2]Department of Rehabilitation Medicine, Graduate School of Medicine, The University of Tokyo, Tokyo, Japan. [3]Department of Orthopaedic Surgery, Fukuoka Children's Hospital, Fukuoka, Japan. [4]Department of Orthopedic Surgery, Nagoya University Graduate School of Medicine, Nagoya, Japan. [5]Department of Orthopaedic Surgery, National Center for Child Health and Development, Tokyo, Japan. [6]Department of Pediatrics, Hamamatsu University School of Medicine, Hamamatsu, Japan. [7]Department of Hygiene, Fujita Health University School of Medicine, Toyoake, Japan.

References
1. Alexander PG, Clark KL, Tuan RS. Prenatal exposure to environmental factors and congenital limb defects. Birth Defects Res C Embryo Today. 2016;108: 243–73.
2. Bonafe L, Cormier-Daire V, Hall C, Lachman R, Mortier G, Mundlos S, Nishimura G, Sangiorgi L, Savarirayan R, Sillence D, et al. Nosology and classification of genetic skeletal disorders: 2015 revision. Am J Med Genet A. 2015;167A:2869–92.
3. Castilla EE, Cavalcanti DP, Dutra MG, Lopez-Camelo JS, Paz JE, Gadow EC. Limb reduction defects in South America. Br J Obstet Gynaecol. 1995;102: 393–400.
4. Bedard T, Lowry RB, Sibbald B, Kiefer GN, Metcalfe A. Congenital limb deficiencies in Alberta-a review of 33 years (1980-2012) from the Alberta congenital anomalies surveillance system (ACASS). Am J Med Genet A. 2015;167A:2599–609.
5. Vasluian E, van der Sluis CK, van Essen AJ, Bergman JE, Dijkstra PU, Reinders-Messelink HA, de Walle HE. Birth prevalence for congenital limb defects in the northern Netherlands: a 30-year population-based study. BMC Musculoskelet Disord. 2013;14:323.
6. International Clearinghouse for Birth Defects Monitoring Systems. International clearinghouse for birth defects surveillance and research annual report 2014. Rome: The International Centre on Birth Defects–ICBDSR Centre; 2014.
7. Ogino T, Minami A, Fukuda K, Kato H. Congenital anomalies of the upper limb among the Japanese in Sapporo. J Hand Surg Br. 1986;11(3):364–71.
8. Kuyper MA, Breedijk M, Mulders AH, Post MW, Prevo AJ. Prosthetic management of children in the Netherlands with upper limb deficiencies. Prosthetics Orthot Int. 2001;25(3):228–34.
9. Colen DL, Lin IC, Levin LS, Chang B. Radial longitudinal deficiency: recent developments, controversies, and an evidence-based guide to treatment. J Hand Surg Am. 2017;42(7):546–63.
10. Westberry DE, Davids JR. Proximal focal femoral deficiency (PFFD): management options and controversies. Hip Int. 2009;19(Suppl 6):S18–25.
11. Simmons ED Jr, Ginsburg GM, Hall JE. Brown's procedure for congenital absence of the tibia revisited. J Pediatr Orthop. 1996;16:85–9.
12. Spiegel DA, Loder RT, Crandall RC. Congenital longitudinal deficiency of the tibia. Int Orthop. 2003;27:338–42.
13. Naudie D, Hamdy RC, Fassier F, Morin B, Duhaime M. Management of fibular hemimelia: amputation or limb lengthening. J Bone Joint Surg Br. 1997;79:58–65.
14. McCarthy JJ, Glancy GL, Chnag FM, Eilert RE. Fibular hemimelia: comparison of outcome measurments after amputation and lengthening. J Bone Joint Surg Am. 2000;82-A:1732–5.
15. Ohno Y, Kawamura T, Tamakoshi A, Wakai K, Aoki R, Kojima M, Lin Y, Hashimoto T, Nagai M, Minowa M. Epidemiology of diseases of unknown etiology, specified as "intractable diseases". J Epidemiol. 1996;6:S87–94.
16. Migita K, Uehara R, Nakamura Y, Yasunami M, Tsuchiya-Suzuki A, Yazaki M, Nakamura A, Masumoto J, Yachie A, Furukawa H, et al. Familial Mediterranean fever in Japan. Medicine (Baltimore). 2012;91:337–43.
17. Kuriyama S, Kusaka Y, Fujimura M, Wakai K, Tamakoshi A, Hashimoto S, Tsuji I, Inaba Y, Yoshimoto T. Prevalence and clinicoepidemiological features of moyamoya disease in Japan: findings from a nationwide epidemiological survey. Stroke. 2008;39:42–7.
18. Wakai K, Tamakoshi A, Ikezaki K, Fukui M, Kawamura T, Aoki R, Kojima M, Lin Y, Ohno Y. Epidemiological features of moyamoya disease in Japan: findings from a nationwide survey. Clin Neurol Neurosurg. 1997;99(Suppl 2):S1–5.
19. Sada KE, Amano K, Uehara R, Yamamura M, Arimura Y, Nakamura Y, Makino H. A nationwide survey on the epidemiology and clinical features of eosinophilic granulomatosis with polyangiitis (Churg-Strauss) in Japan. Mod Rheumatol. 2014;24:640–4.

20. Wakai K, Ohta A, Tamakoshi A, Ohno Y, Kawamura T, Aoki R, Kojima M, Lin Y, Hashimoto S, Inaba Y, et al. Estimated prevalence and incidence of adult Still's disease: findings by a nationwide epidemiological survey in Japan. J Epidemiol. 1997;7:221–5.

21. Tsuboi H, Asashima H, Takai C, Hagiwara S, Hagiya C, Yokosawa M, Hirota T, Umehara H, Kawakami A, Nakamura H, et al. Primary and secondary surveys on epidemiology of Sjogren's syndrome in Japan. Mod Rheumatol. 2014;24: 464–70.

22. Yamaguchi Y, Torisu H, Kira R, Ishizaki Y, Sakai Y, Sanefuji M, Ichiyama T, Oka A, Kishi T, Kimura S, et al. A nationwide survey of pediatric acquired demyelinating syndromes in Japan. Neurology. 2016;87:2006–15.

23. Masamune A, Kikuta K, Nabeshima T, Nakano E, Hirota M, Kanno A, Kume K, Hamada S, Ito T, Fujita M, et al. Nationwide epidemiological survey of early chronic pancreatitis in Japan. J Gastroenterol. 2017;52(8):992–1000.

24. Hamada S, Masamune A, Kikuta K, Hirota M, Tsuji I, Shimosegawa T. Nationwide epidemiological survey of acute pancreatitis in Japan. Pancreas. 2014;43:1244–8.

25. Hashimoto S, Fukutomi K, Sasaki R, Ohno Y, Aoki K, Nagai M, Nakamura Y, Yanagawa H. Nationwide epidemiological survey for estimating annual number of patients treated for intractable diseases in Japan: its significance and methodology. In: Yanagawa H, Sasaki R, Nagai M, Ohno Y, Hirohata T, Hashimoto T, Inaba Y, Nakamura K, editors. Recent progress of epidemiologic study of intractable diseases in Japan. Tokyo: The Epidemiology of Intractable Diseases Research Committee, the Ministry of Health and Welfare of Japan; 1992. p. 9–14.

26. Ohno Y, Suzuki S, Tamakoshi A, Sasaki R, Yanagawa H, Shibazaki H. Methodological issues in nationwide epidemiological survey for estimating annual number of patients treated for intractable diseases. In: Yanagawa H, Sasaki R, Nagai M, Ohno Y, Hirohata T, Hashimoto T, Inaba Y, Nakamura K, editors. Recent progress of epidemiologic study of intractable diseases in Japan. Tokyo: The Epidemiology of Intractable Diseases Research Committee, the Ministry of Health and Welfare of Japan; 1992. p. 15–22.

27. Krebs DE, Edelstein JE, Thornby MA. Prosthetic management of children with limb deficiencies. Phys Ther. 1991;71(12):920–34.

28. Mano H, Fujiwara S, Haga N. Adaptive behaviour and motor skills in children with upper limb deficiency. Prosthetics Orthot Int. 2017; 309364617718411

29. Nagata E, Kano H, Kato F, Yamaguchi R, Nakashima S, Takayama S, Kosaki R, Tonoki H, Mizuno S, Watanabe S, et al. Japanese founder duplications/triplications involving BHLHA9 are associated with split-hand/foot malformation with or without long bone deficiency and Gollop-Wolfgang complex. Orphanet J Rare Dis. 2014;9:125.

17

A comparison of one-year treatment utilization for shoulder osteoarthritis patients initiating care with non-orthopaedic physicians and orthopaedic specialists

Sarah B Floyd[1,2,5*] (iD), Cole G Chapman[1,2], Ellen Shanley[2,3], Lauren Ruffrage[2], Eldon Matthia[4], Peter Cooper[4] and John M Brooks[1,2]

Abstract

Background: In this paper we investigate patients seeking care for a new diagnosis of shoulder osteoarthritis (OA) and the association between a patient's initial physician specialty choice and one-year surgical and conservative treatment utilization.

Methods: Using retrospective data from a single large regional healthcare system, we identified 572 individuals with a new diagnosis of shoulder OA and identified the specialty of the physician which was listed as the performing physician on the index shoulder visit. We assessed treatment utilization in the year following the index shoulder visit for patients initiating care with a non-orthopaedic physician (NOP) or an orthopaedic specialist (OS). Descriptive statistics were calculated for each group and subsequent one-year surgical and conservative treatment utilization was compared between groups.

Results: Of the 572 patients included in the study, 474 (83%) received care from an OS on the date of their index shoulder visit, while 98 (17%) received care from a NOP. There were no differences in baseline patient age, gender, BMI or pain scores between groups. OS patients reported longer symptom duration and a higher rate of comorbid shoulder diagnoses. Patients initiating care with an OS on average received their first treatment much faster than patients initiating care with NOP (16.3 days [95% CI, 12.8, 19.7] vs. 32.3 days [95% CI, 21.0, 43.6], $Z = 4.9$, $p < 0.01$). Additionally, patients initiating care with an OS had higher odds of receiving surgery (OR = 2.65, 95% CI: 1.42, 4.95) in the year following their index shoulder visit.

Conclusions: Patients initiating care with an OS received treatment much faster and were treated with more invasive services over the year following their index shoulder visit. Future work should compare patient-reported outcomes across patient groups to assess whether more expensive and invasive treatments yield better outcomes for patients with shoulder OA.

Keywords: Shoulder, Osteoarthritis, Treatment, Surgery, Injections, Physical therapy

* Correspondence: floydsb@mailbox.sc.edu
[1]Department of Health Services Policy and Management, University of South Carolina, Columbia, SC, USA
[2]Center for Effectiveness Research in Orthopaedics, Greenville, SC, USA
Full list of author information is available at the end of the article

Background

The shoulder is the third most common large joint affected by the degenerative condition osteoarthritis (OA) [1], and OA of the shoulder may affect as many as one-third of patients over the age of 60 [2]. Shoulder OA is associated with significant pain and reduction in mobility and quality of life [2, 3], yet treatment for shoulder OA is not definitive and includes both conservative and surgical modalities [2]. Current recommendations favor conservative management as initial treatment for shoulder OA [4]. Patients with symptomatic shoulder OA can choose from a wide range of physicians to treat their condition, and patients may initially visit a primary care practitioner or a specialist such as an orthopaedic surgeon to begin their treatment. There is no consensus on the optimal provider to initiate care and the specialty of the first provider contact for OA may shape each patient's treatment course [5–7].

Shoulder OA is a common orthopaedic complaint in primary care medicine [8–10]. Yet, research suggests that primary care physicians receive limited training in musculoskeletal diseases [11, 12] compared to orthopaedic specialists who receive comprehensive training on the diagnosis and treatment of complex musculoskeletal conditions [13]. The healthcare literature lacks consensus as to the type of physicians who should care for patients with particular medical conditions [14, 15]. Specialists have been shown to achieve better clinical outcomes for some conditions such as myocardial infarction, stroke, asthma, and rheumatoid arthritis [16–22]. In most cases specialists know more about [22, 23] and are more likely to use optimal treatments their areas of expertise [24]. However, at times the treatment regimens provided by specialists have been shown to be more expensive and wasteful [16, 19, 24–27]. While others have assessed the factors affecting treatment utilization post OA diagnosis for patients initiating care with orthopaedic specialists [28], this will be the first to compare orthopaedic treatment utilization for patients initiating care with non-orthopaedic physicians and orthopaedic specialists. We hypothesized that patients initially seeking care from an orthopaedic specialist would be more likely to receive invasive treatment such as surgical care and less likely to receive conservative treatment for shoulder OA.

Methods

Data sources and overview

Data for this study included standard billing records from 2012 to 2014 for patients diagnosed with shoulder OA in 2013 from a single large regional healthcare system. The health system where the study was performed is one of the largest integrated healthcare systems in the Southeastern US, with over 15,000 employees across 7 medical campuses and 155 affiliated practice sites.

Standard billing records included service-line level information such as the date of service, billing physician, service facility, Current Procedural Terminology (CPT) and International Classification of Disease, Ninth Revision (ICD-9-CM) diagnostic codes associated with each healthcare service provided as well as patient age, sex and insurance status. These data were used for cohort identification and measurement of treatment utilization. In addition, medical charts were abstracted for a subset of the study sample. Medical chart data included clinical data not available in the standard billing records such as body mass index (BMI), smoking status, pain score and symptom duration. This study was approved by the Health System Institutional Review Board where the study was conducted (intentionally blinded).

Patient sample

We identified all patients with an Evaluation and Management visit (E/M visit: CPT codes 992XX) in the health system that had at least 1 of 192 ICD-9-CM diagnosis codes related to shoulder pain or dysfunction in 2013. The date of the first visit with a shoulder-related diagnosis was designated, and is henceforth referred to as the index shoulder visit. Patients with any shoulder-related diagnosis, as defined above, in the period of 365 days prior to their index shoulder visit were excluded to allow researchers to make comparisons across patients seeking care for a new shoulder problem. Patients with shoulder OA were then identified as those with a diagnosis code from a clinical exam confirming shoulder OA in the period of 90-days after their index shoulder visit (ICD-9 codes 715.11, 715.21, 715.31, 715.91); all other patients without a diagnosis of shoulder OA were excluded. Patients who were less than 18-years old at index or who had incomplete data (e.g. patient age, gender, visit date, etc.) for creating study measures were excluded. The final cohort meeting all inclusion criteria included 572 patients. A patient sample flow chart is included in Fig. 1.

A retrospective chart review was conducted to compare patient and clinical variables that were not available in standard billing data. Due to inconsistencies in charting practices, clinical data such as pain scores and symptom duration were often missing from patient charts in the non-orthopaedic setting. Multiple rounds of stratified simple random sampling were used to identify and select complete patient charts for review. Only 24 out of 98 patient charts from non-orthopaedic physicians contained complete clinical information. Therefore, we selected and reviewed all 24 complete non-orthopaedic physician patient charts and selected a matched sample of 24 complete orthopaedic specialist patient charts to conduct the retrospective chart review.

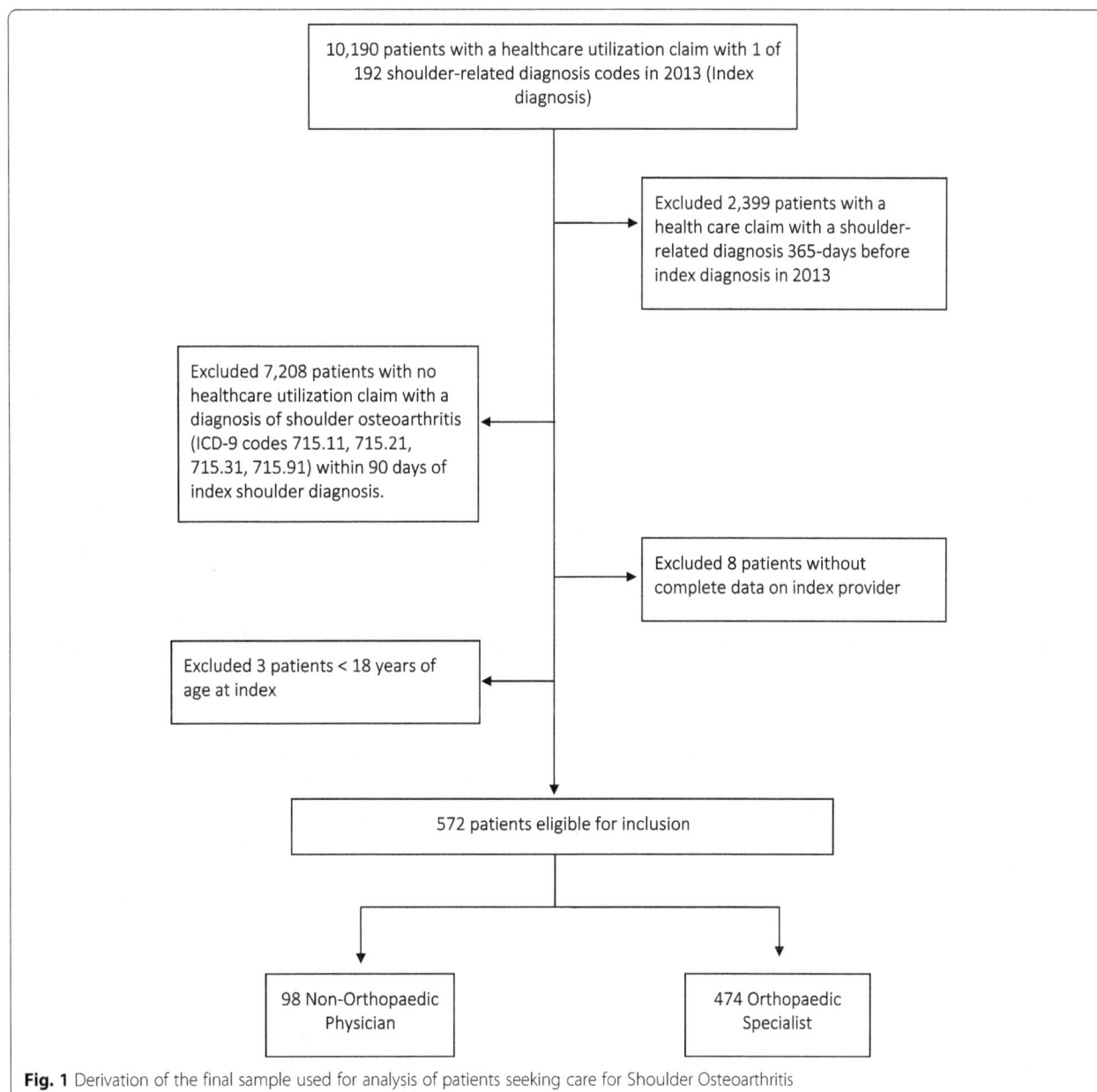

Fig. 1 Derivation of the final sample used for analysis of patients seeking care for Shoulder Osteoarthritis

Measures

Physician specialty designation

The specialty of the physician or health care provider which was listed as the billing physician on the index shoulder visit for each patient was identified by linking providers to the National Plan and Provider Enumeration System files, which contain specialty information as taxonomy codes, by unique National Provider Identification (NPI) numbers [29]. Physician specialty was defined based upon the taxonomy code designated as most current. Physicians and health care providers (nurse practitioners) were then classified, based on specialty, as being either non-orthopaedic physicians (NOP) or orthopaedic specialists (OS). NOP included mainly family and internal medicine physicians (65.3%), rheumatologists (21.4%) and other non-orthopaedic specialties (13.3%). Other specialties included pain management specialists (7.1%), neurosurgeons (3.1%), physical medicine and rehabilitation specialists (2.0%) and general surgeons (1.0%). OS included orthopaedic surgeons (80.4%) and sports medicine trained primary care physicians (19.6%). Sports medicine primary care physicians were classified as OS because they are fellowship trained in musculoskeletal conditions and practice alongside orthopaedic surgeons in the local health system.

Treatment utilization variables

Treatments were grouped into four modalities and ranked in order of invasiveness. The hierarchy of invasiveness was established through clinical discussion with a practicing physical therapist and was assessed through evaluation of treatment time and potential complications. Physical therapy was considered the lowest level of treatment, followed by corticosteroid injections, arthroscopic surgery and finally total joint replacement. Treatment consisted of four separate modalities, defined as follows:

1. Physical therapy (CPT code: 29240, 76,881 76,942, 970XX, 971XX, 975XX)
2. Corticosteroid injections (CPT code: 205XX, 206XX, J3301, J0702)
3. Arthroscopic surgery (CPT code: 298XX, 23,020, 23,130, 23,430, 23,700)
4. Total joint replacement (CPT code: 23470, 23,472)

The treatment period was defined as 365-days following the index shoulder visit. Patients receiving no treatment during the treatment period were classified in a period of watchful waiting. Time to OA diagnosis from index shoulder visit and time from index shoulder visit to first treatment received were assessed for each patient, and measured in days. The first treatment modality received by each patient, if a treatment modality was ever received, and the number of physical therapy (PT) sessions and injections received during the treatment period were assessed for each patient. The first treatment received was defined as the first treatment received after the index shoulder visit. If multiple treatment modalities were used on the same date, the first treatment received was recorded as the most invasive treatment modality of those used on the same day. If more than one treatment was received throughout the treatment period; both treatment modalities were recoded and included in the analysis of treatments ever received. We assessed differences in treatment utilization variables between patients grouped by the provider specialty of their index shoulder visit.

Covariates

It is well established that comorbidity burden is a patient factor that is expected to influence treatment choices and treatment outcomes for patients [30, 31]. To control for differences in comorbidity burden across patients at index, billing data were used to assess healthcare utilization in the 365 days prior to the index shoulder visit for measures of baseline patient health. General comorbidity burden was measured using the Charlson Comorbidity Index (CCI) [32]. CCI is a validated measure of burden of disease. Comorbidities are weighted from 1 to 6 for mortality risk and disease severity, and then summed to form the total CCI score. Additionally, the number and type of healthcare visits by type (e.g. non-orthopaedic physician visits and orthopaedic specialist

visits) in the year preceding the index shoulder visit were measured under the theory that higher use reflects poorer health status. Shoulder-specific health was assessed using concomitant shoulder diagnoses received within 90 days following the index shoulder visit.

Medical chart data extraction was performed by a team of two medical students. Patient charts from the index shoulder visit were reviewed and clinical data including body mass index (BMI), smoking status, pain score and symptom length, were extracted and recorded for each patient.

Analyses

Patient characteristics at baseline and treatment utilization were compared between patient groups. Conservative baseline patient comparisons were based on 95% confidence intervals. The Shapiro Wilk test was used to assess normality of continuous variables. Treatment utilization was compared between patient groups using the Wilcoxon rank-sum test for continuous variables and Pearson's chi-square and Fisher's exact test for categorical data. Significance was established at $p < 0.05$. Multivariable logistic regression was used to estimate the independent influence of specialty of first provider seen and probability of receiving surgical treatment for shoulder OA. Models were adjusted for patient's age, gender, insurance type, previous healthcare utilization, and concurrent shoulder diagnoses. The primary independent variable, specialty of first provider, was modeled as a dichotomous variable (1 = OS, 0 = NOP). Patient age was modeled as dummy variable with age categories of 18–34, 35–49, 50–64, 65–79 and 80 and above. Patient sex was a dichotomous variable of 1 = male and 0 = female. Insurance status was modeled as a dummy variable for public, private, other insurance and workers compensation. Previous health care visits and shoulder diagnoses were included as dichotomous variables (1 = yes, 0 = no). Concurrent shoulder diagnoses were specified in the model using two variables: one indicating whether the patient had any diagnosis of rotator cuff tear within 90 days following the index shoulder visit and another indicating whether the patient had any diagnosis of rheumatoid arthritis, humerus fracture, adhesive capsulitis or instability. The grouping of these conditions was based on their near-zero variance, each was present in less than 4% of the sample. Results are presented as adjusted Odds Ratios (OR) with accompanying 95% confidence intervals (95% CI). SAS software (Version 9.4) and R (Version 1.0.153) were used for data cleaning and statistical analyses.

Results

Study sample by physician specialty

Of the 572 patients included in the study, 474 (83%) were provided care from an OS on the date of index

Table 1 Measures of shoulder health and general health from billing data for shoulder osteoarthritis patients by physician specialty ($N = 572$)

Patient Characteristics		Total Study Sample ($N = 572$)	Non-Orthopaedic Physician ($N = 98$)	Orthopaedic Specialist ($N = 474$)
Age	Mean	60.3	61.5	60.1
	(95% CI)	(59.2, 61.4)	(58.9, 64.1)	(58.9, 61.3)
Male Sex	n (%)	302 (52.8)	44 (44.9)	258 (54.4)
	(95% CI)	(48.6, 56.9)	(34.8, 55.3)	(49.8, 59.0)
Insurance type				
Public	n (%)	307 (53.7)	45 (45.9)	262 (55.3)
	(95% CI)	(49.5, 57.8)	(35.8, 56.3)	(50.7, 59.8)
Private	n (%)	219 (38.3)	48 (48.9)	171 (36.1)
	(95% CI)	(34.3, 42.4)	(38.7, 59.3)	(31.7, 40.6)
Worker's compensation	n (%)	35 (6.1)	2 (2.0)	33 (7.0)
	(95% CI)	(4.3, 8.4)	(0.2, 7.2)	(4.8, 9.6)
Other	n (%)	11 (1.9)	3 (3.1)	8 (1.7)
	(95% CI)	(0.9, 3.4)	(0.6, 8.7)	(0.7, 3.3)
Concurrent Shoulder Diagnoses[a]				
Rotator Cuff Tear	n (%)	173 (30.2)	16 (16.3)	157 (33.1)
	(95% CI)	(26.5, 34.2)	(9.6, 25.2)	(28.9, 37.6)
Rheumatoid Arthritis	n (%)	7 (1.2)	7 (7.1)	0 (0.0)
	(95% CI)	(0.6, 2.7	(2.9, 14.2)	(0.0, 1.2)
Humerus Fracture	n (%)	6 (1.0)	0 (0.0)	6 (1.3)
	(95% CI)	(0.4, 2.3)	(0.0, 3.7)	(0.5, 2.7)
Instability	n (%)	9 (1.6)	0 (0.0)	9 (1.9)
	(95% CI)	(0.7, 3.0)	(0.0, 3.7)	(0.9, 3.6)
Adhesive capsulitis	n (%)	19 (3.3)	1 (1.0)	18 (3.8)
	(95% CI)	(2.0, 5.1)	(0.03, 5.5)	(2.2, 5.9)
Charlson Comorbidity Index[b]				
Score 0	n (%)	223 (69.0)	55 (68.0)	168 (69.4)
	(95% CI)	(63.7, 74.0)	(56.6, 77.8)	(63.2, 75.2)
Score 1	n (%)	54 (16.7)	15 (18.5)	39 (16.1)
	(95% CI)	(12.8, 21.2)	(10.7, 28.7)	(11.7, 21.4)
Score 2	n (%)	38 (11.8)	7 (8.6)	31 (12.8)
	(95% CI)	(8.5, 15.8)	(3.5, 17.0)	(8.9, 17.7)
Score 3	n (%)	4 (1.2)	2 (2.5)	2 (0.8)
	(95% CI)	(0.3, 3.1)	(0.3, 8.6)	(0.1, 2.9)
Score 4	n (%)	2 (0.6)	1 (1.2)	1 (0.4)
	(95% CI)	(0.08, 2.2)	(0.03, 6.7)	(0.01, 2.3)
Healthcare utilization in the 365 days prior to index shoulder visit				
Patients who visited a NOP	n (%)	221 (38.6)	70 (71.4)	151 (31.9)
	(95% CI)	(34.6, 42.7)	(61.4, 80.1)	(27.7, 36.3)
Number of visits to NOP[c]	Mean	4.1	4.3	4.0
	(95% CI)	(3.6, 4.7)	(3.6, 5.0)	(3.3, 4.8)

Table 1 Measures of shoulder health and general health from billing data for shoulder osteoarthritis patients by physician specialty (N = 572) (Continued)

Patient Characteristics		Total Study Sample (N = 572)	Non-Orthopaedic Physician (N = 98)	Orthopaedic Specialist (N = 474)
Patients who visited an OS	n (%)	88 (15.4)	18 (18.4)	70 (14.8)
	(95% CI)	(12.5, 18.6)	(11.3, 27.5)	(11.7, 18.3)
Number of visits to OS[d]	Mean	2.2	2.1	2.3
	(95% CI)	(1.9, 2.6)	(1.5, 2.7)	(1.9, 2.7)

[a]Among all OA patients
[b]Among patients with healthcare utilization in previous 365 days
[c]Among patients having one or more visit with non-orthopaedic physician
[d]Among patients having one or more visit with an orthopaedic specialist

shoulder visit, while 98 (17%) initiated care with a NOP (Table 1). Patients in the study ranged from 20 to 95 years of age. There was no difference in the mean age or proportion of male patients initiating care with an OS compared to a NOP. A larger proportion of patients initiating care with an OS had a concurrent diagnosis of rotator cuff tear (33.1% [95% CI, 28.9, 37.6] vs. 16.3% [95% CI, 9.6, 25.2]) and a smaller proportion had a concurrent diagnosis of a chronic joint problem requiring ongoing management, such as rheumatoid arthritis (0.0% [95% CI, 0.0, 1.2] vs. 7.1% [95% CI, 2.9, 14.2]), compared to patients initiating care with an NOP. A higher proportion of OS patients were publicly insured (55.3% [95% CI, 50.7, 59.8] vs. 45.9% [95% CI, 35.8, 56.3]) or had a worker's compensation claim (7.0% [95% CI, 4.8, 9.6] vs. 2.0% [95% CI, 0.2, 7.2]), compared to NOP patients. There were no meaningful differences in Charlson Comorbidity Index scores among NOP and OS patients, although a larger proportion of patients of NOP visited a NOP in the year prior to their index shoulder visit (71.4% [95% CI, 61.4, 80.1] vs 31.9% [95% CI, 27.7, 36.3]).

Treatment utilization by physician specialty
Table 2 shows additional comparisons of treatment utilization by initiating physician group. There was no significant difference in the time from index shoulder visit to OA diagnosis across patients by specialty of the initiating physician. However, patients initiating care with an OS received their first treatment in significantly less time (16.3 days [95% CI, 12.8, 19.7] vs. 32.3 days [95% CI, 21.0, 43.6] Z = 4.9, $p < 0.01$) compared to patients initiating care with a NOP. Injection was the most common first treatment modality for both NOP (33.7% [95% CI, 24.4, 43.9]) and OS patients (53.4% [95% CI, 48.8, 57.9]). A significantly larger proportion of OS patients received arthroscopic surgery (15.2% [95% CI, 12.1, 18.7]) or total joint replacement (4.8% [95% CI, 3.1, 7.2]) as their first treatment modality compared to NOP patients, of whom 7.1% [95% CI, 2.9, 14.2] received arthroscopic surgery and 2.0% [95% CI, 0.2, 7.1] received

total joint replacement as their first treatment (p-value < 0.001 by Fisher's exact test).

During the 365-day treatment period, 64.3% [95% CI, 59.8, 68.7] of patients initiating care with OS and 46.9% [95% CI, 36.8, 57.3] of those initiating care with NOP received injections (X^2 (1, N = 572) = 10.4, p-value < 0.01). A larger proportion of NOP patients utilized physical therapy (21.4% [95% CI, 13.8, 30.9]) than OS patients (15.4% [95% CI: 12.3, 19.0]; X^2 (1, N = 572) = 2.1, p-value 0.14), but there was no significant difference in the average number of physical therapy visits (1.2 PT visits [95% CI, 1.0, 1.4] for NOP; 1.2 PT visits [95% CI, 1.1, 1.3] for OS) or injections (1.6 injections [95% CI, 1.4, 1.9] for NOP; 1.6 injections [95% CI, 1.5, 1.7] for OS) received across groups. Thirty-seven percent [95% CI, 33.2, 42.1] of orthopaedic patients received arthroscopic surgery at some time during the treatment period, compared to only 18.4% [95% CI, 11.3, 27.5] of non-orthopaedic patients (X^2 (1, N = 572) = 13.3, p-value< 0.01). Among the 43% (N = 248) of patients receiving arthroscopic or arthroplasty surgery during the treatment period, patients initiating care with an OS received surgical treatment in significantly less time (62.5 days [95% CI, 55.1, 69.8] vs. 96.9 days [95% CI, 62.6, 131.1] Z = 2.9, $p < 0.01$) than NOP patients. Forty-three percent [95% CI, 33.9, 54.3] of NOP patients received none of the specified treatments during the 365-day treatment period, compared to only 15.4% [95% CI, 12.3, 19.0] of patients initiating care with an OS (X^2 (1, N = 572) = 40.7, p-value < 0.01).

Table 3 shows results from a logistic regression model predicting surgical treatment in the year following index shoulder visit. The adjusted odds of surgery were significantly higher for patients visiting an orthopaedic specialist on their index shoulder visit (OR = 2.65 [95% CI, 1.42, 4.95]) compared to non-orthopaedic patients.

Comparison of key variables from charts
Complete detail on characteristics of the chart abstraction sample is provided in Table 4.

Table 2 Treatment utilization for shoulder osteoarthritis patients by physician specialty ($N = 572$)

		Total Study Sample ($N = 572$)	Non-Orthopaedic Physician ($n = 98$)	Orthopaedic Specialist ($n = 474$)	p value
Days from index shoulder visit to OA diagnosis	Mean	19.6	21.6	19.2	0.25*
	(95% CI)	(17.5, 21.8)	(16.3, 26.9)	(16.9, 21.6)	
Days from index shoulder visit to first treatment	Mean	18.2	32.3	16.3	< 0.01*
	(95% CI)	(14.8, 21.5)	(21.0, 43.6)	(12.8, 19.7)	
First Treatment Initiated					
Physical therapy	n (%)	66 (11.5)	13 (13.3)	53 (11.2)	< 0.01[‡]
	(95% CI)		(7.3, 21.6)	(8.5, 14.4)	
Injection	n (%)	286 (50.0)	33 (33.7)	253 (53.4)	
	(95% CI)		(24.4, 43.9)	(48.8, 57.9)	
Arthroscopic surgery	n (%)	79 (13.8)	7 (7.1)	72 (15.2)	
	(95% CI)		(2.9, 14.2)	(12.1, 18.7)	
Total joint replacement	n (%)	25 (4.4)	2 (2.0)	23 (4.8)	
	(95% CI)		(0.2, 7.1)	(3.1, 7.2)	
Watchful Waiting	n (%)	116 (20.3)	43 (43.9)	73 (15.4)	
	(95% CI)		(33.9, 54.3)	(12.3, 19.0)	
Treatment ever received[a]					
Physical therapy	n (%)	94 (16.4)	21 (21.4)	73 (15.4)	0.14[†]
	(95% CI)		(13.8, 30.9)	(12.3, 19.0)	
Injection	n (%)	351 (61.4)	46 (46.9)	305 (64.3)	< 0.01[†]
	(95% CI)		(36.8, 57.3)	(59.8, 68.7)	
Arthroscopic surgery	n (%)	196 (34.3)	18 (18.4)	178 (37.5)	< 0.01[†]
	(95% CI)		(11.3, 27.5)	(33.2, 42.1)	
Total joint replacement	n (%)	52 (9.1)	4 (4.1)	48 (10.1)	0.08[‡]
	(95% CI)		(1.1, 10.1)	(7.5, 13.2)	
Watchful Waiting	n (%)	116 (20.3)	43 (43.8)	73 (15.4)	< 0.01[†]
	(95% CI)		(33.9, 54.3)	(12.3, 19.0)	
Number of PT sessions over treatment period[c]	Mean	1.2	1.2	1.2	0.81*
	(95% CI)	(1.1, 1.3)	(1.0, 1.4)	(1.1, 1.3)	
Number of injections over treatment period[b]	Mean	1.6	1.6	1.6	0.42*
	(95% CI)	(1.5, 1.7)	(1.4, 1.9)	(1.5, 1.7)	
Days from index shoulder visit to surgery[d]	Mean	65.4	96.9	62.5	< 0.01*
	(95% CI)	(58.0, 72.8)	(62.6, 131.1)	(55.1, 69.8)	

[a]Groups are not mutually exclusive and will sum to greater than 100 %
[b]Among patients receiving at least one injection in the treatment period
[c]Among patients receiving at least one physical therapy session in the treatment period
[d]Among patients receiving arthroscopic surgery or total joint replacement in the treatment period
*p-value produced from Wilcoxon rank-sum test
[†]p-value produced from Pearson's chi-square test
[‡]p-value produced from Fisher's exact test

Patients initiating care with an OS reported longer symptom duration (17.9 months [95% CI, 8.3, 27.5]) compared to patients initiating care with NOP (3.5 months [95% CI, 0.3, 6.8]). However, there was no difference in the BMI, pain score, or proportion of smokers at the index visit between patient groups.

Discussion

To our knowledge, this study is the first to investigate the relationship between a patient's initial provider choice and their orthopaedic treatment utilization in the year following a shoulder diagnosis. Results from this study show that patients initially seeing an OS for OA

Table 3 Adjusted odds ratios of surgical treatment (N = 572)

	Model
	Surgery within 1 year$^{\pm}$
Index visit with Non-Orthopaedic Physician	Reference
Index visit with Orthopaedic Specialist	2.65** [1.42, 4.95]
Male	1.40 [0.93, 2.11]
Age	
18–34	Reference
35–49	1.00 [0.27, 3.62]
50–64	0.72 [0.20, 2.57]
65–79	0.44 [0.12, 1.70]
80+	0.18* [0.04, 0.92]
Insurance Type	
Private	Reference
Public	1.08 [0.61, 1.90]
Other	1.45 [0.34, 6.25]
Worker's Comp	2.54* [1.05, 6.17]
Previous Healthcare Utilization	
Family Medicine visit	0.94 [0.61, 1.46]
Orthopaedic Specialist visit	1.35 [0.76, 2.39]
Concurrent Shoulder Diagnoses	
Rotator Cuff Tear	10.69*** [6.76, 16.93]
Other shoulder diagnosis	2.16* [0.99, 4.71]

Exponentiated coefficients interpreted as Odds Ratio; 95% confidence interval in parentheses
$^{\pm}$Total joint replacement or arthroscopic surgery received within 1-year of index shoulder visit
$^{+}p < .1$, $^{*}p < .05$, $^{**}p < .01$, $^{***}p < .001$

have a higher proportion of concurrent shoulder diagnoses and report longer symptom duration than NOP patients, although they do not differ in Charlson comorbidity index scores, age, sex, BMI, smoking status or pain scores. Across patient groups, time from initial shoulder visit to diagnosis of OA was not clinically or statistically different. However, patients initiating care with an OS received their first treatment on average much faster and were more likely to receive surgery in

the year following their index shoulder visit than patients initiating care with a NOP.

Our findings suggest there are clear differences in shoulder OA treatment utilization for patients initially receiving care from NOP and OS. The shorter time to treatment suggests that patients may receive more immediate symptom relief if care is initiated with an OS. Additionally, a larger proportion of OS patients received surgical treatment, including arthroscopic surgery and total joint replacement compared to patients seeing a NOP. Patients of OS did report longer symptom duration and more concurrent shoulder diagnoses, suggesting that their overall shoulder health may be more severe than that of patients seeing a NOP.

While our results show differences in treatment utilization across patients initiating care with different physician specialties, they do not provide evidence as to appropriateness of care or which type of physician provided "better" care for shoulder OA. Our study can't conclude whether higher use of surgical treatment resulted in improved patient outcomes for patients receiving care from OS. Although, in a study among patients with shoulder pain, Kuijpers and colleagues found that patients reporting persistent symptoms generated more than twice as much costs compared to patients reporting recovery after 6 months [33]. This supports the theory that early intervention, if effective in slowing the disease progression or removing the degenerative bone and cartilage, may eliminate the need for ongoing shoulder treatment. Furthermore, chronic shoulder pain lasting longer than 3 months has been shown to increase depression, anxiety and sleep disruptions [34]. Therefore, early, effective treatment may have wide ranging positive effects on a patient's physical as well as mental health. Inference on effectiveness of early and more aggressive treatment paths can best be assessed with information on long-term orthopaedic treatment utilization and patient-reported outcomes. Future work needs to compare patient-reported outcomes across physician and treatment groups to more completely answer questions surrounding comparative risks and

Table 4 Clinical characteristics from retrospective chart review for shoulder osteoarthritis patients by physician specialty (N = 48)

		Total Study Sample (N = 48)	Non-Orthopaedic Physician (n = 24)	Orthopaedic Specialist (n = 24)
BMI	Mean	34.4	36.3	32.6
	(95% CI)	(30.1, 38.8)	(28.1, 44.5)	(30.0, 36.2)
Number of current smokers	n (%)	5 (10.4)	2 (8.3)	3 (12.5)
	(95% CI)	(3.5, 22.7)	(1.0, 27.0)	(2.7, 32.4)
Symptom duration in months	Mean	10.7	3.5	17.9
	(95% CI)	(5.4, 16.0)	(0.3, 6.8)	(8.3, 27.5)
Pain scale score	Mean	5.7	5.7	5.7
	(95% CI)	(5.0, 6.4)	(4.4, 7.0)	(4.8, 6.6)

benefits of receiving care from OS versus other provider types. Furthermore, given the heterogeneity of treatment effects across patients, the observed variation in treatment across patients and entry points may reflect the effective mix for this population and treatments are properly distributed across patients.

Several important limitations of this study must be acknowledged more completely. The health system in which the study was conducted has a well-known orthopaedic practice led by a well-known shoulder specialist. It is possible that the proportion of patients seeking care from OS is higher than might be expected elsewhere and the treatment courses observed may also be unique to the health system. Moreover, because the data used for this study comes from a single healthcare system, it is possible that patients in the sample received care from other outside providers that we do not observe which could result in misclassification bias. It is possible that patients may have visited a NOP provider and been referred to an OS provider. This would result in the more severe shoulder cases appearing in the OS provider group. However, the health system where the study was performed is one of the largest integrated healthcare systems in the Southeastern US which increases the likelihood that we captured a patient's first touch with the healthcare system. In efforts to ensure we captured the first shoulder visit, we included shoulder diagnosis codes which occurred in any diagnosis position. To confirm our findings we would recommend a larger study be conducted across many healthcare sites and systems. Similarly, administrative billing records did not contain pharmacologic treatment information, so we could not include pain medication utilization in our results. Unfortunately, due to inconsistent radiologic documentation we could not assess the stage of OA for each patient. However, because there were no observed differences in age or pain scale across patients, we do not expect meaningful differences in OA stage across patient groups.

We acknowledge that our sampling strategy for the selection of patient charts could potentially result in patient samples which were not representative of the larger patient populations of each physician group. Unfortunately we were limited by the number of charts which contained complete clinical information in the NOS setting and it is possible that patients with complete charts were systematically different than those without complete charts, and therefore are not representative of the larger NOS population. Furthermore, a sample of more than 24 charts should be reviewed from the larger OS group to ensure the sample is not biased. In order to confirm our results, a larger chart review should be conducted. If the patient populations do indeed differ in meaningful ways, the differences in treatment utilization we observed may

be justified. We selected a parsimonious model for our logistic regression analysis; however we did not have patient information on underlying condition severity, patient socioeconomic status, or granularity surrounding patient insurance structure which may affect referral patterns. Lastly, it is possible that differences in treatment utilization were due to differences in patient preferences for treatment. More work is needed to compare patient preferences for treatment across provider types.

Conclusions

This study is the first to explore differences in shoulder OA treatment utilization for patients who enter the healthcare system through different physician channels. Results show that patients initiating care with an OS received treatment faster and were treated with more invasive services over the year following their index shoulder visit. However, this study did not assess the effectiveness or appropriateness of different treatment utilization. Future work should compare patient-reported outcomes across physician and treatment groups in larger patient samples which contain multiple health systems.

Abbreviations

BMI: Body Mass Index; CCI: Charlson Comorbidity Index; CPT: Current Procedural Terminology; E/M: Evaluation and Management; ICD-9-CM: International Classification of Disease, Ninth Revision; NOP: Non-orthopaedic physician; NPI: National Provider Identification; OA: Osteoarthritis; OS: Orthopaedic specialist; PT: Physical Therapy

Funding

This study was funded by the Center for Effectiveness Research in Orthopaedics.

Authors' contributions

SF, CC, ES, LR, and JB made substantial contributions to conception and design, acquisition of data, and analysis and interpretation of study findings. SF and CC analyzed and interpreted the results regarding treatment utilization. ES was involved in drafting the manuscript and revising it critically for important clinical contributions. EM, PC and LR performed the chart abstraction, and were major contributors in writing the manuscript. All authors read and approved the final manuscript.

Competing interests

The authors declare that they have no competing interests.

Author details

[1]Department of Health Services Policy and Management, University of South Carolina, Columbia, SC, USA. [2]Center for Effectiveness Research in Orthopaedics, Greenville, SC, USA. [3]ATI Physical Therapy, Greenville, SC, USA. [4]University of South Carolina School of Medicine Greenville, Greenville, SC, USA. [5]Arnold School of Public Health, University of South Carolina, 915 Greene St., Suite 303C, Columbia, SC 29208, USA.

References

1. Gross C, Dhawan A, Harwood D, Gochanour E, Romeo A. Glenohumeral joint injections: a review. Sports Health. 2013;5(2):153–9.
2. Chillemi C, Franceschini V. Shoulder osteoarthritis. Arthritis. 2013;2013:370231.
3. Millett PJ, Gobezie R, Boykin RE. Shoulder osteoarthritis: diagnosis and management. Am Fam Physician. 2008;78(5):605–11.

4. Denard PJ, Wirth MA, Orfaly R. Management of glenohumeral arthritis in the young adult. e Journal of Bone & Joint Surgery A. 2011;93(9):885–92.

5. Horn ME, George SZ, Fritz JM. Influence of initial provider on health care utilization in patients seeking Care for Neck Pain. Mayo Clinic Proceedings: Innovations, Quality & Outcomes. 2017;1(3):226–33.

6. Hurwitz EL, Li D, Guillen J, et al. Variations in patterns of utilization and charges for the care of neck pain in North Carolina, 2000 to 2009: a statewide claims' data analysis. J Manip Physiol Ther. 2016;39(4):240–51.

7. Fritz JM, Kim J, Dorius J. Importance of the type of provider seen to begin health care for a new episode low back pain: associations with future utilization and costs. J Eval Clin Pract. 2016;22(2):247–52.

8. Wofford J, Mansfield RJ, Watkins RS. Patient characteristics and clinical management of patients with shoulder pain in U.S. primary care settings: secondary data analysis of the national ambulatory medical care survey. BMC Musculoskelet Disord. 2005;6(4):1–6.

9. Katz JN, Solomon DH, Schaffer JL, Horsky J, Burdick E, Bates DW. Outcomes of care and resource utilization among patients with knee or shoulder disorders treated by general internists, rheumatologists, or orthopedic surgeons. Am J Med. 2000;108(1):28–35.

10. MacKay C, Canizares M, Davis AM, Badley EM. Health care utilization for musculoskeletal disorders. Arthritis Care Res (Hoboken). 2010;62(2):161–9.

11. Meenan RF, Goldenberg DL, Allaire SH, Anderson JJ. The rheumatology knowledge and skills of trainees in internal medicine and family practice. J Rheumatol. 1988;15:1693–700.

12. Renner BR, DeVellis BM, Ennett ST, et al. Clinical rheumatology training of primary care physicians: the resident perspective. J Rheumatol. 1990;17:666–72.

13. Donohoe M. Comparing generalist and specialty care. Archives Internal Medicine. 1998;158:1596–608.

14. Smetana GWLB, Bindman AB, Burstin H, Davis RB, Tija J, Rich EC. A comparison of outcomes resulting from generalist vs specialist care for a single discrete medical condition. Archives Internal Medicine. 2007;167:10–20.

15. Turner BJLC. Differences between generalists and specialists. J Gen Intern Med. 2001;16:422–4.

16. Jollis JG, DeLong ER, Peterson ED, et al. Outcome of acute myocardial infarction according to the specialty of the admitting physician. NEJM. 1996;335:1880–7.

17. Horner RD, Landsman PB, Feussner JR. Patterns of care associated with improved stroke outcomes: preliminary evidence from VA medical centers. AHSR FHSR Annu Meet Abstr Book. 1995;12:49–50.

18. Kaste MPH, Sarna S. Where and how should elderly stroke patients be treated? A randomized trial. Stroke. 1995;26:249–53.

19. Freund DASJ, Hurley R, et al. Specialty differences in the treatment of asthma. J All Clin Immunol. 1989;84:401–6.

20. Ward MMLP, Fried JF. Progression of functional disability in patients with rheumatoid arthritis. Arch Intern Med. 1993;153:2229–37.

21. Criswell LASC, Yelin EH. Differences in use of second-line agents and prednisone for treatment of rheumatoid arthritis by rheumatologists and non-rheumatologists. J Rheumatol. 1997;24:2283–90.

22. Harrold LRFT, Gurwitz JH. Knowledge, patterns of care and outcomes of Care for Generalists and Specialists. J Gen Intern Med. 1999;14:499–511.

23. Ayanian JZHP, Guadagnoli E, et al. Knowledge and practices of generalists and specialist physicians regarding drug therapy for acute myocardial infarction. NEJM. 1994;331:1136–42.

24. Mazzuca SABK, Katz BP, Li W, Stewart K. Therapeutic strategies distinguish community based primary care physicians from rheumatologists in the management of osteoarthritis. J Rheumatol. 1993;20:80–6.

25. Carey TS, Garrett J, Jackman A, McLaughlin C, Fryer J, Smucker DR, Curtis P, Darter J, Defriese G, Evans A, et al. The outcomes and costs of care for acute low-back-pain among patients seen by primary-care practitioners, chiropractors, and orthopedic surgeons. N Engl J Med. 1995;333(14):913–7.

26. Shekelle PGMM, Louie R. Comparing the costs between provider types of episodes of back pain. Spine. Spine. 1995;20:221–7.

27. Post P, Wittenberg J, Burgers J. Do specialized centers and specialists produce better outcomes for patients with chronic diseases than primary care generalists? A systematic review. Int J Qual Health Care. 2009;21(6):387–96.

28. Badley EM, Canizares M, MacKay C, Mahomed NN, Davis AM. Surgery or consultation: a population-based cohort study of use of orthopaedic surgeon services. PLoS One. 2013;8(6):e65560.

29. National Plan & Provider Enumeration System. NPI Registry. [Internet. Accessed 3 May 2017]; Available from https://nppes.cms.hhs.gov/NPPES/Welcome.do

30. Gagnier JJ, Allen B, Watson S, Robbins CB, Bedi A, Carpenter JE, Miller BS. Do medical comorbidities affect outcomes in patients with rotator cuff tears? Orthop J Sports Med. 2017;5(8):2325967117723834.

31. Menzies IB, Mendelson DA, Kates SL, Friedman SM. The impact of comorbidity on perioperative outcomes of hip fractures in a geriatric fracture model. Geriatr Orthop Surg Rehabil. 2012;3(3):129–34.

32. Charlson M, Pompei P, Ales K, Mac Kenzie C. A new method of classifying prognostic comorbidity in longitudinal studies: development and validation. Journal of Chronic Disease. 1987;40(5):373–83.

33. Kuijpers T, van Tulder MW, van der Heijden GJMG, Bouter LM, van der Windt DAWM. Costs of shoulder pain in primary care consulters: a prospective cohort study in the Netherlands. BMC Musculoskelet Disord. 2006;7:83.

34. Cho CH, Jung SW, Park JY, Song KS, Yu KI. Is shoulder pain for three months or longer correlated with depression, anxiety, and sleep disturbance? J Shoulder Elb Surg. 2013;22(2):222–8.

18

Self-recordings of upper arm elevation during cleaning – comparison between analyses using a simplified reference posture and a standard reference posture

Camilla Dahlqvist[1]* ⓘ, Catarina Nordander[1], Mikael Forsman[2] and Henrik Enquist[1]

Abstract

Background: To reduce ergonomic risk factors in terms of awkward and constrained postures and high velocities, it is important to perform adequate risk assessments. Technical methods provide objective measures of physical workload. These methods have so far mainly been used by researchers. However, if written instructions how to apply the sensors and how to adopt the reference posture are provided, together with triaxial accelerometers, it may be possible for employees to record their own physical workload. The exposure in terms of e.g. upper arm elevations could then easily be assessed for all workers in a workplace. The main aims of this study were: 1) to compare analyses for self-recording of upper arm elevation during work using a simplified reference posture versus using a standard reference posture, and 2) to compare the two reference postures.

Methods: Twenty-eight cleaners attached an accelerometer to their dominant upper arm and adopted a simplified reference according to a written instruction. They were thereafter instructed by a researcher to adopt a standard reference. Upper arm elevations were recorded for 2 or 3 days. Each recording was analysed twice; relative to the simplified reference posture and relative to the standard reference posture. The group means of the differences in recorded upper arm elevations between simplified and standard reference analyses were assessed using Wilcoxon signed ranks test. Furthermore, we calculated the group mean of the differences between the simplified reference posture and the standard reference posture.

Results: For arm elevation during work (50th percentile), the group mean of the differences between the two analyses was 0.2° (range -7 – 10°). The group mean of the differences between the two references was 9° (range 1 – 21°). The subjects were able to follow the instructions in the protocol and performed self-recording of upper arm elevation and velocity.

Conclusions: The small difference between the two analyses indicates that recordings performed by employees themselves are comparable, on a group level, with those performed by researchers. Self-recordings in combination with action levels would provide employers with a method for risk assessment as a solid basis for prevention of work-related musculoskeletal disorders.

Keywords: Inclinometry, Zero position, Self-measurement, Physical workload, Angular velocity, Arm elevation, Hotel housekeeping

* Correspondence: camilla.dahlqvist@med.lu.se
[1]Division of Occupational and Environmental Medicine, Department of Laboratory Medicine, Lund University, SE-221 85 Lund, Sweden
Full list of author information is available at the end of the article

Background

Many jobs involve repetitive work, prolonged muscular load and work performed in awkward and constrained postures. Such work are known to be risk factors for developing work-related musculoskeletal disorders (WMSDs) in the neck/shoulder region, arms, and hands [1–4]. To reduce these risks, it is important to perform risk assessments, and to implement organisational and technical measures when necessary [5]. The reliability of risk assessments is important as this affects the decisions made and the priorities afforded different interventions [6].

Several kinds of risk assessment methods are available, such as self-reporting, observational methods and technical methods, all of which have advantages and disadvantages [7]. For example, in self-reporting, which has the advantage of being practical in large groups, overestimation of the workload is common among individuals with pain [8]. Observational methods are often easy to use and interpret, and give a rough estimate of postures during work, but results vary between observers [9]. As observational methods have no common references, they tend to give different results when assessing the risk of developing WMSDs [10, 11]. Technical methods, on the other hand, provide exact numerical values for both postures and movements during work, i.e. upper arm elevation and velocity [12].

There is a commonly held belief that technical methods require expensive equipment, technical understanding and are time-consuming [13]. However, low-cost sensors for recording of elevations and velocities during work are now commercially available [14, 15]. These sensors have also made it feasible to measure the workload over several days [16]. Many studies have been performed previously in which the workload on a few individuals has been recorded during 1 day [17, 18]. With the advent of low-cost sensors, it is now possible to monitor the entire workforce over several days.

Measurements over extended periods of time are important in planning job rotation as a measure for the prevention of WMSDs [19]. Furthermore, measurements made over several days will give a better idea of the loads experienced on an average working day [20]. Such an average measurement is likely to be more strongly correlated with the prevalence of WMSDs than those from one-day recordings. So far, the number of technical recordings has been limited, mainly due to the need for researchers.

If self-recording of physical workload was possible, all the employees' workload at almost any workplace could be explored for several days. Such recordings would be invaluable when performing risk assessments. However, it would be necessary to develop easily understandable instructions so that the employees can attach the equipment and calibrate it, i.e. adopt a reference posture. The reference posture should have a high reproducibility, and this can be studied if recordings are performed over several days. The reference posture should also be easy to adopt, and without the need of extra material. Such a reference would rule out our standard reference posture, which we have used in many studies, as the latter requires a chair and a dumbbell [17, 21–23]. A self-recording method also requires a reliable method of identifying the reference, as this defines 0 degrees of inclination. Furthermore, the starting and stopping times of work and breaks should be noted, to distinguish between working time and leisure time.

One occupation with a high physical workload and a high risk of WMSDs is cleaning [24]. As an example, the prevalence of complaints and diagnoses in neck/shoulders has been reported to be 48% among female hospital cleaners working in a traditional work organisation [25]. Around the world there are many employees working as cleaners and it is important to perform risk assessments of their work in a cost-effective manner. Therefore, we would like to test the self-recording method in the cleaning industry.

The main aims of this study were: 1) to compare analyses for self-recording of upper arm elevation during work using a simplified reference posture versus using a standard reference posture, and 2) to compare the two reference postures. Other aims were to study the between-day repeatability in the simplified reference posture, and to assess the suitability of a protocol for self-recording. Furthermore, we aimed to compare the physical workload, the between-day repeatability of the workload, and to assess the risk of musculoskeletal disorders among different types of cleaning.

Subjects and methods
Study design

This was a field study including two parts. In part one (self-recordings), workers received a protocol with instructions on how to attach a triaxial accelerometer (GC inclinometer) to the upper arm, and how to adopt a reference posture. It was adopted by the cleaners themselves, without the need of extra material, and referred to as the simplified reference posture. A researcher then instructed each of them to adopt the standard reference posture. The workers wore the GC inclinometer continuously, both day and night, for 2 or 3 days. They repeated the simplified reference posture each morning and noted starting and stopping times of work and lunch breaks for each day in a provided form.

In part two (researchers' recordings), which was conducted on different days than the self-recordings, the researchers attached the GC inclinometer to the worker's right upper arm and instructed each subject to perform the standard reference posture. The researchers followed each worker during the one-day recording and noted exact starting and stopping times for work and breaks.

Subjects
Self-recordings
Twenty-eight subjects, 24 women and 4 men, participated in the study (Table 1). Their mean age was 43 years (range 22–58). Twenty-four of the subjects (20 women and 4 men) worked as hotel cleaners and 4 (all women) as office cleaners. Three of the 28 subjects were native Swedish speakers, while the other 25 spoke English and Swedish of varying quality. All the hotel cleaners cleaned hotel rooms (denoted hotel housekeeping). Some of them (eleven subjects) also had other tasks such as cleaning corridors, conference rooms, pool areas and/or dining rooms (denoted hotel housekeeping+). The office cleaners cleaned mainly offices, but also toilets, changing rooms, corridors and dining rooms.

Researchers' recordings
Fourteen right-handed female hotel cleaners participated in standard one-day recordings performed by professionals (Table 1). Their mean age was 42 years (range 22–57). They all cleaned hotel rooms. Five of these also performed self-recording, on separate occasions.

Materials
Triaxial accelerometers with an integrated data logger (USB Accelerometer Model X16-mini, Gulf Coast Data Concepts, LLC, Waveland, MS, USA, "GC inclinometer") with a sampling frequency of 25 Hz were used. This frequency is sufficient as it has been shown that 99.5% of the signal power for wrist (and it is not expected to be higher for the upper arms) was contained in the 0–5 Hz band in occupational repetitive work [26]. The size was $5 \times 2.4 \times 1.3$ cm and they contained a 2 GB memory for data logging, a female micro USB-connector and a rechargeable battery [14]. The accelerometer was attached to the upper arm, just below the insertion of the deltoid muscle, with double-sided adhesive tape and fixed with plastic film (Tegaderm™, 3 M Health Care, St Paul, MN, USA) to secure them from falling off.

Procedures
Standard reference posture
The researcher instructed the subject to sit on a chair and lean towards the backrest with the arm hanging vertically over the backrest, holding a dumbbell in the hand (Fig. 1a) [21].

Simplified reference posture
The subject followed the instructions in the protocol and leaned to the right with the arm alongside the body and with an extended elbow for about 20 s (Fig. 1b) [14].

Table 1 Anthropometric characteristics

	Self-recording			Researchers' recording		
	Height (cm)	Weight (kg)	BMI	Weight (cm)	Height (kg)	BMI
	160	50	20	160	50	20
	170	73	25	170	73	25
	172	61	21	172	61	21
	–	–	–	–	–	–
	169	70	25	169	70	25
	–	82	–			
	168	65	23			
	176	73	24			
	168	66	23			
	167	54	19			
	168	80	28			
	150	42	19			
	174	106	35			
	168	80	28			
	153	50	21			
	–	–	–			
	159	82	32			
	155	59	25			
	–	–	–			
	154	50	21			
	160	50	20			
	158	62	25			
	169	74	26			
	167	65	23			
	146	51	24			
	163	63	24			
	148	48	22			
	168	75	27			
				177	69	22
				160	50	20
				165	–	–
				162	–	–
				158	63	25
				160	61	24
				160	60	23
				157	52	21
				172	65	22
Mean	163	65	24	165	61	22.5
SD	8.4	15	4	6.5	8.0	2.1

Height, weight and BMI for the 37 subjects participating in the study. Twenty-eight subjects participated in the self-recording and fourteen subjects participated in the researchers' recording. Five subjects participated in both types of recordings
- missing data

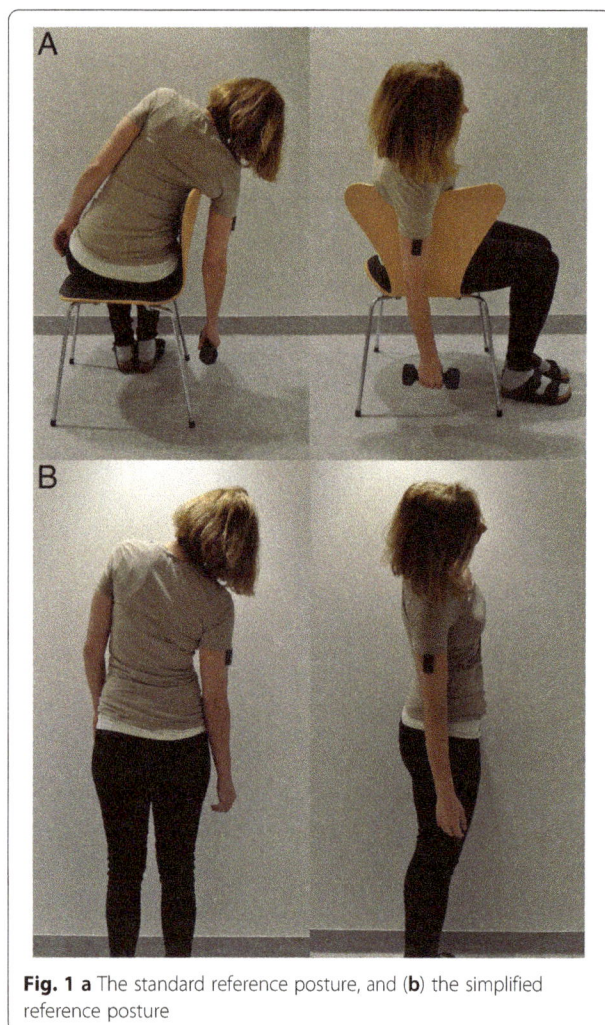

Fig. 1 a The standard reference posture, and (**b**) the simplified reference posture

The protocol

The self-recording method was tested in the cleaning industry. We made one Swedish and one English version of the protocol, as it is known to be a high proportion of immigrants among the employees [27]. Twenty-five subjects chose to use the Swedish version, while three subjects chose the English version. The protocol with instructions for using the GC inclinometer consisted mainly of pictures with short explanations how to attach the GC inclinometer and how to perform the simplified reference posture (see Additional file 1). The researcher noted that the first subjects seemed to have some difficulties in understanding the Swedish and English instructions properly, due to language barriers. Therefore, we improved the protocol in steps during the study. The first change (version 2) was to add instructions on how to start the GC inclinometer (which for the first subjects had been performed by the researcher), to obtain a complete instruction for self-recording of upper arm elevation and velocity. We also simplified the part on how

to attach the inclinometer. The second change (version 3) was to add a second series of toe jumps after the simplified reference posture to improve our ability to determine which part of the recording corresponded to it. To make it easier for the subjects to perform the self-recording, minor changes were made throughout the study, such as highlighting the most important steps (starting the device and performing the simplified reference posture), numbering the various steps in the protocol and simplifying the language in the text boxes. Three versions of the protocol were used. Version 1 was used by four subjects, version 2 was used by five, and version 3 was used by 19 subjects. A few subjects needed help to start the GC inclinometer and some of them had to be reminded to adopt the simplified reference posture. However, the need for help decreased with improved versions of the protocol.

Self-recordings

Each subject was given a GC inclinometer and a protocol with instructions. Nineteen subjects (at twelve different times) individually followed the protocol and attached the GC inclinometer, performed five toe jumps and adopted the simplified reference posture by themselves. The toe jumps were later used to find this part of the recording. At one occasion, nine subjects were helped by their supervisor, due to lack of time. The supervisor started and attached the GC inclinometer, and instructed each subject how to perform the simplified reference posture. The supervisor had not used the protocol previously.

For each subject, the researcher did a brief visual inspection of that the GC inclinometer was attached properly. The researcher then instructed each of the subjects to perform the standard reference posture.

The subjects were instructed to perform the simplified reference posture every morning and to note the time for this and the starting and stopping times of work and lunch breaks in the provided form. They were instructed to apply more plastic film if needed and they were also told to remove the GC inclinometer if they experienced itching or irritation of the skin. Nineteen of the subjects wore the GC inclinometer for 3 days and nine subjects wore it for 2 days. At the end of the second or third working day, the researcher instructed the subject to perform the standard reference posture again, and then removed the GC inclinometer. In four cases the supervisor removed the GC inclinometer, and one subject removed it herself. The stop time was noted.

Researchers' recordings

Researchers experienced in technical methods attached the GC inclinometer to the subject's right upper arm, one subject at a time, on different days from the self-recordings. Each subject was instructed to adopt the standard reference posture for the right upper arm. The researchers followed each subject during their working day, noting the exact starting and stopping times for work, breaks, and different work tasks.

Questionnaire

To further assess the suitability of the protocol and the self-recording method, all subjects were asked, after the recording, to answer six questions about their perceptions of the self-recording.

Data processing and analyses

The data were processed with the EMINGO software suite, developed by the Division of Occupational and Environmental Medicine in Lund, Sweden using MATLAB (version 2016b, Math Works INC., Natick, MA, USA). The data were resampled at 20 Hz, anti-aliased, low-pass filtered (5 Hz), and visually inspected.

Self-recording

Upper arm elevations and velocities were recorded continuously but only the data on work were analysed. Lunch breaks were excluded according to the times noted in the provided form. The data were analysed twice; once using the simplified reference posture as reference (henceforth referred to as the simplified reference analysis) and once using the standard reference as reference (henceforth referred to as the standard reference analysis). The 1st, 10th, 50th, 90th and 99th percentiles of the angular distribution (°) and the percentage of time the arm was elevated above 30°, 60° and 90° were calculated. Furthermore, the median generalised angular velocity (°/s) was derived for each subject. 1 °/s = 0.017 rad s^{-1} and 1 rad s^{-1} = 57.3 °/s. Group means of upper arm elevations and velocities were calculated for comparisons between the simplified reference analysis and the standard reference analysis. Further, for each subject we calculated the differences between the results derived from the two different analyses, as well as the absolute differences (i.e. the non-negative difference, regardless of sign). Then the group means of the differences and the group means of the absolute differences were calculated.

Furthermore, for each subject, we calculated the difference between the simplified reference posture and the standard reference posture (°). In most cases we used the references from day 1. In one case, the GC inclinometer fell off during day 1. The subject attached it again, and the researcher (who was still there) instructed her, during her lunch break, to perform the standard reference posture again. Another subject appeared to have replaced the GC inclinometer upside down after it had fallen off during the morning day 1 (detected during

data analysis), and therefore this part of the recording was discarded. For this subject, the standard reference posture from day 3 was used. The simplified reference posture from day 2 was used for both these subjects.

The first and second simplified reference posture were used to investigate the reliability of the reference. Nine of the subjects performed the simplified reference posture on one occasion only and were therefore excluded when analysing the within-subject variation of the reference.

The within-subject variation in workload between the first and second working days was also calculated among the hotel cleaners. Then, two recordings were excluded because the subjects removed their GC inclinometer while showering after day 1. They had replaced the device after showering, but did not repeat the simplified reference posture, and therefore, the data for the remaining days had to be rejected. The remaining 22 recordings were divided into hotel housekeeping and hotel housekeeping+, with eleven subjects in each group.

When comparing upper arm elevations and velocities between the specific types of cleaning (hotel housekeeping, hotel housekeeping+, and office cleaning), as well as when comparing with the researchers' one-day recordings of hotel housekeeping, the standard reference analysis was used. The four men were excluded from these calculations, to be able to compare them with previous and future recordings, where the results for women and men are separated [28].

Researchers' recordings

Upper arm elevations and velocities during the working day were analysed, lunch breaks excluded. The same measures as for the self-recordings were calculated; the percentiles of the angular distribution (°) and the percentage of time the arm was elevated above 30°, 60° and 90° were calculated for each subject. The median generalised angular velocity (°/s) was also derived, and group means of both elevations and velocities were calculated.

Statistical analyses

The statistical analyses were carried out with IBM SPSS Statistics Version 22 (SPSS, Chicago, IL, USA). The alpha level was set at 0.05. Comparisons between group means of upper arm elevations for the two reference analyses were performed using Wilcoxon signed ranks test. The within-subject variation was calculated using one-way ANOVA for the simplified reference posture and for the upper arm elevations and velocities during work. The 50th and 90th percentiles of upper arm elevation and the median generalised angular velocity were the dependent variables, and subject was the independent variable. To investigate the repeatability of the simplified reference posture and of the workload between working days, the repeatability coefficient (°) and the intraclass correlation coefficient (ICC) were calculated [29, 30]. We used ICC (1,1) i.e. one-way random effects model, absolute agreement, single measures. ICC estimates less than 0.5, between 0.5 and 0.75, between 0.75 and 0.9, and greater than 0.90 indicate poor, moderate, good, and excellent reliability, respectively [31]. The difference between the simplified reference posture and the standard reference posture of two following occasions, respectively, as well as upper arm elevations (50th and 90th percentiles) and the median angular velocity of two working days were the input variables in the model. Comparisons between group means of different types of cleaning were performed using Kruskal-Wallis one-way analysis of variance. Post hoc analyses for p-values < 0.05 was performed using Mann-Whitney U-test. The non-parametric tests were used since the data were not normally distributed.

Results
Simplified reference analysis versus standard reference analysis
Recordings of workload
The group means of upper arm elevation and the percentage of time above 30°, 60° and 90° during work were very similar between the simplified reference analysis and the standard reference analysis (Table 2). The upper arm velocity was identical (data not shown), as this is not dependent on the reference.

The individual differences between the simplified reference analysis and the standard reference analysis at the 50th percentile of arm elevation during work are shown in Fig. 2. The group mean difference was 0.2° (range -7 – 10°).

Table 2 Group means of upper arm elevations during work for the simplified and the standard reference analyses

	Simplified reference analysis	Standard reference analysis	
	Mean (range)	Mean (range)	p-value
Percentile (°)			
1st	5 (2 – 8)	5 (2 – 10)	0.68
10th	14 (7 – 21)	13 (8 – 20)	0.98
50th	30 (20 – 47)	30 (22 – 38)	0.98
90th	64 (45 – 91)	64 (50 – 86)	0.95
99th	109 (88 – 132)	110 (94 – 134)	0.30
Percentage of time			
> 30°	49 (27 – 78)	49 (34 – 63)	0.95
> 60°	13 (4 – 35)	12 (5 – 24)	0.95
> 90°	4 (1 – 10)	3 (1 – 8)	0.98

Group means (°) for the simplified reference analysis and the standard reference analysis at the 1st, 10th, 50th, 90th and 99th percentiles of upper arm elevation and the percentage of time above 30°, 60° and 90° for the 28 subjects during work. P-values for difference calculated with Wilcoxon signed rank tests

The group mean of the absolute differences in the 50th percentile of arm elevation was 4° (range 0 – 10°; Table 3), and for the percentage of time above 30° it was 9% (range 0 – 21%), for 60° 2% (0 – 11%), and for 90° 1% (0 – 3%).

Simplified reference posture versus standard reference posture
The differences (°) between the simplified reference posture and the standard reference posture on days 1, 2, and 3 for each subject are shown in Fig. 3. The group mean of the differences for day 1 (day 2 for two subjects) was 9° (range 1 – 21°). The individual arm position in the simplified reference posture relative to the arm position during the standard reference posture from day 1 (day 2 for two subjects) are shown in Fig. 4. They deviated in all directions (flexion, extension, adduction and/ or abduction) without any obvious pattern.

Within-subject variation of simplified reference posture
The within-subject variation in the simplified reference posture was poor, with an ICC of 0.2 (Table 4). The repeatability coefficient was 16°.

The protocol
No subjects were excluded due to an incorrect placement of the GC inclinometer. Nevertheless, we improved the protocol during the study. These changes appeared to make it easier for the subjects to follow, as the help needed decreased with improved versions of the protocol. An additional change (version 4) was made after the analyses, with instructions not to replace the GC inclinometer if it falls off.

The protocol includes three parts (see Additional file 1):

1) Starting the GC inclinometer.
2) Attaching the GC inclinometer to the upper arm.
3) Performing the simplified reference posture.

Comparing different types of cleaning
Concerning self-recordings, the median upper arm velocity was higher in hotel housekeeping than in hotel housekeeping+ (82 vs 63 °/s; Table 5). There were no differences between self-recordings and researchers' recordings of hotel housekeeping (Table 5).

Five individuals participated in both the researchers' recordings and the self-recordings. The 90th percentile of upper arm elevation and the median generalised angular velocity for these individuals are shown in Figure 5. For them, the group mean difference for the 90th percentile of upper arm elevation between the researchers' recording on 1 day and the self-recording on several days, using the standard reference, was 1° (range -2 – 8°). The group mean difference for the upper arm velocity was -7 °/s (range -21 °/s – 2 °/s).

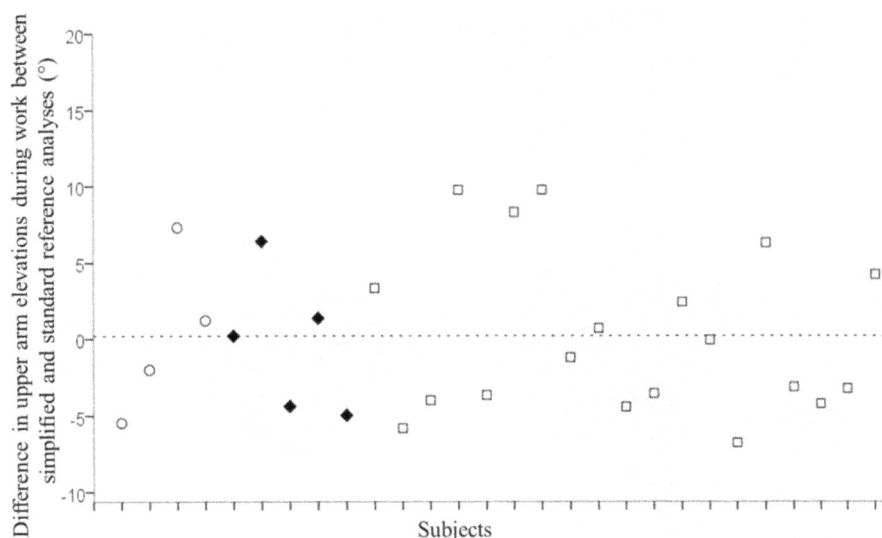

Fig. 2 Individual difference (°) between the simplified reference analysis and the standard reference analysis from day 1 at the 50th percentile of upper arm elevation during work for the 28 subjects. The dashed line indicates the group mean difference (0.2°). Version 1 of the self-recording protocol was used by four subjects (o), version 2 was used by five (♦) and version 3 was used by 19 subjects (□)

Within-subject variation in workload between days

The repeatability coefficient for hotel housekeeping was 1.6° with an ICC of 0.98 for the 50th percentile of upper arm elevation (Table 6). Corresponding values for hotel housekeeping+ were 4.8° and 0.86, respectively. The individual variations in upper arm velocities during the different working days are shown in Fig. 6.

The subjects' perception of self-recording

The subjects' perceptions are reported in Table 7. One subject answered "Bad" to one of the questions. All other answers were positive. Additionally, 87% of the subjects stated that the GC inclinometer had not interfered during work or leisure time during the three-day recording, and 96% were willing to wear the GC inclinometer again.

Discussion

On group level, the recordings of upper arm elevation during work using the simplified reference posture were almost identical to the same recordings using the standard reference posture. The subjects were able to follow the instructions in the protocol and performed self-recording of upper arm elevations and velocities for several days.

Simplified reference posture and standard reference posture

For recordings of arm elevations, it has been suggested that it is sufficient to attach an inclinometer with one of its axes aligned with the upper arm (humerus) without adopting a reference posture [15, 32]. However, since the humerus may not be parallel to the line of gravity, for example in subjects with voluminous upper arms (strong or obese), we believe that it is important to perform a reference posture to define 0° inclination. When using the standard reference posture the arm hangs out from the body (see Fig. 1a). Thus, this should be a minor problem. In the simplified reference posture the arm is closer to the body (see Fig. 1b). We therefore plotted the difference between the two reference postures from day 1 (Fig. 4) versus BMI. We saw no correlation, and do not suspect a major influence of BMI.

Table 3 Group means of the absolute differences of upper arm elevations during work between the simplified and the standard reference analyses

	Mean absolute difference (range)
Percentile (°)	
1st	1.8 (0.0 – 4.4)
10th	3.8 (0.2 – 9.1)
50th	4.2 (0.1 – 9.8)
90th	4.2 (0.0 – 12)
99th	4.7 (0.3 – 18)
Percentage of time	
> 30°	9.3 (0.2 – 21)
> 60°	2.3 (0.0 – 11)
> 90°	0.6 (0.1 – 2.9)

The group mean of the absolute differences (°; Mean absolute difference) at the 1st, 10th, 50th, 90th and 99th percentiles of the angular distributions (°) and the percentage of time above 30°, 60° and 90° for the 28 subjects during work, between the simplified reference analysis and the standard reference analysis

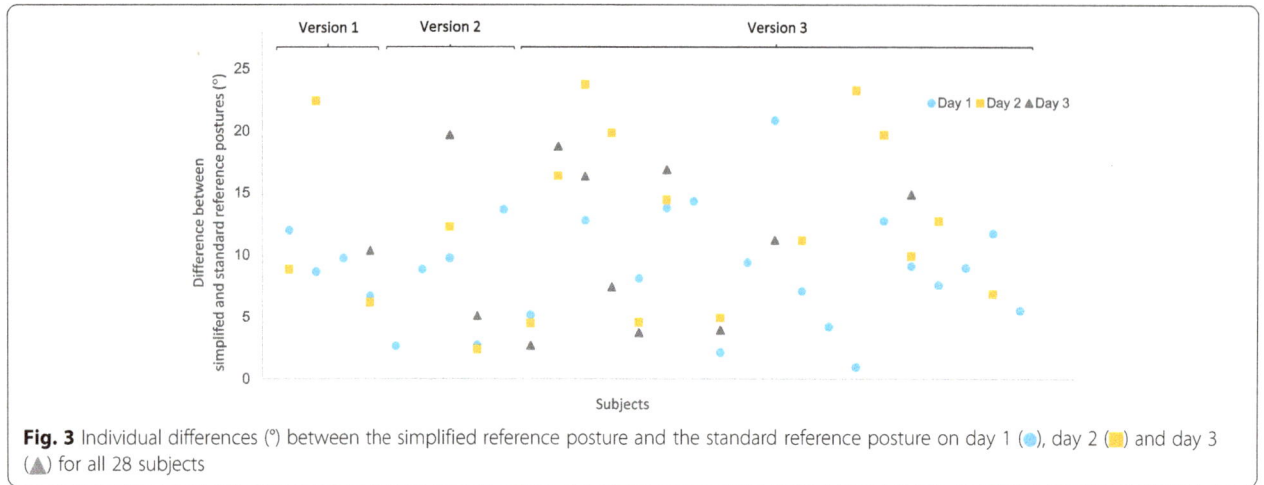

Fig. 3 Individual differences (°) between the simplified reference posture and the standard reference posture on day 1 (●), day 2 (■) and day 3 (▲) for all 28 subjects

For each individual, the difference in upper arm elevation during work between the two analyses was lower than the difference between the two references, and may be explained by the triangle inequality (see Fig. 7). The distance between the two reference points can be seen as the length of one side of a triangle (a). The distance between one of the reference points and a specific elevation point during work can then be seen as the length of a second side of the triangle (b), while the distance between the other reference point and the same specific elevation point can be seen as the length of the third side of the triangle (c). Thus, as the length of one side in a triangle is less than the difference (Δ) of the lengths of the two other sides, the difference between

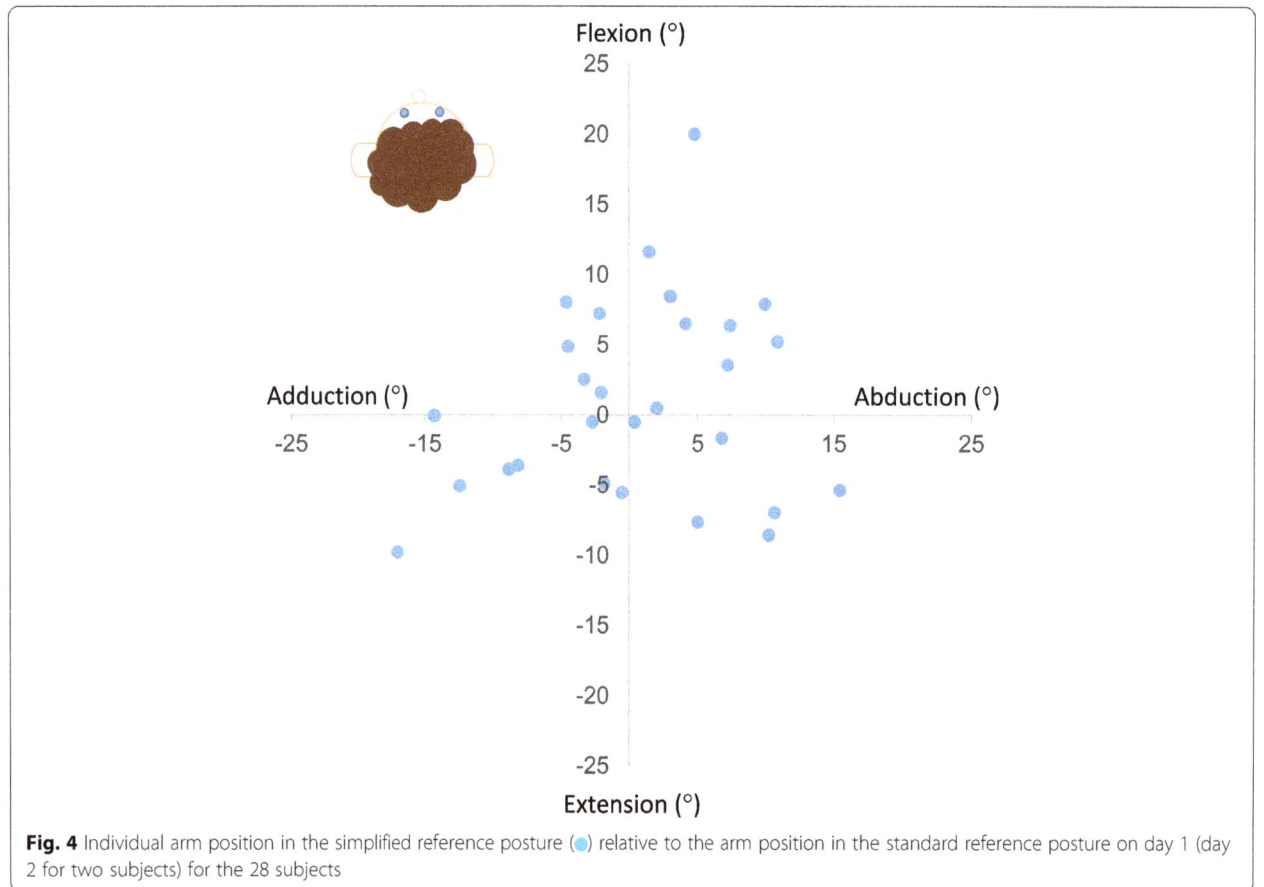

Fig. 4 Individual arm position in the simplified reference posture (●) relative to the arm position in the standard reference posture on day 1 (day 2 for two subjects) for the 28 subjects

Self-recordings of upper arm elevation during cleaning – comparison between analyses using a simplified...

219

Table 4 The within-subject variation of the simplified reference posture

Simplified reference posture		
Within-subject variation	Repeatability coefficient	ICC
SD (95% CI)		
5.6 (3.7 – 7.5)	16	0.2

The within-subject variation (°; standard deviation (SD) and 95% confidence interval (95% CI)), the repeatability coefficient (°) and the intraclass correlation coefficient (ICC) of the simplified reference posture

the two reference analyses will be less than the difference between the two references ($\Delta = b - c < a$). For an elevation point that is equally far from the two reference points, the triangle becomes isosceles and the difference between the two reference analyses will be zero ($\Delta = b - c = 0$). If the elevation point is in line with the two references, the triangle becomes a line and the difference between the two reference analyses will be the same as the difference between the two references ($\Delta = b - c = a$). In this study, the difference during work was never more than 10°, while the difference between the two references was up to 21°. In addition, the group mean difference during work was as low as 0.2° (range -7 – 10°). We therefore consider, on group level, the simplified reference posture sufficient for recording of elevations of the upper arm, given that it is the same work tasks and a low degree of freedom in work performance for all individuals [33]. In the current group of cleaners, the simplified reference posture deviated from the standard reference in a uniform pattern (i.e. in all directions, see Fig. 4). Consequently, deviations during work were balanced on group level. However, this may not be the case in other populations. A non-uniform deviation pattern will introduce a systematic error. Concerning upper arm velocity, the self-recording method can be used on individual level, as this measure is not dependent on the reference.

Within-subject variation of simplified reference posture

In a previous study of natural head posture recorded with inclinometer, the individual overall variability (standard deviation) was 1.6° [34]. In our study, the standard deviation of the within-subject variation was 5.6° for the simplified reference posture, i.e. somewhat higher. We speculate that this difference may be because it is more difficult to repeat an arm posture (without support) than a head posture, as in the latter the sight angle serves as a reference. The repeatability coefficient for the simplified reference posture was 16°. Thus, in 95% of measurements, the absolute difference between two simplified reference measurements on one subject is not expected to exceed 16°. Therefore, a recording of upper arm elevations analysed with the simplified reference posture at only one occasion should be interpreted with some caution.

The protocol and the subjects' perceptions of self-recording

The protocol was continuously improved during the study. Thereby, the problems that occurred during the study were resolved. Most importantly, if the GC inclinometer falls off it should not be replaced. Further, toe jumps are performed before *and* after the simplified reference posture. We believe that version 4 is easy to use. Still, for subjects that do not speak Swedish or English, one might consider to translate it into the language in question.

According to the questionnaire which the subjects answered after the study, all but one of the subjects were positive to self-recordings of upper arm elevations and velocities. Only one person answered "Bad" to the question "How did you experience to put on more plastic film?" Since eight subjects reported that it had not been necessary, we think this negative answer was due to language barriers, and this subject also meant that it had not been necessary.

Table 5 Group means of upper arm elevation and velocity during different types of cleaning

	Self-recordings during 3 days			Standard one-day recordings
	Hotel housekeeping (n = 9)	Hotel housekeeping+ (n = 11)	Office cleaning (n = 4)	Hotel housekeeping (n = 14)
	Mean (range)	Mean (range)	Mean (range)	Mean (range)
Elevation (°)				
50th	30 (25 – 36)	28 (22 – 35)	33 (29 – 38)	28 (21 – 38)
90th	65 (50 – 79)	62 (50 – 77)	64 (54 – 83)	61 (47 – 75)
Velocity (°/s)				
50th	82[a] (53 – 114)	63[a] (37 – 89)	56 (37 – 75)	92 (66 – 129)

Group means at the 50th and 90th percentiles of upper arm elevation (°) and the median generalised upper arm angular velocity (°/s) during different types of cleaning when using the standard reference posture as reference. (Data from the four men are excluded). The generalised angular velocity is not dependent on the reference posture. Hotel housekeeping = cleaning hotel rooms, hotel housekeeping+ = cleaning hotel rooms and other tasks such as cleaning corridors. The standard recordings were performed by researchers. Differences calculated by Kruskal-Wallis analysis of variance. Post hoc analysis with Mann-Whitney U-test
[a]$p = 0.05$

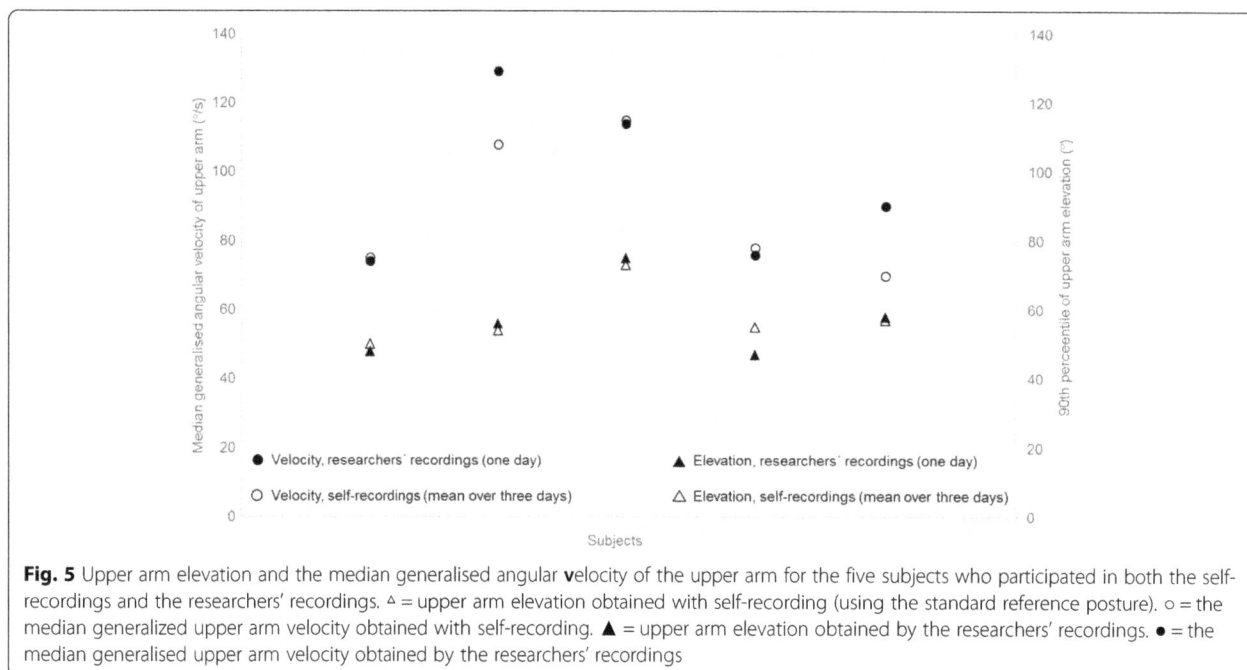

Fig. 5 Upper arm elevation and the median generalised angular **v**elocity of the upper arm for the five subjects who participated in both the self-recordings and the researchers' recordings. △ = upper arm elevation obtained with self-recording (using the standard reference posture). ○ = the median generalized upper arm velocity obtained with self-recording. ▲ = upper arm elevation obtained by the researchers' recordings. ● = the median generalised upper arm velocity obtained by the researchers' recordings

Risk of musculoskeletal disorders among cleaning staff

Our research group has performed technical measurements of upper arm elevations and velocities for about thirty years in about sixty different occupations. Most of these occupational groups have also been clinically examined using the standardised Health Surveillance in Adverse Ergonomics Conditions (HECO) method [35, 36] which quantifies the prevalence of WMSDs and diagnoses of the neck and upper extremities. Exposure-response relationships were obtained by compiling the data from the technical measurements and the clinical examinations, and we found strong associations between upper arm velocity and several diagnoses [2]. Based on this knowledge, we have recently proposed action levels for the prevention of WMSDs. The proposed action level for the median generalised angular velocity is 60 °/s [37]. This is well in line with the findings in a recent study

by Dalbøge et al., where it was indicated that a median generalised angular velocity of the upper arm below 45 °/s was safe [38]. Based on previous studies [2, 39–42], we have proposed an action level of 60° for the 90th percentile of upper arm elevation. The action level for elevation was exceeded in office cleaning, while the action levels for both elevation and angular velocity were exceeded in hotel housekeeping (both self-recordings and researchers' recordings) and hotel housekeeping+, indicating the need for preventive actions. Hence, it was highly relevant to test the self-recording method among cleaners.

Within-subject variation of workload between working days

The within-subject variation in upper arm elevation and velocity between working days in hotel housekeeping was low. This indicates that the work is monotonous and repetitive. The between days variation differed

Table 6 The group means and the within-subject variations of upper arm elevation and velocity between working days

Percentile	Hotel housekeeping (*n* = 11)				Hotel housekeeping+ (*n* = 11)			
	Group mean (° or °/s)	Within-subject variation SD (95% CI)	Repeatability coefficient (° or °/s)	ICC	Group mean (° or °/s)	Within-subject variation SD (95% CI)	Repeatability coefficient (° or °/s)	ICC
50th (°)	29	0.6 (0.3 – 0.9)	1.6	0.98	28	1.7 (0.9 – 2.5)	4.8	0.86
90th (°)	64	1.5 (0.8 – 2.2)	4.1	0.97	62	4.4 (2.3 – 6.4)	12	0.80
Vel. (°/s)	81	4.7 (2.5 – 6.9)	13	0.93	63	12 (6.4 – 18)	33	0.66

The group mean, the within-subject variation (° or °/s; standard deviation (SD) and 95% confidence intervals (95% CI)), the repeatability coefficient (° or °/s) and the intraclass correlation coefficient (ICC) of upper arm elevations (°; 50th and 90th percentiles of the angular distribution) and median upper arm velocity (°/s; Vel.) between working days for 22 subjects. Self-recordings of hotel housekeeping and hotel housekeeping+. Hotel housekeeping = cleaning hotel rooms and hotel housekeeping+ = cleaning hotel rooms and other tasks such as cleaning corridors. The standard reference posture was used as reference

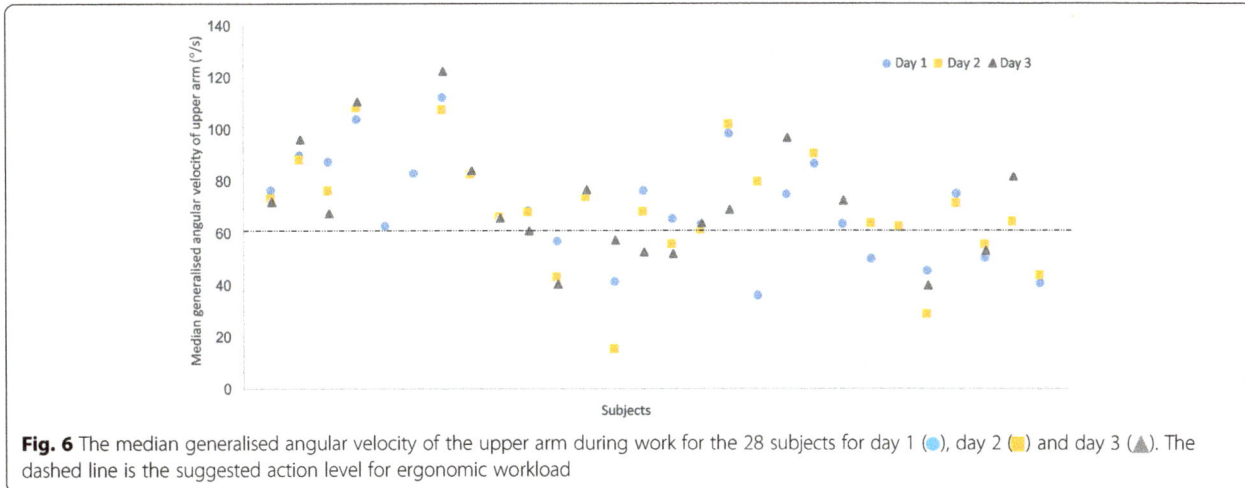

Fig. 6 The median generalised angular velocity of the upper arm during work for the 28 subjects for day 1 (●), day 2 (■) and day 3 (▲). The dashed line is the suggested action level for ergonomic workload

between hotel housekeeping + and hotel housekeeping, and one explanation could be that there were additional and more varied work tasks in hotel housekeeping+, such as for example cleaning corridors, conference rooms and pool areas.

Methodological considerations

To the best of our knowledge, this is the first time self-recordings have been made of upper arm elevation and velocity. This required a protocol explaining how to perform the self-recording. A strength of the study was that the protocol was tested and improved in an occupation with a high proportion of immigrants. Even if the

Table 7 Questionnaire responses after the self-recording

	Bad	Rather bad	Rather good	Good
How did you experience to wear the GC-inclinometer during several days?			4 (17%)	20 (83%)
How did you experience to sleep with the GC-inclinometer on?			5 (22%)	18 (78%)
How did you experience to shower with the sensor?			3 (15%)	17 (85%)
How did you experience to attach more plastic film?[a]	1 (7%)		1 (7%)	12 (86%)
How did you experience to perform the toe jumps and the reference position each morning?			1 (5%)	21 (95%)
How did you experience to fill in the diary?			7 (32%)	15 (68%)

Distribution of questionnaire responses from 24 subjects after self-recording of upper arm elevation and velocity during 3 days. The response rate (proportion within brackets) are given for the different options
[a] eight subjects reported that this was not necessary

subjects spoke poor Swedish and English, they were able to perform self-recordings. This indicates that the protocol is easy to follow and may be used by most employees. A weakness is that we did not improve the protocol systematically and did not evaluate the different steps of improvements in a systematic manner. Instead, we made changes in the protocol based on how comfortable and secure the subjects appeared to be when they attached the GC inclinometer and performed the simplified reference posture. On a visual inspection of Fig. 2 we did not see any improvement concerning the individual differences between the two analyses. Thus, we do not think that different versions of the protocol impacted on our data.

Considering recordings of upper arm elevation, we judge a difference of 5° to be clinically relevant. Prior to the study we did not know the distribution of the differences between the analyses with the two different reference postures. As this was about 5° for both the 50th and the 90th percentiles we would have needed 11 subjects to be able to detect a 5° difference between the two analyses with an 80% power. As 28 cleaners were included, we could detect a difference of 3°.

Conclusions

The small difference between the simplified reference analysis and the standard reference analysis indicates that recordings performed by employees themselves are comparable, on group level, with those performed by researchers. The subjects in this study were able to perform self-recording of upper arm elevations and velocities using the protocol provided. The simplified reference posture is sufficient on group level, with the assumption that it is the same work tasks and a high similarity in work performance for all individuals. The self-recording method can be used at an individual level

$\Delta = b - c < a$

Elevation point

b   c

Standard reference posture point   a   Simplified reference posture point

Elevation point

$\Delta = b - c = 0$

b   c

Standard reference posture point   a   Simplified reference posture point

$\Delta = b - c = a$

b

Standard reference posture point   a   c   Elevation point

Simplified reference posture point

Fig. 7 The triangle inequality may be used to explain that the average difference in upper arm elevation between the two analyses was lower than the difference between the two reference postures. The upper triangle illustrates the case that is likely to occur most of the work time. In that case the difference $\Delta = b - c < a$, where a is the difference between the two reference posture points, and b – c is the difference between the two analyses. In the (unusual) middle case $\Delta = b - c = 0$; the elevation point is equally far from the two reference posture points, and in the (unusual) lower case, $\Delta = b - c = a$, the elevation point is in line with and outside the two reference posture points, and the difference between the two reference analyses will be the same as the difference between the two reference postures. So Δ is always less or equal to the difference between the two reference posture points

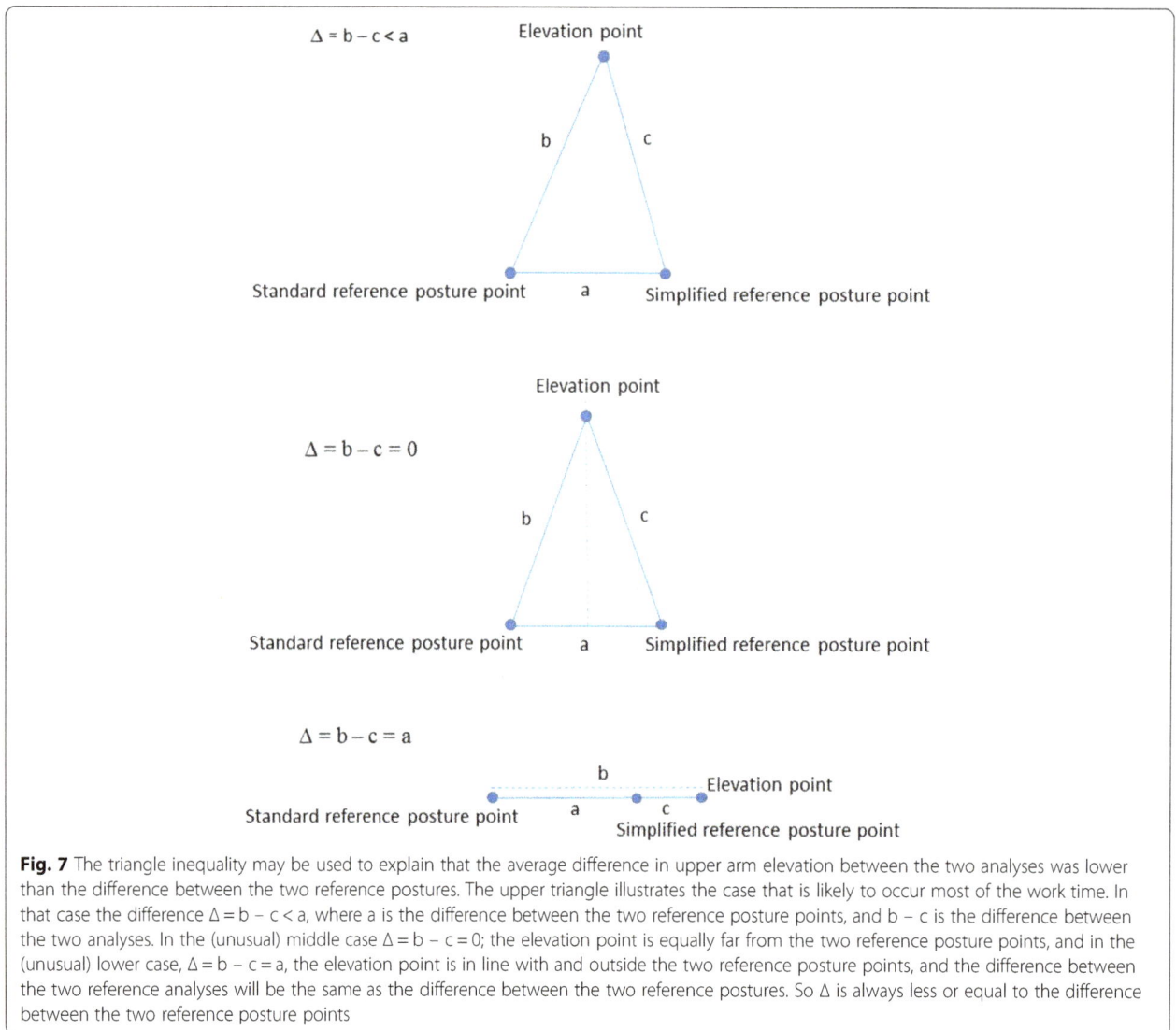

for recording of upper arm velocity. Self-recording could increase the use of technical methods when performing risk assessments and, in combination with action levels for the prevention of WMSDs, increase the accuracy of risk assessments. In addition, self-recording in combination with action levels would provide employers with a method of assessing the risk of developing WMSDs among employees, which would be an important improvement of prevention. Hotel cleaning implies a high risk of musculoskeletal disorders due to a high upper arm velocity.

Abbreviations
GC inclinometer: Gulf Coast triaxial accelerometer X16-mini; WMSDs: Work-related musculoskeletal disorders

Acknowledgements
The authors wish to thank all the subjects, the hotels, and cleaning companies participating in the study.

Funding
The current study was supported by AFA Insurance (No. 150181). AFA Insurance had no role in the design of the study, collection, analysis, interpretation of data, and in writing the manuscript.

Authors' contributions
CD and CN were responsible for the concept and design of the study. CD was responsible for the data collection and performed the data analyses and the statistical analyses. CD drafted the manuscript. HE was responsible for development of the software for data analyses. CD, CN, MF and HE were responsible for the interpretation of the results. CD, CN, MF and HE have contributed to, read, and approved the final manuscript.

Competing interests
The authors declare that they have no competing interests.

Author details
[1]Division of Occupational and Environmental Medicine, Department of Laboratory Medicine, Lund University, SE-221 85 Lund, Sweden. [2]Division of Ergonomics, KTH Royal Institute of Technology, SE-141 57 Huddinge, Sweden.

References

1. da Costa BR, Vieira ER. Risk factors for work-related musculoskeletal disorders: a systematic review of recent longitudinal studies. Am J Ind Med. 2010;53:285–323.
2. Nordander C, Hansson G-Å, Ohlsson K, Arvidsson I, Balogh I, Strömberg U, Rittner R, Skerfving S. Exposure–response relationships for work-related neck and shoulder musculoskeletal disorders – analyses of pooled uniform data sets. Appl Ergon. 2016;55:70–84.
3. Nordander C, Ohlsson K, Åkesson I, Arvidsson I, Balogh I, Hansson G-Å, Strömberg U, Rittner R, Skerfving S. Exposure–response relationships in work-related musculoskeletal disorders in elbows and hands – a synthesis of group-level data on exposure and response obtained using uniform methods of data collection. Appl Ergon. 2013;44:241–53.
4. van Rijn RM, Huisstede BM, Koes BW, Burdorf A. Associations between work-related factors and the carpal tunnel syndrome--a systematic review. Scand J Work Environ Health. 2009;35:19–36.
5. Phillips K, Bills J, Gare J. Developing modified equipment and work practices to reduce the risk of work-related musculoskeletal disorders from conservation treatment. AICCM Bulletin. 2016;37:42–8.
6. Spielholz P, Silverstein B, Morgan M, Checkoway H, Kaufman J. Comparison of self-report, video observation and direct measurement methods for upper extremity musculoskeletal disorder physical risk factors. Ergonomics. 2001;44:588–613.
7. Li G, Buckle P. Current techniques for assessing physical exposure to work-related musculoskeletal risks, with emphasis on posture-based methods. Ergonomics. 1999;42:674–95.
8. Hansson GA, Balogh I, Bystrom JU, Ohlsson K, Nordander C, Asterland P, Sjolander S, Rylander L, Winkel J, Skerfving S. Questionnaire versus direct technical measurements in assessing postures and movements of the head, upper back, arms and hands. Scand J Work Environ Health. 2001;27:30–40.
9. Eliasson K, Palm P, Nyman T, Forsman M. Inter- and intra- observer reliability of risk assessment of repetitive work without an explicit method. Appl Ergon. 2017;62:1–8.
10. Chiasson M-È, Imbeau D, Aubry K, Delisle A. Comparing the results of eight methods used to evaluate risk factors associated with musculoskeletal disorders. Int J Ind Ergon. 2012;42:478–88.
11. Takala EP, Pehkonen I, Forsman M, Hansson GA, Mathiassen SE, Neumann WP, Sjogaard G, Veiersted KB, Westgaard RH, Winkel J. Systematic evaluation of observational methods assessing biomechanical exposures at work. Scand J Work Environ Health. 2010;36:3 24.
12. Hansson G-Å, Balogh I, Ohlsson K, Granqvist L, Nordander C, Arvidsson I, Åkesson I, Unge J, Rittner R, Strömberg U, Skerfving S. Physical workload in various types of work: part II. Neck, shoulder and upper arm. Int J Ind Ergon. 2010;40:267–81.
13. David GC. Ergonomic methods for assessing exposure to risk factors for work-related musculoskeletal disorders. Occup Med. 2005;55:190–9.
14. Dahlqvist C, Hansson G-Å, Forsman M. Validity of a small low-cost triaxial accelerometer with integrated logger for uncomplicated measurements of postures and movements of head, upper back and upper arms. Appl Ergon. 2016;55:108–16.
15. Korshøj M, Skotte JH, Christiansen CS, Mortensen P, Kristiansen J, Hanisch C, Ingebrigtsen J, Holtermann A. Validity of the Acti4 software using ActiGraph GT3X+accelerometer for recording of arm and upper body inclination in simulated work tasks. Ergonomics. 2014;57:247–53.
16. Villumsen M, Madeleine P, Jørgensen MB, Holtermann A, Samani A. The variability of the trunk forward bending in standing activities during work vs. leisure time. Appl Ergon. 2017;58:273–80.
17. Åkesson I, Balogh I, Hansson GÅ. Physical workload in neck, shoulders and wrists/hands in dental hygienists during a work-day. Appl Ergon. 2012;43:803–11.
18. Arvidsson I, Balogh I, Hansson G-Å, Ohlsson K, Åkesson I, Nordander C. Rationalization in meat cutting – consequences on physical workload. Appl Ergon. 2012;43:1026–32.
19. Balogh I, Ohlsson K, Nordander C, Bjork J, Hansson GA. The importance of work organization on workload and musculoskeletal health--grocery store work as a model. Appl Ergon. 2016;53(Pt A):143–51.
20. Jørgensen MB, Korshøj M, Lagersted-Olsen J, Villumsen M, Mortensen OS, Skotte J, Søgaard K, Madeleine P, Thomsen BL, Holtermann A. Physical activities at work and risk of musculoskeletal pain and its consequences: protocol for a study with objective field measures among blue-collar workers. BMC Musculoskelet Disord. 2013;14:213.
21. Hansson GA, Arvidsson I, Ohlsson K, Nordander C, Mathiassen SE, Skerfving S, Balogh I. Precision of measurements of physical workload during standardised manual handling. Part II: Inclinometry of head, upper back, neck and upper arms. J Electromyogr Kinesiol. 2006;16:125–36.
22. Simonsen JG, Dahlqvist C, Enquist H, Nordander C, Axmon A, Arvidsson I. Assessments of physical workload in sonography tasks using Inclinometry, goniometry, and Electromyography. Saf Health Work. 2018;9:326–33.
23. Heilskov-Hansen T, Wulff Svendsen S, Frølund Thomsen J, Mikkelsen S, Hansson G-Å. Sex differences in task distribution and task exposures among Danish house painters: an observational study combining questionnaire data with biomechanical measurements. PLoS One. 2014;9:1–10.
24. Buchanan S, Vossenas P, Krause N, Moriarty J, Frumin E, Shimek JAM, Mirer F, Orris P, Punnett L. Occupational injury disparities in the US hotel industry. Am J Ind Med. 2010;53:116–25.
25. Unge J, Ohlsson K, Nordander C, Hansson GA, Skerfving S, Balogh I. Differences in physical workload, psychosocial factors and musculoskeletal disorders between two groups of female hospital cleaners with two diverse organizational models. Int Arch Occup Environ Health. 2007;81:209–20.
26. Hansson GÅ, Balogh I, Ohlsson K, Rylander L, Skerfving S. Goniometer measurement and computer analysis of wrist angles and movements applied to occupational repetitive work. J Electromyogr Kinesiol. 1996;6:23–35.
27. Thörnquist A. East-West Labour Migration and the Swedish Cleaning Industry : A matter of immigrant competition? In: ThemES - Themes on Migration and Ethnic Studies. Linköping: Linköping University Electronic Press; 2015. p. 43.
28. Messing K, Punnett L, Bond M, Alexanderson K, Pyle J, Zahm S, Wegman D, Stock SR, de Grosbois S. Be the fairest of them all: challenges and recommendations for the treatment of gender in occupational health research. Am J Ind Med. 2003;43:618–29.
29. McGraw KO, Wong SP. Forming inferences about some intraclass correlation coefficients. Psychol Methods. 1996;1:30–46.
30. Martin Bland J, Altman D. Statistical methods for assessing agreement between two methods of clinical measurement. Lancet. 1986;327:307–10.
31. Koo TK, Li MY. A guideline of selecting and reporting Intraclass correlation coefficients for reliability research. J Chiropr Med. 2016;15:155–63.
32. Hallman DM, Jørgensen MB, Holtermann A. Objectively measured physical activity and 12-month trajectories of neck–shoulder pain in workers: a prospective study in DPHACTO. Scand J Public Health. 2017;45:288–98.
33. Balogh I, Hansson G-Å, Ohlsson K, Strömberg U, Skerfving S. Interindividual variation of physical load in a work task. Scand J Work Environ Health. 1999;25:57–66.
34. Üşümez S, Orhan M. Reproducibility of natural head position measured with an inclinometer. Am J Orthod Dentofac Orthop. 2003;123:451–4.
35. Jonker D, Gustafsson E, Rolander B, Arvidsson I, Nordander C. Health surveillance under adverse ergonomics conditions – validity of a screening method adapted for the occupational health service. Ergonomics. 2015;58:1519–28.
36. Nordander C, Ohlsson K, Akesson I, Arvidsson I, Balogh I, Hansson GA, Stromberg U, Rittner R, Skerfving S. Risk of musculoskeletal disorders among females and males in repetitive/constrained work. Ergonomics. 2009;52:1226–39.
37. Arvidsson I, Dahlqvist C, Enquist H, Nordander C. Action levels for prevention of work related musculoskeletal disorders. Lund: Occupational and Environmental Medicine; 2017. http://sodrasjukvardsregionen.se/download/rapport-182017-atgardsnivaer-mot-belastningsskada
38. Dalbøge A, Frost P, Andersen JH, Svendsen SW. Surgery for subacromial impingement syndrome in relation to intensities of occupational mechanical exposures across 10-year exposure time windows. Occup Environ Med. 2017.
39. Svendsen SW, Bonde JP, Mathiassen SE, Stengaard-Pedersen K, Frich LH. Work related shoulder disorders: quantitative exposure-response relations with reference to arm posture. Occup Environ Med. 2004;61:844–53.
40. Bodin J, Ha C, Petit Le Manac'h A, Sérazin C, Descatha A, Leclerc A, Goldberg M, Roquelaure Y. Risk factors for incidence of rotator cuff syndrome in a large working population. Scand J Work Environ Health. 2012;38:436–46.
41. Dalbøge A, Frost P, Andersen JH, Svendsen SW. Cumulative occupational shoulder exposures and surgery for subacromial impingement syndrome: a nationwide Danish cohort study. Occup Environ Med. 2014;71:750–6.
42. Mayer J, Kraus T, Ochsmann E. Longitudinal evidence for the association between work-related physical exposures and neck and/or shoulder complaints: a systematic review. Int Arch Occup Environ Health. 2012;85:587–603.

19

Sleep problems and fatigue as predictors for the onset of chronic widespread pain over a 5- and 18-year perspective

Katarina Aili[1,2,7*] (iD), Maria Andersson[1,3], Ann Bremander[1,3,4,5,6], Emma Haglund[1,4], Ingrid Larsson[1,7] and Stefan Bergman[1,7,8]

Abstract

Background: Previous research suggests that sleep problems may be an important predictor for chronic widespread pain (CWP). With this study we investigated both sleep problems and fatigue as predictors for the onset of CWP over a 5-year and an 18-year perspective in a population free from CWP at baseline.

Methods: To get a more stable classification of CWP, we used a wash-out period, including only individuals who had not reported CWP at baseline (1998) and three years prior baseline (1995). In all, data from 1249 individuals entered the analyses for the 5-year follow-up and 791 entered for the 18-year follow-up. Difficulties initiating sleep, maintaining sleep, early morning awakening, non-restorative sleep and fatigue were investigated as predictors separately and simultaneously in binary logistic regression analyses.

Results: The results showed that problems with initiating sleep, maintaining sleep, early awakening and non-restorative sleep predicted the onset of CWP over a 5-year (OR 1.85 to OR 2.27) and 18-year (OR 1.54 to OR 2.25) perspective irrespective of mental health (assessed by SF-36) at baseline. Also fatigue predicted the onset of CWP over the two-time perspectives (OR 3.70 and OR 2.36 respectively) when adjusting for mental health. Overall the effect of the sleep problems and fatigue on new onset CWP (over a 5-year perspective) was somewhat attenuated when adjusting for pain at baseline but remained significant for problems with early awakening, non-restorative sleep and fatigue. Problems with maintaining sleep predicted CWP 18 years later irrespective of mental health and number of pain regions (OR 1.72). Reporting simultaneous problems with all four aspects of sleep was associated with the onset of CWP over a five-year and 18-yearperspective, irrespective of age, gender, socio economy, mental health and pain at baseline. Sleep problems and fatigue predicted the onset of CWP five years later irrespective of each other.

Conclusion: Sleep problems and fatigue were both important predictors for the onset of CWP over a five-year perspective. Sleep problems was a stronger predictor in a longer time-perspective. The results highlight the importance of the assessment of sleep quality and fatigue in the clinic.

Keywords: Musculoskeletal pain, Insomnia, CWP, Prospective study, Longitudinal study, Population study

* Correspondence: katarina.aili@fou-spenshult.se
[1]Spenshult Research and Development Center, FoU Spenshult, Bäckagårdsvägen 47, SE-302 74 Halmstad, Sweden
[2]Unit of occupational medicine, Institute of Environmental Medicine, Karolinska Institutet, Stockholm, Sweden
Full list of author information is available at the end of the article

Introduction

Experiencing musculoskeletal pain is common [1], however, the clinical presentation vary substantially.

One way of classifying musculoskeletal pain is by the number and localization of pain-sites. Localized pain is rather uncommon [2] and probably represent a different type of disorder than multisite or widespread pain. Individuals with localized pain report better general health, less pain severity and less problems with sleep than individuals with widespread pain [3]. The number of pain sites has shown to have an almost linear relationship to reduced functional ability [2] and an inverse linear relationship to general health, sleep quality and mental health [4]. If localized pain represents the one end of a pain spectra with overall better general health, chronic widespread pain (CWP) and fibromyalgia represent the other end of the spectra, having a large impact on health. Primary care patients with CWP have more comorbidities with other somatic diseases and mental illness than patients with localized chronic low back pain [5].

Population-based studies have described a CWP-prevalence of 10–17% among adult men and women [6–10]. Between 34 and 57% of those reporting CWP at baseline still reported CWP 1 to 11 years later [6–8, 10]. For early identification of patients at risk for CWP it is important to find predictors so that interventions could be directed more efficiently. Number of painful regions at baseline, age and family history of pain have been found to predict the onset of CWP [7]. Other predictors found in population-based prospective studies are somatization, illness behaviour [11, 12] and sleep disturbances [12].

Sleep problems are common among individuals reporting musculoskeletal pain. The causal sleep-pain relationship is complex and reciprocal [13, 14]. Previous studies indicate that sleep predict pain prognosis, [15–17]. The underlying mechanisms for why disturbed sleep would predict pain prognosis is not yet fully established, however there are studies indicating that sleep disturbances influence pain sensitization and pain inhibitory systems [18].

CWP, where pain is present above and below the waist, on the right and left side of the body and the axial skeleton (according to the ACR 1990 criteria for fibromyalgia [19]), is a condition commonly associated to disturbed pain systems. Prospective studies have found that sleep problems predict the onset of CWP [12, 20, 21] and resolution from CWP [17]. Sleep problems are typically assessed by (self-reported) items referring to initiating sleep, maintaining sleep and non-restorative sleep. Not feeling rested when waking up (non-restorative sleep) seems from previous studies to be the perhaps most prominent predictor out of the different types of sleep problems [17, 20]. Although this parameter ought to be closely related to fatigue, none of the studies have tried to separate the effect of fatigue from the sleep problems.

Chronic fatigue and CWP is known to common co-occur, and the disorders have been suggested to at least partly share pathogenetic pathways [22]. Sleep quality and sleep loss is related to fatigue [23, 24], but the concept of fatigue also refers to a state of mental or physical energy deprivation, rather than actual sleepiness. Although the co-occurrence of fatigue and CWP is well established, little is known about the association between fatigue and CWP prospectively.

Prospective studies of sleep and CWP share some methodological issues to handle. Musculoskeletal pain conditions, including CWP, are recurrent and regardless of using an established definition (e.g. ACR 1990 criteria for fibromyalgia), you will end up with some "border-line-cases" who move in and out of fulfilling criteria for CWP. This migration in and out of CWP has previously been reported, where almost half of those with CWP at baseline no longer reported CWP at one- or three-year follow-up [7, 8]. Although these subjects most likely have disturbances in pain regulation systems, intensity and locations of pain fluctuates, and they could falsely be categorized as "no CWP" when studied at a single time point. Studying predictors for the onset of CWP is thus complicated by that pain tend to be recurrent over time and there is a need for studies with more stable baseline classifications of individuals free from CWP at baseline.

The aim of this population-based study was to investigate if sleep problems and fatigue predicted the onset of CWP over a 5-year and up to 18-year perspective in a cohort who had not reported CWP 3 years prior to baseline.

Method

Population and design

This study is based on data from the EPIPAIN study, a prospective population study that was initiated in 1995 in order to investigate the prevalence and risk factors for long term musculoskeletal pain in south of Sweden. The target population for EPIPAIN was all of the 70,704 inhabitants aged 20–74, living in two municipalities and healthcare districts on the southern west coast of Sweden. For inclusion to EPIPAIN, a representative sample of subjects was selected from the official computerised population register. The register is categorised by date of birth, and the selection of subjects was made by choosing every 18th man and women respectively for each of the municipalities. A postal questionnaire was sent out in May 1995 to the 3928 selected individuals. After two postal reminders, 2425 subjects had responded to the postal survey in 1995.

Follow-up questionnaires were sent out to the subjects in 1998, 2003 and 2016. The cohort included in this study was formed out of the 1922 subjects who responded the survey in 1995 and 1998. Baseline was set to 1998 in this study with a three-year wash-out period between 1995 and 1998. Only individuals who had not reported CWP in 1995 and 1998 were included in the study. The chosen times to follow-up were 5 years (year 2003); and 18 years (year 2016).

Chronic widespread pain

Chronic musculoskeletal pain was assessed by an overall key question: Have you experienced pain lasting more than 3 months during the last 12 months? An introduction to the question explained that the pain should be persistent or regularly recurrent in the musculoskeletal system. Pain was considered to be chronic if it had been persistent or recurrent for more than 3 months during the last 12 months.

In addition, if chronic pain was reported, the location and distribution of the pain was reported by a manikin with 18 predefined regions. Head and abdomen were not included amongst the predefined regions [7, 25].

A distinction was made between chronic regional pain (CRP) and chronic widespread pain (CWP) according to the ACR 1990 criteria for fibromyalgia [19]. According to the 1990 ACR criteria, pain was classified as widespread when present in both the left and right side of the body and also above and below the waist. In addition, axial skeletal pain (i.e. in the cervical spine, the anterior chest, the thoracic spine or the lower back) should be present. When chronic pain was present but criteria for a widespread condition were not met, the subject was classified as having CRP.

Subjects who did not report any chronic pain were labelled as "no chronic pain" (NCP).

Sleeping problems

Problems related to sleep were assessed by four items adopted from the Uppsala Sleep Inventory (USI), which has been used in several previous epidemiological studies [26, 27]: How much of a problem do you have with: (1) Falling asleep at night? (2) Waking up during the night? (3) Waking up too early in the morning? (4) Not feeling rested after sleep?

The problems were recorded on a five-point Likert scale: [1]=no problems, [2]=minor problems, [3]=moderate problems, [4]=severe problems, and [5]=very severe problems. Those who had responded "moderate problems", "severe problems" or "very severe problems" were considered to have sleep problems.

The sleep problems were treated as four separate variables of sleep, 1) Difficulties initiating sleep; 2) Difficulties maintaining sleep; 3) Early morning awakening; and 4) Non-restorative sleep.

Fatigue was estimated by the vitality subscale from the SF-36 questionnaire [28, 29]. The items from the subscale assess how great part of the time the last 4 weeks one have felt 1) alert and strong; 2) full of energy; 3) worn out; 4) tired. The response rates range from [1] "All the Time" to [6] "None of the time". The scale was converted according to the SF-36 manual into a scale ranging from 0 to 100, were a higher score indicate less problem with fatigue. Three levels of fatigue (low, intermediate, high) was constructed by dividing the included cohort's scoring into tertiles. "Low fatigue" then represented scorings of 85–100; "intermediate fatigue" represent scorings of 70–84 and "high fatigue" represent scorings between 0 and 69. The vitality subscale from SF-36 has been widely used in studies of populations with musculoskeletal pain, including fibromyalgia, and is a validated measure of fatigue [30].

Potential confounders

Mental health [20, 31] and socio-economy [21] as well as baseline pain [20] has previously been found to be associated to both sleep problems and CWP. The potential confounders considered in this study were age, gender, number of musculoskeletal pain sites, socio economy and mental health at baseline.

Number of (chronic) musculoskeletal pain sites were reported by a manikin, as described above, with eighteen possible regions.

Mental Health was assessed by the subscale MH from SF-36, including five items referring to the last 4 weeks: How much of the time during the last 4 weeks have you... 1) been a very nervous person?; 2) felt so down in the dumps that nothing could cheer you up?; 3) felt calm and peaceful; 4) felt downhearted and blue?; 5) been a happy person? Three levels of mental health (poor, intermediate, good) was constructed by dividing the included cohort's scoring into tertiles. "good mental health" then represent scores between 93 and 100; "intermediate mental health" scores between 84 and 92; and "poor mental health" scores between 0 and 83.

Socio economy as measured by Socio economic groups according to Statistics Sweden was based on self-reported occupation in 1995. Four groups of socio-economic classes were formed; Manual workers, assistant non-manual employees, intermediate/higher non-manual employees and others (including self-employed, farmers, housewives, students).

Ethics

All study participants signed an informed consent before entering the study. The study was approved by the Regional Ethical Review Board, Faculty of Medicine, University of Lund, Sweden (Dnr LU 389–94; Dnr 2016/132).

Statistics

The included cohort and the subjects that had been excluded due to reporting CWP in 1995 and/or 1998 were compared with respect to age, gender, the four sleep parameters, fatigue, number of pain regions, mental health and socio economy (based on type of occupation) at baseline. The prevalence of exposed to each sleep problem and fatigue respectively within the different categories of gender, pain regions, mental health and socio economy were compared. Pearson's chi-square test and independent t-test were used in the analyses for difference.

Odds ratios for CWP were calculated using binary logistic regression analysis. The effect of the four different sleep problems and fatigue were tested separately, for each year of follow-up.

Firstly, the four different sleep parameters and fatigue were tested in separate models in order to see if the different sleep problems or fatigue were of different importance. The predictors and the potential confounders were tested in binary logistic regression analysis, adjusting for age and gender. Multivariate analyses were then performed. Due to the complex relationship between pain, sleep and mental ill health [13], the analyses were presented in three models: 1) adjusting for age, gender, socio economy and mental health and 2) adjusting for age, gender socio economy and number of pain sites; and 3) adjusting for age, gender, socio economy, mental health and number of pain sites. The decision to let either number of pain sites or mental health enter models 1 and 2 and to let them act together in model 3 was made based on an attempt to be transparent in how the two affect the results, separately and together.

Secondly, the independent effect of sleep and fatigue on CWP was tested, and the two variables were included in the same model. To get one sleep variable instead of four separate sleep variables, sleep problems were categorized into having 0–4 of the (4) sleep problems. Again, number of pain sites and mental health were included in different models, and simultaneously. The effect of number of sleep problems, mental health and socio-economy were analysed in a "Model A", including also age and gender. In separate analyses Model A was tested when including fatigue, and number of pain sites.

All logistic regression analyses were performed twice, one for CWP at the five-year follow-up, and once for CWP at the 18-year follow-up.

The analyses were performed with the SPSS 21 Statistical Package.

Results

In all, 1922 subjects responded to the survey in 1995 and 1998. Missing data on pain questions were found in 49 cases in 1995, and 22 cases in 1998. In all, 1852 subjects had data from both 1995 and 1998 and could thus enter the analysis. Among these, 340 individuals had reported CWP in either 1995 or 1998 and were excluded from the analysis.

The excluded subjects were significantly older, were more likely to be female, to have problems with sleep and differed in socio economy from the included individuals. Further, the excluded individuals generally rated higher fatigue, poorer mental health and more pain severity. See Table 1.

Out of the 1512 individuals who fulfilled the inclusion criteria, 1249 had responded to the pain items in 2003, and were thus eligible for the analysis referring to the 5-year follow up; and 791 responded to the items in 2016 and were thus eligible for the analysis referring to the 18-year follow-up. See flow-chart in Fig. 1.

Out of the included subjects, 89 (7%) had CWP in the 5-year follow-up and 103 (13%) had CWP in the 18-year follow-up. There was no difference in proportion of men and women reporting CWP in the 5-year follow up (8% vs 6%, $p = 0.14$). However, there were significantly larger proportion of females than men reporting CWP in the 18-year follow-up (16% vs 10%, $p = 0.01$). There was a significantly larger proportion who reported CWP 5- and 18 years later among those with sleeping problems and fatigue compared to those without sleeping problems and fatigue at baseline. See Table 2. The same was seen for differences in number of pain regions and level of mental health. Data not shown.

One fourth of those who reported all four sleep problems (concurrently) at baseline had CWP 5 years later, and one third had CWP 18 years later. Among those reported none of the sleeping problems at baseline, 4% reported CWP 5 years later and 8% 18 years later.

In all, 769 individuals had data on pain at all three time points. Looking at changes in pain between the 5-year follow-up and the 18-year follow-up, 59% stayed in the same pain group (NCP, CRP or CWP). Out of the 52 who reported CWP in the 5-year follow-up (and who had data also at the 18-year follow-up), 56% ($n = 29$) reported CWP also in the 18-year follow-up. In all, 100 participants reported CWP in the 18-year follow-up. See Fig. 1.

Exposed at baseline

As presented in Fig. 2, there was a significantly higher proportion of females reporting problems with initiating sleep and problems with maintaining sleep at baseline. No gender differences were seen for problems with early awakening, non-restorative sleep or fatigue.

There were a larger proportion among individuals reporting more number of pain regions who reported problems with sleeping (significant for all sleep parameters) and fatigue. The same trend was seen for mental health, where subjects reporting poor mental health were more likely to also report problems with sleep (all sleep parameters) and fatigue.

Predictors for CWP in crude analysis

After adjusting for age and gender, all sleep parameters, fatigue (SF-36 Vitality), number of pain regions and

Table 1 Presenting baseline characteristics of the cohort with baseline stable NCP or CRP and individuals excluded from the study due to reporting CWP in − 95 and/or − 98. Prevalence of baseline exposures and covariates in included and excluded subjects, and history of CWP in excluded individuals. Significance of differences between included and excluded subjects are presented as p-values (tested with t-test and chi²-test respectively)

	Included cohort (stable NCP or CRP) (n = 1512)	Excluded subjects (CWP in 1995 and/or 1998) (n = 340)	p-value for diff. Incl. vs excl.
Age (1998)			< 0.01
Mean (sd)	49 (15)	56 (13)	
Gender; n (%)			<.01
Male	729 (48)	111 (33)	
Female	783 (52)	229 (67)	
Initiating sleep; n (%)			<.01
No Problem	1211 (81)	175 (53)	
Problem	282 (19)	158 (47)	
Maintaining sleep; n (%)			<.01
No Problem	1024 (69)	109 (33)	
Problem	461 (31)	220 (67)	
Early awakening; n (%)			<.01
No Problem	1149 (78)	145 (44)	
Problem	331 (22)	186 (56)	
Non restorative sleep; n (%)			<.01
No Problem	1075 (73)	123 (37)	
Problem	404 (27)	207 (63)	
Fatigue[a]			<.01
Mean (sd)	72 (21)	44 (25)	
Number of Regions			<.01
0	1096 (73)	42 (12)	
1–2	204 (13)	10 (3)	
3–5	177 (12)	80 (24)	
6–11	35 (2)	152 (45)	
12–18	0	56 (17)	
Mental Health[b]			< .01
Mean (sd)	84 (17)	69 (23)	
Socio economy[c]			< .01
High non manual work	440 (29)	48 (14)	
Ass non manual	212 (14)	55 (16)	
Manual	664 (44)	196 (58)	
Others	196 (13)	41 (13)	
CWP history at baseline			
CWP in −95 only	−	103 (30)	
CWP in −98 only	−	101 (30)	
CWP in both −95 and − 98	−	136 (40)	

[a]Assessed by SF-36 vitality scale; [b]Assessed by SF-36 Mental health scale; [c]Classified by occupation – intermediate/higher non-manual employees, Assistant non-manual employees, Manual workers and "others"

mental health (SF-36) predicted the onset of new CWP in the 5-year- and 18-year follow-up. Being a manual worker in 1995 predicted the onset of new CWP in the 5-year follow-up. See Table 3.

The effect of sleep as a predictor for CWP in multivariate models

Over a five-year perspective, all sleep parameters and fatigue predicted the onset of CWP, irrespective of age,

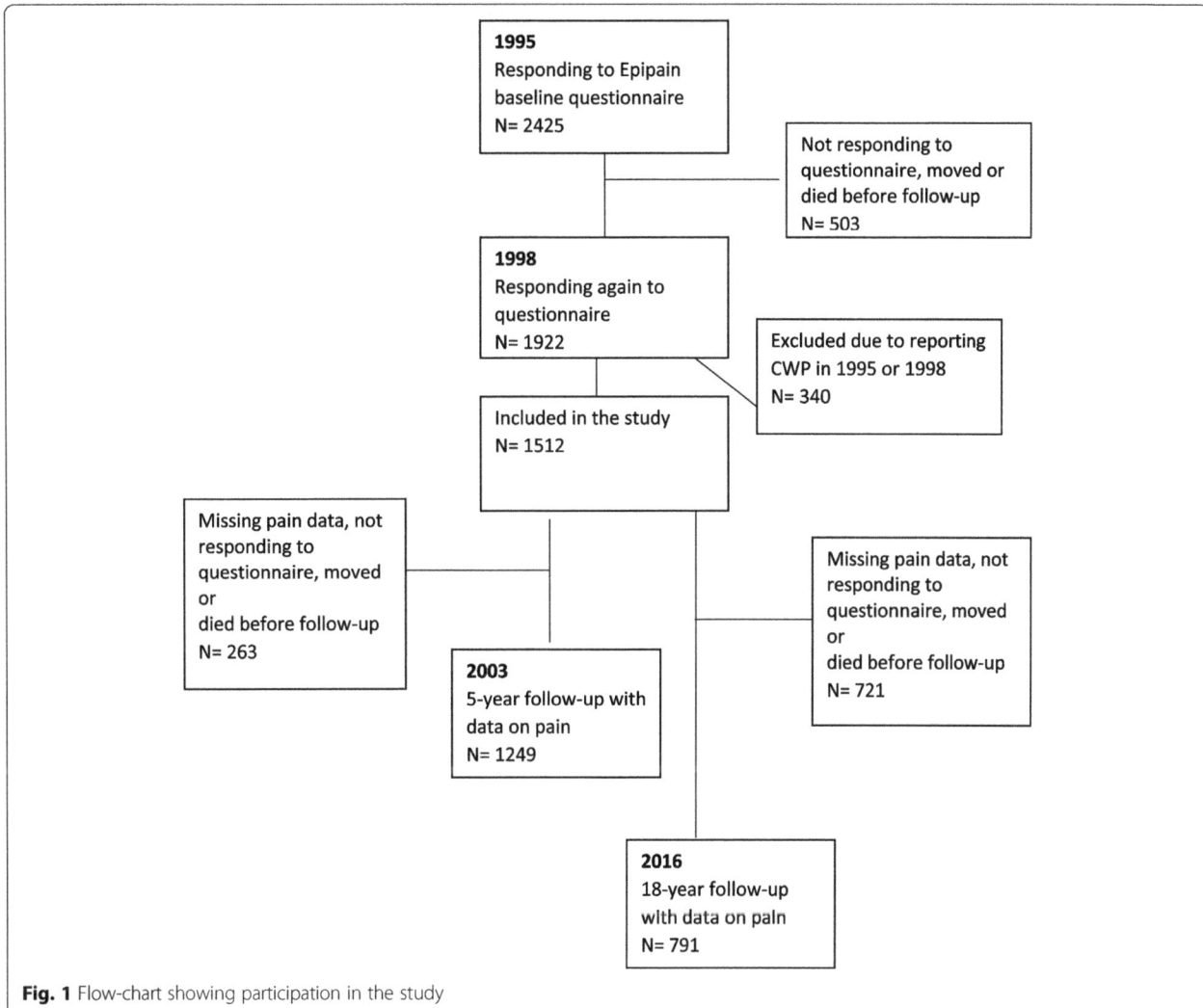

Fig. 1 Flow-chart showing participation in the study

gender, mental health and socio-economy (model 1). When adjusting for number of pain sites at baseline instead of mental health (model 2), fatigue and all sleep parameters except maintaining sleep predicted the onset of CWP. Finally, adjusting for age, gender, socio-economy, mental health and number of pain sites (model 3), none of the sleep parameters or fatigue significantly predicted the onset of CWP 5 years later.

Over the 18-year perspective, fatigue and all sleep parameters except early awakening significantly predicted CWP when adjusting for age, gender, socio-economy and mental health. However, when including number of pain sites at baseline in the model separately (model 2) and simultaneously with mental health (model 3), maintaining sleep was the only parameter that remained significant in the 18-year follow-up.

Results are presented in Table 4.

In all, 785 individuals did not report any of the sleeping problems at baseline (fatigue not included), 268

reported one of the problems, 167 two, 128 three and 117 subjects reported to have all four sleep problems.

In a multivariate model (Model A) including age, gender, mental health, socio-economy and number of sleep problems, reporting four sleep problems, reporting poor mental health and the socio-economy-parameter manual work were all associated with the onset of CWP 5 years later. Adding fatigue to the model showed that sleep problems, fatigue and manual work predicted CWP independently from each other, however mental health did not remain significant in the model. When, instead, including number of pain sites to Model A, reporting four sleep problems, reporting at least three pain-sites and manual work predicted the onset of CWP. Reporting at least three pain sites at baseline and manual work were the only parameters that remained significant when adding also fatigue to the model. See Table 5.

Over an 18-year perspective, sleep problems were stronger independent predictor for CWP. Out of the

Table 2 Presenting prevalence of baseline sleep problems and fatigue. Cross tabulation of baseline sleep problems and CWP at respective follow-up. Differences between no CWP and CWP cases in respective year for follow-up have been tested with chi^2-test

	5-year follow-up($N = 1249$)			18-year follow-up ($N = 791$)		
	No CWP	CWP	p	No CWP	CWP	p
	$N = 1160$	$N = 89$		$N = 688$	$N = 103$	
Initiating sleep; n (%)			< 0.01			< 0.01
No Problem	950 (95)	53 (5)		580 (89)	70 (11)	
Problem	198 (85)	34 (15)		103 (76)	32 (24)	
Maintaining sleep; n (%)			< 0.01			< 0.01
No Problem	811 (95)	41 (5)		500 (91)	52 (9)	
Problem	330 (88)	46 (12)		183 (78)	50 (22)	
Early awakening; n (%)			< 0.01			< 0.01
No Problem	909 (95)	49 (5)		556 (89)	70 (11)	
Problem	228 (86)	37 (14)		124 (80)	32 (20)	
Non restorative sleep; n (%)			< 0.01			< 0.01
No Problem	856 (95)	42 (5)		525 (90)	56 (10)	
Problem	283 (87)	44 (13)		159 (78)	45 (22)	
Fatigue; n (%)			< 0.01			< 0.01
Low	455 (97)	14 (3)		285 (91)	27 (9)	
Intermediate	355 (94)	21 (6)		230 (90)	26 (10)	
High	346 (87)	53 (13)		173 (78)	50 (22)	

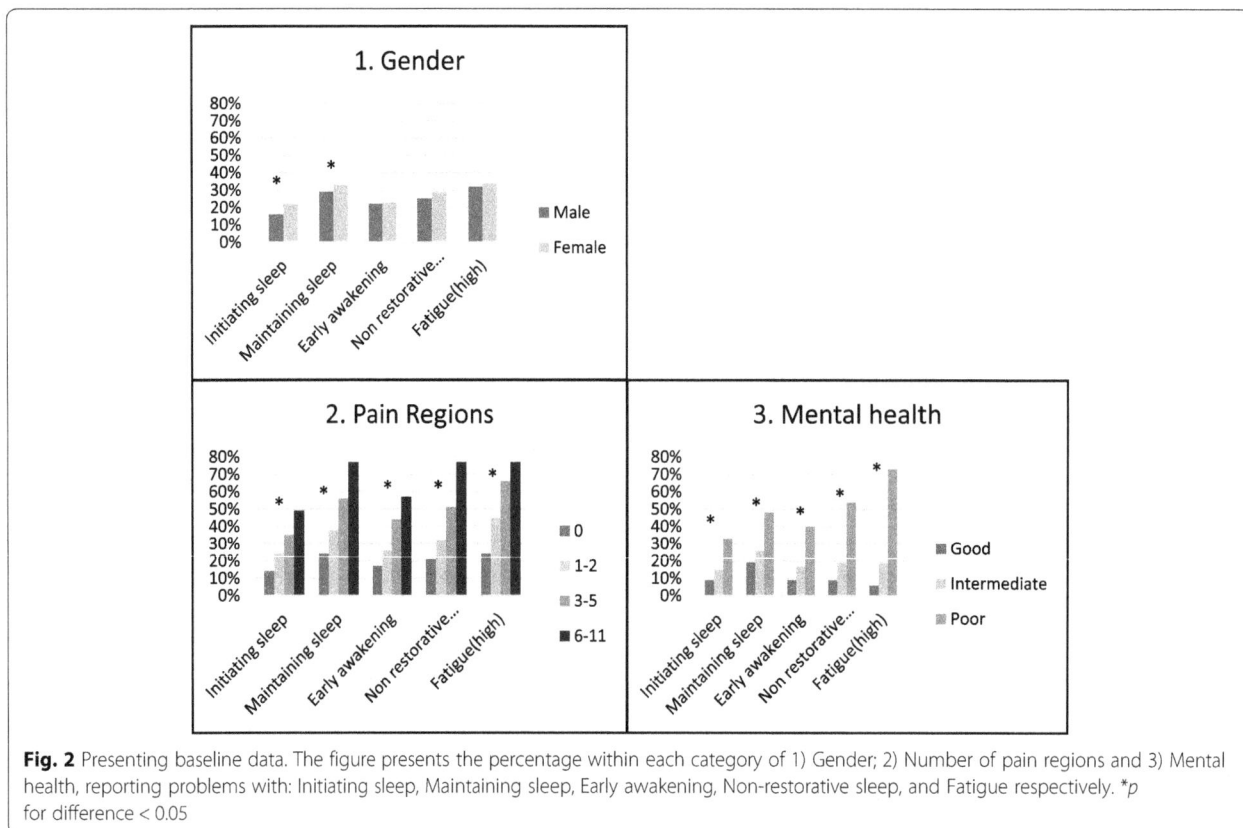

Fig. 2 Presenting baseline data. The figure presents the percentage within each category of 1) Gender; 2) Number of pain regions and 3) Mental health, reporting problems with: Initiating sleep, Maintaining sleep, Early awakening, Non-restorative sleep, and Fatigue respectively. *p for difference < 0.05

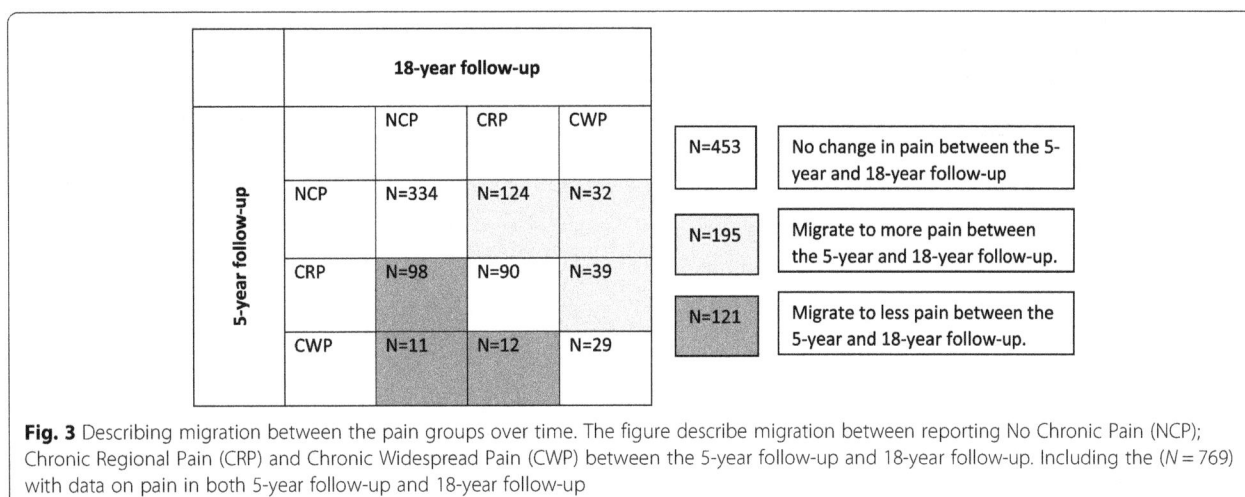

Fig. 3 Describing migration between the pain groups over time. The figure describe migration between reporting No Chronic Pain (NCP); Chronic Regional Pain (CRP) and Chronic Widespread Pain (CWP) between the 5-year follow-up and 18-year follow-up. Including the (N = 769) with data on pain in both 5-year follow-up and 18-year follow-up

included parameters, only sleep problems and number of pain regions at baseline significantly and independently, predicted CWP. See Table 6.

Discussion

The aim of this study was to investigate if sleep problems and fatigue predict the onset of CWP five- and 18 years later. The results from this study indicate that in a cohort free from CWP at baseline, difficulties initiating sleep, maintaining sleep, early morning awakening, non-restorative sleep and fatigue respectively predicted the onset of CWP in a 5-year perspective irrespective of age, gender, socio-economy and mental health. This was true also over an 18-year perspective, except for the sleep parameter early morning awakening. When adding number of pain sites in the model none of the sleep parameters or fatigue predicted the onset of CWP in the 5-year follow-up. However, problems with maintaining sleep consistently predicted the onset of CWP 18 years later in all models.

When adding all sleep problems together, receiving a parameter measuring 0–4 sleep problems, sleep problems predicted the onset of CWP 5 years later irrespective of age, gender, mental health and socio-economy. Further, sleep problems and fatigue predicted the onset of CWP 5 years later irrespective of each other. However, in a full model including the parameters mentioned above plus sleep problems, fatigue and number of pain sites, only ≥3 pain sites at baseline and having manual work at baseline significantly predicted the onset of CWP 5 years later. Over an 18-year perspective however, reporting 4 sleep problems at baseline and reporting pain at baseline (at least 1–2 pain sites) were the only predictors that remained significant when included in a full multivariate model.

The over-all results, that sleep is a predictor for CWP, is in line with what previous studies have found

[12, 21, 31, 32]. These studies have used follow-ups of 15 months, 6 years and 11 years. Our findings, that sleep seems to be an important predictor also over very long time-spans are supported by prospective studies showing that insomnia predict chronic widespread musculoskeletal pain 11 years later [32]. Although the previous studies have used a study design where following a cohort free from CWP at baseline, this study is the first study being able to exclude also those who had had CWP 3 years prior to baseline.

The mechanistic relationship between sleep problems and chronic pain is not yet clear. One suggested mechanism is that insufficient sleep alters the processes of pain habituation and sensitization, and increase vulnerability to chronic pain [18]. The purpose of using a wash-out period was to distinguish between regional pain (presumably without central sensitization) and CWP (where disturbed pain systems are common). We then found that over a five-year perspective, the sleep-CWP relationship was not explained by pain regions at baseline or mental health. Further, fatigue predicted the onset of CWP independently from mental health and sleep problems, but not independently from number of pain regions at baseline. This implies that the association between fatigue and CWP is explained by number of pain sites rather than mental health and sleep problems. In the longer time-perspective of 18 years however, fatigue did not predict the onset of CWP independently from sleep problems. Possibly, this could be interpreted as fatigue being more associated with disturbances in pain systems, whereas sleep problems not only are associated with disturbed pain systems, but also indicates a vulnerability to chronic pain, preceding disturbances of the system.

Using the wash-out period, allowing only those who had not reported CWP both at baseline and 3 years prior to baseline, we attended to capture *new* onset CWP. This is however more likely to be true for the results

Table 3 Presenting results from univariate model (adjusted for age and gender). Odds ratio (OR), 95% confidence intervals (95% CI) and p-value (p) for reporting CWP in the 5-year and 18-year follow-up respectively. Number of individuals per category of exposure at baseline are presented as N for the 5-year follow-up and 18-year follow-up respectively

	N	CWP 5-year OR (95% CI)	p	N	CWP 18-year OR (95% CI)	p
Gender						
Male	586	1		345	1	
Female	663	1.44 (0.92–2.24)	.107	446	1.77 (1.14–2.75)	.011
Initiating sleep[a]						
No problem	1003	1		650	1	
Problem	232	2.82 (1.77–4.50)	<.001	135	2.49 (1.55–4.00)	<.001
Maintaining sleep[a]						
No problem	852	1		552	1	
Problem	376	2.53 (1.61–3.98)	<.001	233	2.74 (1.75–4.28)	<.001
Early awakening[a]						
No problem	958	1		626	1	
Problem	265	2.83 (1.79–4.46)	<.001	156	1.97 (1.23–3.15)	.005
Non-restorative[a]						
No problem	898	1		581	1	
Problem	327	3.15 (2.02–4.92)	<.001	204	2.62 (1.70–4.04)	<.001
Fatigue[b]						
Low	469	1		312	1	
Intermediate	376	1.99 (1.00–3.99)	.051	256	1.20 (0.68–2.11)	.533
High	399	4.93 (2.69–9.05)	<.001	223	2.96 (1.78–4.92)	<.001
Pain regions						
0	904	1		571	1	
1–2	167	1.61 (0.78–3.32)	.202	113	3.03 (1.72–5.31)	<.001
3–5	146	7.40 (4.40–12.42)	<.001	89	5.33 (3.05–9.31)	<.001
6–11	32	12.40 (5.50–28.02)	<.001	18	13.38 (4.99–35.89)	<.001
Mental health[c]						
Good	365	1		234	1	
Intermediate	487	1.89 (0.96–3.73)	.065	326	1.37 (0.77–2.45)	.288
Poor	388	3.87 (2.05–7.34)	<.001	229	2.70 (1.53–4.75)	.001
Socio economy[d]						
High non manual	384	1		285	1	
Ass non manual	178	1.98 (0.93–5.21)	.076	107	1.17 (0.59–2.96)	.660
Manual	537	2.74 (1.51–4.94)	.001	321	1.45 (0.89–2.36)	.136
Others	150	1.45 (0.61–3.55)	.395	78	1.25 (0.58–2.68)	.574

[a]*Problem* = [Moderate problems - very severe problems]; *No Problems* = [no problems - minor problems]. [b] Based on scorings on SF-36 vitality scale [Low = 85–100; Intermediate = 70–84; High = 0–69]
[c]Based on scorings on SF-36 Mental Health scale [Good = 93–100; Intermediate = 84–92; Poor = 0–83]; [d] Classified by occupation – intermediate/higher non-manual employees, Assistant non-manual employees, Manual workers and "others"

found in the 5-year follow-up than the 18-year follow-up. One of the reasons for why sleep problems predict CWP also over longer time periods may be that sleep problems [6] and fatigue [8] predict persistence of CWP. At the 18-year follow-up it is reasonable to believe that what we see is the combined effect of sleep problems on the onset of CWP, as well as persistence of CWP. As shown in Fig. 3, a large part of the study participants stayed in the same pain group between the 5-year and 18-year follow-up. However, 44% of those reporting CWP in the 5-year follow-up reported "No Chronic Pain" or "Chronic Regional Pain" in the 18-year follow-up and the mere part of those reporting CWP in the 18-year follow-up (70%) did not report CWP in the 5-year

Table 4 Results from multivariate analysis. Presenting the effect of difficulties initiating sleep, difficulties maintaining sleep, early morning awakening, non-restorative sleep and fatigue on the odds ratio (OR) for reporting CWP in the 5-year and 18-year follow-up respectively. The OR, 95% confidence intervals (95% CI) and p-value (p) are presented in model 1–3. N = 1249 entered the 5-year follow-up analyses; N = 791 entered in the 18-year follow-up analyses

	Adjusted for age gender, mental health[c], socio-economy[d]		Adjusted for age, gender, socio-economy[d] and number of pain sites		Adjusted for age, gender, socio-economy[d], mental health[c] and number of pain sites	
	CWP 5-year	CWP 18-year	CWP 5-year	CWP 18-year	CWP 5-year	CWP 18-year
	OR (95% CI)	OR (95% CI)	OR (95% CI)	OR (95% CI)	OR (95% CI)	OR (95% CI)
Initiating sleep[a]						
No Problem	1	1	1	1	1	1
Problem	1.91 (1.16–3.14)*	1.93 (1.18–3.18)*	1.71 (1.03–2.85)*	1.68 (1.00–2.81)	1.37 (0.81–2.34)	1.51 (0.89–2.57)
Maintaining Sleep[a]						
No problem	1	1	1		1	1
Problem	1.85 (1.14–3.01)*	2.25 (1.40–3.61)*	1.60 (0.98–2.63)	1.88 (1.16–3.05)*	1.32 (0.79-2.21)	1.72 (1.05–2.84)*
Early awakening[a]						
No problem	1	1			1	
Problem	2.00 (1.23–3.27)*	1.54 (0.94–2.54)	1.71 (1.04–2.83)*	1.32 (0.79–2.21)	1.45 (0.86–2.43)	1.18 (0.69–2.01)
Non-restorative[a]						
No problem	1	1			1	1
Problem	2.27 (1.37–3.75)*	2.04 (1.26–3.29)*	1.90 (1.15–3.13)*	1.57 (0.97–2.56)	1.51 (0.88–2.58)	1.39 (0.83–2.34)
Fatigue[b]						
Low	1	1	1	1	1	1
Intermediate	1.75 (0.83–3.66)	1.09 (0.60–2.00)	1.71 (0.84–3.45)	1.05 (0.59–1.89)	1.48 (0.70–3.15)	0.97 (0.52–1.79)
High	3.70 (1.76–7.84)*	2.36 (1.24–4.50)*	2.59 (1.34–3.47)*	1.62 (0.92–2.85)	1.93 (0.87–4.26)	1.34 (0.69–2.68)

[a]*Problems* = [Moderate problems - very severe problems]; *No Problems* = [no problems - minor problems]. [b] Based on scorings on SF-36 vitality scale [Low = 85–100; Intermediate = 70–84; High = 0–69]; [c]Based on scorings on SF-36 Mental Health scale [Good = 93–100; Intermediate = 84–92; Poor = 0–83]; [d]Classified by occupation – intermediate/higher non-manual employees, Assistant non-manual employees, Manual workers and "others"
*p < 0.05

follow-up. We have not found any previous prospective studies investigating the effect of predictors for CWP both over a "shorter" time span (5 years) and a very long time-span (18 years) simultaneously.

In this study we found that difficulties maintaining sleep, and possibly difficulties initiating sleep, seems to be stronger independent predictors for CWP in a long-term perspective (18 years) than in a 5-year perspective. The opposite trend was seen for early morning awakening, non-restorative sleep and fatigue. Other studies of sleep and CWP that has specified single component of sleep in their analysis [17, 20] point out non-restorative sleep and trouble initiating sleep as the two important components, when investigating the onset of CWP 3 years later (among older adults) [20] and resolution from CWP 15 months later [17]. A previous study [31] suggest that difficulties initiating or maintaining sleep, could worsen a person's depressive symptoms over time, which may explain some of our findings. A recent review concludes that deterioration in sleep is associated with an increased risk for developing a pain condition [33]. Future studies should investigate the variance of both sleep and CWP over time for better

understanding of the clinical meaning of the findings in the present study.

We chose to include mental health and number of pain regions in separate models in the analysis. Pain, sleep problems and mental health are known to commonly co-occur. It was not under the scope of this study to unravel the different pathways through which sleep, pain, fatigue and mental health interact. However, knowing that the relationship is complex, we wanted to be as transparent as possible when exploring the effect of sleep and fatigue on CWP. A recent review [13] investigating the relationship between sleep and pain suggest that sleep, pain and negative mood share variance after presenting studies that suggest sleep to be a mediator between the relationship between pain and depression [34]; pain to mediate the relationship between sleep and depression [35]; and negative mood to mediate the relationship between sleep and pain [36]. Sleep problems have further been found to predict the development of depression among individuals with persistent pain [37]. Another recent study found that insomnia and sleep duration are risk factors for developing chronic multisite pain and that the mediation effect of depressive symptoms, at least partially explained the increased risk

Table 5 Presenting odds ratios (OR) and 95% confidence intervals (95% CI) for CWP 5 years later. Model A includes age, gender, mental health, socio economy and number of sleep problems

	Model A	Model A + fatigue	Model A + number of pain regions	Model A + number of pain regions and fatigue
	OR (95% CI)	OR (95% CI)	OR (95% CI)	OR (95% CI)
No of sleep problems				
0	1	1	1	1
1	1.13 (0.57–2.27)	1.00 (0.50–2.03)	0.93 (0.45–1.89)	0.88 (0.43–1.80)
2	1.01 (0.44–2.32)	0.84 (0.36–1.96)	0.73 (0.31–1.72)	0.68 (0.29–1.62)
3	1.71 (0.77–3.81)	1.39 (0.62–3.15)	1.14 (0.49–2.63)	1.05 (0.45–2.45)
4	4.00 (2.03–7.91)**	3.06 (1.51–6.21)**	2.18 (1.04–4.56)*	1.99 (0.93–4.24)
Fatigue[a]				
Low		1		1
Intermediate		1.62 (0.76–3.45)		1.47 (0.69–3.16)
High		2.68 (1.21–5.96)*		1.59 (0.68–3.71)
Pain regions at baseline				
0			1	1
1–2			1.39 (0.64–3.02)	1.34 (0.62–2.91)
3–5			4.89 (2.73–8.76)**	4.53 (2.47–8.30)**
>6			8.24 (3.37–20.15)**	7.78 (3.13–19.26)**
Mental health[b]				
Good	1	1	1	1
Intermediate	1.60 (0.79–3.23)	1.26 (0.60–2.66)	1.42 (0.70–2.90)	1.23 (0.58–2.62)
Poor	2.41 (1.17–4.93)*	1.42 (0.62–3.24)	1.93 (0.93–4.02)	1.54 (0.67–3.56)
Socio economy (work)[c]				
High non-manual	1	1	1	1
Ass non-manual	1.69 (0.75–3.82)	1.69 (0.75–3.84)	1.87 (0.81–4.32)	1.86 (0.80–4.28)
Manual	2.75 (1.47–5.13)**	2.73 (1.46–5.12)**	2.34 (1.23–4.44)*	2.34 (1.23–4.46)*
Other	1.40 (0.56–3.49)	1.35 (0.54–3.39)	1.27 (0.50–3.27)	1.26 (0.49–3.23)

[a]Based on scorings on SF-36 vitality scale [Low = 85–100; Intermediate = 70–84; High = 0–69];[b]Based on scorings on SF-36 Mental Health scale [Good = 93–100; Intermediate = 84–92; Poor = 0–83]; [c]Classified by occupation – intermediate/higher non-manual employees, Assistant non-manual employees, Manual workers and "others"
*$p < 0.05$; **$p < 0.01$

[31]. Further, CWP and fatigue commonly co-exist, and it has been shown that many of those reporting both fatigue and CWP also report anxiety or depression [38].

Having had pain previously is an important predictor for reporting more pain sites at follow-up [39]. In this study, individuals who had reported CWP 3 years prior to baseline were excluded from entering the analyses to get a more stable baseline classification of "no CWP". Most other studies do not include a wash-out period when studying the onset of CWP. As shown in Tables 1, 30% of the excluded reported CWP in 1995, but not in 1998, which means that if we had chosen to not use a wash-out period, we would have classified them as "no CWP" at baseline (– 98). The included cohort differed significantly from the excluded group in all parameters of interest in this study; age, gender, the four sleep parameters, fatigue, number of pain regions, pain severity,

mental health and socio economy and the excluded group were with respect to these parameters supposedly a more vulnerable group of individuals in general. These differences strengthen our hypothesis that these factors are of importance. When interpreting the result, it is important to bear in mind that they are based on a cohort that due to the wash-out period include a higher proportion of individuals who are supposedly less vulnerable to CWP than a random sample from a general population would be.

Previous population-based studies have established a higher CWP-prevalence among women than men [11, 40]. Unexpectedly, in this study, female gender predicted the onset of CWP in the 18-year follow-up, but not in the 5-year follow-up. One explanation for this may be the use of a wash-out period for CWP, as discussed above. The effect of gender that was seen in the 18-year follow-up may

Table 6 Presenting odds ratios (OR) and 95% confidence intervals (95% CI) for CWP 18 years later. Model A includes age, gender, mental health, socio economy and number of sleep problems

	Model A	Model A + fatigue	Model A + number of pain regions	Model A + number of pain regions and fatigue
	OR (95% CI)	OR (95% CI)	OR (95% CI)	OR (95% CI)
No of sleep problems				
0	1	1	1	1
1	1.82 (1.00–3.34)	1.73 (0.93–3.20)	1.57 (0.84–2.95)	1.57 (0.83–2.96)
2	1.38 (0.65–2.91)	1.27 (0.59–2.71)	1.03 (0.48–2.22)	1.02 (0.47–2.23)
3	2.44 (1.19–5.00)*	2.17 (1.03–4.56)*	1.78 (0.84–3.80)	1.75 (0.81–3.82)
4	3.95 (1.90–8.20)**	3.33 (1.55–7.13)**	2.36 (1.06–5.23)*	2.29 (1.01–5.18)*
Fatigue[a]				
Low		1		1
Intermediate		0.96 (0.51–1.79)		0.89 (0.47–1.67)
High		1.79 (0.89–3.60)		1.13 (0.54–2.37)
Pain regions at baseline				
0			1	1
1–2			2.83 (1.57–5.12)**	2.76 (1.52–5.02)**
3–5			4.03 (2.20–7.37)**	3.84 (2.05–7.20)**
> 6			8.63 (3.05–24.43)**	8.24 (2.88–23.63)**
Mental health[b]				
Good	1	1	1	1
Intermediate	1.22 (0.67–2.25)	1.15 (0.61–2.18)	1.21 (0.65–2.24)	1.21 (0.63–2.31)
Poor	1.75 (0.92–3.13)	1.25 (0.59–2.66)	1.36 (0.70–2.63)	1.27 (0.59–2.72)
Socio economy (work)[c]				
High non-manual	1	1	1	1
Ass non-manual	1.22 (0.61–2.47)	1.25 (0.62–2.54)	1.21 (0.58–2.49)	1.22 (0.59–2.53)
Manual	1.49 (0.90–2.48)	1.50 (0.90–2.51)	1.40 (0.83–2.38)	1.41 (0.83–2.38)
other	1.24 (0.56–2.77)	1.26 (0.56–2.83)	1.29 (0.56–3.00)	1.31 (0.56–3.04)

[a]Based on scorings on SF-36 vitality scale [Low = 85–100; Intermediate = 70–84; High = 0–69]
[b]Based on scorings on SF-36 Mental Health scale [Good = 93–100; Intermediate = 84–92; Poor = 0–83]; [c]Classified by occupation – intermediate/higher non-manual employees, Assistant non-manual employees, Manual workers and "others"
*$p < 0.05$; **$p < 0.01$

reflect that females have higher risk for persistent CWP than men. A previous study on the cohort [7] found that women had higher risk for developing CWP, and higher risk (however non-significant) than men for persistent CWP. The gender difference in risk for long-term persistence of CWP has been seen also in other cohorts [6]. However, a British study with one-year follow-up did not find any gender difference in persistence of CWP [8].

There are some methodological issues to be considered when interpreting the results from this study. The results rely upon self-reported data from questionnaires. Individuals classified as CWP in this study may have differed if they were diagnosed by a physician. By the criterion used in this study, subjects could have reported up to 11 sites without fulfilling the criteria for CWP. One could fulfil the CWP criteria if reporting pain from

only three sites, thus the individuals classified as CWP may be heterogeneous. This approach for classifying CWP [19] is however the most commonly used in population-studies, and our results are therefore comparable to other studies [6, 8–12, 17, 20, 21, 40].

The parameter indicating socio economy may have some problems. The classification was made based on occupation according to a classification system by Statistics Sweden, 1982. In 1998, when data was assessed from which the socio-economy parameter was classified in this study, this classification was considered accurate to use. We chose to use this parameter in this study to get an idea of the impact of socio economy and/or type of work, although we are aware it is not a perfect estimation.

Another issue worth mentioning is the repeated analysis, due to our decision to perform separate analysis in models including mental health and number of pain sites, separately and simultaneously. The multiple analysis increases the risk for false positive associations. In the age-gender adjusted analysis (presented as crude analysis) of the predictors, the *p*-values were very low (below 0.001). This imply that there is a very small risk for false positive results in the "crude" relationship between the investigated predictors and CWP. However, as moving on and analysing the predictors in several models, with less convincing p-values, the risk for false positive results increase. This is a limitation with the study.

Another issue is the potential nonparticipation bias. In the five-year follow-up, the response rate was 90% and in the 18-year follow-up, the response rate was 63%. Especially the response rate of the latter follow-up could potentially have caused bias. However, in comparison to other studies with this long-term follow-up, the response rate is within a range one would expect.

Conclusions

This prospective populations study showed that all the investigated sleep problems, (initiating sleep, maintaining sleep, early awakening and non-restorative sleep) as well as fatigue are important predictors for the future development of CWP both over a 5-year, and 18-year perspective. Problems with maintaining sleep was a weaker predictor in the five-year follow-up but was the only sleep parameter that predicted the onset of CWP over an 18-year perspective irrespective of both mental health and number of pain sites.

Reporting all four sleep problems simultaneously was a strong predictor for CWP 5 years- and 18-years later. Fatigue predicted the onset of CWP 5 years later irrespective of sleep problems, age, gender, socio-economy and mental health, but not independently from pain sites. The results from this study are in line with what previous prospective studies have shown, and with this study we add knowledge of the importance of fatigue as predictor over a shorter perspective. This highlights the importance of the assessment of sleep quality and fatigue in the clinic. This study suggests that the fatigue-CWP association is explained by number of pain sites (and possibly disturbed pain systems) rather than mental health or sleep problems. This study also suggests that sleep problems may indicate a vulnerability to chronic pain at an earlier stage.

Abbreviations
CI: Confidence interval; CRP: Chronic regional pain; CWP: Chronic widespread pain; NCP: No chronic pain

Acknowledgements
Not applicable

Funding
The Epipain study was supported from a grant from Swedish AFA insurance.

Authors' contributions
KA and SB have taken the lead of the work with the study and has shared the responsibility for the integrity of the study as a whole and for taking the progress forward with analysing data and writing the manuscript. MA, AB, EH and IL has actively contributed to the work of formulating the conception and design, data assessments, analysing and interpretation of data and critical review of the manuscript. All authors have approved the final version of the article.

Competing interest
The authors declare that they have no competing interests.

Author details
¹Spenshult Research and Development Center, FoU Spenshult, Bäckagårdsvägen 47, SE-302 74 Halmstad, Sweden. ²Unit of occupational medicine, Institute of Environmental Medicine, Karolinska Institutet, Stockholm, Sweden. ³Department of Clinical Sciences, Section of Rheumatology, Lund University, Lund, Sweden. ⁴School of Business, Engineering and Science, Halmstad University, Halmstad, Sweden. ⁵Department of Regional Health Research, University of Southern Denmark, Odense, Denmark. ⁶Syddansk Universitet Research Unit, King Christian X Hospital for Rheumatic Diseases, Hospital of Southern Jutland, Copenhagen, Graasten, Denmark. ⁷School of Health and Welfare, Halmstad University, Halmstad, Sweden. ⁸Primary Health Care Unit, Department of Public Health and Community Medicine, Institute of Medicine, The Sahlgrenska Academy, University of Gothenburg, Gothenburg, Sweden.

References
1. Hagen K, Svebak S, Zwart JA. Incidence of musculoskeletal complaints in a large adult Norwegian county population. The HUNT Study. Spine (Phila Pa 1976). 2006;31:2146–50.
2. Kamaleri Y, Natvig B, Ihlebaek CM, Bruusgaard D. Localized or widespread musculoskeletal pain: does it matter? Pain. 2008;138:41–6.
3. Natvig B, Bruusgaard D, Eriksen W. Localized low back pain and low back pain as part of widespread musculoskeletal pain: two different disorders? A cross-sectional population study. J Rehabil Med. 2001;33:21–5.
4. Kamaleri Y, Natvig B, Ihlebaek CM, Benth JS, Bruusgaard D. Number of pain sites is associated with demographic, lifestyle, and health-related factors in the general population. Eur J Pain. 2008;12:742–8.
5. Viniol A, Jegan N, Leonhardt C, Brugger M, Strauch K, Barth J, Baum E, Becker A. Differences between patients with chronic widespread pain and local chronic low back pain in primary care--a comparative cross-sectional analysis. BMC Musculoskelet Disord. 2013;14:351.
6. Mundal I, Grawe RW, Bjorngaard JH, Linaker OM, Fors EA. Prevalence and long-term predictors of persistent chronic widespread pain in the general population in an 11-year prospective study: the HUNT study. BMC Musculoskelet Disord. 2014;15:213.
7. Bergman S, Herrstrom P, Jacobsson LT, Petersson IF. Chronic widespread pain: a three year followup of pain distribution and risk factors. J Rheumatol. 2002;29:818–25.
8. McBeth J, Macfarlane GJ, Hunt IM, Silman AJ. Risk factors for persistent chronic widespread pain: a community-based study. Rheumatology (Oxford). 2001;40:95–101.
9. Mansfield KE, Sim J, Jordan JL, Jordan KP. A systematic review and meta-analysis of the prevalence of chronic widespread pain in the general population. Pain. 2016;157:55–64.
10. Papageorgiou AC, Silman AJ, Macfarlane GJ. Chronic widespread pain in the population: a seven year follow up study. Ann Rheum Dis. 2002;61:1071–4.
11. McBeth J, Macfarlane GJ, Benjamin S, Silman AJ. Features of somatization predict the onset of chronic widespread pain: results of a large population-based study. Arthritis Rheum. 2001;44:940–6.
12. Gupta A, Silman AJ, Ray D, Morriss R, Dickens C, MacFarlane GJ, Chiu YH, Nicholl B, McBeth J. The role of psychosocial factors in predicting the onset of chronic widespread pain: results from a prospective population-based study. Rheumatology (Oxford). 2007;46:666–71.

13. Finan PH, Goodin BR, Smith MT. The association of sleep and pain: an update and a path forward. J Pain. 2013;14:1539–52.

14. McBeth J, Wilkie R, Bedson J, Chew-Graham C, Lacey RJ. Sleep disturbance and chronic widespread pain. Curr Rheumatol Rep. 2015;17:469.

15. Aili K, Nyman T, Hillert L, Svartengren M. Sleep disturbances predict future sickness absence among individuals with lower back or neck-shoulder pain: a 5-year prospective study. Scand J Public Health. 2015;43:315–23.

16. Aili K, Nyman T, Svartengren M, Hillert L. Sleep as a predictive factor for the onset and resolution of multi-site pain: a 5-year prospective study. Eur J Pain. 2015;19:341–9.

17. Davies KA, Macfarlane GJ, Nicholl BI, Dickens C, Morriss R, Ray D, McBeth J. Restorative sleep predicts the resolution of chronic widespread pain: results from the EPIFUND study. Rheumatology (Oxford). 2008;47:1809–13.

18. Simpson NS, Scott-Sutherland J, Gautam S, Sethna N, Haack M. Chronic exposure to insufficient sleep alters processes of pain habituation and sensitization. Pain. 2018;159:33–40.

19. Wolfe F, Smythe HA, Yunus MB, Bennett RM, Bombardier C, Goldenberg DL, Tugwell P, Campbell SM, Abeles M, Clark P, et al. The American College of Rheumatology 1990 criteria for the classification of fibromyalgia. Report of the Multicenter Criteria Committee. Arthritis Rheum. 1990;33:160–72.

20. McBeth J, Lacey RJ, Wilkie R. Predictors of new-onset widespread pain in older adults: results from a population-based prospective cohort study in the UK. Arthritis Rheumatol. 2014;66:757–67.

21. Davies KA, Silman AJ, Macfarlane GJ, Nicholl BI, Dickens C, Morriss R, Ray D, McBeth J. The association between neighbourhood socio-economic status and the onset of chronic widespread pain: results from the EPIFUND study. Eur J Pain. 2009;13:635–40.

22. Kato K, Sullivan PF, Evengard B, Pedersen NL. Chronic widespread pain and its comorbidities: a population-based study. Arch Intern Med. 2006;166: 1649–54.

23. Akerstedt T, Axelsson J, Lekander M, Orsini N, Kecklund G. Do sleep, stress, and illness explain daily variations in fatigue? A prospective study. J Psychosom Res. 2014;76:280–5.

24. Theorell-Haglow J, Lindberg E, Janson C. What are the important risk factors for daytime sleepiness and fatigue in women? Sleep. 2006;29:751–7.

25. Bergman S, Herrstrom P, Hogstrom K, Petersson IF, Svensson B, Jacobsson LT. Chronic musculoskeletal pain, prevalence rates, and sociodemographic associations in a Swedish population study. J Rheumatol. 2001;28:1369–77.

26. Mallon L, Broman JE, Hetta J. Sleep complaints predict coronary artery disease mortality in males: a 12-year follow-up study of a middle-aged Swedish population. J Intern Med. 2002;251:207–16.

27. Lindberg E, Janson C, Gislason T, Svardsudd K, Hetta J, Boman G. Snoring and hypertension: a 10 year follow-up. Eur Respir J. 1998;11:884–9.

28. Ware JE Jr, Gandek B. Overview of the SF-36 health survey and the international quality of life assessment (IQOLA) project. J Clin Epidemiol. 1998;51:903–12.

29. Sullivan M, Karlsson J, Ware JE Jr. The Swedish SF-36 health survey–I. evaluation of data quality, scaling assumptions, reliability and construct validity across general populations in Sweden. Soc Sci Med. 1995;41:1349–58.

30. Hewlett S, Dures E, Almeida C. Measures of fatigue: Bristol rheumatoid arthritis fatigue multi-dimensional questionnaire (BRAF MDQ), Bristol rheumatoid arthritis fatigue numerical rating scales (BRAF NRS) for severity, effect, and coping, Chalder fatigue questionnaire (CFQ), checklist Individual Strength (CIS20R and CIS8R), Fatigue Severity Scale (FSS), Functional Assessment Chronic Illness Therapy (Fatigue) (FACIT-F), Multi-Dimensional Assessment of Fatigue (MAF), Multi-Dimensional Fatigue Inventory (MFI), Pediatric Quality Of Life (PedsQL) Multi-Dimensional Fatigue Scale, Profile of Fatigue (ProF), Short Form 36 Vitality Subscale (SF-36 VT), and Visual Analog Scales (VAS). Arthritis Care Res (Hoboken). 2011;63(Suppl 11):S263–86.

31. Generaal E, Vogelzangs N, Penninx BW, Dekker J. Insomnia, Sleep Duration, Depressive Symptoms, and the Onset of Chronic Multisite Musculoskeletal Pain. Sleep. 2017;40:1.

32. Uhlig BL, Sand T, Nilsen TI, Mork PJ, Hagen K. Insomnia and risk of chronic musculoskeletal complaints: longitudinal data from the HUNT study, Norway. BMC Musculoskelet Disord. 2018;19:128.

33. Afolalu EF, Ramlee F, Tang NKY. Effects of sleep changes on pain-related health outcomes in the general population: a systematic review of longitudinal studies with exploratory meta-analysis. Sleep Med Rev. 2018;39:82–97.

34. Miro E, Martinez MP, Sanchez AI, Prados G, Medina A. When is pain related to emotional distress and daily functioning in fibromyalgia syndrome? The mediating roles of self-efficacy and sleep quality. Br J Health Psychol. 2011; 16:799–814.

35. Hamilton NA, Pressman M, Lillis T, Atchley R, Karlson C, Stevens N. Evaluating evidence for the role of sleep in fibromyalgia: a test of the sleep and pain diathesis model. Cognit Ther Res. 2012;36:806–14.

36. O'Brien EM, Waxenberg LB, Atchison JW, Gremillion HA, Staud RM, McCrae CS, Robinson ME. Negative mood mediates the effect of poor sleep on pain among chronic pain patients. Clin J Pain. 2010;26:310–9.

37. Campbell P, Tang N, McBeth J, Lewis M, Main CJ, Croft PR, Morphy H, Dunn KM. The role of sleep problems in the development of depression in those with persistent pain: a prospective cohort study. Sleep. 2013;36:1693–8.

38. Creavin ST, Dunn KM, Mallen CD, Nijrolder I, van der Windt DA. Co-occurrence of pain and fatigue in a community sample of Dutch adults. Eur J Pain. 2010;14:327–34.

39. Kamaleri Y, Natvig B, Ihlebaek CM, Benth JS, Bruusgaard D. Change in the number of musculoskeletal pain sites: a 14-year prospective study. Pain. 2009;141:25–30.

40. Coggon D, Ntani G, Palmer KT, Felli VE, Harari R, Barrero LH, Felknor SA, Gimeno D, Cattrell A, Vargas-Prada S, et al. Patterns of multisite pain and associations with risk factors. Pain. 2013;154:1769–77.

20

Contributions of symptomatic osteoarthritis and physical function to incident cardiovascular disease

Michela Corsi[1], Carolina Alvarez[2], Leigh F. Callahan[2,3], Rebecca J. Cleveland[2,3], Yvonne M. Golightly[2,4,5], Joanne M. Jordan[2,3], Amanda E. Nelson[2,3], Jordan Renner[2,6], Allen Tsai[1] and Kelli D. Allen[2,3,7*]

Abstract

Background: Osteoarthritis (OA) is associated with worsening physical function and a high prevalence of comorbid health conditions. In particular, cardiovascular disease (CVD) risk is higher in individuals with OA than the general population. Limitations in physical function may be one pathway to the development of CVD among individuals with OA. This study evaluated associations of symptomatic knee OA (sxKOA), baseline physical function and worsening of function over time with self-reported incident CVD in a community-based cohort.

Methods: Our sample consisted of individuals from the Johnston County Osteoarthritis Project who did not report having CVD at baseline. Variables used to evaluate physical function were the Health Assessment Questionnaire (HAQ), time to complete 5 chair stands, and the 8-ft walk. Worsening function for these variables was defined based on previous literature and cutoffs from our sample. Logistic regression analyses examined associations of sxKOA, baseline function and worsening of function over time with self-reported incident CVD, unadjusted and adjusted for relevant demographic and clinical characteristics.

Results: Among 1709 participants included in these analyses, the mean age was 59.5 ± 9.5 years, 63.6% were women, 15% had sxKOA, and the follow up time was 5.9 ± 1.2 years. About a third of participants reported worsening HAQ score, about two-fifths had worsened chair stand time, half had worsened walking speed during the 8-ft walk, and 16% self-reported incident CVD. In unadjusted analyses, sxKOA, baseline function, and worsening function were all associated with self-reported incident CVD. In multivariable models including all of these variables, sxKOA was not associated with incident CVD, but worsening function was significantly associated with increased CVD risk, for all three functional measures: HAQ odds ratio (OR) = 2.49 (95% confidence interval (CI) 1.90–3.25), chair stands OR = 1.58 (95% CI 1.20–2.08), 8-ft walk OR = 1.53 (95%CI 1.15–2.04). These associations for worsening function remained in models additionally adjusted for demographic and clinical characteristics related to CVD risk.

Conclusions: The association between symptomatic knee osteoarthritis and cardiovascular disease risk was explained by measures of physical function. This highlights the importance of physical activity and other strategies to prevent functional loss among individuals with symptomatic knee osteoarthritis.

Keywords: Osteoarthritis, Function, Cardiovascular disease

* Correspondence: kdallen@email.unc.edu
[2]Thurston Arthritis Research Center, University of North Carolina at Chapel Hill, 3300 Thurston Bldg., CB# 7280, Chapel Hill, NC 27599, USA
[3]Department of Medicine, University of North Carolina at Chapel Hill, 125 MacNider Hall CB# 7005, Chapel Hill, NC 27599, USA
Full list of author information is available at the end of the article

Background

Osteoarthritis (OA) is a key contributor to functional disability that is becoming increasingly prevalent worldwide [1]. Symptomatic knee OA (sxKOA) is associated with functional limitations, which tend to worsen over time [2, 3]. Individuals with OA also have a significantly increased risk of cardiovascular disease (CVD) [4–6]. Individuals with OA tend to have multiple risk factors for CVD, including increased body mass index (BMI), hypertension, physical inactivity, and nonsteroidal anti-inflammatory drug (NSAID) use [5, 7]. For this reason, many hypotheses have been proposed regarding underlying pathophysiological mechanisms connecting OA and CVD, including the role of common molecular or metabolic pathways, chronic low-grade inflammation leading to both conditions, and the development of functional limitations from OA that in turn leads to a lack of physical activity, exacerbating both conditions [7, 8].

Recently, a number of studies have shown an association between physical function and CVD among individuals with OA. Schieir et al. showed that there was a greater risk of CVD in women with arthritis (with participants primarily having OA), compared to women without arthritis; the risk of CVD was further increased in women with both arthritis and physical limitations [9]. Among men in this study, there was only an increased risk of incident CVD for those who reported both arthritis and physical limitations. Together these results suggest that physical function may play a significant role in the development of CVD in patients with arthritis. While this study focused broadly on arthritis, another cohort study found that the relationship between sxKOA and CVD was sustained when controlling for age, obesity, and metabolic factors, yet became insignificant when controlling for functional limitations [10]. However, this was a cross-sectional study, so a causal relationship could not be established. Another cohort study found that individuals with hip or knee OA who used a walking aid due to functional disability had a 30% greater risk of developing CVD than those who did not use a walking aid [11]. Another recent longitudinal cohort study found a dose-response relationship between the number of joints with OA and CVD risk; however, this relationship became non-significant when controlling for difficulty walking [12].

The purpose of this study was to examine associations of sxKOA, baseline physical function and worsening of function over time with self-reported incident CVD in a community-based cohort. In particular, we were interested in understanding whether different measures of physical function explained any relationship between sxKOA and CVD risk. This study adds to the literature in several important ways. First, it is one of few studies to examine the association between OA and CVD risk in a longitudinal analysis. Second, this study has multiple measures of function, including performance-based measures, which to our knowledge have not been used in other longitudinal studies of this topic. This deepens our understanding of how various functional measures may serve as predictors of CVD among individuals with OA. Third, this study examined not only baseline function but also change in function over time; prior studies have not assessed the role of worsening function over time and how this may play in the development of CVD in individuals with OA.

Methods

Participants

This study involved participants in the Johnston County Osteoarthritis Project (JoCo OA), an ongoing community-based study focusing on hip and knee OA in a rural population [13]. Participants were civilian, non-institutionalized African-American and Caucasian adults aged 45 years and older selected from six townships within Johnston County, North Carolina. Initial enrollment occurred from 1991 to 1997 (Original Cohort), with first follow-up of this cohort occurring from 1999 to 2003. A second wave of enrollment occurred in 2003–2004 (Enrichment Cohort), aimed at enriching the sample for AA and younger individuals. First follow-up of this group occurred from 2006 to 2011. This research was reviewed and approved by the Institutional Review Board of the University of North Carolina, Chapel Hill; all participants provided written informed consent.

From participants enrolled in the Original Cohort ($N = 3249$) and Enrichment Cohort ($N = 1141$), we excluded individuals who did not have baseline clinic data, follow-up clinic data (due to loss to follow-up), and baseline and follow-up knee OA and CVD status. Then those who self-reported having CVD at baseline were excluded (Fig. 1). Finally, we excluded individuals who were missing baseline or follow-up data for functional tests or covariates, leading to a final sample size of 1709. Complete case analysis (CCA) was used so that only participants with non-missing baseline covariates and physical function status at baseline and follow-up were analyzed. This proportion of participant with missing baseline or follow-up data for analyses was 4.9%, so the impact of bias from their removal is likely to be small and CCA can be conducted regardless of the missing data pattern (Fig. 1) [14].

Measures

Outcome: Incident self-report CVD

Incident CVD was assessed at first follow-up through self-report. The definition of CVD was based on the World Health Organization criteria; due to changes in these criteria, self-report items differed slightly at different time points. For the Original Cohort, CVD at first follow-up was defined as having a heart attack, stroke, circulation or other heart problem. For the Enrichment

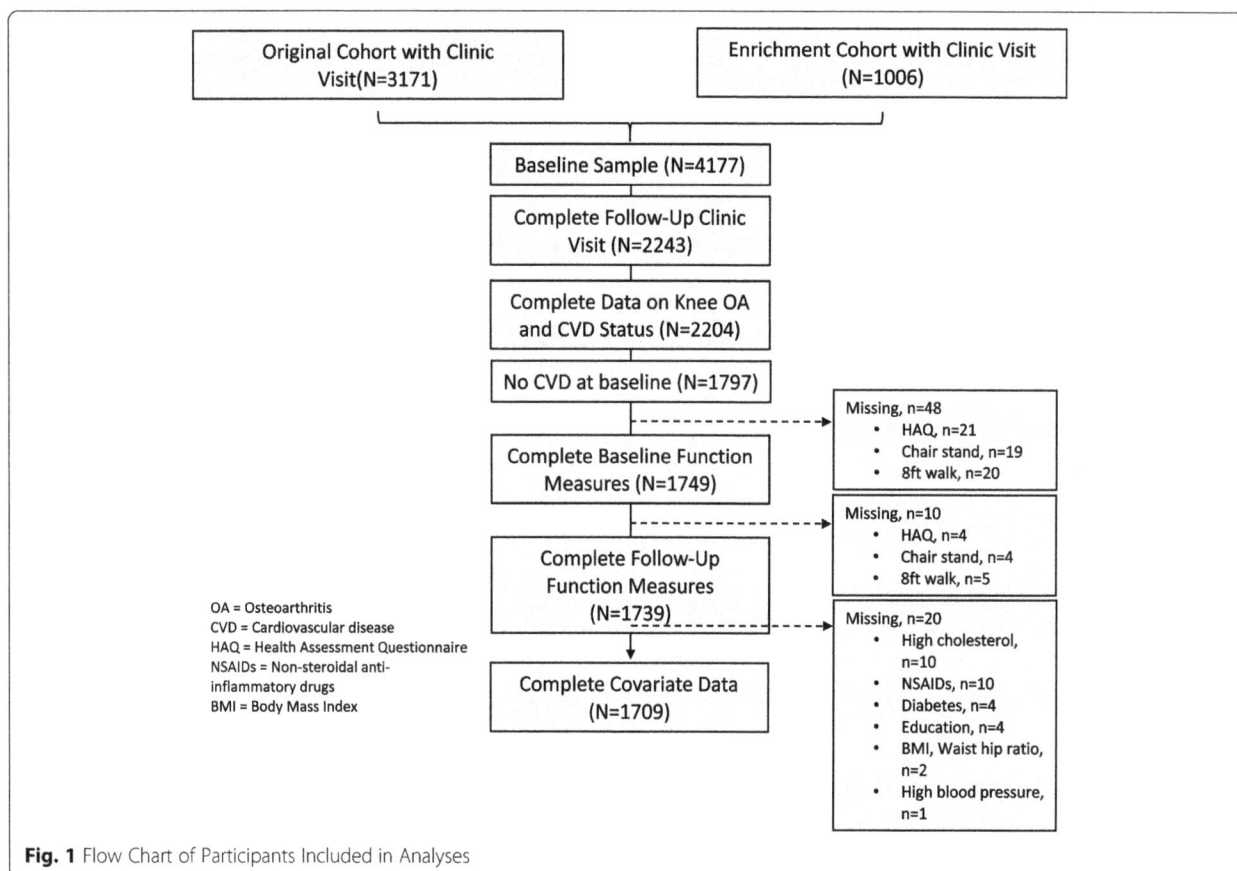

Fig. 1 Flow Chart of Participants Included in Analyses

Cohort, the incident CVD definition at first follow-up was expanded to include angina and congestive heart failure.

Symptomatic knee OA

JoCo OA participants had anteroposterior (Original Cohort enrollment) or posteroanterior (Enrichment Cohort enrollment) radiographs taken of both knees while weight-bearing using a Synaflexer® positioning device. All radiographs were read for Kellgren-Lawrence (K-L) score by a single bone and joint radiologist (JBR) without regard to participant's clinical status. Intrarater reliability and inter-rater reliability, assessed with another trained radiologist, were both high (weighted kappas were 0.89 and 0.86, respectively). For the purpose of this study, radiographic KOA was defined as a K-L grade ≥ 2. To assess joint symptoms, participants were asked: "On most days, do you have pain, aching, or stiffness in your...right/left knee." Participants responding "yes" to this question for a joint with radiographic OA were considered to have sxKOA.

Function measures

We included three measures of physical function: chair stands, 8-ft walk, and the Health Assessment Questionnaire Disability Index (HAQ).

Health assessment questionnaire The HAQ is a measure of self-reported disability, assessing ability to perform typical eight daily tasks (dressing, arising, eating, walking, reaching, gripping, chores, and hygiene) during the past 7 days [15]. Answers for each question are scored from 0 to 3, with 0 being no disability and 3 being complete disability. Per scoring guidelines, mean HAQ score was calculated for each participant if six or more of the eight categories were non-missing. We categorized baseline mean HAQ as follows: HAQ = 0, 0 < HAQ < 1, or HAQ ≥ 1, based on definitions previously used with JoCo OA data [16]. Based on the previously established minimum clinically important difference in HAQ score [15, 17, 18], we defined a clinically significant change as baseline +/– 0.22; individuals whose baseline scores rose by 0.22 or more were classified as worsening, and those whose baseline scores fell by 0.22 or more were classified as improving. If change in speed did not meet these values, participants were classified as having stayed the same. The groups were then dichotomized into improved/stayed the same, or worsened.

Chair stands Based on previously established protocols [19, 20], we assessed time for participants to complete 5 chair stands. Participants were seated in a chair with feet touching the floor and asked to rise without the use of arms as support. To ensure this, participants were asked to cross their arms at their wrists and hold them tight to their chests throughout the test. Participants who were unable to rise from a chair by themselves or scoot forward or stand up without using their arms were classified being unable to complete this test. For those able to perform this task, time taken to complete the 5 chair stands was recorded in seconds. We then categorized times into quartiles, based on baseline scores of those without sxKOA in our study sample. These thresholds were also determined separately for males and females due to evidence of differences in performance between these two groups [21]. For males, these cutoffs were time < 8.4 s (quartile 1, Q1), 8.4 s < time < 10.2 s (quartile 2, Q2), 10.2 s < time < 12.9 s (quartile 3, Q3), 12.9 s < time (quartile 4, Q4), or unable to complete all five chair stands. For females, these cutoffs were time < 9.0 s (Q1), 9.0 s < time < 11.3 s (Q2), 11.3 s < time < 14.1 s (Q3), 14.1 s < time (Q4), or unable to complete all five chair stands. We then categorized participants as either having worsened (moved up a quartile from baseline) or stayed the same / improved (remained in the same quartile or moved down a quartile from baseline) at the time of first follow-up. Participants unable to complete the chair stands at baseline were categorized as follows: staying the same / improving if they became able to complete at follow-up and worsening if they remained unable to complete at follow-up.

8-foot walk Using previously established procedures [20, 22], participants were asked to perform two trials in which they walked the 8-ft at their normal pace; times of the two trials were averaged and converted to gait speed (m/s) and kept continuous for the baseline measure. We categorized participants as either worsening or staying the same/improving in gait speed at follow-up. We defined worsening as a decrease of 0.1 m/s based on previous literature suggesting this may be a clinically relevant decline [23, 24].

Covariates Variables that could potentially confound the associations between sxKOA, function and CVD were included in multivariable models. These included: baseline enrollment group (Original vs. Enrichment cohort), age, gender, race (African American vs. Caucasian), education (< high school vs. ≥ high school), body mass index (BMI), waist to hip ratio (WHR), self-reported presence of diabetes, hypertension, or high cholesterol, and self-reported nonsteroidal anti-inflammatory drugs (NSAIDs) use at baseline. BMI, diabetes mellitus, hypertension and high cholesterol are often considered aspects of metabolic syndrome. These variables were included in our model as previous research has indicated

there may be underlying metabolic contributions to the development of comorbid CVD in individuals with OA [8]. NSAID use was also chosen as a possible confounder as it too has been indicated as a possible contributor to increased CVD risk in individuals with OA [7].

Statistical analysis

Descriptive statistics were calculated for all participants in the final analytic sample. Logistic regression models were used to model the odds of incident CVD. These population-averaged models for non-normal (binomial) measures were fit to each of the three physical function measure analyses. First, unadjusted odds ratios (OR) and 95% confidence intervals (CI) were computed to examine associations of sxKOA, baseline function, and worsening function with incident CVD. Second, multivariable models that jointly examined associations of sxKOA, baseline function and worsening function with incident CVD (Model 1) were conducted. Third, multivariable models that included Model 1 variables along with relevant demographic and health covariates (Model 2) were conducted. Models 1 and 2 were assessed for the interaction of sxKOA with physical function (both the baseline measure and the follow-up worsening indicator) at the 0.05 significance level. All statistical computations were performed using SAS, version 9.4 (Cary, NC).

Results

Participant characteristics are summarized in Table 1. Almost a quarter of our sample consisted of the Enrichment cohort, and overall mean time to follow-up was 5.9 ± 1.2 years. The sample comprised 63.6% women, 27.8% African Americans, and 25.9% with less than a high school education, while mean age of participants was 59.5 ± 9.5 years. The mean BMI was 29.3 ± 6.0 kg/m², with over three quarters of participants being overweight (38.2%) or obese (38.4%). At baseline, approximately a tenth of participants had diabetes, a third had hypertension, a fifth had high blood cholesterol, and almost a third reported NSAID use. Baseline sxKOA was present for approximately 15% of participants, and approximately 16% of participants developed CVD by their first follow-up. Individuals with sxKOA at baseline had 1.50 times the unadjusted odds of incident CVD (95% CI 1.08–2.08).

HAQ

Regarding mean HAQ scores, over half of participants (58.6%) had a score of zero, almost a third (30.8%) had 0 < HAQ < 1, and about a tenth (10.6%) had 1 ≤ HAQ at baseline. About a third (33.0%) of participants worsened by 0.22 units or more in mean HAQ score by first follow-up (which corresponds to the minimum clinically important difference), with the remainder staying the same or improving.

Table 1 Descriptive Characteristics of Study Sample ($N = 1709$)

Characteristic	Mean (SD) or %
Baseline	
% Original cohort	75.6
Demographic	
Mean (SD) Age	59.5 (9.5)
% Women	63.6
% African American	27.8
% with < 12 Years Education	25.9
Health Related	
Mean (SD) Body Mass Index (kg/m^2)	29.3 (6.0)
Mean (SD) Waist to Hip Ratio	0.87 (0.09)
% Hypertension	32.9
% Diabetes	8.7
% High cholesterol	20.8
OA Related	
% Non-steroidal Anti-inflammatory Drug Use	31.5
% Symptomatic Osteoarthritis	15.4
Function Related	
Mean Health Assessment Questionnaire; HAQ (SD)	0.27 (0.47)
% 0 = HAQ	58.6
% 0 < HAQ < 1	30.8
% 1 ≤ HAQ	10.6
Mean (SD) Speed During 8 ft. Walk (m/s)	0.87 (0.26)
Mean (SD) Chair Stand Times (s)	12.2 (4.8)
% Q1[a]	20.5
% Q2	23.1
% Q3	23.5
% Q4	27.5
% Unable to Complete	5.4
Follow-up	
Mean (SD) years to follow-up	5.9 (1.2)
% Worsened HAQ	33.0
% Worsened 8 ft. Walk speed	49.6
% Worsened Chair Stand Time	42.2
% Incident Cardiovascular Disease	15.9

[a] 5 Chair stand time quartlies defined from the non-exposure subsample without sxKOA at baseline: Males: Q1 (time < =8.4 s), Q2 (8.4 s < time < =10.2 s), Q3 (10.2 s < time < =12.9 s), Q4 (12.9 s < time)"; Females: Q1 (time < =9.0 s), Q2 (9.0 s < time < =11.3 s), Q3 (11.3 s < time < =14.1 s), Q4 (14.1 s < time)
SD standard deviation, *OA* Osteoarthritis

There were no significant interactions of sxKOA with baseline or worsening HAQ scores, so overall main effects are reported (Table 2). In unadjusted analyses, participants with baseline HAQ scores > 0 had 30–90% higher odds of incident CVD compared to those with HAQ = 0; those with worsening HAQ scores over time

had 2.5 times greater odds of incident CVD. In multivariable Model 1, baseline HAQ score ≥ 1 and worsening HAQ continued to have significantly greater odds of incident CVD, but sxKOA was no longer significantly associated with CVD risk in this model. These associations were similar in the fully adjusted model (Model 2), in which age and self-reported diabetes were also associated with incident CVD.

Chair stands

For chair stands, 5.4% of participants were unable to complete the test at baseline, and the quartile cutoff distribution (fastest to slowest times) was 20.5%, 23.1%, 23.5 and 27.5%. About 42% of participants worsened by moving up a quartile (or becoming unable) in chair stand performance at follow-up, with the remaining staying the same or improving.

There were no significant interactions of sxKOA with baseline or worsening chair stand time and so overall main effects are reported (Table 3). Compared to participants in the lowest quartile (Q1) of chair stand time, those in higher quartiles (Q2, Q3, and Q4) and those unable to complete the test had significantly elevated unadjusted odds of incident CVD; worsening chair stand performance over time was also associated with increased incident CVD. In multivariable Model 1, similar associations with incident CVD remained for baseline chair stand quartiles and worsening chair stand time, but sxKOA was no longer significantly associated with incident CVD risk in this model. These associations were similar in the fully adjusted model (Model 2), although inability to complete chair stands was no longer significantly associated with incident CVD risk; sex and diabetes were also associated with increased CVD risk.

8-foot walk

The mean baseline gait speed during the 8-ft walk was 0.87 m/s (SD = 0.26). About half (49.6%) of participants worsened by decreasing 0.1 m/s or more in mean gait speed by first follow-up. The measure of baseline gait speed showed a significant interaction with baseline sxKOA status, so effects of baseline gait speed are shown separately for participants without and with sxKOA (Table 4). Results for baseline gait speed are presented in units of 0.3 m/s difference; this was selected because it approximated 1 standard deviation for the distribution of baseline gait speeds. For participants without sxKOA, unadjusted odds of incident CVD were higher for those with a slower gait speed at baseline. In contrast, for participants with sxKOA, baseline gait speed was not associated with incident CVD. In unadjusted analyses, there was no association between worsening gait speed and incident CVD.

Table 2 Unadjusted and Adjusted Associations of sxKOA and HAQ Scores with Incident CVD

Variable	Unadjusted OR (95% CI)	Model 1[a] OR (95% CI)	Model 2[a] OR (95% CI)
sxKOA vs. no sxKOA at baseline	**1.50 (1.08, 2.08)**	1.14 (0.80, 1.61)	1.10 (0.76, 1.61)
Baseline 0 < HAQ < 1 vs. HAQ = 0	1.29 (0.97, 1.72)	1.17 (0.87, 1.57)	1.08 (0.79, 1.47)
Baseline 1 ≤ HAQ vs. HAQ = 0	**1.94 (1.32, 2.85)**	**1.91 (1.27, 2.86)**	**1.82 (1.18, 2.79)**
Worsened HAQ vs. unchanged or improved	**2.51 (1.93, 3.27)**	**2.49 (1.90, 3.25)**	**2.35 (1.79, 3.10)**
Age: 1 year increase			**1.02 (1.00, 1.03)**
Gender: Female vs. Male			1.28 (0.91, 1.80)
Race: Black vs. White			1.13 (0.83, 1.54)
Education: <HS vs. HS or greater			0.89 (0.65, 1.24)
Cohort: Enrichment vs. Original			0.96 (0.69, 1.33)
BMI: 1 kg/m^2 increase			0.98 (0.95, 1.00)
WHR: 0.1 unit increase			1.15 (0.98, 1.36)
Diabetes vs. not			**1.84 (1.21, 2.80)**
Hypertension vs. not			1.10 (0.81, 1.48)
High cholesterol vs. not			1.03 (0.74, 1.44)
NSAIDs vs. not			1.27 (0.94, 1.71)

CI confidence interval, sxKOA symptomatic knee osteoarthritis, HAQ health assessment questionnaire, HS high school, BMI body mass index, WHR waist-to-hip ratio, NSAIDs non-steroidal anti-inflammatory drugs
[a]Models 1 and 2 are adjusted for all variables with data listed in the column

Table 3 Unadjusted and Adjusted Associations of sxKOA and Chair Stands with Incident CVD

Variable	Unadjusted OR (95% CI)	Model 1[a] OR (95% CI)	Model 2[a] OR (95% CI)
sxKOA vs. no sxKOA at baseline	**1.50 (1.08, 2.08)**	1.28 (0.90, 1.80)	1.24 (0.86, 1.79)
Baseline 5 chair stand time Q2 vs. Q1**	**1.77 (1.14, 2.75)**	**1.82 (1.17, 2.83)**	**1.77 (1.13, 2.78)**
Baseline 5 chair stand time Q3 vs. Q1**	**1.93 (1.25, 2.98)**	**2.04 (1.31, 3.16)**	**1.79 (1.14, 2.81)**
Baseline 5 chair stand time Q4 vs. Q1**	**1.85 (1.21, 2.82)**	**2.02 (1.30, 3.15)**	**1.65 (1.02, 2.65)**
Baseline 5 chair stand time unable vs. Q1**	**2.50 (1.36, 4.58)**	**2.14 (1.16, 3.98)**	1.71 (0.89, 3.27)
Worsened 5 Chair stand time vs. unchanged or improved	**1.50 (1.15, 1.94)**	**1.58 (1.20, 2.08)**	**1.45 (1.09, 1.93)**
Age: 1 year increase			1.01 (1.00, 1.03)
Gender: Female vs. Male			**1.46 (1.05, 2.04)**
Race: Black vs. White			1.11 (0.82, 1.52)
Education: <HS vs. HS or greater			0.95 (0.68, 1.31)
Cohort: Enrichment vs. Original			1.06 (0.77, 1.47)
BMI: 1 kg/m^2 increase			0.98 (0.96, 1.01)
WHR: 0.1 unit increase			1.16 (0.99, 1.36)
Diabetes vs. not			**1.91 (1.26, 2.89)**
Hypertension vs. not			1.13 (0.84, 1.52)
High cholesterol vs. not			1.03 (0.74, 1.44)
NSAIDs vs. not			1.30 (0.97, 1.74)

CI confidence interval, Q quarter, sxKOA symptomatic knee osteoarthritis, HS high school, BMI body mass index, WHR waist-to-hip ratio, NSAIDs non-steroidal anti-inflammatory drugs
[a]Models 1 and 2 are adjusted for all variables with data listed in the column

Table 4 Unadjusted and Adjusted Associations of sxKOA and 8-Foot Walk with Incident CVD

Variable	Unadjusted OR (95% CI)	Model 1[a] OR (95% CI)	Model 2[a] OR (95% CI)
Baseline 0.3 m/s (1SD) decrease in mean 8 ft. walk speed among those without sxKOA	**1.46 (1.23, 1.74)**	**1.64 (1.35, 1.99)**	**1.46 (1.17, 1.82)**
Baseline 0.3 m/s (1SD) decrease in mean 8 ft. walk speed among those with sxKOA	0.91 (0.62, 1.33)	0.99 (0.67, 1.47)	0.90 (0.59, 1.36)
Worsened 8 ft. walk vs. unchanged or improved	1.12 (0.87, 1.45)	**1.53 (1.15, 2.04)**	**1.47 (1.07, 2.01)**
Age: 1 year increase			1.01 (0.99, 1.03)
Gender: Female vs. Male			1.35 (0.96, 1.91)
Race: Black vs. White			1.05 (0.77, 1.44)
Education: <HS vs. HS or greater			0.92 (0.66, 1.27)
Cohort: Enrichment vs. Original			1.10 (0.79, 1.54)
BMI: 1 kg/m^2 increase			0.98 (0.96, 1.01)
WHR: 0.1 unit increase			1.15 (0.98, 1.36)
Diabetes vs. not			**1.80 (1.19, 2.71)**
Hypertension vs. not			1.11 (0.83, 1.49)
High cholesterol vs. not			1.09 (0.79, 1.52)
NSAIDs vs. not			**1.34 (1.00, 1.80)**

CI confidence interval, *Q* quarter, *sxKOA* symptomatic knee osteoarthritis, *HS* high school, *BMI* body mass index, *WHR* waist-to-hip ratio, *NSAIDs* non-steroidal anti-inflammatory drugs
[a]Models 1 and 2 are adjusted for all variables with data listed in the column

In multivariable Model 1, slower baseline gait speed remained associated with incident CVD only for those without sxKOA. Worsening gait speed was also associated with incident CVD in Model 1. These associations were similar in the fully adjusted Model 2, in which NSAID use and self-reported diabetes were also associated with incident CVD.

Discussion

In this analysis, we examined the unique contributions of sxKOA, baseline function and worsening of function with incident CVD risk. With respect to sxKOA, we found significant associations with incident CVD risk in unadjusted analyses, but not in multivariable analyses adjusting for functional variables. There were significant associations of functional variables with incident CVD risk, and in particular, worsening of function variables over time was consistently associated with CVD risk in multivariable models. The association of one function variable, 8-ft walk, differed between those with and without sxKOA, being important only in the latter group.

The finding of a significant bivariate association of sxKOA with CVD risk is in agreement with results of prior studies [5, 10–12, 25]. Importantly, the longitudinal nature of this association supports that sxKOA predicts development of future CVD. In multivariable analyses including function variables, even prior to adjustment for other confounders, sxKOA was no longer significantly associated with CVD risk. This confirms another recent longitudinal study in which the association of number of joints with OA with CVD risk was

explained by self-reported difficulty walking at baseline [12]. These studies indicate that function is at least one key contributor to CVD risk among individuals with sxOA. Knowledge of this underlying mechanism is extremely important, as it points to a potential intervention approach. In particular, physical activity programs can significantly improve functional outcomes among individuals with sxKOA [26] and therefore may confer an important benefit regarding downstream CVD risk, particularly since physical activity also improves a number of metabolic factors leading to CVD.

There were a number of interesting findings regarding associations of functional measures with CVD risk. First, it is notable that all of the function measures (with the exception of 8-ft walk for people with sxKOA) were associated with increased CVD risk, suggesting that both performance-based measures and self-report measures (e.g., HAQ) may be helpful markers of CVD risk; this adds to prior studies that have shown positive associations with self-report function measures. Second, even when baseline function and change in function were included in the same model, change in function consistently remained significantly associated with incident CVD risk. This also adds to prior studies, which have focused on functional status at a single time point. These results illustrate the importance of functional decline in the prediction of CVD, regardless of baseline functional status, and further illustrates the importance of physical activity programs that can slow the progression of functional decline. Third, functional measures (particularly change in function over time) continued to have significant associations with CVD risk even in fully adjusted models that included a number of factors related to metabolic syndrome (e.g, BMI, WHR, diabetes). This is important since metabolic syndrome has been another proposed mechanism underlying the association between OA and CVD [7, 8]. Kendzerska et al. also found that self-reported walking-related disability continued to predict CVD risk even when adjusting for BMI and other metabolic factors [12]. This evidence supports that function plays a unique role in the relationships between sxKOA and CVD risk. Fourth, there was an interaction between sxKOA and the 8-ft walk variable: those without sxKOA who had worse baseline 8-ft walk speed were at a greater risk of developing incident CVD, but for those with sxKOA, baseline 8-ft walk performance was not a predictor of incident CVD risk. We hypothesize this result may be due to the fact that our sxKOA group had worse baseline walking speeds than the non-OA group at baseline (.75 m/s vs. 89 m/s), which confirms prior studies [27, 28]. Since walking speed was low overall among those with sxKOA, the variability within that lower range may not have been associated with differential CVD risk.

The association of between baseline chair stand time categories and increased CVD risk was non-linear. Relative to participants in the best baseline chair stand category (Q1), odds of CVD risk were elevated more for middle categories (Q2, Q3) than for those in the worst categories (Q4, unable to complete). However, the odds ratios were still relatively similar (1.65–1.79 in fully adjusted models). The lack of completely linear relationship may be due to the relatively small number of participants in each baseline chair stand group.

Strengths of this study include a community-based cohort including African American and Caucasian men and women, the use of both self-reported and performance-based measures of physical function, the longitudinal approach, and the inclusion of worsening variables for physical function measures. However, there are several limitations to note. First, CVD and function measures at follow-up were assessed at a single time point; therefore, we could not ascertain the specific time of occurrence, and it is possible that functional decline occurred after a CVD diagnosis or event within the follow-up period. Second, incident CVD was assessed via self-report. Although this method allows data for large samples to be obtained readily and cost-effectively, this can result in less accurate representation of true CVD. Strategies were employed in data collection in order to maximize self-report accuracy of CVD. These included impartial and standardized phrasing of the National Health Interview Survey question, ensuring that respondents understood the question completely, and that adequate amount of time for recall was given. However, there may still be instances of inaccurate reporting (either over-reporting or under-reporting).

Third, the incident CVD variable definition differed somewhat between cohorts, with angina and congestive heart only being included for the Enrichment Cohort. Fourth, some data were missing due to loss-to-follow-up, and it is possible that individuals with missing follow-up data were less healthy and had more functional limitations than those with complete data.

Conclusion

Overall, our study indicates that function is a key contributor to the association between symptomatic knee osteoarthritis and cardiovascular disease risk. Further, worsening of function over time seems to have a particularly important role. Physical activity and structured exercise programs can substantially improve function and are already key recommendations for OA management [26]. Unfortunately, many people with symptomatic knee osteoarthritis remain physically inactive [29], placing them at risk for functional loss, and perhaps subsequent elevation of cardiovascular disease risk as a result. These results further elevate the importance of efforts to enhance physical activity among individuals with symptomatic knee osteoarthritis and also highlight the importance of regular physical function assessment.

Abbreviations
BMI: Body Mass Index; CCA: Complete case analysis; CI: Confidence interval; CVD: Cardiovascular disease; HAQ: Health Assessment Questionnaire; JoCo OA: Johnston County Osteoarthritis Project; K-L: Kellgren Lawrence; NSAID: Non-steroidal Anti-Inflammatory Drug; OA: Osteoarthritis; OR: Odds ratio; Q: Quartile; SD: Standard deviation; SxKOA: Symptomatic knee osteoarthritis; WHR: Waist to Hip Ratio

Acknowledgements
We are thankful to the participants and staff in the Johnston County Osteoarthritis Project. Their efforts and dedication to the project made this research possible.

Funding
JoCo OA is supported by the Centers for Disease Control and Prevention / Association of Schools of Public Health cooperative agreements S043, S1734 and S3486 and U01DP003206 and U01DP006266. Further funding was supplied by NIAMS Multipurpose Arthritis and Musculoskeletal Disease Center grant 5-P60-AR3070, NIAMS Multidisciplinary Clinical Research Center grant 5 P60 AR49465–03 and P60AR30701, and NIA 5-T35-AG038047–07 UNC-CH Summer Research in Aging for Medical Students (MSTAR) and the Center for Health Services Research in Primary Care, Durham VA Health Care System (CIN 13–410). The findings and conclusions in this report are those of the authors and do not necessarily represent the official position of the Centers for Disease Control and Prevention. The authors retained full independence with respect to design of the study, data collection, analysis, interpretation of data and writing the manuscript.

Authors' contributions
MC, CA, AT and KDA contributed to initial planning of these secondary analyses and drafting of the manuscript. CA and RC contributed to plans for and conduct of statistical analyses. LFC, RC, YMG, JMJ, AEN, and JR contributed to the design and conduct of the parent study. All authors reviewed, edited and approved the final manuscript.

Competing interests

The authors declare that they have no competing interests.

Author details

[1]College of Medicine, Northeast Ohio Medical University, 4209 OH-44, Rootstown, OH 44272, USA. [2]Thurston Arthritis Research Center, University of North Carolina at Chapel Hill, 3300 Thurston Bldg., CB# 7280, Chapel Hill, NC 27599, USA. [3]Department of Medicine, University of North Carolina at Chapel Hill, 125 MacNider Hall CB# 7005, Chapel Hill, NC 27599, USA. [4]Injury Prevention Research Center, University of North Carolina at Chapel Hill, CB# 7505, 137 E Franklin St, Chapel Hill, NC 27599, USA. [5]Department of Epidemiology, University of North Carolina at Chapel Hill, 170 Rosenau Hall, CB#7400, Chapel Hill, NC 27599, USA. [6]Department of Radiology, University of North Carolina at Chapel Hill, 2006 Old Clinic, CB, Chapel Hill, NC #7510, USA. [7]Center for Health Services Research in Primary Care, Department of Veterans Affairs Healthcare System, 508 Fulton Street, Durham, NC, USA.

References

1. Cross M, Smith E, Hoy D, Nolte S, Ackerman I, Fransen M, Bridgett L, Williams S, Guillemin F, Hill CL, et al. The global burden of hip and knee osteoarthritis: estimates from the global burden of disease 2010 study. Ann Rheum Dis. 2014;73(7):1323–30.
2. Oiestad BE, White DK, Booton R, Niu J, Zhang Y, Torner J, Lewis CE, Nevitt M, LaValley M, Felson DT. Longitudinal course of physical function in people with symptomatic knee osteoarthritis: data from the multicenter osteoarthritis study and the osteoarthritis initiative. Arthritis Care Res (Hoboken). 2016;68(3):325–31.
3. White DK, Zhang Y, Niu J, Keysor JJ, Nevitt MC, Lewis CE, Torner JC, Neogi T. Do worsening knee radiographs mean greater chances of severe functional limitation? Arthritis Care Res (Hoboken). 2010;62(10):1433–9.
4. Hall AJ, Stubbs B, Mamas MA, Myint PK, Smith TO. Association between osteoarthritis and cardiovascular disease: systematic review and meta-analysis. Eur J Prev Cardiol. 2016;23(9):938–46.
5. Veronese N, Trevisan C, De Rui M, Bolzetta F, Maggi S, Zambon S, Musacchio E, Sartori L, Perissinotto E, Crepaldi G, et al. Association of Osteoarthritis with Increased Risk of cardiovascular diseases in the elderly: findings from the Progetto Veneto Anziano study cohort. Arthritis Rheumatol. 2016;68(5):1136–44.
6. Rahman MM, Kopec JA, Anis AH, Cibere J, Goldsmith CH. Risk of cardiovascular disease in patients with osteoarthritis: a prospective longitudinal study. Arthritis Care Res (Hoboken). 2013;65(12):1951–8.
7. Fernandes GS, Valdes AM. Cardiovascular disease and osteoarthritis: common pathways and patient outcomes. Eur J Clin Investig. 2015;45(4):405–14.
8. Le Clanche S, Bonnefont-Rousselot D, Sari-Ali E, Rannou F, Borderie D. Inter-relations between osteoarthritis and metabolic syndrome: a common link? Biochimie. 2016;121:238–52.
9. Schieir O, Hogg-Johnson S, Glazier RH, Badley EM. Sex variations in the effects of arthritis and activity limitation on first heart disease event occurrence in the Canadian general population: results from the longitudinal National Population Health Survey. Arthritis Care Res (Hoboken). 2016;68(6):811–8.
10. King L, Kendzerska T, Hawker G. The Relationship Between Osteoarthritis and Cardiovascular Disease: Results from a Population-Based Cohort. American College of Rheumatology Annual Scientific Meeting. 2015;67:954.
11. Hawker GA, Croxford R, Bierman AS, Harvey PJ, Ravi B, Stanaitis I, Lipscombe LL. All-cause mortality and serious cardiovascular events in people with hip and knee osteoarthritis: a population based cohort study. PLoS One. 2014; 9(3):e91286.
12. Kendzerska T, Juni P, King LK, Croxford R, Stanaitis I, Hawker GA. The longitudinal relationship between hand, hip and knee osteoarthritis and cardiovascular events: a population-based cohort study. Osteoarthr Cartil. 2017;25(11):1771–80.
13. Jordan JM, Helmick CG, Renner JB, Luta G, Dragomir AD, Woodard J, Fang F, Schwartz TA, Abbate LM, Callahan LF, et al. Prevalence of knee symptoms and radiographic and symptomatic knee osteoarthritis in African Americans and Caucasians: the Johnston County osteoarthritis project. J Rheumatol. 2007;31(4):172–80.
14. Allison PD. Quantitative applications in the social sciences: missing data. Thousand Oaks, CA: Sage Publications Ltd; 2002.
15. Bruce B, Fries JF. The Stanford health assessment questionnaire: dimensions and practical applications. Health Qual Life Outcomes. 2003;1:20.
16. Elliott AL, Kraus VB, Fang F, Renner JB, Schwartz TA, Salazar A, Huguenin T, Hochberg MC, Helmick CG, Jordan JM. Joint-specific hand symptoms and self-reported and performance-based functional status in African Americans and Caucasians: the Johnston County osteoarthritis project. Ann Rheum Dis. 2007;66(12):1622–6.
17. Bijsterbosch J, Scharloo M, Visser AW, Watt I, Meulenbelt I, Huizinga TW, Kaptein AA, Kloppenburg M. Illness perceptions in patients with osteoarthritis: change over time and association with disability. Arthritis Rheum. 2009;61(8):1054–61.
18. Kosinski M, Zhao SZ, Dedhiya S, Osterhaus JT, Ware JE Jr. Determining minimally important changes in generic and disease-specific health-related quality of life questionnaires in clinical trials of rheumatoid arthritis. Arthritis Rheum. 2000;43(7):1478–87.
19. Dobson F, Hinman RS, Roos EM, Abbott JH, Stratford P, Davis AM, Buchbinder R, Snyder-Mackler L, Henrotin Y, Thumboo J, et al. OARSI recommended performance-based tests to assess physical function in people diagnosed with hip or knee osteoarthritis. Osteoarthr Cartil. 2013;21(8):1042–52.
20. Guralnik JM, Simonsick EM, Ferrucci L, Glynn RJ, Berkman LF, Blazer DG, Scherr PA, Wallace RB. A short physical performance battery assessing lower extremity function: association with self-reported disability and prediction of mortality and nursing home admission. J Gerontol. 1994;49(2):M85–94.
21. Cleveland RJ, Schwartz TA, Renner J, Jordan JM, Callahan LF. Physical function and mortality: the Johnston County osteoarthritis project. Boston, MA: American college of rheumatology annual scientific meeting; 2014.
22. Purser JL, Golightly YM, Feng Q, Helmick CG, Renner JB, Jordan JM. Association of slower walking speed with incident knee osteoarthritis-related outcomes. Arthritis Care Res (Hoboken). 2012;64(7):1028–35.
23. Hardy SE, Perera S, Roumani YF, Chandler JM, Studenski SA. Improvement in usual gait speed predicts better survival in older adults. J Am Geriatr Soc. 2007;55(11):1727–34.
24. Middleton A, Fritz SL, Lusardi M. Walking speed: the functional vital sign. J Aging Phys Act. 2015;23(2):314–22.
25. Ong KL, Wu BJ, Cheung BM, Barter PJ, Rye KA. Arthritis: its prevalence, risk factors, and association with cardiovascular diseases in the United States, 1999 to 2008. Ann Epidemiol. 2013;23(2):80–6.
26. Roddy E, Zhang W, Doherty M. Aerobic walking or strengthening exercise for osteoarthritis of the knee? A systematic review. Ann Rheum Dis. 2005; 64(4):544–8.
27. Pisters MF, Veenhof C, van Dijk GM, Heymans MW, Twisk JW, Dekker J. The course of limitations in activities over 5 years in patients with knee and hip osteoarthritis with moderate functional limitations: risk factors for future functional decline. Osteoarthr Cartil. 2012;20(6):503–10.
28. Queen RM, Sparling TL, Schmitt D. Hip, knee, and ankle osteoarthritis negatively affects mechanical energy exchange. Clin Orthop Relat Res. 2016; 474(9):2055–63.
29. Song J, Hochberg MC, Chang RW, Hootman JM, Manheim LM, Lee J, Semanik PA, Sharma L, Dunlop DD, Osteoarthritis Initiative I. Racial and ethnic differences in physical activity guidelines attainment among people at high risk of or having knee osteoarthritis. Arthritis Care Res (Hoboken). 2013;65(2):195–202.

21

Does improvement towards a normal cervical sagittal configuration aid in the management of cervical myofascial pain syndrome

Ibrahim M. Moustafa[1,2]* (iD), Aliaa A. Diab[2], Fatma Hegazy[1] and Deed E. Harrison[3]

Abstract

Background: There is a growing interest concerning the understanding of and rehabilitation of the sagittal configuration of the cervical spine as a clinical outcome. However, the literature on the topic specific to conservative treatment outcomes of patients with chronic myofascial cervical pain syndrome (CMCPS) has not adequately addressed the relationship between cervical sagittal alignment and improved pain, disability and range of motion.

Methods: A randomized controlled study with a 1-year follow-up. Here, 120 (76 males) patients with chronic CMCPS and defined cervical sagittal posture abnormalities were randomly assigned to the control or an intervention group. Both groups received the Integrated neuromuscular inhibition technique (INIT); additionally, the intervention group received the denneroll cervical traction device. Alignment outcomes included two measures of sagittal posture: cervical angle (CV), and shoulder angle (SH). Patient relevant outcome measures included: neck pain intensity (NRS), neck disability (NDI), pressure pain thresholds (PPT), cervical range of motion using the CROM. Measures were assessed at three intervals: baseline, 10 weeks, and 1 year after the 10 week follow up.

Results: After 10 weeks of treatment, between group statistical analysis, showed equal improvements for both the intervention and control groups in NRS ($p = 0.36$) and NDI ($p = 0.09$). However, at 10 weeks, there were significant differences between groups favoring the intervention group for PPT ($p<0.001$) and all measures of CROM ($p<0.001$). Additionally, at 10 weeks the sagittal alignment variables showed significant differences favoring the intervention group for CV $p<0.001$ and SH ($p<0.001$) indicating improved CSA. Importantly, at the 1-year follow-up, between group analysis identified a regression back to baseline values for the control group for the non-significant group differences (NRS and NDI) at the 10-week mark. Thus, all variables were significantly different between groups favoring the intervention group at 1-year follow up: NRS ($p<0.001$), NDI ($p<0.001$), PPT $p<0.001$), CROM ($p<0.001$), CV ($p<0.001$), SH ($p<0.001$).

(Continued on next page)

* Correspondence: iabuamr@sharjah.ac.ae; ibrahiem.mostafa@pt.cu.edu.eg
[1]Department of Physiotherapy, College of Health Sciences, University of Sharjah, Sharjah, United Arab Emirates
[2]Basic Science Department, Faculty of Physical Therapy, Cairo University, 7 Mohamed Hassan El gamal Street-Abbas El Akaad, Nacer City, Egypt
Full list of author information is available at the end of the article

(Continued from previous page)

Conclusion: The addition of the denneroll cervical orthotic to a multimodal program positively affected CMCPS outcomes at long term follow up. We speculate the improved sagittal cervical posture alignment outcomes contributed to our findings.

Keywords: Randomized controlled trial, Cervical lordosis, Cervical posture, Cervical pain, Myofascial pain, Traction

Background

Chronic myofascial pain syndrome (CMPS) is a musculoskeletal condition or syndrome that is typically associated myofascial trigger points (MTrP). CMPS has a lifetime prevalence of up to 85% with variations as low as 15% for a point prevalence [1, 2]. CMPS significantly impacts a patient's health related quality of life outcomes with studies including: disability, financial status, depression, anxiety, and generalized neck pain [3, 4].

Myofascial pain syndrome remains one of the most common sources of pain in chronic non-specific neck pain. Factors commonly cited as predisposing to MPS among subjects with chronic non-specific neck pain include abnormal postural, inadequate rest, overstretching, over-shortening or more generally, repetitive mechanical stress [1, 2]. In clinical practice, different approaches such as massage, acupuncture and electro-thermotherapy are quite commonly used in the treatment of CMPS [3, 4]. However, the effectiveness of many of these approaches did not appear to be superior to placebo [3]. A recent systematic review found that functional exercise protocols have very low quality evidence for a positive small-to-moderate effect on pain intensity in patients suffering from MPS [5].

Identification of causative variables for MTrPs is a first step to prevent development and secondarily to develop potential treatments preventing recurrence. Although the exact mechanisms are still unknown, [6, 7] it is accepted that mechanical factors are thought to be factors associated in the development of MTrPs [1, 2, 8]. In this regard, various studies have confirmed that prolonged abnormal postures have been regarded as one of the causes of MPS [9, 10].

In the cervical region, various studies point to the fact that altered sagittal plane alignment of the cervical spine such as straightened, s-curves, reversed curves, and anterior head translation can result in abnormal stresses and strains leading to premature and acceleration of degenerative changes in the muscles, ligaments, bony structures and neural elements [11–13]. Furthermore, preliminary randomized trials have demonstrated improved neck pain, dizziness, disability, positioning sense, flexion / extension kinematics, arm pain, and somatosensory evoked potentials in patient groups receiving devices aimed at

restoration of the cervical curve and posture [14–17]. One such device for the rehabilitation of sagittal cervical alignment is the cervical denneroll spine orthotic out of Sydney, Australia. Two previous clinical trials have demonstrated the denneroll is a reliably placed three-point bending extension traction device that is relatively easy to use by both the patient and treating therapist, and it is effective at improving cervical lordosis (10°-14° improvement) and reducing anterior head translation (10-25 mm reduction) [15, 16].

Although the previously mentioned studies make a significant contribution to understanding the important role of a normal cervical lordotic curve and rehabilitation tools to enhance correction, the literature on the topic specific to conservative treatment outcomes of patients with MPS has not adequately addressed the relationship between cervical sagittal alignment and improved pain and disability at short and at long term follow up.

Accordingly, the present randomized controlled trial was undertaken to investigate the functional and pain response outcomes of denneroll cervical extension traction compared to standard care in patient cases with chronic MPS, with a verified hypo-lordosis and anterior translation of the cervical spine. Two primary hypotheses were tested: 1) that denneroll cervical traction will improve the sagittal alignment of the cervical spine. 2) The secondary hypothesis tested was whether restoration of normal cervical sagittal alignment will improve both short and long-term outcomes in cervical myofascial pain syndrome patients.

Methods

Patients

A prospective, investigator-blinded, parallel-group, randomized clinical trial was conducted at one of our university's research departments, the trial was registered with the Clinical Trial Registry PACTR201801002968301. Cairo university institutional review board approval was obtained prior to the study and all subjects were recruited from our institutions local outpatient clinic. Patients with cervical MPS were recruited from our university's rehabilitation clinic. Patients were recruited and treated from March 2016 to October 2017 including a 1-year of follow-up.

Participants were screened prior to inclusion for alterations in two primary cervical alignment variables: loss of the cervical lordosis and anterior head translation. As part of our University's IRB approved protocol, each participant was only to receive initial cervical spine radiography (with no follow up spine radiography) because a primary goal of the cervical denneroll orthotic is to restore the cervical lordosis, thus participants were necessarily screened for hypo-lordosis. Participants were included if their cervical lordosis was less than 25° as measured using the intersection of two lines drawn along the posterior body margins of C2 and C7 [12]. Initial cervical radiological assessment was important to identify the cervical curve apex to determine where a subject should properly place the apex of the denneroll in their cervical spine [16, 18].

Concerning anterior head translation, the participant had to have significant anterior head translation as measured by the craniovertebral angle (CVA). If the CVA was less than 50°, then a participant was referred to the study. Our selection of 50° as a reference angle was guided by the study of Yib et al. [19]. Consecutive patients were included if they had active, palpable MTrPs on a single side or both sides of the upper trapezius muscle. Diagnosis was made according to Travell and Simons' criteria, whereby five major and at least one minor criteria are required for clinical diagnosis [20]. The major criteria are (1) localized neck pain; (2) pain or altered sensations in expected referred pain area for given trigger point; (3) taut band within the muscle; (4) exquisite tenderness in a point along taut band; (5) restricted range of motion. The minor diagnostic criteria for MPS are (1) reproduction of the patient's chief pain complaint by manual pressure on MTrP nodule; (2) a local twitch response; and (3) pain relief obtained by muscular treatment. Participants were excluded if any signs or symptoms of medical "red flags" were present: tumor, fracture, rheumatoid arthritis, osteoporosis, and prolonged steroid use. Additionally, subjects were excluded with previous spine surgery and any exam findings consistent with neurological diseases and vascular disorders.

An independent research assistant performed a concealed permuted block randomization using a computer-generated randomization schedule with a random block size.

Randomization

Our study design randomly assigned eligible participants to 1 of 2 groups: an intervention group ($n = 60$) or control group (n = 60). Examiner blinding was obtained through an independent research assist; not knowing the study design and not specifically involved in any aspect of the trial. This research assistant created a concealed permuted block randomization for subject group allocation; where equal numbers were placed in each group using a permuted block design of different sizes.

Treatment methods

Both the control group and the intervention groups received the treatment interventions including: Integrated neuromuscular inhibition technique (INIT), Ischemic Compression, Strain Counterstrain (SCS), and muscle energy technique (MET). Additionally, the participants in the intervention group received the denneroll cervical traction. The control group was treated also with a placebo treatment using a small cervical towel applied in the supine position located in the mid cervical spine as an intervention to mimic the denneroll traction time; but without applying significant extension bending of the cervical spine.

Following 30 sessions, participants were re-evaluated a minimum of 24 h after their last session and then each subject was again followed for an additional 1-year time frame with no supervised treatment. The treating therapist (F.H), for both the control and intervention groups, was un-blinded to the treatment method but the subjects and assessor (A.I.M.M. and A.A.D.) who conducted the measurements were blinded.

Denneroll extension traction for the intervention group

The participants in the intervention group additionally received the denneroll cervical extension traction (Denneroll Industries, Sydney Australia; http://www.denneroll.com) following previously published protocols [18, 21]. The patients were instructed to lie supine and keep their legs extended. Based on the apex of each participant's cervical curvature on the initial radiograph, the therapist positioned the apex of the denneroll in one of two regions (mid cervical placement or lower cervical placement). The duration of the traction session started at 2–3 min and increased 1 min per session until reaching the goal of 20 min, the traction was repeated three times per week for 10 weeks. See Fig. 1.

Integrated neuromuscular inhibition technique (INIT)

The treating therapist first identified the TrPs to be treated within the upper trapezius muscle. The practitioner evaluated the fibers of the upper trapezius, making note of any active TrPs, by firmly pinching using the thumb and the forefinger. Ischemic compression was applied by placing the thumb and index finger over the active TrP. The therapist applied slow, increasing levels of sustained pressure to the area until a relaxation of the tissue barrier was felt. Following a release of pressure, the therapist again applied increased pressure until a new barrier was felt. This process was repeated until the patient indicated the area was no longer tender or until 90 s had elapsed; whichever came first. All identified

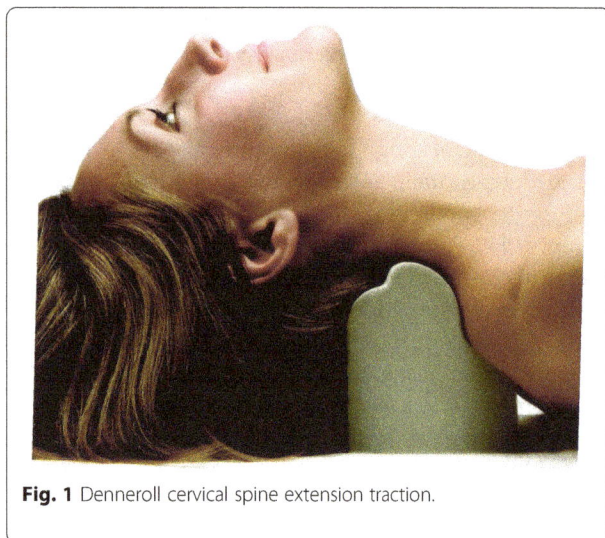

Fig. 1 Denneroll cervical spine extension traction.

TrPs were treated in the above manner per generally accepted methodology reported in the literature [6–8].

Ischemic compression and strain Counterstrain (SCS)

Here, moderate pressure was applied by the therapist to the identified MTrP while each patient rated their level of pain on a scale from 1 to 10. Once the patient's pain was reproduced, the therapist maintained pressure over the active MTrP and located a position that eased the patient's perception of pain. This position of ease was generally identified as positioning the affected muscle in a shortened/relaxed state; where a reduction in pain intensity of 70% was indicated by the patient. Once identified, the position of ease was held for 20–30 s and this was repeated for three to five repetitions by the therapist; similar to other generally accepted methodology reported in the literature [6–8].

Muscle energy technique (MET)

Following SCS, the participants received MET applied to the affected upper trapezius. Here, an isometric contraction was held for 7–10 s and was followed by further cervical spine contralateral side bending, flexion, and ipsilateral rotation to maintain and increase the soft tissue stretch as the muscle belly relaxes. The MET stretch position was repeated three to five times per treatment session and was maintained for 30 s. This protocol is similar to other generally accepted methodology reported in the literature [6–8].

All the participant received the treatment by the same physiotherapist, who had 15 years of experience in manual therapy.

Home exercise protocol

Participants were advised to perform a home exercise program once daily. The program included strengthening exercises for scapular retractors, deep cervical flexors, and neck extensors. This protocol has been previously reported [18, 21]. The participants were instructed to practice the same home exercise program at least twice a week during the 1 year follow up period. During the follow up period, participants were followed up by telephone interviews every 3 months.

Outcome measures

The participants underwent a series of assessments at three time intervals: prior to treatment, after 10 weeks of intensive treatment, and at 1 year of follow-up. The order of measurements was the same for all participants.

Primary outcome measure

- The Neck Disability Index (NDI), consisting of 10 items related to daily living activities, was our primary patient-reported outcome measure. The reliability, construct validity, and responsiveness to change of the NDI have all been assessed [18, 21].

Secondary outcome measures

- Cervical sagittal alignment, neck pain on a numerical rating scale, cervical ROM and pain pressure thresholds via an algometric score were secondary outcome measures.

Postural cervical sagittal alignment

Standing cervical and shoulder posture was measured with photogrammetry, which provide valid and reliable indicators of the spine [16]. Two angles of measurement were used cervical angle (CV), and shoulder angle (SH) (Fig. 2) - and obtained in the sagittal view as follows:

Cervical angle - The cervical angle is highly reliable to assess forward head translation [17]. It is defined as the angle between the true horizontal line through the spinous process of C7 and a line connecting spinous process of C7 with the tragus. In this study, if the angle was less than 50°, the participant was considered to have forward head posture; where subjects with FHP have a significantly smaller CV when compared with normal subjects [22].

Shoulder angle - A line was drawn between the midpoint of the humerus and spinous process of C7, and the angle of this line to the horizontal line through the midpoint of the humerus was calculated in degrees. In the present study, we considered 52° as the reference angle based on Brink et al. [23].

Pain intensity Neck pain intensity was measured using the numerical pain rating scale (NPRS) [24]. The patients

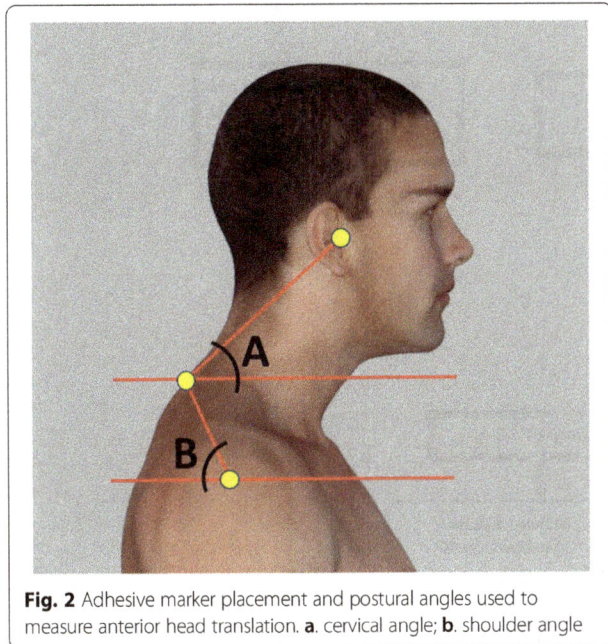

Fig. 2 Adhesive marker placement and postural angles used to measure anterior head translation. **a**. cervical angle; **b**. shoulder angle

were asked to place a mark along the line indicating their current pain intensity; 0 reflecting "no pain" and 10 reflecting the "worst pain".

Pressure-pain threshold (PPT) algometric measurement

A pressure threshold algometer (Lutron electronic, FG5005, RS232) was used to measure PPT in the most tender point (MTP) of the upper trapezius muscle before and after treatment. The average value of 3 repetitive measurements with an interval of 30 to 60 s (expressed as kilograms per square centimeter) was taken for data analysis of the PPT [25].

Cervical ROM

Cervical spine global range-of-motion was measured using the valid and reliable cervical range-of-motion (CROM) device [26]. The participant was instructed to perform flexion, extension, right/left lateral flexion, right/left rotation in upright sitting. The patient was instructed to perform each movement when he/she attained the maximum active range of motion. Three trials were conducted for each direction of movement, and the average of the three measurements were recorded for analysis. All measurements were taken by the same researcher who has postgraduate qualifications and 15 years of clinical experience in musculoskeletal physiotherapy.

Data analysis

Descriptive statistics were calculated including mean ± standard deviation (SD) for age, height and weight. The outcome measures of NDI, pain intensity, algometric

score, CROM, CV angle and SH angle were measured using repeated measures one-way analysis of variances (ANOVA) to compare measurements made before treatment, after the 10 weeks of treatment, and at 1-year follow up. Tukey's post-hoc multiple comparisons was implemented when necessary. The baseline score for outcomes were used as covariates in a one-way analysis of covariance (ANCOVA) when baseline differences are substantial enough to influence the study outcomes. We considered a mean difference of more than 10.5 points on the NDI as a MCID. Effect sizes measured using Cohen's d were calculated to examine the average impact of the intervention [27]. According to the method of Cohen, $d \approx 0.2$ indicates a small effect and negligible clinical importance, $d \approx 0.5$ indicates a medium effect and moderate clinical importance and $d \approx 0.8$ indicates a large effect and high clinical importance [24]. For all statistical tests the level of significance was set at $p < 0.05$. Correlations (Pearson's r) were used to examine the relationships between the amount of changes in CV and SH (in the study group) and the amount of change in NDI, pain intensity, ROM, and pressure algometry.

Sample size

A sample size of 100 patients provided a 90% power of detecting minimal clinically important change (MCIC) on the Neck Disability Index (NDI) of 10.5 points (scale range 0–50. To account for possible participant drop-outs, the sample size was increased by 20% in each group.

Missing values were addressed by using multiple regression models. Model parameters were estimated with multiple regression applied to each imputed data set separately. These estimates and their standard errors were combined into one overall estimate using Rubin's rules.

Results

A diagram of patient flow and randomization for our study is shown in Fig. 3. Two hundred and fifteen patients were initially screened with 120 of them being eligible to participate in the study. In total 120 (100%) completed the first study follow up after 30 visits or 10 weeks of treatment. At the 1-year follow up, 102 (85%) participants completed the entire study duration. At baseline, both groups were comparable with regard to all variables and had no statistically or clinically relevant differences, except for the cervical rotation ROM and Algometric pressure (Table 1).

Primary outcome measure
NDI

The difference between the intervention group and the control group was not significant after 10 weeks ($p = .09$; 95% CI [− 1.59 to .131]), however, it was significant at 1-year follow up ($< 0.001^*$; 95% CI [− 11.9–10.23]). The

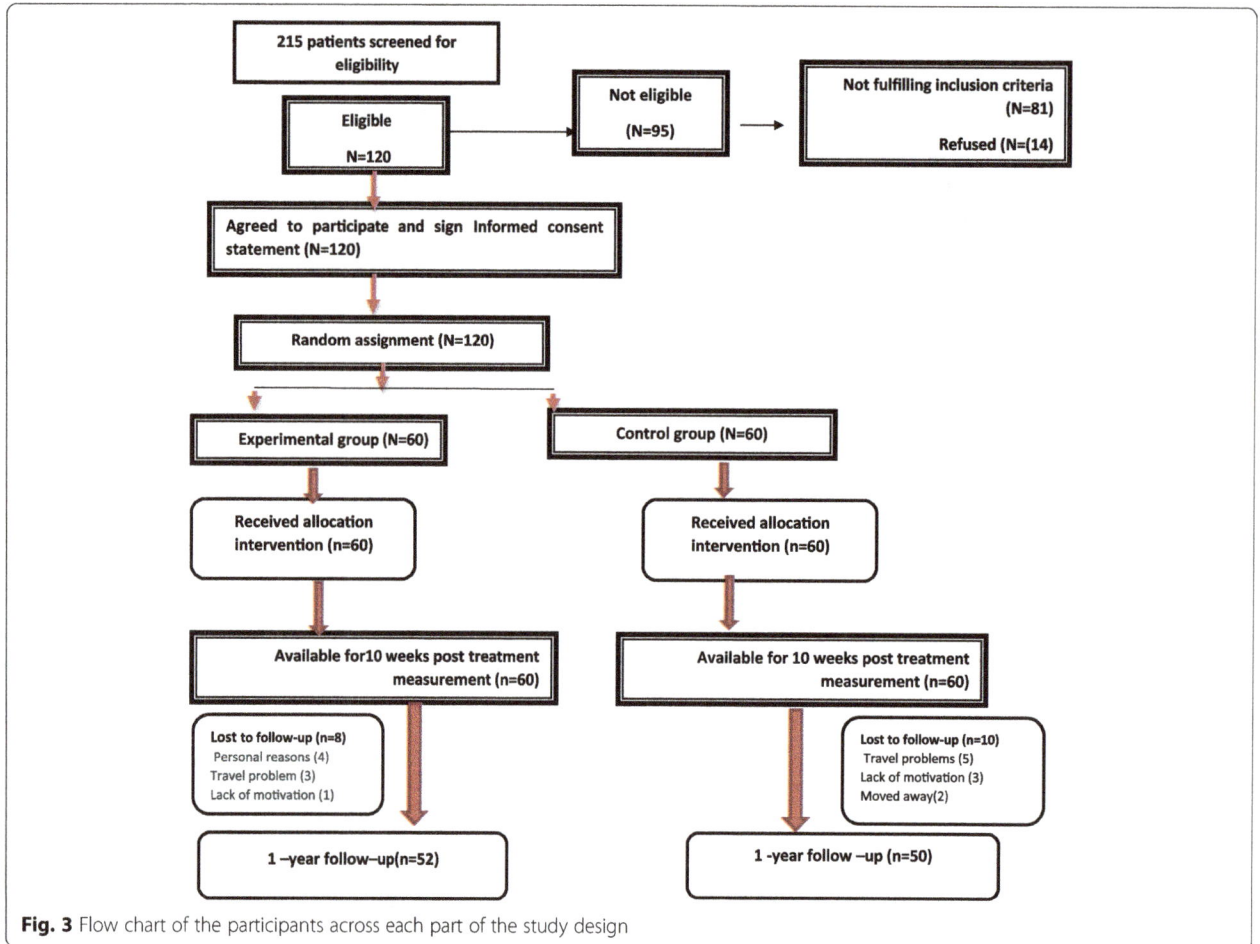

Fig. 3 Flow chart of the participants across each part of the study design

effect size (Cohen's d) was 0.9 (Table 2). These findings indicated a greater improvement in the interventional group in the NDI and a regression back to baseline-pre-treatment values in the NDI for the control subjects.

Secondary outcome measures
Pain intensity and algometric pressure
Subsequent analyses depending on the presence of interactions for main effects, revealed that after 10 weeks of treatment, the two arms of treatment (both interventional and control groups) seemed roughly equally successful in improving the pain intensity, and pressure algometry outcome measures. At 10 weeks, the unpaired t test analysis revealed insignificant differences between the experimental and control groups for pain intensity ($p = 0.36$), while there was a significant difference for algometry (p<0.001). In contrast, at the 1-year follow-up, the between group analysis showed that there were statistically significant differences in the interventional and control groups for neck pain intensity [0.4 vs. 4.2], $p < .001$), and pressure algometry [3.9 vs. 2], $p < .001$). Table 3 presents this data. The difference between groups at 1-year follow up period reached the MCID for

pain intensity and algometric pressure. The effect sizes were 0.67 and .9 respectively (Table 3).

Cervical angle and shoulder angle
The general linear model with repeated measures indicated significant group x time effects at both the 10 weeks of treatment mark and the 1-year follow up in favor of the interventional group on measures of cervical angle ($p<0.001$) and shoulder angle ($p<0.001$). Table 4 presents group means and standard deviations for each of these variables at each evaluation period. Also, the between group differences with 95% confidence intervals (CI) are presented. The difference between groups after 10 weeks and at 1-year follow up period reached the MCID for all cervical alignment parameters; cervical angle and shoulder angle. The effect sizes on the cervical and shoulder parameters varied from 3.7 to 5.7.

Cervical range of motion
Similarly, all measures of cervical spine range of motion indicated greater improvement in the interventional group compared to the control group at both the 10-week and 1-year follow up points: flexion ($p<0.001$),

Table 1 Baseline participant demographics

	Experimental group (n = 60)	Control group (n = 60)
Age(y)	33.1 ± 8	31.9 ± 7
Weight(kg)	76 ± 10	78 ± 11
Male	40(67%)	36(60%)
Female	20(33%)	24(40%)
Education level		
Primary school	4	3
Secondary school	8	8
Advanced technical colleague	21	20
University diploma	15	13
Others	12	16
Employment status		
Full-time	47	49
Part-time	8	7
Unemployed	5	4
NDI	35.7 ± 2.6	35.1 ± 3.2
Cervical angle	44.8 ± 3.5	45.03 ± 3.1
Shoulder angle	48.2 ± 2.1	48.3 ± 1.7
Pain intensity	5.3 ± .7	5.1 ± .8
Algometric pressure	1.9 ± .2	1.7 ± .3
Cervical flexion	53.2 ± 1	52.8 ± 2.1
Cervical extension	68.1 ± 1.2	67.6 ± 2.5
Right cervical rotation	72.3 ± 2.4	73.7 ± 2.6
Left cervical rotation	72.3 ± 2.4	74.3 ± 2.8
Right lateral flexion	42.3 ± 2	41.9 ± 2.1
Left lateral flexion	42.5 ± 2.1	42.2 ± 2.1

extension ($p<0.001$), right rotation ($p<0.001$), left rotation ($p<0.001$), right tilting ($p<0.001$), left tilting ($p<0.001$). Table 4 presents the group means and standard deviations for each of the ROM variables at each evaluation period. Also, the between group differences with 95% confidence interval (CI) values for each variable are presented for the 10 week vs. baseline evaluations and the 1 year follow up vs. baseline evaluations in

Table 4. The difference between groups after 10 weeks and at 1-year follow up period reached the MCID for all cervical ROM parameters. The effect sizes varied from 1.7 to 3.8 (Table 4).

Correlation of posture parameters to primary and secondary outcomes

The amount of change in the CV angle (anterior head translation) at baseline vs. 10 weeks in the intervention group receiving the denneroll significantly correlated with the amount of change in NDI ($p<0.032$), pain intensity ($p<0.05$), pressure algometry ($p<0.033$) and all ROM measures. Whereas, the amount of change in the SH angle at baseline vs. 10 weeks in the intervention group correlated only with pain intensity ($p<0.015$), and algometry ($p<0.012$). The significant correlations were maintained at 1-year follow up with no significant differences in the findings from 10-weeks to 1-year indicating stability. Table 5 presents this data.

Discussion

Our primary study hypothesis was that reduction or correction of abnormal sagittal cervical posture alignment would impact the short and long-term outcomes of subjects suffering from chronic cervical myofascial pain syndrome (CMPS). Following 30 treatment sessions, our 10-week re-examination findings indicated that there were significant differences between groups favoring the intervention group for sagittal posture alignment, pain pressure thresholds (PPT) and all measures of cervical range of motion (CROM). Further, at the 1-year follow-up, the between group analysis identified a regression back to baseline values for the control group's neck pain and disability, while the intervention groups variables remained stable where all measures showed statistically significant improvements favoring the intervention group: NRS ($p<0.001$), NDI ($p<0.001$), PPT $p<0.001$), CROM ($p<0.001$), CV ($p<0.001$), SH ($p<0.001$). The above findings confirm our primary study hypothesis.

Regarding improvement in sagittal cervical posture alignment in subjects using the cervical denneroll orthotic, our intervention group's outcomes are similar to

Table 2 The changes in primary outcomes (NDI) in experimental and control groups vs time

Outcome	Experimental group	Control group	Mean difference (95% CI)	P value	effect size (Cohen's d)	Effect size r
NDI						
Baseline	35.7 ± 2.6	35.1 ± 3.2	[−.5 1.7]	.2		
After 10 weeks	23.3 ± 2.8	24 ± 1.8	[−1.59 .13]	.09		
1-year follow up	17.4 ± 1.3	28.5 ± 1.2	[−11.9-10.2]	< 0.001	8.8	.9
G	< 0.001					
T	< 0.001					
G*T	< 0.001					

NDI Neck disability index, G group T: time G vs T: group versus time

Table 3 The changes in secondary outcomes; pain intensity and algometry in experimental and control groups vs time

Outcome	Experimental group	Control group	Mean difference (95% CI)	P value	effect size (Cohen's d)	Effect size r
Pain intensity						
Baseline	5.3 ± .7	5.1 ± .8	[−.05 .5]	.11		
After 10 weeks	1.4 ± .9	1.6 ± .8	[−.5 .17]	.36		
1-year follow up	.4 ± .4	4.2 ± .7	[−4.1-3.6]	< 0.001	.6	.9
G	< 0.001					
T	< 0.001					
G*T	< 0.001					
Algometric pressure						
Baseline	1.9 ± .2	1.71 ± .3	[.15.3]	< 0.001		
After 10 weeks	3.6 ± .3	3.3 ± .5	[.13.5]	< 0.001	.7	.8
1-year follow up	3.9 ± .2	2 ± .4	[1.8 2.1]	< 0.001	.9	.9
G	< 0.001					
T	< 0.001					
G*T	< 0.001					

G: group T: time G vs T: group versus time

those reported in two earlier trials using this patient prescribed orthotic device [15, 16]. Devices such as the denneroll, act as three-point-bending cervical extension traction devices; where structures located anterior to the axis of extension rotation will be exposed to significant tension loads and structures posterior will experience compression. The anterior tension loading likely unloads the intervertebral disc, causing tension on the anterior cervical spine muscles, and anterior longitudinal ligament, leading to visco-elastic creep deformation resulting in increasing the cervical lordosis and reducing anterior head translation [16, 18, 28].

Anterior head translation and protraction or rounding of the shoulders are likely two postures that are coupled together. In our current study, we identified that the intervention group receiving the cervical denneroll was found to have a reduction in both anterior head posture and a more retracted shoulder / scapular position following treatment. Reduction in anterior head translation is likely responsible for the improvement in shoulder alignment. Similarly, Diab et al., identified that reduction in sagittal head posture was an effective means for improving 3-D spinal posture of the thoracic region and pelvis [29]. Collectively, the finding that rehabilitation of cervical sagittal posture may subtly improve full spine posture measures indicates that there must exist a top down neurophysiological regulation of upright human posture that is driven by the sagittal alignment of the cervical lordosis and forward head posture [30, 31].

Forward head posture and neck disability index

It is interesting that the application of an integrated neuromuscular inhibition technique alone or in conjunction with an intervention program for forward head

posture reduction (denneroll orthotic) seem roughly equally successful in improving neck disability status after 10 weeks of treatment. However, our 1-year follow up data revealed a significant decline in the neck disability index for the control group. The temporal improvement in the control group may be attributed to the strong association between pain relief in both groups and functional status. However, over time, the continuous increased and / or asymmetrical loading from forward head posture may be the possible explanation for the decline in functional disability status for the control group at 12 months follow up. This concept of biomechanical dysfunction resulting from anterior head translation is supported by predictions from experimental and biomechanical spine-posture modeling studies [15, 19, 32, 33] as well as from post-surgical outcomes [34, 35] and large scale cross-sectional investigations [36].

Specifically, Tang et al. [34] identified that anterior translation distance of C2 relative to C7 (termed the SVA) on lateral cervical radiographs positively correlated with the neck disability index in 113 patients receiving posterior cervical spine fusions. Similar results were identified in a prospective sample of 49 patients by Roguski et al. [35]. In a large cross sectional analysis of 656 subjects, Oe et al. [36] identified strong correlations between activities of daily living on the EuroQOL questionnaire and the C2-C7 SVA. These three studies [34–36] are supported by the results of the current investigation where we identified a statistically significant correlation between our experimental groups improvement in their anterior head translation (CV angle) and their consequent improvement in NDI 10-weeks post treatment and at long term follow up.

Table 4 Changes in secondary outcomes; cervical ROM and posture parameters

Cervical angle (CV)						
	Experimental group	Control group	Mean difference (95% CI)	P value	effect size (Cohen's d)	Effect size r
Baseline	44. 8 ± 3.5	45 ± 3.2	[−1.5 .94]	.6		
After 10 weeks	54.8 ± 2.5	45 ± 3.3	[8.8 10.9]	< 0.001	5.2	.9
1-year follow up	54.2 ± 2.7	44.5 ± 3.1	[8.7 10.8]	< 0.001	5.7	.9
G	< 0.001					
T	< 0.001					
G*T	< 0.001					
Shoulder angle						
Baseline	48.2 ± 2.1	48.3 ± 1.7	[−.77 .6]	.8		
After 10 weeks	57.7 ± 2.9	48.06 ± 1.6	[8.7 10.4]	< 0.001	4.1	.9
1-year follow up	56.9 ± 3.1	48.3 ± 1.4	[7.71 9.4]	< 0.001	3.7	.9
G	< 0.001					
T	< 0.001					
G*T	< 0.001					
Flexion						
Baseline	42.3 ± 2	41.9 ± 2.1	[−.31 1.2]	.2		
After 10 weeks	46.7 ± 1.5	43.3 ± 1.7	[2.8 4.1]	< 0.001	2.5	.7
1-year follow up	46.3 ± 1.4	42.9 ± 2.3	[2.7 4.1]	< 0.001	1.7	.7
G	< 0.001					
T	< 0.001					
G*T	< 0.001					
Extension						
Baseline	68.1 ± 1.2	67.6 ± 2.5	[−.14 1.3]	.1		
After 10 weeks	75.2 ± 1.8	68.2 ± 2.4	[6.3 7.8]	< 0.001	3.2	.9
1-year follow up	74.4 ± 1.7	67.6 ± 1.9	[6.2 7.3]	< 0.001	3.0	.9
G	< 0.001					
T	< 0.001					
G*T	< 0.001					
Right rotation						
Baseline	72.3 ± 2.4	73.7 ± 2.6	[−2.3 -.4]	< 0.001		
After 10 weeks	79.7 ± 1.4	74.8 ± 2.3	[4.2 5.5]	< 0.001	2.6	.8
1-year follow up	78.8 ± .9	74.8 ± 2.1	[3.4 4.6]	< 0.001	2.5	.8
G	< 0.001					
T	< 0.001					
G*T	< 0.001					
Left rotation						
Baseline	72.3 ± 2.4	74.3 ± 2.8	[−2.94-1.05]	< 0.001		
After 10 weeks	79.6 ± 1.4	74.8 ± 2.3	[4.21 5.4]	< 0.001	2.6	.8
1-year follow up	78.8 ± .9	74.8 ± 2.1	[3.4 4.6]	< 0.001	2.5	.8
G	< 0.001					
T	< 0.001					
G*T	< 0.001					
Right tilt						
Baseline	42.3 ± 2	41.9 ± 2.1	[−.31 1.18]	.2		

Table 4 Changes in secondary outcomes; cervical ROM and posture parameters *(Continued)*

Cervical angle (CV)

	Experimental group	Control group	Mean difference (95% CI)	P value	effect size (Cohen's d)	Effect size r
After 10 weeks	46.7 ± 1.5	43.3 ± 1.7	[2.8 4.05]	< 0.001	2.5	.7
1-year follow up	46.3 ± 1.4	42.9 ± 2.3	[2.724 4.1]	< 0.001	1.7	.7
G	< 0.001					
T	< 0.001					
G*T	< 0.001					
Left Right tilt						
Baseline	42.5 ± 2.1	42.2 ± 2.1	[−.42 1.12]	.3		
After 10 weeks	46.7 ± 1.6	43.45 ± 1.8	[2.6 3.9]	< 0.001	2.5	.7
1-year follow up	46.4 ± 1.4	43.15 ± 2.3	[2.5 3.9]	< 0.001	1.7	.7
G	< 0.001					
T	< 0.001					
G*T	< 0.001					

G: group T: time G vs T: group versus time

Pain intensity and algometric pressure

Overall, our findings revealed a significant and stable decrease in pain intensity for the study group. This long lasting improvement of pain for the study group seems attributable to the restoration of normal posture. It is generally accepted that spinal function is directly related to spinal structure. Abnormal posture elicits abnormal stresses and strains in many structures, including bones, intervertebral discs, facet joints, musculotendinous tissues, and neural elements [13, 27, 32, 33], that can be considered as a predisposing factor for pain from an alteration in mechanical loading. Of interest, in FHP, reciprocal postural compensation was observed in the upper and lower cervical spine to maintain horizontal gaze. FHP caused flexion in the lower segments and extension in the atlanto-occipital and atlantoaxial segments. The transition between flexion and extension occurred in the C2–C4 region. These compensations have implications towards increased abnormal stresses and strains [37]. Thus, restoring the normal sagittal configuration is likely to minimize the abnormal stresses.

This mechanical relationship between prolonged abnormal postures and MPS has previously been identified in different studies [9, 10]. However, few studies have directly evaluated the relationship between forward head posture and MPS in neck and shoulder. Sun et al., examined the correlation between the presence of MPS and abnormal cervical sagittal alignment concluding that "there was no relationship between the forward head position and the presence, location, and number of trigger points" [38]. While Penas et al., highlighted the positive relationship between forward head posture and the presence of active trigger points [39].

The discrepancy and conflict regarding the relationship between abnormal forward head posture with MPS

identified by earlier authors cannot be directly compared with our current study because earlier studies are cross-sectional correlation studies without an ability to ascribe cause and effect. In the current study, the significant correlations between the amount of change in the CV angle in the intervention group and neck disability, pain intensity, and algometry outcomes indicates that forward head posture reduction improves the outcomes of MPS.

Concerning the pain level outcomes in the control group, the temporal reduction of pain may be attributed to short term effects of integrated neuromuscular inhibition technique. For example, Hu et al. [40] reported that pain reduction, improvement of MTrP sensitivity, and increase in ROM after various modalities for cervical myofascial pain and trigger-point sensitivity may not be maintained long term. Similarly, the systematic review of Vernon and Schneider [41] provides moderately strong evidence to support the use of some manual therapies in the immediate relief of TrP tenderness. However, only limited evidence to support the use of manual therapies over longer courses of treatments in the management of TrPs and MPS was found.

Cervical ROM

One might speculate that the improvement of ROM is attributed to a decrease of pain intensity. However, the significant differences between our study and control groups at the two measurement intervals favoring the study group indicate that the loss in ROM is not or not only driven by the presence of myofascial pain [34, 42]. Other factors associated with restricted ROM besides increased muscle tension and pain need considered. Mechanically though, forward head translation alters the anatomic alignment of the cervical spine joints in the

Table 5 Pearson's r correlation matrix for outcome variables in the intervention group

	Δ cervical angle 0-10w	Δ cervical angle 10-1Y	Δ shoulder angle 0-10w	Δ shoulder angle 10w -1Y
Δ pain 0-10 W	−.2 P = .05		−.2 P = .015	
Δ pain 10 W-1Y		−.1 P = .2		−.05 P = .3
Δ NDI 0-10w	−.24 P = .032		−.11 P = .196	
Δ NDI 10 w-1Y		.2 P = .0		.07 P = .2
Δ algometric 0–10 w	.24 P = .033		.29 P = .012	
Δ algometric 10w-1 Y		−.027 P = .4		−.002 P = .4
ROM flexion 0–10 w	.2 P = .028		.15 P = .1	
ROM flexion 10w-1 Y		−.16 P = .1		−.007 P = .4
ΔROM extension 0–10 w	.34 P = .003		−.06 P = .3	
ΔROM extension 10w-1 Y		.06 P = .3		.053 P = .3
ΔROM RT rotation 0–10 w	.25 P = .026		.14 P = .1	
ΔROM RT rotation 10w-1 Y		−.11 P = .1		.033 P = .4
ΔROM left rotation 0–10 w	.4 P = .036		.03 P = .4	
ΔROM rotation lt 10w-1 Y		−.1 P = .1		.013 P = .4
ΔROM RT lateral flex 0–10 w	.2 P − .020		.12 P = .1	
ΔROM RT lateral flex 10w-1 Y		.14 P = .1		
ΔROM left lateral flex 0–10 w	.2 P = .021		.05 P = .3	
ΔROM left lateral flex 10w-1 Y		.04 P = .3		−.1 P = .2

sagittal plane, alters the lever arms of the cervical spine muscles and thus this is the most plausible explanation for altered cervical spine ROM [35]. This statement is further supported by the significant correlation between the amount of change in the CV angle in the intervention group and all ROM outcomes. The current study results are logical and agree with those of four other studies [35, 36, 43, 44], each of which investigated the association between forward head and cervical ROM.

Limitations

The current study has some potential limitations. First, our study lacked blinding of participants and treatment providers. Due to the nature of the interventions, it was not be possible to blind participants and treatment providers to the interventions provided. Second, we used a sample of convenience from 1 clinic; which may not be representative of the entire population of patients with CMCPS. Additionally, we chose selective but relevant patient outcome measures (NDI, pain scale, pain pressure thresholds, range of motion) to identify if changes in sagittal plane posture deviations are related to CMCPS improvement. It is possible that other measures of CMCPS outcomes would have different relationships (greater or less improved) with posture alignment changes and that different interventions than those tested herein may improve patients with CMCPS more considerably.

Third, although the correlations identified between our postural measures and patient outcomes were statistically significant, they would be classified in the moderate range. This indicates that there are other variables, not accounted for in the current study design, which have determining effects on neck disability, pain, and range of motion outcomes. Along this line, we were unable to obtain follow-up lateral cervical radiographs. Thus, we do not if know the cervical lordosis was improved in the experimental group receiving the denneroll and if this may have added any significance to the correlation to patient outcomes.

Within these limitations, the unique contribution of this study is that it evaluated the independent effect of structural rehabilitation of the cervical spine sagittal posture on the short and long term severity of the signs and symptoms associated with CMCPS; which to our knowledge has not been previously reported. A major strength of the present study is the information as to how long pain relief lasted after treatment; up to 1-year. Whereas additional post-treatment measurements with longer than a 1-year interval might have identified a waning effectiveness of treatment.

Conclusion

This study identified that restoring a more normal cervical sagittal alignment with denneroll traction has a strong positive impact on pain, function, and ROM in patients with myofascial pain syndrome. Our one-year follow-up revealed stable improvement in all measured variables. The findings provide objective evidence that biomechanical dysfunction in terms of abnormal head and cervical posture influences the outcome measures of MPS. These observed effects should be of value to clinicians and health professionals involved in the treatment of MPS where cervical spine alignment rehabilitation can be added to the interventions for MPS patients who present with significant posture abnormality.

Abbreviations

CMCPS: Chronic myofascial cervical pain syndrome; CV: Cervical angle; INIT: Neuromuscular inhibition technique; NDI: Neck disability index; NRS: Neck pain intensity; PPT: Pressure pain thresholds; SH: Shoulder angle

Acknowledgements
We thank the CBP NonProfit, Inc. for supplying the Dennerolls used is this study.

Funding
This study was financially supported by funding from the Chiropractic Biophysics Non-profit, Inc., Inc. The contribution in terms of supplying the Dennerolls used is this study.Chiropractic Biophysics Non-profit, Inc. is a nonprofit corporation dedicated to the advancement of chiropractic principles through scientific research.

Authors' contributions
IMM and AAD, involved in study conception and design, as well as implementation, analysis and interpretation of data, and manuscript preparation FH made substantial contributions to the conception and design of the study and the drafting of the article, DEH made substantial contributions to the conception and design of the study, the analysis and interpretation of the data and the revision of the article. All authors have reviewed and approved the final manuscript.

Competing interests
DEH is the president of a company that distributes the cervical Denneroll product to health care providers in North America. IMM and AAD and FH have no conflicts of interest related to this project.

Author details
[1]Department of Physiotherapy, College of Health Sciences, University of Sharjah, Sharjah, United Arab Emirates. [2]Basic Science Department, Faculty of Physical Therapy, Cairo University, 7 Mohamed Hassan El gamal Street-Abbas El Akaad, Nacer City, Egypt. [3]CBP Nonprofit (a spine research foundation), Eagle, ID, USA.

References

1. KADEFORS R, Forsman M, Zoéga B, Herberts P. Recruitment of low threshold motor-units in the trapezius muscle in different static arm positions. Ergonomics. 1999;42:359–75 [cited 2018 Jul 4] Available from: http://www.ncbi.nlm.nih.gov/pubmed/10024852.
2. Kostopoulos D, Rizopoulos K. The manual of trigger point and myofascial therapy: Slack; 2001.
3. Rickards LD. The effectiveness of non-invasive treatments for active myofascial trigger point pain: A systematic review of the literature. Int J Osteopath Med. 2006;9:120–36 Elsevier; [cited 2018 Jan 11] Available from: https://www.sciencedirect.com/science/article/pii/S1746068906000952.
4. Dommerholt J, Grieve R, Layton M, Hooks T. An evidence-informed review of the current myofascial pain literature – January 2015. J Bodyw Mov Ther. 2015;19:126–37 Churchill Livingstone [cited 2018 Jan 11] Available from: https://www.sciencedirect.com/science/article/pii/S1360859214001922.
5. Mata Diz JB, de Souza JRLM, Leopoldino AAO, Oliveira VC. Exercise, especially combined stretching and strengthening exercise, reduces myofascial pain: a systematic review. J Physiother. 2017;63:17–22 [cited 2017 May 21] Available from: http://www.sciencedirect.com/science/article/pii/S1836955316300911.
6. Fernández-de-las-Peñas C, Dommerholt J. Myofascial trigger points: peripheral or central phenomenon? Curr Rheumatol Rep. 2014;16:395 [cited 2017 Dec 2] Available from: http://www.ncbi.nlm.nih.gov/pubmed/24264721.
7. Pace MC, Mazzariello L, Passavanti MB, Sansone P, Barbarisi M, Aurilio C. Neurobiology of pain. J Cell Physiol. 2006;209:8–12 [cited 2017 Dec 2] Available from: http://www.ncbi.nlm.nih.gov/pubmed/16741973.
8. Gerwin R. Myofascial pain syndrome: Here we are, where must we go? J Musculoskelet Pain. 2010;18:329–47 Taylor & Francis [cited 2017 Dec 2] Available from: http://www.tandfonline.com/doi/full/10.3109/10582452.2010.502636.
9. Yoo W-G. Effect of the Neck Retraction Taping (NRT) on Forward Head Posture and the Upper Trapezius Muscle during Computer Work. J Phys Ther Sci. 2013;25:581–2 Society of Physical Therapy Science [cited 2017 Dec 2] Available from: http://www.ncbi.nlm.nih.gov/pubmed/24259806.
10. Gupta BD, Aggarwal S, Gupta B, Gupta M, Gupta N. Effect of deep cervical flexor training vs. conventional isometric training on forward head posture, pain, neck disability index in dentists suffering from chronic neck pain. J Clin Diagnostic Res. 2013;7:2261–4 [cited 2017 Dec 2] Available from: http://www.ncbi.nlm.nih.gov/pubmed/24298492.
11. McAviney J, Schulz D, Bock R, Harrison DE, Holland B. Determining the relationship between cervical lordosis and neck complaints. J Manipulative Physiol Ther. 2005;28:187–93 [cited 2016 Apr 25] Available from: http://www.ncbi.nlm.nih.gov/pubmed/15855907.
12. Harrison DD, Janik TJ, Troyanovich SJHB. Comparisons of lordotic cervical spine curvatures to a theoretical ideal model of the static sagittal cervical spine. Spine (Phila Pa 1976). 1996;21:667–75.
13. Harrison DDE, Cailliet R, Harrison DDE, Troyanovich SJ, Harrison SO. A review of biomechanics of the central nervous system--part II: spinal cord strains from postural loads. J Manipulative Physiol Ther. 1999;22:322–32 [cited 2016 Apr 25] Available from: http://www.ncbi.nlm.nih.gov/pubmed/10395435.
14. Diab AA, Moustafa IM. The efficacy of forward head correction on nerve root function and pain in cervical spondylotic radiculopathy: a randomized trial. Clin Rehabil. 2012;26:351–61 [cited 2016 Apr 30] Available from: http://www.ncbi.nlm.nih.gov/pubmed/21937526.
15. Moustafa IM, Diab AA, Taha S, Harrison DE. Addition of a sagittal cervical posture corrective orthotic device to a multimodal rehabilitation program improves short- and long-term outcomes in patients with discogenic cervical radiculopathy. Arch Phys Med Rehabil. 2016;97:2034–44 [cited 2017 Dec 2] Available from: http://www.ncbi.nlm.nih.gov/pubmed/27576192

16. Singla D, Veqar Z, Hussain ME. Photogrammetric assessment of upper body posture using postural angles: a literature review. J Chiropr Med. 2017;16: 131–8 Elsevier [cited 2018 Jul 4] Available from: http://www.ncbi.nlm.nih. gov/pubmed/28559753.

17. Shumway-Cook A, Woollacott MH. Motor control : theory and practical applications [Internet]. Lippincott Williams & Wilkins; 2001 [cited 2018 Jan 11]. Available from: https://books.google.ae/books/about/Motor_Control. html?id=301hQgAACAAJ&redir_esc=y

18. Juul T, Søgaard K, Davis AM, Roos EM. Psychometric properties of the neck outcome score, neck disability index, and short form–36 were evaluated in patients with neck pain. J Clin Epidemiol. 2016;79:31–40 [cited 2018 Jan 11] Available from: http://linkinghub.elsevier.com/retrieve/pii/S0895435616300270.

19. Yip CHT, Chiu TTW, Poon ATK. The relationship between head posture and severity and disability of patients with neck pain. Man Ther. 2008;13:148–54 [cited 2016 Apr 30] Available from: http://www.ncbi.nlm.nih.gov/pubmed/17368075.

20. Institute of Medicine (US) Committee on Pain, Disability and CIB, Osterweis M, Kleinman A, Mechanic D. Appendix myofascial pain syndromes due to trigger points. National Academies Press (US); 1987 [cited 2017 Dec 6]; Available from: https://www.ncbi.nlm.nih.gov/books/NBK219241/

21. MacDermid JC, Walton DM, Avery S, Blanchard A, Etruw E, McAlpine C, et al. Measurement properties of the neck disability index: a systematic review. J Orthop Sports Phys Ther. 2009;39:400–17 [cited 2016 Apr 30] Available from: http://www.ncbi.nlm.nih.gov/pubmed/19521015.

22. Falla D, Jull G, Russell T, Vicenzino B, Hodges P. Effect of neck exercise on sitting posture in patients with chronic neck pain. Phys Ther. 2007;87:408–17 [cited 2017 Dec 6] Available from: http://www.ncbi.nlm.nih.gov/pubmed/17341512.

23. Brink Y, Crous LC, Louw QA, Grimmer-Somers K, Schreve K. The association between postural alignment and psychosocial factors to upper quadrant pain in high school students: a prospective study. Man Ther. 2009;14:647–53 [cited 2017 Dec 6] Available from: http://linkinghub.elsevier.com/retrieve/pii/S1356689X09000411.

24. Cohen J. Statistical power analysis for the behavioral sciences (2nd ed.) New York: Academic Press; 1977.

25. Tsai C-T, Hsieh L-F, Kuan T-S, Kao M-J, Chou L-W, Hong C-Z. Remote effects of dry needling on the irritability of the myofascial trigger point in the upper trapezius muscle. Am J Phys Med Rehabil. 2010;89:133–40 [cited 2018 Jan 11] Available from: http://www.ncbi.nlm.nih.gov/pubmed/19404189.

26. Audette I, Dumas J-P, Côté JN, De Serres SJ. Validity and between-day reliability of the Cervical Range of Motion (CROM) device. J Orthop Sport Phys Ther. 2010;40:318–23 [cited 2018 Feb 8] Available from: http://www. ncbi.nlm.nih.gov/pubmed/20436238.

27. Harrison DE, Harrison DD, Harrison SOTS. A review of biomechanics of the central nervous system. Part 1: spinal canal deformations caused by changes in posture. J Manip Physiol Ther. 2000;23:217–20.

28. Kourtis D, Magnusson ML, Smith F, Hadjipavlou A, Pope MH. Spine height and disc height changes as the effect of hyperextension using stadiometry and MRI. Iowa Orthop J. 2004;24:65–71 [cited 2016 Apr 30] Available from: http://www.ncbi.nlm.nih.gov/pubmed/15296209.

29. Diab AA. The role of forward head correction in management of adolescent idiopathic scoliotic patients: a randomized controlled trial. 2012 [cited 2016 may 10];26. Available from: http://www.ncbi.nlm.nih.gov/pubmed/22801470.

30. Morningstar MW, Strauchman MN, Weeks DA. Spinal manipulation and anterior headweighting for the correction of forward head posture and cervical hypolordosis: a pilot study. J Chiropr Med. 2003;2:51–4 Elsevier [cited 2018 Jan 11] Available from: http://www.ncbi.nlm.nih.gov/pubmed/19674595.

31. Ledin T, Hafström A, Fransson PA, Magnusson M. Influence of neck proprioception on vibration-induced postural sway. Acta Otolaryngol. 2003; 123:594–9 [cited 2018 Jan 11] Available from: http://www.ncbi.nlm.nih.gov/ pubmed/12875581.

32. Harrison DE, Colloca CJ, Harrison DD, Janik TJ, Haas JW, Keller TS. Anterior thoracic posture increases thoracolumbar disc loading. Eur Spine J. 2005;14: 234–42 Springer [cited 2018 Jan 11] Available from: http://www.ncbi.nlm. nih.gov/pubmed/15168237.

33. Keller TS, Colloca CJ, Harrison DE, Harrison DD, Janik TJ. Influence of spine morphology on intervertebral disc loads and stresses in asymptomatic adults: implications for the ideal spine. Spine J. 2005;5:297–309 [cited 2018 Jan 11] Available from: http://www.ncbi.nlm.nih.gov/pubmed/15863086.

34. Gerwin RD, Dommerholt J, Shah JP. An expansion of Simons' integrated hypothesis of trigger point formation. Curr Pain Headache Rep. 2004;8:468–75 [cited 2018 Jan 11] Available from: http://www.ncbi.nlm.nih.gov/pubmed/ 15509461.

35. Walmsley RP, Kimber P, Culham E. The effect of initial head position on active cervical axial rotation range of motion in two age populations. Spine (Phila Pa 1976). 1996;21:2435–42 [cited 2018 Jan 11] Available from: http://www.ncbi.nlm.nih.gov/pubmed/8923628.

36. Fernández-de-las-Peñas C, Alonso-Blanco C, Cuadrado M, Pareja J. Forward head posture and neck mobility in chronic tension-type headache. Cephalalgia. 2006;26:314–9 [cited 2017 may 14] Available from: http://www. ncbi.nlm.nih.gov/pubmed/16472338.

37. Patwardhan AG, Havey RM, Khayatzadeh S, Muriuki MG, Voronov LI, Carandang G, et al. Postural consequences of cervical sagittal imbalance: a novel laboratory model. Spine (Phila Pa 1976). 2015;40:783–92 [cited 2018 Jan 11] Available from: http://content.wkhealth.com/linkback/openurl?sid= WKPTLP:landingpage&an=00007632-201506010-00006.

38. Sun A, Yeo HG, Kim TU, Hyun JK, Kim JY. Radiologic assessment of forward head posture and its relation to myofascial pain syndrome. Ann Rehabil Med. 2014;38:821–6 [cited 2018 Jan 11] Available from: https://synapse. koreamed.org/DOIx.php?id=10.5535/arm.2014.38.6.821.

39. Fernandez-de-las-Penas C, Alonso-Blanco C, Cuadrado ML, Gerwin RD, Pareja JA. Trigger points in the suboccipital muscles and forward head posture in tension-type headache. Headache J Head Face Pain. 2006;46: 454–60 [cited 2018 Jan 11] Available from: http://www.ncbi.nlm.nih.gov/ pubmed/16618263.

40. Hou C-R, Tsai L-C, Cheng K-F, Chung K-C, Hong C-Z. Immediate effects of various physical therapeutic modalities on cervical myofascial pain and trigger-point sensitivity. Arch Phys Med Rehabil. 2002;83:1406–14 [cited 2018 Jan 11] Available from: http://www.ncbi.nlm.nih.gov/pubmed/ 12370877.

41. Vernon H, Schneider M. Chiropractic management of myofascial trigger points and myofascial pain syndrome: a systematic review of the literature. J Manipulative Physiol Ther. 2009;32:14–24 [cited 2018 Jan 11] Available from: http://www.ncbi.nlm.nih.gov/pubmed/19121461.

42. Simons DG. Understanding effective treatments of myofascial trigger points. J Bodyw Mov Ther. 2002;6:81–8 Churchill Livingstone [cited 2018 Jan 11] Available from: https://www.sciencedirect.com/science/article/pii/ S1360859202902718.

43. De-La-Llave-Rincón AI, Fernández-De-Las-Peñas C, Palacios-Ceña D, Cleland JA. Increased forward head posture and restricted cervical range of motion in patients with carpal tunnel syndrome. J Orthop Sport Phys Ther. 2009;39: 658–64 [cited 2018 Jan 11] Available from: http://www.ncbi.nlm.nih.gov/ pubmed/19721213.

44. Yoo W-G, An D-H. The relationship between the active cervical range of motion and changes in head and neck posture after continuous VDT work. Ind Health. 2009;47:183–8 [cited 2018 Jan 11] Available from: http://www. ncbi.nlm.nih.gov/pubmed/19367048.

22

On the influence of surface coating on tissue biomechanics – effects on rat bones under routine conditions with implications for image-based deformation detection

Aqeeda Singh[1], Mario Scholze[1,2] and Niels Hammer[1,3,4*] (iD)

Abstract

Background: Biomechanical testing using image-based deformation detection techniques such as digital image correlation (DIC) offer optical contactless methods for strain and displacement measurements of biological tissues. However, given the need of most samples to be speckled for image correlation using sprays, chemical alterations with impact on tissue mechanicals may result. The aim of this study was to assess the impact of such surface coating on the mechanical properties of rat bones, under routine laboratory conditions including multiple freeze-thaw cycles.

Methods: Two groups of rat bones, highly-uniform and mixed-effects, were assigned to six subgroups consisting of three types of surface coating (uncoated, commercially-available water- and solvent-based sprays) and two types of bone conditions (periosteum attached and removed). The mixed-effects group had undergone an additional freeze-thaw cycle at -20 degrees. All bones underwent a three-point bending test ranging until material failure.

Results: Coating resulted in similar and non-significantly different mechanical properties of rat bones, indicated by elastic moduli, maximum force and bending stress. Scanning electron microscopy showed more pronounced mechanical alterations related to the additional freeze-thaw cycle, with fewer cracks being present in a bone from the highly-uniform group.

Conclusions: This study has concluded that surface coating with water- or solvent-based sprays for enhancing image correlation for DIC and having an additional freeze-thaw cycle do not significantly alter mechanical properties of rat bones. Therefore, this method may be recommended as an effective way of obtaining a speckled pattern.

Keywords: 3-point bending test, Biomechanical experiment, Chemical fixation, Digital image correlation, Tensile test

* Correspondence: nlshammer@googlemail.com
[1]Department of Anatomy, University of Otago, Lindo Ferguson Building, 270 Great King St, Dunedin 9016, New Zealand
[3]Department of Orthopedic and Trauma Surgery, University Clinics of Leipzig, Leipzig, Germany
Full list of author information is available at the end of the article

Background

Biomechanical testing is a frequently used tool to assess load deformation behaviour of tissue samples in the field of medicine. The information gathered is utilised for clinical purposes, for example, understanding the mechanical performance of bones allows researchers to predict the effects of pathological processes. It also allows researchers to identify areas of stress that may result in fractures during intense activity [1]. The exact measurement of displacements and strain during deformation is a key point for the determination of accurate material properties. To facilitate this, digital image correlation (DIC) is being used to measure displacement and strain of different materials [2]. This is a contactless optical method of imaging the deformations occurring at the surface of the tissue when loaded, which avoids measurement inaccuracies arising from material slippage with tension tests [3]. Furthermore, DIC measures displacements without the influence of the mechanical properties (and elasticity) of the testing device itself.

The method of DIC typically involves software-based algorithms, which facilitate tracking discrete points on the sample and analysing their relative displacement that has been captured in a series of images during the deformation [3]. DIC is dependent on surfaces which have distinct surface characteristics that can serve as natural speckles. Surfaces which do not have natural contrasts, e.g. tendons and ligaments, need to be speckled and this is commonly done using commercially-available sprays. Using sprays that deposit paint dots randomly is quick and effective method to achieve such speckled appearance [4]. As a consequence of this surface pre-treatment, alterations to the mechanical properties of the biological tissues may result.

It is hypothesised that these changes in properties may be the result of chemical, or osmotic changes in the tissues. The solvent-based spray may increase the elastic modulus and strength of the bones due to chemically and osmotically changing the periosteum. The effect may be explained by the ingredients in the solvent-based spray; acetone and xylene are two key ingredients used in the spray that are also used for tissue fixation. As such, the periosteum of the bone may become a target of the denaturation and dehydration induced by the fixatives as it is a cellular connective tissue. Acetone is commonly used as a dehydrating agent for preparing histological sections, as it physically exchanges with water [5]. Xylene is a nonpolar solvent that is used as a 'clearing agent' in preparation of tissue sections, and leads to tissue shrinkage and increases stiffness [6, 7]. The combination of these two ingredients may affect the periosteum (soft tissue) on the bones and consequently result in changes in the mechanical properties.

A second issue may be introduced by using DIC in samples which have been frozen in a non-standardized manner for storage purposes. Freezing avoids the use of fixatives such as formaldehyde or ethanol to prevent autolysis and bacterial contamination [8]. It furthermore helps in acquiring an adequate sample size over a longer period, resulting in tissues with similar properties [9]. However, in 'real-life' scenarios, samples that have been gathered may have already undergone additional freeze-thaw cycles beyond the required protocol. It may be that the bones that have undergone additional freeze-thaw cycles show a greater difference between the coated and uncoated conditions due to the formation of ice needles; ice needles can cause structural damage by growing rapidly at -15 and -30 °C. This can lead to the deterioration of the mechanical properties in the slow-freezing femora especially if they are frozen at -20 °C after being thawed, as was the case in a previous study [9, 10]. Commonly also, tests are performed with more than a one-day interval, and therefore require re-freezing between tests as well as the initial freezing for storage [11]. The micro-fractures caused by these ice needles can form pathways for the sprays and consequently result in more marked chemical alterations.

The purpose of this study was to assess the effects of surface coating on the mechanical properties of rat bones (hard tissues), in a standardized scenario and in a second 'real-life' scenario with an additional freeze-thaw cycle. The latter approach involving refreezing of tissues is not ideal for any mechanical testing but may form a scenario which researchers can be faced with. It was hypothesised that (A) solvent-based spray on the bones may lead to altered mechanical properties, indicated by an increased strength and elastic modulus due to tissue changes. The secondary hypothesis (B) was that the coated and uncoated bone samples may show a greater difference in the group which had undergone an additional freeze-thaw cycle due to the effects of freezing.

Methods

Sample preparation

Bilateral femora and humeri were removed from seventeen rats harvested from animals used for another study approved by the ethics committee of University of Otago (ethical approval number: ET23/16). The animals were euthanized prior to this study for teaching purposes as part of an animal surgery laboratory using CO_2; following the culling of the animals, the tissues were subsequently precooled at 4 °C for 12 h and then shock frozen at -80 °C. Thawing was done in the inverted manner: here, the samples were transferred from -80 °C to -18 °C before they were transferred to room temperature. The aim of this approach was to minimize the formation of ice needles, in line with studies on ligament-bone complexes showing unaltered mechanics as a consequence of freeze-thaw cycles [12–14]. Before the experiments, the bones were dissected further to remove the extra soft tissue, leaving the periosteum fully intact, and this was carried out in a rapid manner to circumvent any drying. Following the dissection, the bones were placed in isotonic saline (0.9 mass %).

All seventeen rats were of the same species, *Rattus norvegicus*; ten rats were of the breed Wistar (500–600 g, all male), and seven rats were of the breed Sprague Dawley (~ 250 g, male and female). The two breeds were separated into two different groups: highly-uniform (Wistar) and mixed-effects (Sprague Dawley). The mixed-effects Sprague Dawley rat bones group had undergone an additional freeze-thaw cycle to simulate realistic laboratory conditions, whereas the highly-uniform Wistar rat bone group had not, therefore these labels intend to reflect the difference in pre-experimental storage conditions that may affect the end outcome. The highly-uniform Wistar rat bones group also consisted of only male rats, thereby making it more 'uniform'. The additional freeze-thaw cycle consisted of the mixed-effects group of bones undergoing another cycle of thawing (to room temperature of 21 °C) and freezing (directly at – 20 °C) without any pre-cooling.

Mechanical testing

All samples, from both groups of rat femora and humeri, were assigned to subgroups randomly, as seen in Fig. 1, which shows the division of samples for the experiments. Prior to testing, all bone samples were divided into a group with periosteum attached (PA) and another group with periosteum removed (PR). These samples were further split into three subsamples each, depending on the nature of the surface coating of the tissue. One subsample was left uncoated (UC), a second one was coated using a water-based spray (WB), and a third one with a solvent-based spray (SB).

Five or more femora and five or more humeri were allocated to each of the six subgroups: UC-PA, UC-PR, WB-PA, WB-PR, SB-PA and SB-PR. Each bone was removed from saline, and six diameter measurements (Electronic Digital Vernier Caliper, MechPro, Melbourne, Vic, Australia, +/– 0.02 mm) were made along the axis perpendicular to the shaft of the bone in the mediolateral plane. Always, the maximum diameter was assessed for each area of circumference, and the measurements were taken in 0.5-mm distances before being averaged to calculate a mean diameter and cross-sectional area. To obtain a pattern of dots on the uncoated samples (Fig. 2), a charcoal pencil (Charcoal Pencil Pitt Monochrome, Faber-Castell, Stein, Germany) was used. The water- and solvent-based sprays that were used to create a speckle of dots were provided by Dy-Mark Pty Ltd. (Wacol, QLD, Australia). The ingredients in the sprays are listed in Table 1.

The coated samples were sprayed with the respective white water- or solvent-based spray to create a base coating, then sprayed with the respective blue water- or solvent-based spray to create the distribution of dots to enhance the contrast for image-based deformation detection (Fig. 2). The underlying base coating was spread until a complete coverage of the shaft was reached, followed by the application of small speckles typically with a speckle size of 0.2–0.8 mm in diameter. The spraying was standardised between the samples by placing every sample 20 cm from the spray nozzle and only spraying for a total of ten to fifteen seconds until the bones were sufficiently coated. Each coated sample had a drying period of fifteen minutes after being sprayed before being tested mechanically.

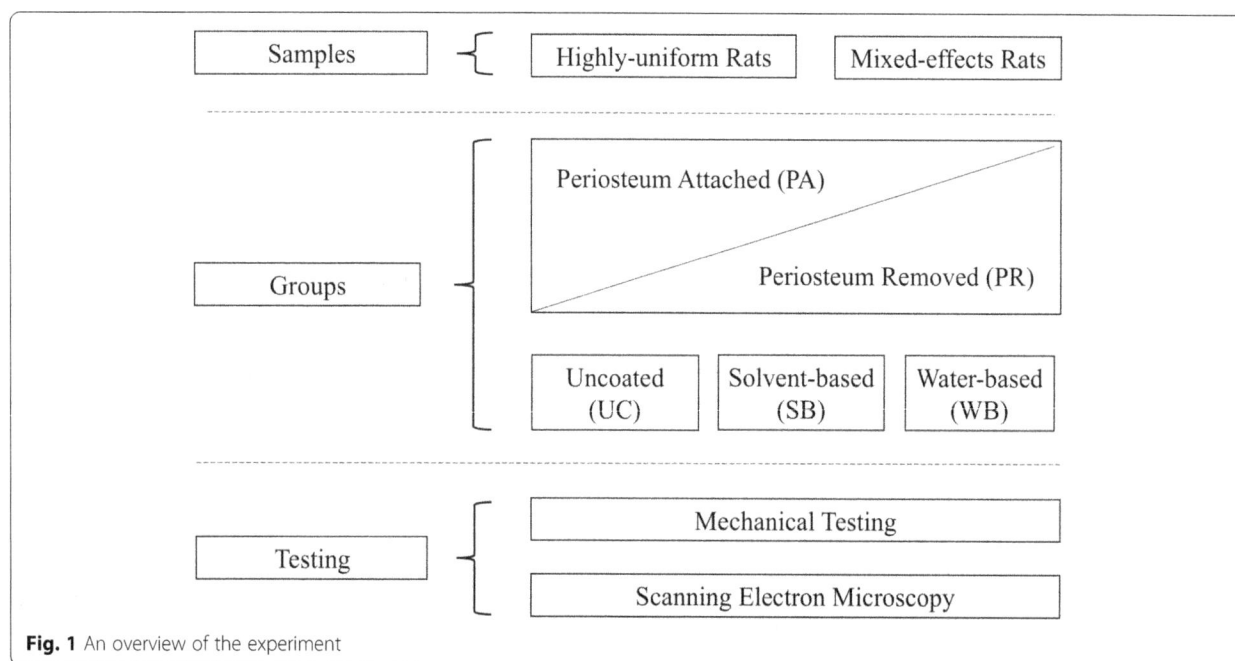

Fig. 1 An overview of the experiment

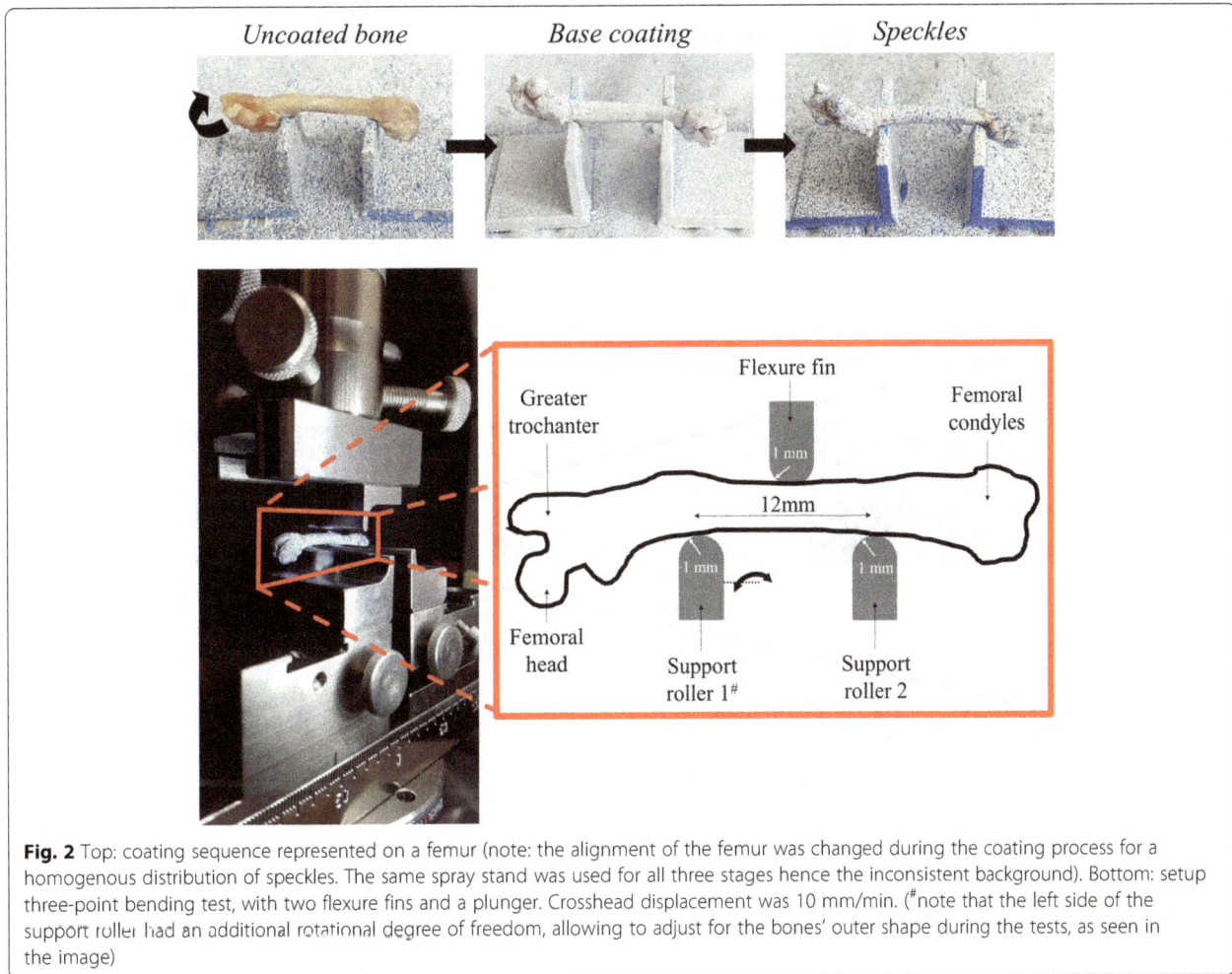

Fig. 2 Top: coating sequence represented on a femur (note: the alignment of the femur was changed during the coating process for a homogenous distribution of speckles. The same spray stand was used for all three stages hence the inconsistent background). Bottom: setup three-point bending test, with two flexure fins and a plunger. Crosshead displacement was 10 mm/min. ([#]note that the left side of the support roller had an additional rotational degree of freedom, allowing to adjust for the bones' outer shape during the tests, as seen in the image)

Tests were conducted using a Z020 universal testing device with a Xforce P 2.5 kN load cell and the TestXpert II software (Zwick Roell Group, Ulm, Germany). The machine displacement system was used for the evaluations of all experiments as the displacement of the sample was assumed to equal the crosshead displacement of the test machine, to prevent influences of the different applied spray patterns itself. Image-based deformation detection was carried out using a method described previously in a paper on biomechanical analysis of stiffness and fracture displacement by Höch et al. (2017), to obtain exemplary image-based evaluations [15].

The bones were subjected to three-point bend testing to failure, where the top-oriented surface of the bone-specimen (touching the plunger) was situated in a state of compression and the bottom-oriented surface was in tension (Fig. 2). For the tests, a preload of 2 N was applied prior to the beginning of data recording. Details on the three-point bending test are given in Fig. 2. Force and vertical displacement were captured over time with a sampling rate of 100 Hz.

The maxima of tensile stress and strain in the sample exist at the bottom-oriented surface directly below the point of load application in the bending plane and thus

Table 1 Ingredients of the sprays used, per the manufacturers' data sheets

Water-based (WB) spray ingredients	Solvent-based (SB) spray ingredients
Isopropanol (10–30%)	Xylene (10–30%)
Water (10–30%)	Acetone (10–30%)
Dimethyl ether (30–60%)	Pigment and filler (10–30%)
Ammonia (< 1%)	Resin (10–30%)
	Dimethyl ether (1–10%)
	Hydrocarbon propellant (10–30%) (less than 0.1% 1, 3 butadiene)

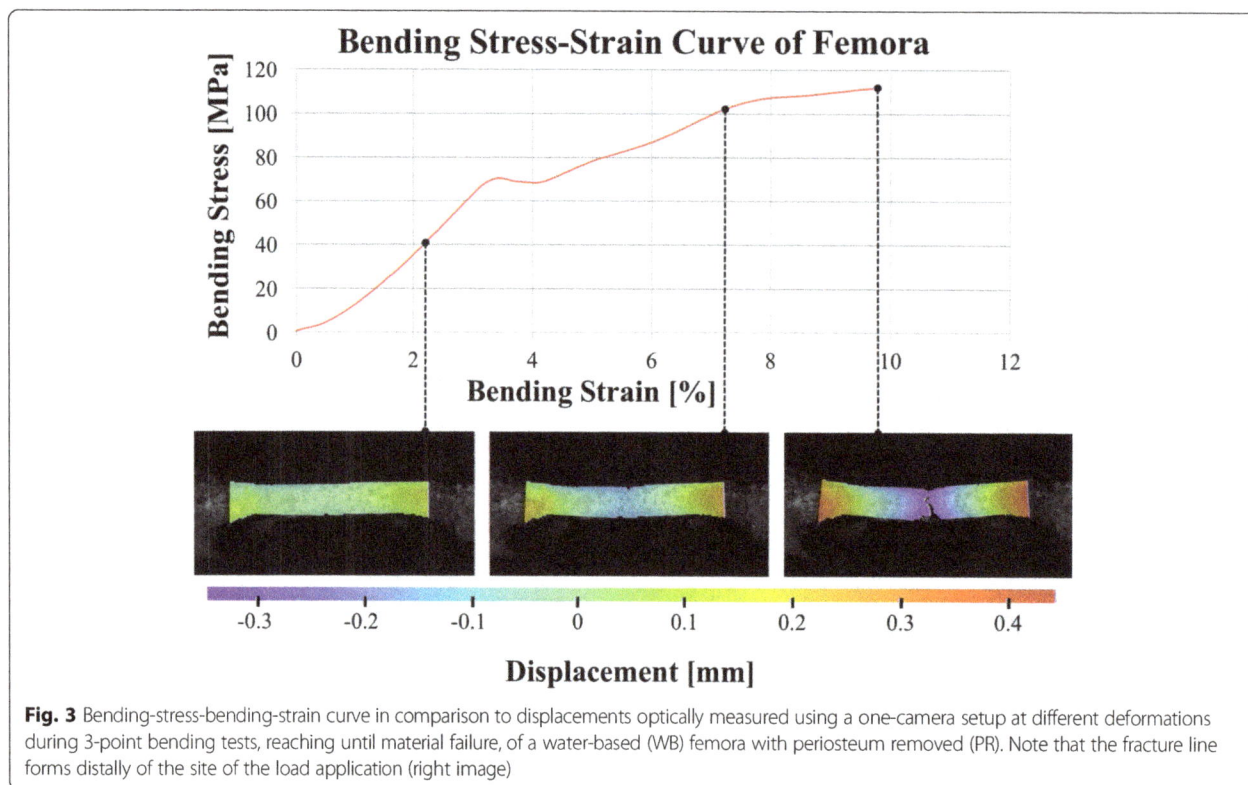

Fig. 3 Bending-stress-bending-strain curve in comparison to displacements optically measured using a one-camera setup at different deformations during 3-point bending tests, reaching until material failure, of a water-based (WB) femora with periosteum removed (PR). Note that the fracture line forms distally of the site of the load application (right image)

were named bending stress and bending strain. The nominal values were calculated with the assumption of a perfect circular cross section according to

$$\sigma_f = \frac{8FL}{\pi d^3}$$

and

$$\epsilon_f = \frac{6Dd}{L^2}$$

respectively [16, 17].

σ_f=stress in the lowermost (highest tensioned) fibres of the bone directly below plunger (MPa), F = load at a given point on the load deflection curve (N), L = support span [8], d = diameter of the bone [8], ϵ_f=strain in the outer surface in the lowermost (highest tensioned) fibres of the bone directly below plunger (mm/mm), D = deflection of the centre of the beam [8]. The elastic modulus was evaluated as the slope of the linear part of the bending-stress-bending-strain curve by regression.

An example of the combined bending stress-strain and image-based deformation detection data is shown in Fig. 3.

Scanning Electron microscopy

Six representative femora were chosen to be prepared for the scanning electron microscopy (SEM). Three samples were randomly chosen from the highly-uniform group and three samples from the mixed-effects group. Subsequent to the three-point bending tests, the bones were fixed in 3% neutral-buffered formaldehyde and then post-fixed in 3% glutaraldehyde/0.1 M phosphate buffer (pH = 7.4). Following this, the bones were dehydrated after being washed in distilled water to allow for the critical point drying process (CPD-030, Bal-Tec AG, Liechtenstein) to take place. The magnifications at which SEM was conducted ranged between 25x and 500x using a JSM-6700F field emission microscope (JEOL Ltd., Tokyo, Japan).

Data evaluation and statistical analysis

A power calculation was not performed to determine an appropriate sample size for the study because, although ideal, it may have been unnecessary given the animals were highly consistent in terms of breed, age and weight. Microsoft Excel (version 15.3, Microsoft Corp., Albuquerque, NM, USA) and Prism 7a (GraphPad Software Inc., Lajolla, CA, USA) were used. The stress-strain data obtained during the femora and humeri experiments were further processed to compute elastic modulus (GPa), maximum force (N), bending strength (MPa), deflection at maximum force [8], strain at maximum force (%), force at break (N) and deflection at break [8] for the bones. Comparisons were made between the six subgroups (UA-PA, UC-PR, WB-PA, WB-PR, SB-PA, SB-PR) in the two different femora and humeri groups. Elastic modulus, maximum force, strength and strain at maximum force were the values being compared statistically. Following assessment for normal distribution, a one-way ANOVA test with post-hoc corrections was used to compare the mean elastic modulus, maximum force, strength and strain at maximum force of each of the six groups within each breed group. The level of significance was set at $p \leq 0.05$.

Results

Stress-strain data were obtained from the 34 rat femora and 32 rat humeri. No tissues were excluded due to macroscopically-evident pathology or for any other reasons.

Coating with water- or solvent-based sprays yielded no significant influence on the mechanical properties of rat bone

The data obtained from both the highly-uniform and mixed-effects bone groups suggested that there was no statistically significant difference between coated and uncoated samples. The only significant difference was between the mean bending strength of UC-PA and WB-PR femora in the highly-uniform group ($p = 0.0354$).

Further qualitative comparison of the bone groups through the graphs showed minute but statistically non-significant changes. In the highly-uniform rats, the elastic modulus and bending strength tended to be slightly higher in the coated than in the uncoated femora. The mean elastic modulus tended to be slightly higher in samples with the periosteum removed in both femora and humeri for the uncoated and the water-based coating group; these values were non-significantly different and the standard deviation outweighed the differences in mean values. An inverted behaviour was found for the solvent-based group. The maximum force also tended to be slightly higher in femora with periosteum removed for only the uncoated and water-based, with the opposite being true for the solvent-based femora group. Also, the values for elastic modulus, maximum force, bending strength and strain at maximum force were mostly higher in the SB-PA subgroup, compared to the UC-PA subgroup, especially in the highly-uniform bone group. These data are summarised in Table 2 and Fig. 4.

In the mixed-effects rats, there were also some statistically non-significant changes found between the six subgroups. In contrast to the highly-uniform group, the elastic modulus and bending strength tended to be higher in uncoated femora and humeri than coated. The SB-PA femora had lower elastic modulus, maximum force and bending strength when compared with SB-PR, which was the opposite in the highly-uniform group. Also, the elastic modulus, bending strength and strain at maximum force were higher in the UC-PR femora subgroup than in the UC-PA femora subgroup. The means for the mixed effect group are summarised in Table 3 and Fig. 5.

Table 2 Summary of the means for the highly-uniform group of rat femora and humeri undergoing three-point bending tests (one standardized snap freezing cycle)

Highly-uniform Group	Elastic Modulus [GPa] Mean ± Standard Deviation	Maximum Force [N]	Bending Strength/ Maximum Stress [MPa]	Strain at Maximum Force [%]
Femora				
UC-PA ($n = 4$)	1.85 ± 0.56	178.25 ± 11.87	82.80 ± 12.04	11.27 ± 1.42
UC-PR ($n = 3$)	1.98 ± 0.45	210.69 ± 5.98	100.33 ± 11.58	12.69 ± 4.48
WB-PA ($n = 3$)	2.06 ± 0.32	185.35 ± 34.44	89.85 ± 14.88	10.55 ± 1.17
WB-PR ($n = 3$)	2.77 ± 0.43	202.02 ± 3.00	114.86 ± 7.98	9.86 ± 1.18
SB-PA (n = 4)	2.18 ± 0.61	204.21 ± 17.97	105.03 ± 20.43	11.27 ± 2.61
SB-PR (n = 3)	1.97 ± 0.23	200.55 ± 19.3	99.36 ± 3.86	10.98 ± 1.69
Humeri				
UC-PA ($n = 3$)	4.93 ± 1.11	111.22 ± 16.77	156.19 ± 19.39	5.02 ± 0.75
UC-PR ($n = 3$)	5.64 ± 1.44	124.12 ± 2.21	162.76 ± 14.61	5.43 ± 1.00
WB-PA ($n = 3$)	4.25 ± 0.43	114.15 ± 10.17	155.95 ± 10.60	5.88 ± 0.61
WB-PR ($n = 3$)	4.67 ± 0.73	105.70 ± 15.37	168.31 ± 25.07	5.01 ± 0.65
SB-PA (n = 3)	5.17 ± 2.81	108.61 ± 15.78	164.81 ± 39.55	6.07 ± 1.96
SB-PR (n = 3)	4.05 ± 0.11	110.70 ± 25.31	162.45 ± 43.98	4.87 ± 1.21

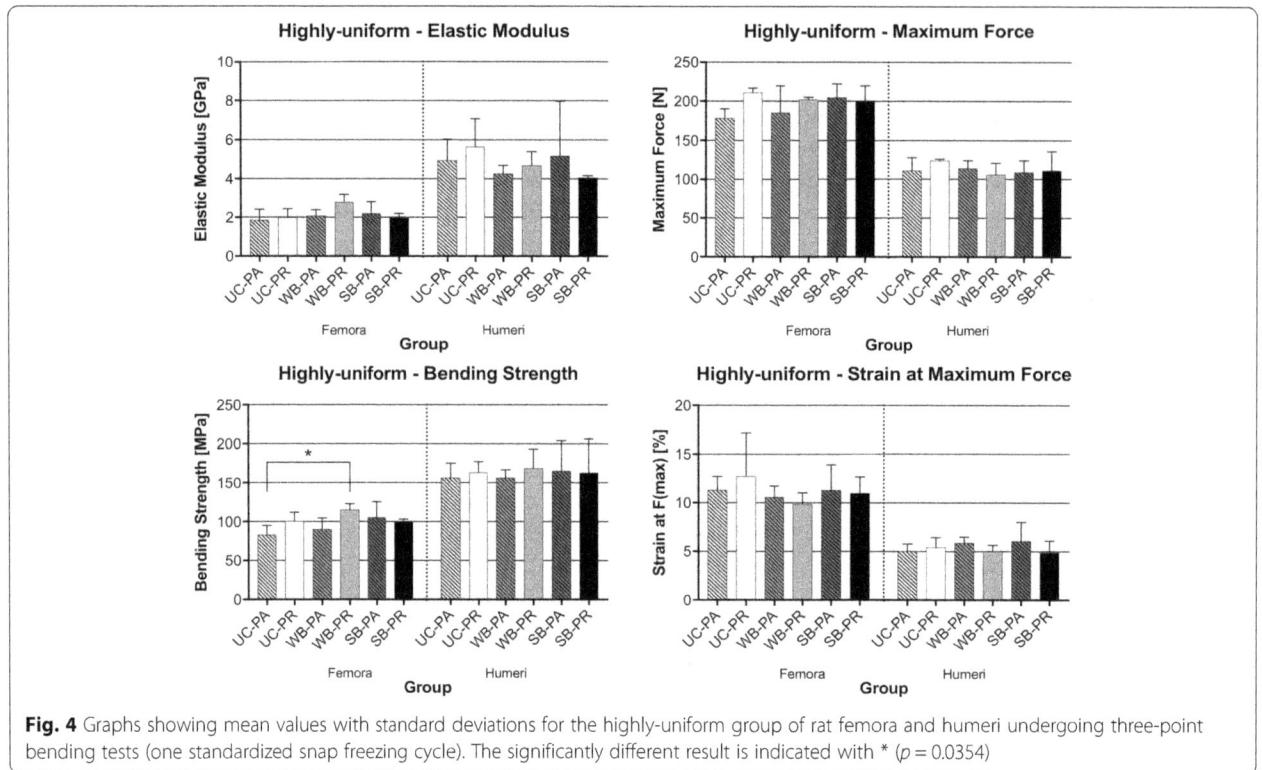

Fig. 4 Graphs showing mean values with standard deviations for the highly-uniform group of rat femora and humeri undergoing three-point bending tests (one standardized snap freezing cycle). The significantly different result is indicated with * ($p = 0.0354$)

SEM has shown more pronounced mechanical alterations related to slow freezing

SEM revealed that there was a qualitative difference in the number and location of cracks found between the mixed-effects and highly-uniform bone groups. As seen in Fig. 6, the femur in the mixed-effects group appeared to have more mechanical damage, which was also located more internally whereas the femur from the highly-uniform group appeared to have fewer cracks, which were located peripherally. It is unclear if these cracks pre-existed prior to the mechanical tests or if they were a consequence of altered behaviour of the pre-weakened tissues.

Table 3 Summary of means for mixed-effects group of rat femora and humeri undergoing three-point bending tests (two freezing cycles)

Mixed-effects Group	Elastic Modulus [GPa]	Maximum Force [N]	Bending Strength/ Maximum Stress [MPa]	Strain at Maximum Force [%]
	Mean ± Standard Deviation			
Femora				
UC-PA (n = 2)	1.89 ± 0.39	180.20 ± 4.94	91.69 ± 12.81	10.24 ± 1.09
UC-PR (n = 2)	2.16 ± 0.51	137.2 ± 19.56	91.82 ± 7.04	12.35 ± 1.60
WB-PA (n = 3)	1.96 ± 1.02	131.40 ± 27.89	83.52 ± 26.11	11.30 ± 4.67
WB-PR (n = 3)	1.61 ± 0.50	150.20 ± 29.09	82.56 ± 21.74	13.46 ± 3.07
SB-PA (n = 1)	0.88	96.33	50.01	15.50
SB-PR (n = 3)	1.37 ± 0.23	140.20 ± 34.77	72.77 ± 13.17	13.4 ± 4.53
Humeri				
UC-PA (n = 2)	5.49 ± 0.26	95.39 ± 2.73	158.50 ± 5.65	5.10 ± 0.28
UC-PR (n = 2)	5.91 ± 1.25	75.64 ± 16.42	170.80 ± 11.40	4.29 ± 0.23
WB-PA (n = 3)	5.56 ± 2.13	78.66 ± 20.35	163.30 ± 29.35	4.69 ± 1.26
WB-PR (n = 3)	3.89 ± 2.41	96.42 ± 17.80	184.40 ± 6.37	6.99 ± 2.76
SB-PA (n = 1)	5.91	79.63	187.50	5.57
SB-PR (n = 3)	4.46 ± 1.24	107.00 ± 23.19	175.90 ± 39.75	5.87 ± 0.93

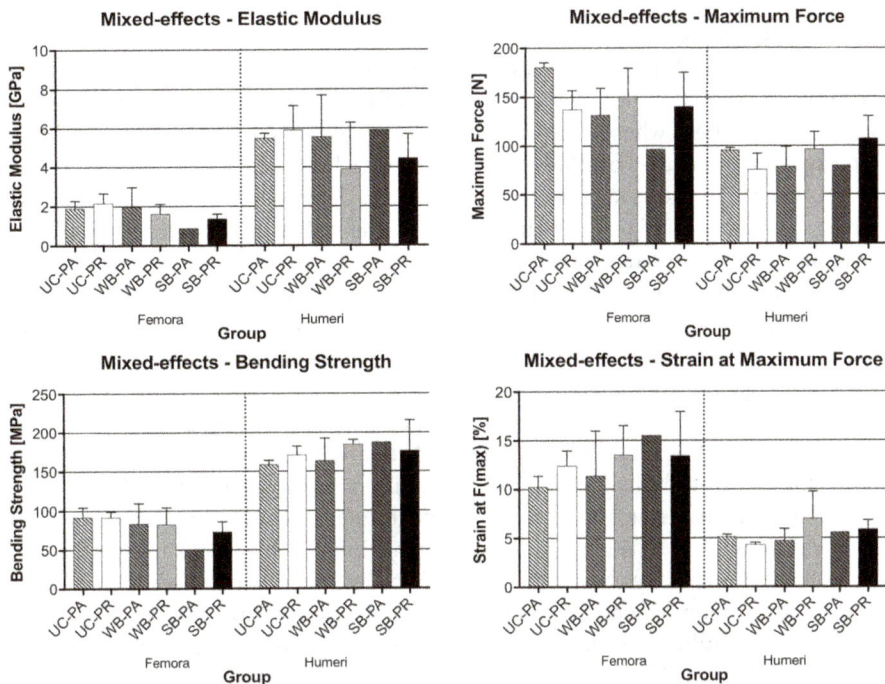

Fig. 5 Graphs showing mean values with standard deviations for the mixed-effects group of rat femora and humeri undergoing three-point bending tests (two freezing cycles)

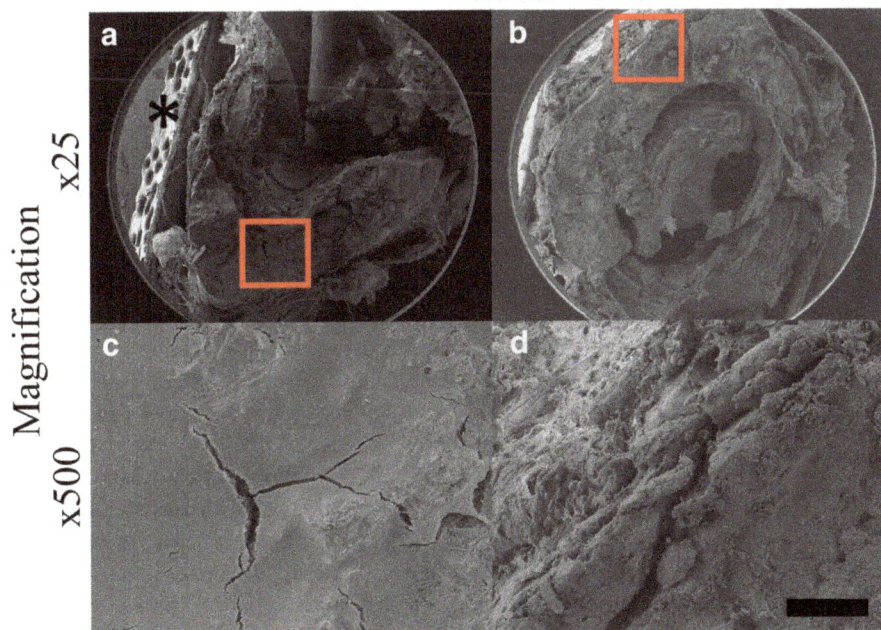

Fig. 6 On the left (**a**, **c**), a femur from the mixed-effect group is shown with partial disruption in cortical bone integrity, indicated by crack-like cavities. On the right (**b**, **d**), a femur is depicted from the highly-uniform group showing fewer cracks, and on the edge of the bone. The asterisk (*) is to indicate the tape used to fix the bones. The bar on the bottom right corner is 1 mm for (**a**, **b**), 68 μm (**c**, **d**)

Discussion

This study has shown that surface coating of rat bones with commercially-available sprays for the purpose of enhancing image correlation for DIC does not significantly alter mechanical properties when tissues are tested within an adequate timeframe after coating. However, some trends were observed in the data collected; in the highly-uniform rats, the elastic modulus, maximum force, bending strength and maximum strain values were higher for the SB-PA subgroup than for UC-PA. One exception was the maximum force measured in humeri. In the mixed-effects rats, the uncoated femora tended to have slightly higher but non-significantly different elastic modulus, maximum force and bending strength.

In this study, rat bones were used as they are a reliable and highly-standardized alternative to human bones [18]. Rat bones are much thinner in diameter and therefore easier to access by chemicals until the tissues are thoroughly diffused. This results in these tissues being affected earlier than samples from larger animal models or human cadavers, thereby allowing chemically or osmotically-induced changes to be observed much quicker.

Efforts were made to have highly standardized samples, allowing inter-individual variation to be outweighed by the differences induced by fixation. This was done by having all the rats as Wistar or Sprague Dawley breeds with the same age and weight. If human samples were used, this would have led to a much greater inter-individual variation due to factors such as gender, age, and size [14]. Weight was used as a measure of maturation, alongside with age. Only male rats were used in the highly-uniform group to achieve the greatest homogeneity, but both male and female rats were used in the mixed-effects group to get close to 'real-life' conditions, with more statistical spread.

It was hypothesized that the solvent-based spray may increase the elastic modulus and strength in bones with periosteum still attached due to chemical or osmotic alterations, which have been discussed above. This effect was confirmed in the highly-uniform femora and humeri that had the periosteum still attached. However, the minor changes in mechanical properties were still statistically non-significant. This phenomenon was not noticed in the mixed-effects rats, but given the small sample size further quantification of this comparison was rendered not useful.

In the mixed-effects rats, the bone group that had undergone the freeze-thaw cycles, trends observed were that the uncoated femora had slightly higher values compared to the coated although still statistically non-significant. The hypothesis that this group may have shown a more pronounced difference between uncoated and coated sample values compared to the highly-uniform group was derived from the concept of ice needle

formation, which has been discussed previously. However, this effect was not noticed in the mechanical experiments quantitatively, but the SEM images did show an increased number of cracks in the bone, though a causal relation at this stage remains unclear. If more cycles of freezing and thawing had occurred, the results could have been different as deterioration of mechanical properties seems to occur after five cycles of freezing and thawing [19, 20].

This is a study that examined the effects of spray coating on rat bones for the purpose of biomechanical testing with image-based deformation detection. A similar study was conducted on porcine collateral ligaments; it concluded that using methylene blue and white paint for speckling did not significantly alter the elastic responses of the soft tissues [21]. Another study investigating mouse carotid arteries with DIC also showed no significant effect on the mechanical properties when using India ink for the speckling pattern [22]. Other studies that have been conducted on bone fixation for preservation purposes have shown different results. A study examining the influence of ethanol and formaldehyde fixation on the mechanical properties of human coxal bones showed irreversible changes to the organic matrix [8]. A different study found a significant influence of chemical fixation with ethanol and formaldehyde on the mechanical properties collagen rich soft tissues such as the iliotibial tract [23]. Though these changes have been found before by these groups, such changes were not evident as a result of surface speckling, which may be a result of different samples being used or that this fixation method involved complete submersion and was long-term. In contrast, another study by the same group investigating the effect of short-term fixation with formalin or ethanol on the mechanics of human cortical bone yielded no vast alterations [11]. This is in accordance with the current study as it examined the effect of short-term fixation with commercial sprays.

Limitations

Firstly, the sample size was relatively small, especially in the mixed-effects group; increasing the sample size may have provided more reliable results in all groups. Increasing the sample size would also have allowed for a control group for the mixed-effects that did not undergo any pre-treatment. Also, the distribution of the samples in the six subgroups could have been done differently so there would be at least two samples in each group. Moreover, this study can be extended by using more types of biological tissues to see alterations across the spectrum of biological tissues that may be used in labs. Secondly, the post-mortem delay must be considered as the samples were frozen for at least two months before they were tested. Controversial evidence suggests that freezing may generally irreversibly alter mechanical properties of unfixed bone. One group found in porcine trabecular bone that after five years, mechanical alteration occurs, whereas no significant difference exists after one year [9]. However, it is unclear if this may also apply to rat and human bone. Also, it may have been beneficial to include samples that were also female in the highly-uniform group to see if sex would affect the results. Third, the calculations for bending stress, bending strain and elastic modulus were carried out with the assumption that the bone is one solid beam with an ideal circular cross-section, and not as a hollow tube. Furthermore, mechanical alterations may possibly also have resulted from the sprays forming a film over the biological tissues. Some aerosol water-based paints contain film-forming polymers, such as acrylate polymers, which have carrier solvents such as isopropanol [24]. These paints may form a 'shell' around the tissues, which thereby mechanically influences the measurements by contributing to the load-bearing structures. However, the ingredients of the sprays used in this study did not contain such film-forming polymers. Even so, it was concluded from SEM that the layers seemed less influential given their minute thickness; it was difficult to even detect the attached layer of the speckling, validating this. Lastly, the exposure time for all experiments in this study was kept constant (fifteen minutes) and the influence of shorter or higher time frames remains unknown. However, there would be a high risk of measuring not only mechanical alterations by the ingredients of the sprays given the nature of ongoing dehydration processes when these tissues are subjected to environmental conditions.

Conclusions
In conclusion, there was found to be no statistically significant difference between coated and uncoated rat femora or humeri – this holds true also for any samples that have undergone an additional freeze-thaw cycle. For the purposes of biomechanical testing using the DIC system, the spray method is recommended as it is an effective and quick method for producing a random speckle pattern [3]. Further research may be done on examining the effects of multiple freeze-thaw cycles with controls when using sprays, and on other kinds of tissues.

Abbreviations
DIC: Digital image correlation; PA: Periosteum attached; PR: Periosteum removed; SB: Solvent based (spray); SEM: Scanning electron microscopy; UC: Uncoated; WB: Water based (spray)

Acknowledgements
The authors would like to thank Elisabeth Girvan for helping with the electron microscopy samples and Fieke Neuman, Rosie Melchers, Natalie Matheson and Greg Anderson for providing the biological samples.

Funding
A University of Otago Divisional Health Science Summer Student Scholarship was awarded to AS. This work was supported by the German Research Foundation (DFG) and Leipzig University within the program of Open Access Publishing.

Authors' contributions
MS and NH planned the experiments, AS and MS carried out the experiments, evaluated the results and drafted the manuscript. NH critically revised the manuscript. All authors read and approved the final manuscript.

Competing interests
The authors declare that they have no competing interests.

Author details
[1]Department of Anatomy, University of Otago, Lindo Ferguson Building, 270 Great King St, Dunedin 9016, New Zealand. [2]Institute of Materials Science and Engineering, Chemnitz University of Technology, Chemnitz, Germany. [3]Department of Orthopedic and Trauma Surgery, University Clinics of Leipzig, Leipzig, Germany. [4]Fraunhofer IWU, Dresden, Germany.

References
1. Sharir A, Barak MM, Shahar R. Whole bone mechanics and mechanical testing. Vet J. 2008;177(1):8–17.
2. McCormick N, Lord J. Digital Image Correlation. Mater Today. 2010; 13(12):52–4.
3. Sichting F, Steinke H, Wagner MF, Fritsch S, Hadrich C, Hammer N. Quantification of material slippage in the iliotibial tract when applying the partial plastination clamping technique. J Mech Behav Biomed Mater. 2015; 49:112–7.
4. Hild F, Roux S. Optical methods for solid mechanics. 1st ed. Weinheim: Wiley-VCH; 2012.
5. Muller LL, Jacks TJ. Rapid chemical dehydration of samples for electron microscopic examinations. J Histochem Cytochem. 1975;23(2):107–10.
6. Metgud R, Astekar MS, Soni A, Naik S, Vanishree M. Conventional xylene and xylene-free methods for routine histopathological preparation of tissue sections. Biotech Histochem. 2013;88(5):235–41.
7. Sermadi W, Prabhu S, Acharya S, Javali S. Comparing the efficacy of coconut oil and xylene as a clearing agent in the histopathology laboratory. J Oral Maxillofac Pathol. 2014;18(Suppl 1):S49–53.
8. Hammer N, Voigt C, Werner M, Hoffmann F, Bente K, Kunze H, Scholz R, Steinke H. Ethanol and formaldehyde fixation irreversibly alter bones' organic matrix. J Mech Behav Biomed Mater. 2014;29:252–8.
9. Lee W, Jasiuk I. Effects of freeze-thaw and micro-computed tomography irradiation on structure-property relations of porcine trabecular bone. J Biomech. 2014;47(6):1495–8.
10. Brown KL, Cruess RL. Bone and cartilage transplantation in orthopaedic surgery. A review. J Bone Joint Surg Am. 1982;64(2):270–9.
11. Linde F, Sorensen HC. The effect of different storage methods on the mechanical properties of trabecular bone. J Biomech. 1993;26(10):1249–52.
12. Mahalingam V, Wojtys EM, Wellik DM, Arruda EM, Larkin LM. Fresh and frozen tissue-engineered three-dimensional bone-ligament-bone constructs for sheep anterior cruciate ligament repair following a 2-year implantation. Biores Open Access. 2016;5(1):289–98.
13. Mahalingam VD, Behbahani-Nejad N, Ronan EA, Olsen TJ, Smietana MJ, Wojtys EM, Wellik DM, Arruda EM, Larkin LM. Fresh versus frozen engineered bone-ligament-bone grafts for sheep anterior cruciate ligament repair. Tissue Eng Part C Methods. 2015;21(6):548–56.
14. Jung HJ, Vangipuram G, Fisher MB, Yang G, Hsu S, Bianchi J, Ronholdt C, Woo SL. The effects of multiple freeze-thaw cycles on the biomechanical properties of the human bone-patellar tendon-bone allograft. J Orthop Res. 2011;29(8):1193–8.
15. Hoch A, Schimpf R, Hammer N, Schleifenbaum S, Werner M, Josten C, Bohme J. Biomechanical analysis of stiffness and fracture displacement after using PMMA-augmented sacroiliac screw fixation for sacrum fractures. Biomed Tech (Berl). 2017;62(4):421 8.
16. ISO B: 178: 2010. Plastics-Determination of flexural properties (ISO 178: 2010) 2010.
17. Callister WD Jr. DGR: Materials science and engineering. New York: John Wiley & Sons, Inc.; 2011.
18. Bagi CM, Berryman E, Moalli MR. Comparative bone anatomy of commonly used laboratory animals: implications for drug discovery. Comp Med. 2011; 61(1):76–85.

19. Boutros CP, Trout DR, Kasra M, Grynpas M. The effect of repeated freeze-thaw cycles on the biomechanical properties of canine cortical bone. VCOT Archive. 2000;(2):59–64.

20. Maiden NR, Byard RW. Unpredictable tensile strength biomechanics may limit thawed cadaver use for simulant research. Aust J Forensic Sci. 2016; 48(1):54–8.

21. Lionello G, Sirieix C, Baleani M. An effective procedure to create a speckle pattern on biological soft tissue for digital image correlation measurements. J Mech Behav Biomed Mater. 2014;39:1–8.

22. Genovese K, Lee YU, Humphrey JD. Novel optical system for in vitro quantification of full surface strain fields in small arteries: II. Correction for refraction and illustrative results. Comput Methods Biomech Biomed Engin. 2011;14(3):227–37.

23. Steinke H, Lingslebe U, Bohme J, Slowik V, Shim V, Hadrich C, Hammer N. Deformation behavior of the iliotibial tract under different states of fixation. Med Eng Phys. 2012;34(9):1221–7.

24. Mark JE. Physical properties of polymers handbook. 2nd ed. Berlin: Springer Science & Business Media; 2007.

Permissions

All chapters in this book were first published in MD, by BioMed Central; hereby published with permission under the Creative Commons Attribution License or equivalent. Every chapter published in this book has been scrutinized by our experts. Their significance has been extensively debated. The topics covered herein carry significant findings which will fuel the growth of the discipline. They may even be implemented as practical applications or may be referred to as a beginning point for another development.

The contributors of this book come from diverse backgrounds, making this book a truly international effort. This book will bring forth new frontiers with its revolutionizing research information and detailed analysis of the nascent developments around the world.

We would like to thank all the contributing authors for lending their expertise to make the book truly unique. They have played a crucial role in the development of this book. Without their invaluable contributions this book wouldn't have been possible. They have made vital efforts to compile up to date information on the varied aspects of this subject to make this book a valuable addition to the collection of many professionals and students.

This book was conceptualized with the vision of imparting up-to-date information and advanced data in this field. To ensure the same, a matchless editorial board was set up. Every individual on the board went through rigorous rounds of assessment to prove their worth. After which they invested a large part of their time researching and compiling the most relevant data for our readers.

The editorial board has been involved in producing this book since its inception. They have spent rigorous hours researching and exploring the diverse topics which have resulted in the successful publishing of this book. They have passed on their knowledge of decades through this book. To expedite this challenging task, the publisher supported the team at every step. A small team of assistant editors was also appointed to further simplify the editing procedure and attain best results for the readers.

Apart from the editorial board, the designing team has also invested a significant amount of their time in understanding the subject and creating the most relevant covers. They scrutinized every image to scout for the most suitable representation of the subject and create an appropriate cover for the book.

The publishing team has been an ardent support to the editorial, designing and production team. Their endless efforts to recruit the best for this project, has resulted in the accomplishment of this book. They are a veteran in the field of academics and their pool of knowledge is as vast as their experience in printing. Their expertise and guidance has proved useful at every step. Their uncompromising quality standards have made this book an exceptional effort. Their encouragement from time to time has been an inspiration for everyone.

The publisher and the editorial board hope that this book will prove to be a valuable piece of knowledge for researchers, students, practitioners and scholars across the globe.

List of Contributors

Yi Zeng, Yuangang Wu and Bin Shen
Department of Orthopaedic Surgery, West China Hospital, West China Medical School, Sichuan University, Chengdu, Sichuan Province 610041, People's Republic of China

Huazhang Xiong
Department of Orthopaedic Surgery, West China Hospital, West China Medical School, Sichuan University, Chengdu, Sichuan Province 610041, People's Republic of China
Department of Orthopedic Surgery, The First Affiliated Hospital of Zunyi Medical College, Zunyi 563003, Guizhou Province, China

Yi Liu
Department of Orthopedic Surgery, The First Affiliated Hospital of Zunyi Medical College, Zunyi 563003, Guizhou Province, China

Nigel C. Hanchard and Helen H. Handoll
School of Health and Social Care, Teesside University, Middlesbrough, UK

Cordula Braun
School of Health and Social Care, Teesside University, Middlesbrough, UK
Present address: Faculty of Health and Physiotherapy, Buxtehude, Germany
Faculty of Health, Harburger Str. 6, 21614 Buxtehude, Germany

Andreas Betthäuser
schulter-zentrum.com, Hamburg, Germany

Jianji Wang, Long Yang, Qingjun Li, Zhanyu Wu, Yu Sun, Qiang Zou, Xuanze Li and Zhe Xu
Department of Orthopedic Surgery, Affiliated Hospital of Guizhou Medical University, Guiyang, China
Center for Bioprinting and Biomanufacturing, Guizhou Medical University, Guiyang, China
Center for Tissue Engineering and Stem Cells, Guizhou Medical University, Guiyang, China

Chuan Ye
Department of Orthopedic Surgery, Affiliated Hospital of Guizhou Medical University, Guiyang, China
Center for Bioprinting and Biomanufacturing, Guizhou Medical University, Guiyang, China
Center for Tissue Engineering and Stem Cells, Guizhou Medical University, Guiyang, China
China Orthopedic Regenerative Medicine Group (CORMed), Guiyang, China

Jennifer L. Keating
Department of Physiotherapy, Monash University, PO Box 527, Frankston, Victoria 3199, Australia

Robert A. Laird
Department of Physiotherapy, Monash University, PO Box 527, Frankston, Victoria 3199, Australia
Superspine, Forest Hills, Melbourne, Australia

Peter Kent
School of Physiotherapy and Exercise Science, Curtin University, Perth, Australia
Department of Sports Science and Clinical Biomechanics, University of Southern Denmark, Odense, Denmark

Hai-Tao Li, Ting Liang, Xi Chen, Jiang-Bo Guo, Hua-Ye Jiang, Zong-Ping Luo and Hui-Lin Yang
Orthopaedic Institute, Department of Orthopaedics, The First Affiliated Hospital of SooChow University, 708 Renmin Rd, Suzhou, Jiangsu 215006, People's Republic of China

Yan-Jun Che
Orthopaedic Institute, Department of Orthopaedics, The First Affiliated Hospital of SooChow University, 708 Renmin Rd, Suzhou, Jiangsu 215006, People's Republic of China
Department of Orthopedics, Peace Hospital Affiliated to Changzhi Medical College, Changzhi, Shanxi, People's Republic of China

Nolan S. Horner, Anthony Habib and Olufemi R. Ayeni
Division of Orthopaedic Surgery, Department of Surgery, McMaster University, 1200 Main St W, Room 4E15, Hamilton, ON L8N 3Z5, Canada

Paul A. Moroz
Faculty of Medicine, University of British Columbia, Vancouver, BC, Canada

Raman Bhullar
Faculty of Medicine, Royal College of Surgeons in Ireland – Medical University of Bahrain, Manama, Bahrain

Nicole Simunovic
Department of Health Research Methods, Evidence and Impact, McMaster University, Hamilton, ON, Canada

Ivan Wong
Department of Orthopaedic Surgery, Dalhousie University and Nova Scotia Health Authority, Halifax, NS, Canada

Asheesh Bedi
MedSport, Department of Orthopaedic Surgery, University of Michigan, Ann Arbor, MI, USA

Alison Rushton
Centre of Precision Rehabilitation for Spinal Pain [CPR Spine] School of Sport, Exercise and Rehabilitation Sciences, University of Birmingham, Birmingham B15 2TT, UK

Konstantinos Zoulas
Polyclinic of Lisieux, Lillebonne, France

Andrew Powell
ARC Physiotherapy, Saffron Walden, UK

JB Staal
Radboud Institute for Health Sciences, IQ healthcare, Radboud UMC, Nijmegen 6500 HB, The Netherlands Research group Musculoskeletal Rehabilitation, HAN University of Applied Sciences, Nijmegen, the Netherlands

Dafang Chen
Department of Epidemiology and Biostatistics, Public Health College, Peking University, 38# Xueyuan Road, Haidian district, Beijing 100191, China

Yanwei Lv
Department of Epidemiology and Biostatistics, Public Health College, Peking University, 38# Xueyuan Road, Haidian district, Beijing 100191, China
Clinical Epidemiology Research Center, Beijing Jishuitan Hospital, 31# Xinjiekou Dongjie, West district, Beijing 100035, China
Department of Spine, Beijing Jishuitan Hospital, 31# Xinjiekou Dongjie, West district, Beijing 100035, China

Lifang Wang and Fangfang Duan
Clinical Epidemiology Research Center, Beijing Jishuitan Hospital, 31# Xinjiekou Dongjie, West district, Beijing 100035, China

Wei Tian
Clinical Epidemiology Research Center, Beijing Jishuitan Hospital, 31# Xinjiekou Dongjie, West district, Beijing 100035, China
Department of Spine, Beijing Jishuitan Hospital, 31# Xinjiekou Dongjie, West district, Beijing 100035, China

Yajun Liu
Department of Spine, Beijing Jishuitan Hospital, 31# Xinjiekou Dongjie, West district, Beijing 100035, China

Owis Eilayyan, Aliki Thomas, Marie-Christine Hallé, Sara Ahmed, Fadi Alzoubi and Andre Bussières
School of Physical and Occupational Therapy, McGill University, 3654 Prom Sir-William-Osler, Montréal, QC H3G 1Y5, Canada
Center for Interdisciplinary Research in Rehabilitation of Greater Montreal (CRIR), Montréal, Canada

Anthony C. Tibbles, Craig Jacobs and Silvano Mior
Canadian Memorial Chiropractic College, North York, Canada

Connie Davis
University of British Columbia, Vancouver, Canada
Centre for Collaboration, Motivation and Innovation, Vancouver, Canada

Roni Evans
University of Minnesota, Minneapolis, USA

Michael J. Schneider
University of Pittsburgh, Pittsburgh, USA

Jan Barnsley
University of Toronto, Toronto, Canada

Cynthia R. Long
Palmer College Davenport, Davenport, USA

Jau-Yih Tsauo
School and Graduate Institute of Physical Therapy, College of Medicine, National Taiwan University, Taipei, Taiwan

Chun-De Liao
School and Graduate Institute of Physical Therapy, College of Medicine, National Taiwan University, Taipei, Taiwan
Department of Physical Medicine and Rehabilitation, Shuang Ho Hospital, Taipei Medical University, Taipei, Taiwan

Hung-Chou Chen
Department of Physical Medicine and Rehabilitation, Shuang Ho Hospital, Taipei Medical University, Taipei, Taiwan
Center for Evidence-Based Health Care, Shuang Ho Hospital, Taipei Medical University, Taipei, Taiwan
Department of Physical Medicine and Rehabilitation, School of Medicine, College of Medicine, Taipei Medical University, No. 250 Wu-Hsing Street, Taipei, Taiwan

Tsan-Hon Liou
Department of Physical Medicine and Rehabilitation, Shuang Ho Hospital, Taipei Medical University, Taipei, Taiwan
Graduate Institute of Injury Prevention and Control, Taipei Medical University, Taipei, Taiwan
Department of Physical Medicine and Rehabilitation, School of Medicine, College of Medicine, Taipei Medical University, No. 250 Wu-Hsing Street, Taipei, Taiwan

Guo-Min Xie
Department of Neurology, Ningbo Medical Center Lihuili Eastern Hospital, Taipei Medical University, Zhejiang, China

Brittney A. Luc-Harkey, Jeffrey N. Katz and Elena Losina
Orthopaedic and Arthritis Center for Outcomes Research, Department of Orthopedic Surgery, Brigham and Women's Hospital, 60 Fenwood Road, Suite 5016, Boston, MA 02115, USA

Clare E. Safran-Norton
Rehabilitation Services, Brigham and Women's Hospital, Boston, MA, USA

Lisa A. Mandl
Weill Cornell Medicine, Hospital for Special Surgery, New York, NY, USA

Liubov Arbeeva and Kimberlea F. Grimm
Thurston Arthritis Research Center, University of North Carolina at Chapel Hill, 3300 Thurston Bldg., CB# 7280, Chapel Hill, NC 27599-7280, USA
Department of Medicine, University of North Carolina at Chapel Hill, 125 MacNider Hall CB# 7005, Chapel Hill, NC 27599, USA

Kelli D. Allen
Thurston Arthritis Research Center, University of North Carolina at Chapel Hill, 3300 Thurston Bldg., CB# 7280, Chapel Hill, NC 27599-7280, USA
Department of Medicine, University of North Carolina at Chapel Hill, 125 MacNider Hall CB# 7005, Chapel Hill, NC 27599, USA
Health Services Research and Development Service, Durham VA Medical Center, Durham, NC, USA

Crystal W. Cené and Caroline T. Nagle
Department of Medicine, University of North Carolina at Chapel Hill, 125 MacNider Hall CB# 7005, Chapel Hill, NC 27599, USA

Cynthia J. Coffman
Health Services Research and Development Service, Durham VA Medical Center, Durham, NC, USA

Department of Biostatistics and Bioinformatics, Duke University Medical Center, Durham, NC, USA

Eugene Z. Oddone
Health Services Research and Development Service, Durham VA Medical Center, Durham, NC, USA
Department of Medicine, Duke University Medical Center, Durham, NC, USA

Erin Haley and Lisa C. Campbell
Department of Psychology, East Carolina University, Greenville, NC, USA

Francis J. Keefe and Tamara J. Somers
6Department of Psychiatry and Behavioral Science, Duke University, Durham, NC, USA

Yashika Watkins
Institute for Health Research and Policy, University of Illinois at Chicago, Chicago, IL, USA

Maurizio Fontana
Orthopaedic Department, Infermi Hospital, Viale Stradone 9, 48018 Faenza, Italy

Marco Cavallo, Graziano Bettelli and Roberto Rotini
Shoulder and Elbow Unit, IRCCS - Istituto Ortopedico Rizzoli, Via G.C. Pupilli 1, Bologna, Italy

Kyu-Jin Cho, Jong-Keun Seon, Won-Young Jang and Chun-Gon Park
Center for Joint Disease, Chonnam National University Hwasun Hospital, 160, Ilsim-Ri, Hwasun-Eup, Hwasun-Gun, Jeonnam 519-809, South Korea

Eun-Kyoo Song
Center for Joint Disease, Chonnam National University Hwasun Hospital, 160, Ilsim-Ri, Hwasun-Eup, Hwasun-Gun, Jeonnam 519-809, South Korea
Department of Orthopaedic Surgery, Chonnam National University Hwasun Hospital, 160 Ilsim-Ri, Hwasun-gun, Jeonnam 519-809, South Korea

Jill Hayden and Mark Asbridge
Department of Community Health and Epidemiology, Dalhousie University, Halifax, NS, Canada

Jordan Edwards
Department of Community Health and Epidemiology, Dalhousie University, Halifax, NS, Canada
Department of Epidemiology and Biostatistics, Schulich School of Medicine and Dentistry, Western University, London, ON, Canada

Kirk Magee
Department of Emergency Medicine, Charles V. Keating Emergency and Trauma Centre, Halifax, NS, Canada

Hiroshi Mano and Sayaka Fujiwara
Department of Rehabilitation Medicine, The University of Tokyo Hospital, Tokyo, Japan

Nobuhiko Haga
Department of Rehabilitation Medicine, The University of Tokyo Hospital, Tokyo, Japan
Department of Rehabilitation Medicine, Graduate School of Medicine, The University of Tokyo, Tokyo, Japan

Kazuyuki Takamura
Department of Orthopaedic Surgery, Fukuoka Children's Hospital, Fukuoka, Japan

Hiroshi Kitoh
Department of Orthopedic Surgery, Nagoya University Graduate School of Medicine, Nagoya, Japan

Shinichiro Takayama
Department of Orthopaedic Surgery, National Center for Child Health and Development, Tokyo, Japan

Tsutomu Ogata
Department of Pediatrics, Hamamatsu University School of Medicine, Hamamatsu, Japan

Shuji Hashimoto
Department of Hygiene, Fujita Health University School of Medicine, Toyoake, Japan

Cole G Chapman and John M Brooks
Department of Health Services Policy and Management, University of South Carolina, Columbia, SC, USA
Center for Effectiveness Research in Orthopaedics, Greenville, SC, USA

Sarah B Floyd
Department of Health Services Policy and Management, University of South Carolina, Columbia, SC, USA
Center for Effectiveness Research in Orthopaedics, Greenville, SC, USA
Arnold School of Public Health, University of South Carolina, 915 Greene St., Suite 303C, Columbia, SC 29208, USA

Lauren Ruffrage
Center for Effectiveness Research in Orthopaedics, Greenville, SC, USA

Ellen Shanley
Center for Effectiveness Research in Orthopaedics, Greenville, SC, USA
ATI Physical Therapy, Greenville, SC, USA

Eldon Matthia and Peter Cooper
University of South Carolina School of Medicine Greenville, Greenville, SC, USA

Camilla Dahlqvist, Catarina Nordander and Henrik Enquist
Division of Occupational and Environmental Medicine, Department of Laboratory Medicine, Lund University, SE-221 85 Lund, Sweden

Mikael Forsman
Division of Ergonomics, KTH Royal Institute of Technology, SE-141 57 Huddinge, Sweden

Maria Andersson
Spenshult Research and Development Center, FoU Spenshult, Bäckagårdsvägen 47, SE-302 74 Halmstad, Sweden
Department of Clinical Sciences, Section of Rheumatology, Lund University, Lund, Sweden

Emma Haglund
Spenshult Research and Development Center, FoU Spenshult, Bäckagårdsvägen 47, SE-302 74 Halmstad, Sweden
School of Business, Engineering and Science, Halmstad University, Halmstad, Sweden

Ingrid Larsson
Spenshult Research and Development Center, FoU Spenshult, Bäckagårdsvägen 47, SE-302 74 Halmstad, Sweden
School of Health and Welfare, Halmstad University, Halmstad, Sweden

Katarina Aili
Spenshult Research and Development Center, FoU Spenshult, Bäckagårdsvägen 47, SE-302 74 Halmstad, Sweden
Unit of occupational medicine, Institute of Environmental Medicine, Karolinska Institutet, Stockholm, Sweden
School of Health and Welfare, Halmstad University, Halmstad, Sweden

Stefan Bergman
Spenshult Research and Development Center, FoU Spenshult, Bäckagårdsvägen 47, SE-302 74 Halmstad, Sweden
School of Health and Welfare, Halmstad University, Halmstad, Sweden
Primary Health Care Unit, Department of Public Health and Community Medicine, Institute of Medicine, The Sahlgrenska Academy, University of Gothenburg, Gothenburg, Sweden

Ann Bremander
Spenshult Research and Development Center, FoU Spenshult, Bäckagårdsvägen 47, SE-302 74 Halmstad, Sweden

Department of Clinical Sciences, Section of Rheumatology, Lund University, Lund, Sweden
School of Business, Engineering and Science, Halmstad University, Halmstad, Sweden
Department of Regional Health Research, University of Southern Denmark, Odense, Denmark
Syddansk Universitet Research Unit, King Christian X Hospital for Rheumatic Diseases, Hospital of Southern Jutland, Copenhagen, Graasten, Denmark

Michela Corsi and Allen Tsai
College of Medicine, Northeast Ohio Medical University, 4209 OH-44, Rootstown, OH 44272, USA

Carolina Alvarez
Thurston Arthritis Research Center, University of North Carolina at Chapel Hill, 3300 Thurston Bldg., CB# 7280, Chapel Hill, NC 27599, USA

Leigh F. Callahan, Rebecca J. Cleveland, Joanne M. Jordan and Amanda E. Nelson
Thurston Arthritis Research Center, University of North Carolina at Chapel Hill, 3300 Thurston Bldg., CB# 7280, Chapel Hill, NC 27599, USA
Department of Medicine, University of North Carolina at Chapel Hill, 125 MacNider Hall CB# 7005, Chapel Hill, NC 27599, USA

Jordan Renner
Thurston Arthritis Research Center, University of North Carolina at Chapel Hill, 3300 Thurston Bldg., CB# 7280, Chapel Hill, NC 27599, USA
Department of Radiology, University of North Carolina at Chapel Hill, 2006 Old Clinic, CB, Chapel Hill, NC #7510, USA

Kelli D. Allen
Thurston Arthritis Research Center, University of North Carolina at Chapel Hill, 3300 Thurston Bldg., CB# 7280, Chapel Hill, NC 27599, USA
Department of Medicine, University of North Carolina at Chapel Hill, 125 MacNider Hall CB# 7005, Chapel Hill, NC 27599, USA
Center for Health Services Research in Primary Care, Department of Veterans Affairs Healthcare System, 508 Fulton Street, Durham, NC, USA

Yvonne M. Golightly
Thurston Arthritis Research Center, University of North Carolina at Chapel Hill, 3300 Thurston Bldg., CB# 7280, Chapel Hill, NC 27599, USA

Injury Prevention Research Center, University of North Carolina at Chapel Hill, CB# 7505, 137 E Franklin St, Chapel Hill, NC 27599, USA
Department of Epidemiology, University of North Carolina at Chapel Hill, 170 Rosenau Hall, CB#7400, Chapel Hill, NC 27599, USA

Fatma Hegazy
Department of Physiotherapy, College of Health Sciences, University of Sharjah, Sharjah, United Arab Emirates

Ibrahim M. Moustafa
Department of Physiotherapy, College of Health Sciences, University of Sharjah, Sharjah, United Arab Emirates
Basic Science Department, Faculty of Physical Therapy, Cairo University, 7 Mohamed Hassan El gamal Street-Abbas El Akaad, Nacer City, Egypt

Aliaa A. Diab
Basic Science Department, Faculty of Physical Therapy, Cairo University, 7 Mohamed Hassan El gamal Street-Abbas El Akaad, Nacer City, Egypt

Deed E. Harrison
CBP Nonprofit (a spine research foundation), Eagle, ID, USA

Aqeeda Singh
Department of Anatomy, University of Otago, Lindo Ferguson Building, 270 Great King St, Dunedin 9016, New Zealand

Mario Scholze
Department of Anatomy, University of Otago, Lindo Ferguson Building, 270 Great King St, Dunedin 9016, New Zealand
Institute of Materials Science and Engineering, Chemnitz University of Technology, Chemnitz, Germany

Niels Hammer
Department of Anatomy, University of Otago, Lindo Ferguson Building, 270 Great King St, Dunedin 9016, New Zealand
Department of Orthopedic and Trauma Surgery, University Clinics of Leipzig, Leipzig, Germany
Fraunhofer IWU, Dresden, Germany

Index

www.ingramcontent.com/pod-product-compliance
Lightning Source LLC
Chambersburg PA
CBHW061331190326
41458CB00011B/3968